ENCYCLOPEDIA OF
FORENSIC AND
LEGAL MEDICINE

ENCYCLOPEDIA OF
FORENSIC AND
LEGAL MEDICINE

EDITED BY

JASON PAYNE-JAMES
ROGER W BYARD
TRACEY S COREY
CAROL HENDERSON

ELSEVIER
ACADEMIC
PRESS

AMSTERDAM • BOSTON • HEIDELBERG • LONDON
NEW YORK • OXFORD • PARIS • SAN DIEGO
SAN FRANCISCO • SINGAPORE • SYDNEY • TOKYO

EDITORS AND EDITORIAL ADVISORY BOARD

FOREWORD – A FORENSIC PERSPECTIVE

To comprehensively encompass the fields of both forensic medicine and legal medicine is an ambitious project indeed, as conventionally, the two disciplines are usually treated separately. Even "forensic medicine" itself is traditionally divided into autopsy pathology and the clinical aspects, so to produce anything more than an overview of the whole spectrum of the subject, is something that has probably never before been attempted in the English language.

The Editors have assembled an impressive array of contributors, each masters of their own topic and the result is an impressive work which deserves the highest praise, both to the authors and to those who have had to labor at editing to achieve a coherent whole – a feat which personal experience has taught me can be a daunting task. Having myself written about ten books on forensic medical topics, as well as contributions to many more, I can vouch for the fact that the most difficult job of all was editing a couple of multi-author volumes.

The content of this encyclopedia is diverse and comprehensive. The actual range can be seen from the very extensive chapter list and covers virtually every sub-discipline in forensic and legal medicine, from anthropology to botany, from malpractice to substance abuse. Some of the subjects dealt with, would be thought of as "forensic science" in the more compartmentalized attitude of Great Britain, but of course in very many countries, there is not the same demarcation of professional interests within their Institutes of Legal Medicine and thus this book avoids geographical restrictions, which in the past have always raised difficulties in writing for different parts of the world, which have markedly diverse medico-legal systems.

Some of the headings in the list of contents would seem unfamiliar to doctors of previous generations – examples might be "accreditation, digital evidence, crime-scene management, profiling, ritualistic crime, terrorism and torture" – but this underlines the evolutionary nature of all medical disciplines, in which legal medicine is no exception. In former years, many textbooks remained relatively static over numerous editions, following a conventional sequence of topics. Whereas forensic science developed almost explosively, the pace of progress in forensic pathology was slow and it seemed hardly worth buying new editions of established manuals. This has all changed and it is timely that such an ambitious work as this encyclopedia should seek to sweep all current knowledge into its grasp for the benefit of those doctors "at the sharp end" of forensic practice, who need to refer to any part of such a broad field of knowledge that now exists.

Professor Bernard Knight, CBE
Cardiff, UK
January 2005.

FOREWORD – A LEGAL PERSPECTIVE

Over my judicial career I have observed a tremendous number of changes in the law, scientific and medical practices, and society in general. DNA evidence is now commonplace in many criminal and family cases, domestic violence and child abuse are unfortunately still prevalent, and the notion of personal rights and freedoms for incapacitated children and adults is now becoming widely accepted. The courts are also becoming increasingly involved in difficult cases concerning individuals who, but for advances in life-prolonging technologies, might have reached a natural death much sooner. I am particularly pleased to see a single work that is relevant to all these topics, and with contributions by distinguished practitioners and authors from many disciplines. I am only disappointed that a work of this importance was not available long ago.

The Encyclopedia will be of use and interest to a wide-ranging audience. Judges, lawyers, medical practitioners, scientists and students will be among the many who will benefit from this single repository of knowledge. I especially welcome, as will many, the electronic version which will receive regular updates. This will ensure that the Encyclopedia remains at the forefront of legal, technological and medical developments and will be of continuing use over the years to come.

The number of cases requiring evidence or advice from medical and other forensic experts has increased over recent years. In some cases as many as nine experts have been involved, providing a variety of viewpoints. The Encyclopedia will be a valuable aid in explaining to judges, lawyers and many others engaged in the court process the technical language of forensic and legal medicine and will assist in elucidating the complex issues which arise for resolution in the courts.

Dame Elizabeth Butler-Sloss, GBE
President of the Family Division
London, UK
January 2005.

PREFACE

The phrase "Forensic and Legal Medicine" may at first appear cumbersome. It does, however, enable all the areas that this Encyclopedia covers to be fully embraced. Global differences in terminology and cross-over with other healthcare and scientific disciplines mean that unlike many other medical specialties such as cardiology or gastroenterology – each with clear boundaries – there may be misunderstanding, both within and without the medical profession as to the vast scope of subject covered. "Forensic medicine" and "legal medicine" are terms that can be used interchangeably, and their specific use may vary from country to country. For many readers, the term "forensic medicine" is synonymous with that of forensic pathology (that specialty of medicine which investigates the cause of death). However, forensic pathology, although part of forensic medicine, is but a small part of the vast range of subjects with which forensic medicine practitioners may be involved. In the broadest terms forensic and legal medicine includes all areas where medicine interacts with the law (including criminal and civil law), judiciary, police bodies, investigative agencies, professional bodies and government or state bodies.

When developing this Enyclopedia the Editors and the Publishers had the objective of providing *the* major reference source of subjects related to forensic and legal medicine. This information is provided in separate chapters generally of about 3–5,000 words. Each chapter gives a source of specific Further Reading to which those requiring even more detailed information can be directed. The degree of interaction of those practising forensic and legal medicine with the law, the judiciary, police bodies, investigative agencies, professional, government and state bodies, will vary from country to country, and from jurisdiction to jurisdiction. Some forensic medicine specialists will be independent of state, government or judiciary, while others will not. Some will work full-time in their field, others part-time. Just a few examples of key areas where differences arise include the investigation of death, approaches to care of detainees in custody, structure of investigative of systems, and interpretation of human rights issues. Clearly it is not possible for a single work, even of this size to illustrate all the differences that exist in our complex world. As Editors, we have sought to identify the most relevant issues and give examples of how such systems, or topics work within a given country or region. There will of course be omissions – and these we apologise for any such in advance. We hope that readers will inform us directly of any information that they feel should have been included. The online version of the Encyclopedia will be updated at timely intervals. Any such suggestions from readers will be assessed and considered as we plan the new material to be included at each update, and will thus help the development and evolution of this work.

The main readership groups of the Encyclopedia are intended to be medical practitioners whose work comprises a forensic element (including forensic pathologists, medical examiners, forensic physicians, forensic odontologists, paediatricians, psychiatrists, psychologists, genitourinary medicine specialists, emergency medicine specialists and primary care physicians), others within the forensic setting (including scientists, toxicologists, anthropologists), legal practitioners (lawyers, advocates, attorneys, coroners, barristers and solicitors), the judiciary, police and related bodies, government and state bodies responsible for – or using the services of – forensic practitioners, research institutes and those undertaking (as educators or students) academic courses or training in medical law, forensic medicine, investigation of crime and related topics. The Editors also hope that those who require authoritative information about the wide range of topics included – such as journalists and campaigning bodies, will find the information contained within as a valuable and indispensable resource.

The Editors have to offer huge thanks to the international spectrum of respected authors of the chapters, for their patience in the production of this substantial work. Each author has been chosen because of their reputation and their expertise in their given topic. Some aspects of some chapters may be controversial – we hope and intend that this is so. Forensic and legal medicine is not a science of absolutes, and its purpose is best served when opinions and approaches to the often complex and sensitive topics of debate can be discussed freely, openly and reasonably without fear of intimidation, retribution or victimisation.

Our thanks must of course go to the publishers – Elsevier – and to the staff of the Major Reference Works Department. In particular, we must congratulate Mark Knowles for his patience and understanding throughout the project, as he as borne the brunt of the development and given the Editors unqualified and unhesitating support. As Editors we have been very grateful for his involvement from shortly after conception, through gestation, to delivery. Assisting Mark have been Tracey Mills, Eleanor Orchard, Sue Stokes, Davinia Hurn-Shanley and Mireille Yanow. Nick Fallon, Mark Listewnik and Carey Chapman were key in establishing and supporting the project through its development. In the production stages Sarah Parkin has been extremely active in identifying any concerns and providing solutions in the production of the work.

Jason Payne-James
Roger W Byard
Tracey S Corey
Carol Henderson
November, 2004

INTRODUCTION

The need for an understanding of the roles, responsibilities and relationships of practitioners of forensic and legal medicine – and those related specialties – in relation to issues outside the specific medical world has never been greater. There are many issues that are of huge relevance today, where the medical and related professions can have a multiplicity of roles. International terrorism is one example. The medical profession may be involved at a number of levels – the investigation of causes of death after an attack; the identification of human remains; the appropriate sampling of substances that may have evidential value; the care and assessment of terrorist suspects and their victims; the presentation of evidence to courts; and at a more local level, issues of consent for treatment of those unable to consent for themselves; and concern for the treatment of prisoners. Each of these issues requires independent, impartial and objective opinions which allow justice to be pursued appropriately and fairly. With this example the skills of forensic pathologists, forensic physicians, forensic anthropologists, forensic odontologists, forensic psychologists, forensic psychiatrists and forensic scientists may be required. Their findings and conclusions need to be given robustly, with emphasis given where facts or scientific research support an opinion, and clear guidance when such facts or research are either equivocal, or not available.

In some ways the forensic and legal medicine specialist may act as one of the gatekeepers within judicial systems. The recognition of the critical importance of such evidence has been highlighted worldwide where expert evidence has been challenged and impartiality has been questioned. Such challenges and questioning have put much focus on attempting to improve and clarify how, when and to what extent expert opinions in the forensic setting can be utilised, and different judicial systems apply a range of tests to such evidence to assess its integrity. This means that for all those working in forensic and legal medicine and its related specialties, and scientific or healthcare specialties, training, update training and audit and assessment has become a *sine qua non*. "Accreditation", "revalidation" and "standard setting" are terms that are used interchangeably worldwide. Training and education in medical law and forensic aspects of medicine are much more widely available and, increasingly, medical practitioners may be dually trained in medicine and law. However, there are few areas of medicine and healthcare now which are untouched by a need to understand certain aspects of forensic and legal medicine. All healthcare professionals need to be aware of, and put into practice, issues such as consent and confidentiality and apply these into their practice. Every medical or healthcare specialty has some aspect that may require specialist forensic and legal medical knowledge. In many areas this knowledge may be available from a forensic practitioner, but all practitioners need to be able to assist their patients in the absence of such a specialist. To give a number of examples: emergency medicine specialists need to be able to document accurately wounds that present for treatment, so that later interpretation in terms of modes of causation may be undertaken; those caring for the elderly need to recognise and document signs of elder abuse; similarly, paediatricians need to recognise and document signs of child abuse; genitourinary medicine specialists and gynaecologists need to be able to assess, document and provide management plans for victims of sexual assault; primary care physicians need to be able to assess and documents signs of domestic or interpersonal violence; psychiatrists and psychologists need to determine whether mentally vulnerable individuals are responsible for their actions; radiologists need to be able to recognise image appearances of non-accidental injury. All may have to present evidence in court to assist a court with their deliberations. The Encyclopedia provides sources of information to assist in all these functions, as well as giving examples of how court and legal systems compare in different jurisdictions worldwide.

The Encyclopedia endeavours to ensure that the cross-over of boundaries between different related but non-medical specialties, such as forensic toxicology, forensic psychology, forensic anthropology and forensic science are understood and defined. The interrelationship between these specialties is complex and the investigation of issues such as war crimes may require the skills of all these specialties and more.

The work undertaken by forensic practitioners must be based on a bedrock of an understanding of human rights and ethical principles. These principles are identified and referred to in the Encyclopedia; the Editors believe that these ethical principles should guide all those whose careers are primarily or even peripherally involved in the forensic and legal medicine setting.

Jason Payne-James
Roger W Byard
Tracey S Corey
Carol Henderson
November, 2004

GUIDE TO USE OF THE ENCYCLOPEDIA

Structure of the Encyclopedia

The material in the Encyclopedia is arranged as a series of entries in alphabetical order. Most entries consist of several articles that deal with various aspects of a topic and are arranged in a logical sequence within an entry. Some entries comprise a single article.

To help you realize the full potential of the material in the Encyclopedia we have provided three features to help you find the topic of your choice: a Contents List, Cross-References and an Index.

1. Contents List

Your first point of reference will probably be the contents list. The complete contents lists, which appears at the front of each volume will provide you with both the volume number and the page number of the entry. On the opening page of an entry a contents list is provided so that the full details of the articles within the entry are immediately available.

Alternatively you may choose to browse through a volume using the alphabetical order of the entries as your guide. To assist you in identifying your location within the Encyclopedia a running headline indicates the current entry and the current article within that entry.

You will find 'dummy entries' where obvious synonyms exist for entries or where we have grouped together related topics. Dummy entries appear in both the contents lists and the body of the text.

Example
If you were attempting to locate material on hair analysis for drugs via the contents list:

HAIR ANALYSIS *See* DNA: Hair Analysis; SUBSTANCE MISUSE: Hair Analysis

The dummy entry directs you to the Hair Analysis article, in the SUBSTANCE MISUSE entry. At the appropriate location in the contents list, the page numbers for articles under Substance Misuse are given.

If you were trying to locate the material by browsing through the text and you looked up Hair Analysis then the following information would be provided in the dummy entry:

Hair Analysis *See* **DNA:** Hair Analysis; **Substance Misuse:** Hair Analysis

---

Alternatively, if you were looking up Substance Misuse the following infrmation would be provided:

SUBSTANCE MISUSE

Contents
Medical Effects
Cocaine and Other Stimulants
Herbal Medicine
Heroin
Substitution Drugs
Sedatives
Miscellaneous Drugs
Urine Analysis
Hair Analysis
Alternative Body Fluids Analysis
Patterns and Statistics
Crime

2. Cross References

All of the articles in the Encyclopedia have been extensively cross-referenced.

The cross-references, which appear at the end of an article, serve three different functions. For example, at the end of the Anthropology: Archeology, Excavation and Retrieval of Remains article, cross-references are used:

i. To indicate if a topic is discussed in greater detail elsewhere.

See Also

Anthropology: Bone Pathology and Ante-mortem Trauma; Cremated Bones; Overview; Role of DNA; Sex Determination; Taphonomy; **Autopsy:** Procedures and Standards; **Deaths:** Trauma, Musculo-skeletal System; **Death Investigation Systems:** United States of America; **Odontology:** Overview; **Post-mortem Changes:** Overview; **War Crimes:** Pathological Investigation; Site Investigation

ii. To draw the reader's attention to parallel discussions in other articles.

See Also

Anthropology: Bone Pathology and Ante-mortem Trauma; Cremated Bones; Overview; Role of DNA; Sex Determination; Taphonomy; **Autopsy:** Procedures and Standards; **Deaths:** Trauma, Musculo-skeletal System; **Death Investigation Systems:** United States of America; **Odontology:** Overview; **Post-mortem Changes:** Overview; **War Crimes:** Pathological Investigation; Site Investigation

iii. To indicate material that broadens the discussion.

See Also

Anthropology: Bone Pathology and Ante-mortem Trauma; Cremated Bones; Overview; Role of DNA; Sex Determination; Taphonomy; **Autopsy:** Procedures and Standards; **Deaths:**

Trauma, Musculo-skeletal System; **Death Investigation Systems:** United States of America; **Odontology:** Overview; **Post-mortem Changes:** Overview; **War Crimes:** Pathological Investigation; Site Investigation

3. Index

The Index will provide you with the page number where the material is located, and the index entries differentiate between material that is a whole article, is part of an article or is data presented in a figure or table. Detailed notes are provided on the opening page of the index.

4. Contributors

A full list of contributors appears at the beginning of each volume.

CONTRIBUTORS

Aggrawal, A
Maulana Azad Medical College, New Delhi, India

Al-Alousi, L M
Leicester Royal Infirmary, Leicester, UK

Allden, K
Dartmouth Medical School, Hanover, NH, USA

Allison, S P
Queen's Medical Centre, Nottingham, UK

Anderson, R A
University of Glasgow, Glasgow, UK

Artecona, J
Tulane University School of Medicine, New Orleans, LA, USA

Asser, S M
Hasbro Children's Hospital, Providence, RI, USA

Baccino, E
Centre Hospitalier Universitaire de Montpellier, Montpellier, France

Baldwin, H B
Forensic Enterprises, Inc., Orland Park, IL, USA

Ballantyne, J
University of Central Florida, Orlando, FL, USA

Barley, V
National Patient Safety Agency, London, UK

Bassindale, C
Lancashire Sexual Assault Forensic Examination Centre, Preston, UK

Becker, R F
Chaminade University of Honolulu, Honolulu, HI, USA

Beh, P S L
University of Hong Kong, Hong Kong, China

Bergeron, C E
American Association of Suicidology, Washington, DC, USA

Berman, A L
American Association of Suicidology, Washington, DC, USA

Betz, P
University of Erlangen-Nuremberg, Erlangen, Germany

Black, S M
University of Dundee, Dundee, UK

Blackwell, S A
The University of Melbourne, Melbourne, NSW, and the Victorian Institute of Forensic Medicine, Southbank, VIC, Australia

Blaho-Owens, K
University of Tennessee College of Medicine, Memphis, TN, USA

Blitzer, H L
Institute for Forensic Imaging, Indianapolis, IN, USA

Bock, J H
University of Colorado at Boulder, CO, USA

Bora, B
Tulane University School of Medicine, New Orleans, LA, USA

Briggs, C A
University of Melbourne, Melbourne, VIC, Australia

Brown, T
University of Leicester, Leicester, UK

Buchino, J J
University of Louisville, Louisville, KY, USA

Burbrink II, D F
Louisville Metropolitan Police Department, Louisville, KY, USA

Burke, A
Armed Forces Institute of Pathology, Washington, DC, USA

Burke, M P
Victorian Institute of Forensic Medicine, Southbank, VIC, Australia

Byard, R W
Forensic Science Centre, Adelaide, SA, Australia

Campbell, W B
Royal Devon and Exeter Hospital, Exeter, UK

Carter, J
Sussex Forensic Medical Services, Brighton, UK

Case, M
St. Louis University Health Sciences Center, St. Louis, MO, USA

Casey, E
Stroz Friedberg LLC, Washington, DC, USA

Cerminara, K L
Nova Southeastern University, Fort Lauderdale, FL, USA

Chaturvedi, A K
Civil Aerospace Medical Institute, Oklahoma City, OK, USA

Chiamvimonvat, N
University of California – Davis ACC, Sacramento, CA, USA

Clark, J
University of Glasgow, Glasgow, UK

Clement, J G
Victorian Institute of Forensic Medicine, Southbank, VIC, Australia

Collier, S G
National Drug Recognition Training Unit, Northampton, UK

Cooper, P N
University of Newcastle upon Tyne, Newcastle upon Tyne, UK

Cordner, S
Victorian Institute of Forensic Medicine, Southbank, VIC, Australia

Corey, T S
University of Louisville School of Medicine and Office of the Chief Medical Examiner, Louisville, KY, USA

Couper, F J
Office of the Chief Medical Examiner, Washington, DC, USA

Cox, A R
West Midlands Centre for Adverse Drug Reaction Reporting, Birmingham, UK

Crane, J
Queen's University, Belfast, UK

Czuzak, M H
University of Arizona, Tucson, AZ, USA

D'Arcy, M
Royal Women's Hospital, Carlton, VIC, Australia

Dada, M A
PathCare, Durban, South Africa

Dargan, P I
National Poisons Information Service, London, UK

Davis, D W
Hennepin County Medical Examiner's Office, Minneapolis, MN, USA

Dean, P
Rochford Police Station, Rochford, UK

DeFreitas, K
McMaster University, Hamilton, ON, Canada

Donald, T
Women's and Children's Hospital, North Adelaide, SA, Australia

Downs, J C U
Georgia Bureau of Investigation, Savannah, GA, USA

Drummer, O H
Victorian Institute of Forensic Medicine, Southbank, VIC, Australia

Dworkin, R
Indiana University School of Law, Bloomington, IN, USA

Edelmann, R J
University of Roehampton, London, UK

El-Fawal, H A N
Mercy College, Dobbs Ferry, NY, USA

Ellen, R L
Monash University, Southbank, VIC, Australia

Eriksson, A
Umeå University, Umeå, Sweden

Ernst, M F
St. Louis University School of Medicine, St. Louis, MO, USA

Evans, V
Ilkley, UK

Farrell, M
National Addiction Centre, London, UK

Fegan-Earl, A W
Forensic Pathology Services, London, UK

Ferner, R E
West Midlands Centre for Adverse Drug Reaction Reporting, Birmingham, UK

Fernie, C G M
University of Glasgow, Glasgow, UK

Ferris, J A J
Auckland Hospital, Auckland, New Zealand

Fisher, R P
Florida International University, North Miami, FL, USA

Flannery, W
National Alcohol Unit, London, UK

Flynn, M
Nova Southeastern University, Fort Lauderdale, FL, USA

Foran, D R
Michigan State University, East Lansing, MI, USA

Fornes, P
University of Paris, Paris, France

Fraser, J
University of Strathclyde, Glasgow, UK

Frazer, J
Cleckheaton, UK

Freckelton, I
Monash University, Melbourne, VIC, Australia

Fung, W K
University of Hong Kong, Hong Kong, China

Gaebler, R
Indiana University School of Law, Bloomington, IN, USA

Gaensslen, R E
University of Illinois at Chicago, Chicago, IL, USA

Gaoling, Z
Peking University, Beijing, China

Gatland, D
Southend Hospital NHS Trust, Essex, UK

Gerostamoulos, J
Victorian Institute of Forensic Medicine, Southbank, VIC, Australia

Glatter, K A
University of California – Davis ACC, Sacramento, CA, USA

Goddard, K
National Fish and Wildlife Services, Ashland, OR, USA

Goff, M L
Chaminade University of Honolulu, Honolulu, HI, USA

Goldberger, B A
University of Florida College of Medicine, Gainesville, FL, USA

Golding, S L
University of Utah, Salt Lake City, UT, USA

Goodwin, W
University of Central Lancashire, Preston, UK

Graffy, E A
Michigan State University, East Lansing, MI, USA

Graham, E A M
University of Leicester, Leicester, UK

Gregersen, M
Institute of Forensic Medicine, University of Århus, Århus, Denmark

Gudjonsson, G H
Institute of Psychiatry, London, UK

Gullberg, R G
Washington State Patrol, Seattle, WA, USA

Haglund, W D
Physicians for Human Rights, Washington, DC, USA

Hall, C M
Great Ormond Street Hospital for Children, London, UK

Hayden-Wade, H
Children's Hospital of San Diego, San Diego, CA, USA

Healy, T E J
University of Manchester, Manchester, UK

Henderson, C
Stetson University College of Law, Gulfport, FL, USA

Henry, M M
Chelsea and Westminster Hospital, London, UK

Herkov, M J
University of North Florida, Jacksonville, FL, USA

Hill, A J
Victorian Institute of Forensic Medicine, Southbank, VIC, Australia

Holck, P
University of Oslo, Oslo, Norway

Horswell, J
Forensic Executives, Upper Mt. Gravatt, QLD, Australia

Houck, M M
West Virginia University, Morgantown, WV, USA

Howard, J D
Tacoma, WA, USA

Hu, Y-Q
University of Hong Kong, Hong Kong, China

Hucker, S J
McMaster University, Hamilton, ON, Canada

Hunsaker, D M
University of Louisville School of Medicine, Louisville, KY, USA

Hunsaker III, J C
University of Kentucky College of Medicine, Frankfort, KY, USA

Hunt, N
Forensic Pathology Services, Abingdon, UK

Imwinkelried, E J
University of California at Davis, Davis, CA, USA

Ives, N K
University of Oxford, Oxford, UK

Jackson, R L
Pacific Graduate School of Psychology, Palo Alto, CA, USA

Jawad, R
King's College Hospital, London, UK

Jennett, B
University of Glasgow, Glasgow, UK

Jenny, C
Brown Medical School, Providence, RI, USA

Jones, A L
National Poisons Information Service, London, UK

Jones, A W
University Hospital, Linköping, Sweden

Jones, G R
Office of the Chief Medical Examiner, Edmonton, AB, Canada

Jordan, C E
University of Kentucky, Lexington, KY, USA

Josse, S E
Formerly University of London, London, UK

Jumbelic, M I
Upstate Medical University, Syracuse, NY, USA

Jureidini, J
Women's and Children's Hospital, Adelaide, SA, Australia

Kahana, T
Division of Identification and Forensic Science, Israel
National Police, Israel

Karch, S B
Berkeley, CA, USA

Keeley, S
Women's and Children's Hospital, North Adelaide,
SA, Australia

Kelliher, T P
Niskayuna, NY, USA

Kennedy, R T
New Mexico Court of Appeals, Albuquerque,
NM, USA

Kerrigan, S
Houston, TX, USA

Keyser-Tracqui, C
Institut de Médecine Légale,
Strasbourg, France

Khanna, A
Sandwell General Hospital, West Bromwich, UK

Kibayashi, K
Saga Medical School, Saga, Japan

Kirk, G M
University of KwaZulu Natal, Durban, South Africa

Koehler, S A
Allegheny County Coroner, Pittsburgh, PA, USA

Krous, H F
Children's Hospital and Health Center, San Diego,
CA, USA

Langford, N J
West Midlands Centre for Adverse Drug Reaction
Reporting, Birmingham, UK

Langlois, N E I
Westmead Hospital, Wentworthville, NSW, Australia

Lau, G
Centre for Forensic Medicine, Health Sciences
Authority, Singapore

Lazarus, N G
Path Care, Durban, South Africa

Lee, H C
Connecticut Forensic Science Laboratory, Meriden,
CT, USA

Leslie, L K
Children's Hospital of San Diego, San Diego, CA, USA

Levin, R J
University of Sheffield, Sheffield, UK

Levine, B
Office of the Chief Medical Examiner, Baltimore,
MD, USA

Levinson, J
John Jay College of Criminal Justice, New York,
NY, USA

Lewis, A
McMaster University, Hamilton, ON, Canada

Liang, B A
California Western School of Law, San Diego, CA, USA

Little, D
Westmead Hospital Wentworthville, NSW, Australia

Liu, R H
Fooyin University, Kaohsiung Msien, Taiwan

Loff, B
Victorian Institute of Forensic Medicine, Southbank,
VIC, Australia

Lord, W D
Serial Killer Unit, FBI Academy, Quantico, VA, USA

Ludes, B
Institut de Médecine Légale, Strasbourg, France

Lunetta, P
University of Helsinki, Helsinki, Finland

Luo, B
Sun Yat Sen Medical School, Gungzhou, China

Lynch, M J
Monash University, Southbank, VIC, Australia

Marc, B
Compiegne Hospital, Compiegne, France

Marks, M K
University of Tennessee, Knoxville, TN, USA

Marks, P
The General Infirmary at Leeds, Leeds, UK

Marrero, L
Shands at Vista, a University of Florida Affiliate, Gainesville, FL, USA

Martrille, L
Centre Hospitalier Universitaire de Montpellier, Montpellier, France

May, C P
Criminal Justice Institute, Little Rock, AR, USA

McKelvie, H
Victorian Institute of Forensic Medicine, Southbank, VIC, Australia

McLay, D
Formerly Strathclyde Police, Glasgow, UK

McNamara, J J
Serial Killer Unit, FBI Academy, Quantico, VA, USA

Meadow, R
University of Leeds, Leeds, UK

Mieczkowski, T
University of South Florida, Tampa, FL, USA

Millward, M J
University of Western Australia, Perth, WA, Australia

Milroy, C M
University of Sheffield, Sheffield, UK

Mimasaka, S
Kumamoto University, Kumamoto, Japan

Miyaishi, S
Okayama University Graduate School of Medicine and Dentistry, Okayama, Japan

Moore, K A
Office of the Chief Medical Examiner, Baltimore, MD, USA

Moriya, F
Kochi University, Nankoku, Japan

Morris, G
Plantation, FL, USA

Morton, R J
Serial Killer Unit, FBI Academy, Quantico, VA, USA

Mossman, D
Wright State University School of Medicine, Dayton, OH, USA

Mura, P
Laboratoire Toxicology/Biochimic, France

Murphy, W A
MD Anderson Cancer Center, Houston, TX, USA

Myers, W C
University of Florida, Gainesville, FL, USA

Nadesan, K
University of Malaya, Kuala Lumpur, Malaysia

Naidoo, S R
University of KwaZulu Natal, Durban, South Africa

Nashelsky, M B
University of Iowa Carver College of Medicine, Iowa City, IA, USA

Natarajan, G A
Chief Medical Examiner's Office, Perth Amboy, NJ, USA

Nathan, R
Merseyside Forensic Psychiatry Service, St Helens, UK

Nathanson, M
Compiegne Hospital, Compiegne, France

Negrusz, A
University of Illinois at Chicago, Chicago, IL, USA

Nordby, J J
Final Analysis Forensics, Tacoma, WA, USA

Nordrum, I
Norwegian University of Science and Technology, Trondheim, Norway

Norfolk, G A
Association of Forensic Physicians, Bristol, UK

Norris, D O
University of Colorado at Boulder, CO, USA

Olle, L
Royal Women's Hospital, Carlton, VIC, Australia

Ong, B B
Queensland Health Scientific Services, Brisbane, QLD, Australia

Orlando, F
Nova Southeastern University, Fort Lauderdale, FL, USA

Pagliaro, E M
Connecticut Forensic Science Laboratory, Meriden, CT, USA

Palmbach, T M
University of New Haven, West Haven, CT, USA

Park, G
Addenbrooke's Hospital NHS Trust, Cambridge, UK

Park, J K
University of California – Davis ACC, Sacramento, CA, USA

Parrish, R N
Office of the Guardian ad Litem, Utah, UT, USA

Patel, M F
Royal Berkshire Hospital, Reading, UK

Payne-James, J
Forensic Healthcare Services Ltd, London, UK

Peel, M
Medical Foundation for the Care of Victims of Torture, London, UK

Perlmutter, D
Institute for the Research of Organized and Ritual Violence LLC, Yardley, PA, USA

Pollak, S
University of Freiburg, Freiburg, Germany

Pounder, D J
University of Dundee, Dundee, UK

Prahlow, J A
South Bend Medical Foundation and Indiana University of Medicine – South Bend Center for Medical Education at the University of Notre Dame, South Bend, IN, USA

Provis, A
Mount Hospital, Perth, WA, Australia

Quatrehomme, G
Laboratoire de Médecine Légale et Anthropologie Médico-légale, and Faculté de Médecine, Nice, France

Rabinovich, R
The Hebrew University of Jerusalem, Jerusalem, Israel

Ratcliff, C
Thames Valley Police, UK

Reavis, J A
Relationship Training Institute, San Diego, CA, USA

Rebmann, A J
Connecticut State Police, Kent, WA, USA

Reeves, R
University of Medicine and Dentistry of New Jersey, Newark, NJ, USA

Ren, L
University of Houston Law Center, Houston, TX, USA

Rittscher, J
General Electric, Niskayuna, NY, USA

Rix, K J B
Leeds Mental Health Teaching Trust, Leeds, UK

Robinson, S
Altrincham, UK

Rogers, R
University of North Texas, Denton, TX, USA

Rognum, T O
University of Oslo, Oslo, Norway

Rosner, R
New York University School of Medicine, and the Forensic Psychiatry Clinic of Bellevue Hospital Center, New York, NY, USA

Rutty, G N
Forensic Pathology Unit, Leicester, UK

Rutty, J E
DeMonfort University, Leicester, UK

Sanchez, T L
New Mexico Court of Appeals, Albuquerque, NM, USA

Saukko, P
University of Turku, Turku, Finland

Saunders, C M
QEII Medical Centre, Perth, WA, Australia

Savage, K A
National Forensic Science Technology Center, Largo, FL, USA

Sawaguchi, T
Tokyo Women's Medical University, Tokyo, Japan

Scheuer, L
Royal Free and University College Medical School,
London, UK

Schreiber, N
University of Miami, Miami, FL, USA

Schuliar, Y
Institut de Recherche Criminelle de la Gendarmerie
Nationale, Rosny-sous-Bois, France

Seals, M
Nova Southeastern University, Fort Lauderdale, FL, USA

Sewell, G J
University of Bath, Bath, UK

Shapiro, L M
Papworth Hospital, Cambridge, UK

Shuttleworth, C
FGI, Ontario, Canada

Simmons, T
University of Central Lancashire, Preston, UK

Simpson, E K
Forensic Science Centre, Adelaide, SA, Australia

Sjøvold, T
Stockholm University, Stockholm, Sweden

Smith, J
Essex, UK

Smock, W S
University of Louisville Hospital, Louisville, KY, USA

Solon, M
Bond Solon, London, UK

Sorg, M H
University of Maine, Orono, ME, USA

Spivack, B S
Office of the Chief Medical Examiner, Louisville,
KY, USA

Stark, M M
St. George's Hospital Medical School, Epsom, UK

Sullivan, J E
University of Louisville, Louisville, KY, USA

Swift, B
Forensic Pathology Unit, Leicester, UK

Synstelien, J A
University of Tennessee, Knoxville, TN, USA

Taylor, R
Royal Cornwall Hospital, Truro, UK

Tersigni, M A
University of Tennessee, Knoxville, TN, USA

Thali, M J
University of Bern, Bern, Switzerland

Thatcher, P J
Forensic Science Center, Darwin, NT, Australia

Thid, M
Umeå University, Umeå, Sweden

Thompson, J W
Tulane University School of Medicine, New Orleans,
LA, USA

Tsokos, M
University of Hamburg, Hamburg, Germany

Tsunenari, S
Kumamoto University, Kumamoto, Japan

Tu, P
General Electric, Niskayuna, NY, USA

Tully, B
Psychologists at Law Group, London, UK

Tunbridge, R
Transport Research Laboratory, Wokingham, UK

Van der Lugt, C
Dutch National Police Selection and Training Institute,
Zutphen, The Netherlands

Vanezis, P
The Forensic Science Service, London, UK

Vayer, J S
University of the Health Sciences, Bethesda,
MD, USA

Vege, Å
University of Oslo, Oslo, Norway

Virmani, R
Armed Forces Institute of Pathology, Washington, DC, USA

Vock, P
University of Bern, Bern, Switzerland

Wagner, G
Medical Examiner's Office, San Diego, CA, USA

Walker, A
University of Sheffield, Sheffield, UK

Wall, I
Ruislip, UK

Weakley-Jones, B
Office of the Chief Medical Examiner, Louisville, KY, USA

Wecht, C H
Allegheny County Coroner, Pittsburgh, PA, USA

Welch, J
King's College Hospital, London, UK

Welner, M
NYU School of Medicine, New York, NY, USA

Wetli, C V
Suffolk County Department of Health Services, Hauppauge, NY, USA

White, J
Women's and Children's Hospital, Adelaide, SA, Australia

Wielbo, D
National Forensic Science Technology Center, Largo, FL, USA

Wilets, J D
Nova Southeastern University, Fort Lauderdale, FL, USA

Williams, G S
Northern Illinois University, DeKalb, IL, USA

Wolff, K
Kings College, London, UK

Wolson, T L
Crime Laboratory Bureau, Miami, FL, USA

Wright, M G
London, UK

Wyatt, J
Royal Cornwall Hospital, Truro, UK

Yonemitsu, K
Kumamoto University, Kumamoto, Japan

Yoshida, K-I
University of Tokyo, Tokyo, Japan

Youyi, H
Peking University, Beijing, China

CONTENTS

VOLUME 1

VOLUME 2

H

VOLUME 3

I

P

R

VOLUME 4

S

T

V

W

Y

ACCREDITATION

Contents

Forensic Specialties Accreditation Board

G R Jones, Office of the Chief Medical Examiner,
Edmonton, AB, Canada

Introduction

The Forensic Specialties Accreditation Board (FSAB) is an independent board established in 2000 to accredit professional bodies that certify forensic scientists and other forensic specialists. The term "specialty" was used because not all forensic disciplines are strictly science-based, but rather they are based on learned knowledge, skills, and abilities. Assistance in developing the FSAB program was provided by the American Academy of Forensic Sciences (AAFS) and the US National Institute of Justice (NIJ).

Accreditation versus Certification

Before going further, it is necessary to clarify the difference between certification and accreditation. In a professional context, the term "certification" is applied to individuals who submit to some process of evaluation and/or examination. It establishes whether individuals have the minimum knowledge, skills, and abilities as defined by the certification body to perform their jobs adequately. In a professional context, certification is often voluntary, although in a regulatory context it may be mandatory to perform a specific task or job.

The term "accreditation" is normally applied to an institution or program. In forensic science that institution is normally a laboratory, but it may be a program such as a professional certification program. An accreditation program evaluates the structure and performance of the institution against a set of standards. If those standards are met or exceeded, accreditation is granted.

Why Accredit the Certifiers?

It is not unreasonable to conclude that a professional certification program should be able to stand on its own without being accredited. Many could. However, there has been a marked increase in the number of forensic certification bodies over the past 10 years or so, some of which apply reasonable program standards, but some of which have few standards. This has become a problem since the courts and the legal system are not readily able to scrutinize every single expert that comes before them in enough detail to establish their credibility as an expert in the field. The courts therefore rely on board-certified credentials; these credentials are a useful baseline if the forensic expert is able to establish that he/she is certified by a reputable certification board and if the standards and reliability of that board can be established. However, determining which certification boards have acceptable programs is not easy.

Many of the mainstream forensic certification boards were established with the help of a US NIJ grant in 1976. However, even though they grew out of the same initiative, some lack components that are considered important today. For example, some have no requirement for a minimum amount of continuing education. Some certification programs do not require periodic recertification. An even greater problem is that some of the less reputable certification programs that have sprung up in recent years do not even have a meaningful examination that evaluates the competency of the individual, but rather are fee-based membership organizations.

Background to FSAB

The FSAB started as a committee of the AAFS in 1996. The AAFS was starting to receive requests to list the certification of forensic boards in its membership directory, but had no means of assessing which certification boards were credible, and which were not. It soon became clear that some type of evaluation or accreditation process needed to be established. At the time, there were only two main programs in North America that accredited certification bodies. The best-known is the American Board of Medical Specialties (ABMS), which is an umbrella organization that accredits most medical certification boards in the USA. These include the American Board of Pathology, which recognizes forensic pathology as a defined subspecialty. In addition, forensic psychiatry is a subspecialty certification under the American Board of Psychiatry and Neurology. However, the ABMS only accredits recognized medical certification boards and cannot accredit nonmedical specialties.

The other accrediting agency offering accreditation of certifying bodies in 1996 was the National Commission for Certifying Agencies (NCCA). The NCCA is a well-established accreditation board with published standards that has accredited over 50 certification boards in various paramedical and other areas. However, most forensic certification boards are very small and would find it difficult or impossible to meet the criteria and financial requirements of NCCA.

More recently, the USA-based American National Standards Institute (ANSI) has offered an accreditation program based on the standard ISO/IEC 17024. However, similar to the NCCA, the ANSI program is cost-prohibitive for the forensic specialty boards, most of which are relatively small. Furthermore, neither the NCCA nor ANSI programs would address some of the difficult issues related to the forensic arena (such as multiple certification boards for the same discipline). While accreditation by NCCA and ANSI remains an option, it was judged that formation of a new accreditation program, based primarily on internationally accepted standards, was the only practical course to follow.

What are the FSAB Accreditation Standards?

The accreditation standards used by FSAB are based primarily on the international ISO/IEC 17024

standards. Additional standards have been added to strengthen the FSAB accreditation program for the forensic specialties, and are readily available. There are two main components to the FSAB program: (1) those standards that apply to the certification body itself; and (2) those that the applicant certification body applies to evaluation and certification of its applicants. Standards applied to the certification body include: (1) a requirement that the certification granting entity be independent and impartial in granting or denying certification; (2) that they have written policies and procedures; (3) that they have a quality management program; and (4) that the structure, scope, and security for examinations are adequate. Standards must be in place that adequately assess the applicant. These are outlined below.

FSAB Standards that Apply to the Certificants

The FSAB program requires that the forensic certifying body have a meaningful credentialing process that stipulates the minimum standards for education, training, and experience, and inquires into the ethics of the applicant. There is also a requirement to conduct a meaningful assessment of the knowledge, skills, and competency of the applicant. Depending on the discipline, part or most of that requirement may be satisfied by a validated examination.

Validation of the examination is required to ensure that the questions are clear, unambiguous, unbiased, and properly cover the scope of the forensic discipline. Part of the examination may be oral or practical. The program must also require mandatory, periodic recertification, not to exceed every five years. Recertification must require continued involvement in the forensic discipline, plus a minimum amount of continuing education (also more broadly called continued competency), and reaffirmation of a commitment to uphold ethical and professional standards.

One other critical feature of the program is that "grandfathering" is not allowed. "Grandfathering" can be defined as the process where people are granted certification by virtue of the fact that they practiced in the profession before or for a defined time after the certification program was instituted.

The Problem of Multiple Certification Boards

One of the biggest problems in accrediting forensic certification bodies is that, for some disciplines, multiple certification boards exist. Different certification programs for the same discipline may be aimed at different levels of forensic practice (e.g., technical versus professional), but in some instances they may have evolved because of differences in philosophy over some aspect of professional practice or qualification.

At the present time, perhaps arguably, true standards for what an individual in a specific professional discipline must know do not exist for any forensic discipline. As a result, arguments abound as to whether the program with the most extensive and stringent standards is the only permissible one. Even if a professional consensus is reached for a given forensic discipline, certification programs may legitimately differ because they are directed at different levels or types of forensic practice. For example, in forensic toxicology, many "bench-level" toxicologists are never required to interpret toxicology results and therefore do not require the education and training in pharmacology that would be required for forensic toxicologists who do give opinion evidence in court. Because of these differences, the FSAB program cannot impose discipline-specific standards (because they do not exist), but does require that each certification program publish and have readily available (e.g., on a website) the standards (including the education, training, knowledge, skills, and abilities) that applicants are required to have to become certified under that program. The rationale is that, even though programs in the same forensic discipline may differ (often for legitimate reasons), anyone can readily determine the nature and scope of the program.

Scope of the FSAB Program

There is no geographic limit to the FSAB program, although for practical reasons it is currently limited to programs that operate in the English language. Any forensic specialty certification program that meets the published FSAB standards can apply for accreditation.

At the time of writing, the FSAB board has representatives from 10 different organizations, covering most of the major forensic disciplines. The first forensic board was accredited in March 2004. A list of current board members and program documents is available through the FSAB website (http://www.thefsab.org).

Further Reading

FSAB *Standards for Accrediting Forensic Specialty Certification Boards.* Available online at: http://www.thefsab.org/standards.html

ISO/IEC 17024 *General Requirements for Bodies Operating Certification Systems of Persons.* Available online at: http://www.iso.ch/iso/en/commcentre/pressreleases/2003/Ref847.html

Crime Scene Investigators

J Horswell, Forensic Executives, Upper Mt. Gravatt, QLD, Australia

History

During the 1980s Australians were subjected to a media frenzy surrounding the disappearance of Azaria Chantel Loren Chamberlain at Ayers Rock in the Northern Territory of Australia on August 17, 1980. The circumstances surrounding the disappearance and the Chamberlain family were subjected to media scrutiny like no case in living criminal history of the Northern Territory, or for that matter many other jurisdictions in Australia.

It was during a Royal Commission of Inquiry conducted by His Honour Justice Trevor Morling that the legal fraternity in Australia and forensic science practitioners sued for changes in the structure, function, and practice of forensic science in Australia. Justice Morling in his report highlighted some deficiencies in forensic science that contributed to the problems encountered in the Chamberlain case and suggested remedies for future practice. Specific areas of concern were the lack of communication between police, experts, and lawyers that resulted in an exaggerated importance being placed on expert evidence. He was also concerned about the absence of uniform and reliable practices throughout Australia which meant that the court could not be sure that "reasonably certain" results were being obtained, reported, and depended upon.

The Commissioner attributed these problems to the lack of infrastructure within forensic science in Australia and advocated the development of a National Institute of Forensic Science (NIFS). His vision for NIFS was to unite experts within Australia and connect them with experts from overseas. The Institute would be responsible for establishing and maintaining standards, facilitating the exchange of information, and research and education. The Commissioner stressed that the onus for funding NIFS should rest with government. It is pleasing to see that NIFS came into operation during the 1990s, funded by the state and federal governments of Australia, with the mandate to do just what the Commissioner had envisaged.

It was during the early 1990s that the Senior Managers of Australian and New Zealand Forensic Laboratories (SMANZFL), representing the forensic science management community in Australia and New Zealand, provided the vital leadership and pressed the newly formed NIFS for the creation of an Australian forensic science accreditation program, which would be managed by the National Association of Testing Authorities (NATA), through its newly formed Forensic Science Accreditation Advisory Committee (FSAAC).

The first third-party forensic science laboratory accreditation program in Australia relied in part on the forensic science laboratory accreditation program already in existence in North America, which was managed by the American Society of Crime Laboratory Directors Laboratory Accreditation Board (ASCLD-LAB), a program ASCLD had been offering to laboratories throughout the world for a number of years. In fact, Melbourne's Victoria Police Forensic Science Center had successfully gained forensic science accreditation through this scheme.

The first Australian program consisted of the American program's forensic science criteria, which basically centered on a quality systems approach to forensic science laboratory management. This, combined with assessment against criteria from the International Guide, International Organization for Standardization (ISO) Guide 25, for testing and calibration laboratories, which had been offered to participating testing and calibration laboratories throughout Australia, by NATA, Australia for some years, was offered as the first Australian program.

With the introduction of ISO 17025 and NATA's new supplementary requirements for forensic science laboratories in Australia, managers of Australian laboratories reviewed the necessity for continuation with ASCLD-LAB's accreditation for their respective laboratories.

It was, however, the foresight of NATA's FSAAC when formulating the classes and subclasses of tests that would come under the umbrella of NATA's forensic science accreditation program that, for the first time anywhere, an accreditation program for forensic science would include crime-scene investigation.

The Field and Identification Specialist Advisory Group (F&ISAG), a committee of SMANZFL, consisting of senior crime-scene investigators, forensic ballistics specialists, and fingerprint specialists, was tasked with coming up with an accreditation program for crime-scene investigators. The F&ISAG formed a smaller group of senior crime-scene investigators into a committee titled the Crime Scene Accreditation Committee (CSAC) to work through the conceptual and development issues surrounding the proficiency testing of crime-scene investigators, which is an integral part of the accreditation process.

Accreditation Criteria for Forensic Science

NATA's ISO 17025 supplementary requirements for accreditation in the field of forensic science application document require that crime-scene investigators be competent in the application of the principles of crime-scene photography, scene examination and exhibit handling, safety, and have an appreciation of the capabilities of other disciplines.

Being part of the overall accreditation regime requires that, even though a facility may go forward seeking accreditation for crime-scene investigation only, it must conform with the International Standard ISO 17025 – general requirements for the competence of testing and calibration laboratories – as well as NATA's supplementary requirements for accreditation in the field of forensic science application document.

The specific aspects of NATA's forensic science accreditation program as it applies to the discipline of crime-scene investigation is outlined below.

Court Testimony Monitoring

The presentation of testimony is the culmination of the work performed by a forensic scientist. It is therefore vitally important that the effectiveness of each examiner in the presentation of oral evidence be reviewed at least once annually. The following are acceptable methods by which monitoring may be carried out:

- observation of the testimony by a supervisor or a peer and completion of the pro-forma testimony evaluation form or
- the completion by officers of the court of a testimony evaluation form or
- a member of the laboratory's technical management team or a supervisor may request responses by telephone from one or more officers of the court. The responses would be used to complete the testimony evaluation form.

The testimony evaluation form allows for personal impressions such as voice volume, tone and fluency, eye contact, demeanor, and etiquette. The testimony of the witness is also evaluated for confidence, responsiveness to questions, preparation and subject knowledge, clarity and conciseness, objectivity, and impartiality. The witness having referenced the case file, diagrams, and photographs as well as the length of time the witness underwent evidence in chief, cross-examination, and reexamination would be included in the evaluation.

The monitoring procedure must also prescribe the remedial action that is to be taken should the evaluation be less than satisfactory and each analyst/examiner must be given timely feedback on the evaluation.

It is a requirement of the accreditation program that there is a documented procedure whereby the testimony of each analyst/examiner is monitored during each year testimony is given. Records of the actual monitoring must be kept for each examiner as a record of the evaluation having taken place.

Figure 1 gives an example of a court testimony monitoring form.

Duties and Competencies of Crime-Scene Investigators

The following is a summary of the main duties of a crime-scene investigator. These seven criteria were developed from information provided to CSAC by each jurisdictional representative on this committee. They were used to develop the competency and internal proficiency testing instrument, and the external proficiency test, which form the crime-scene component of NATA's program.

Initial Assessment of the Scene

1. Assess health and safety risks and take adequate safety precautions.
2. Ascertain the circumstances regarding the incident.
3. Define/redefine the scene boundary to optimize the recovery of physical evidence.

Case Reference Number								

COURTROOM/WITNESS EVALUATION FORM

The purpose of this questionnaire is to provide information that will help staff present more effective court testimony. **Constructive** evaluation of courtroom performance is encouraged.

Name of witness: .... **Date:** ....
Matter of: ....

☐ Coronial: ☐ Magistrates   ☐ Trial:

				1	2	3	4	5
PERSONAL IMPRESSIONS:	1.	VOICE (volume, tone, fluency)						
	2.	EYE CONTACT						
	3.	DEMEANOUR						
	4.	DRESS						
	5.	ETIQUETTE						
TESTIMONY:	1.	CONFIDENT (forceful, direct)						
	2.	RESPONSIVE TO QUESTIONS						
	3.	PREPARED & KNOWLEDGEABLE						
	4.	CLEAR & CONCISE						
	5.	OBJECTIVE						

			1	2	3	4	5
	CASE FILE (referred to in court?)	YES/NO					
	COURTROOM AIDS (diagrams/photos)	YES/NO					

LENGTH OF TIME: EVIDENCE IN CHIEF   ....

CROSS EXAMINATION   ....

COMMENTS:

....

....

Your comments would be appreciated on any of the above aspects of witness performance, which in your view could be improved. As a guide, "5" would be considered improvement needed and "1" no improvement required. If appropriate, indicate how witness performance could be improved.

COMPLETED BY:..   DATE:....................

Figure 1 Courtroom/witness evaluation form. Reproduced with permission from Horswell J (ed.) (2004) *The Practice of Crime Scene Investigation.* Boca Raton, FL: CRC Press.

Control of the Scene

1. Ensure that a log of all persons entering and leaving the scene is established and maintained.
2. Preserve the scene during the examination.
3. Advise those entering and leaving the scene of an access and exit path to minimize loss of evidence.
4. Adopt appropriate procedures to prevent contamination and loss of evidence.

Examination of the Scene

1. Identify and apply an appropriate search pattern.
2. Accurately record details of the scene.
3. Locate physical and trace evidence.
4. Make appropriate arrangements to collect evidence from victims and suspects.
5. Seek assistance from other specialists where appropriate.

Interpretation of the Evidence

1. Establish the possible significance of the evidence.
2. Establish the possible sequence(s) of events, where appropriate.
3. Communicate the significance and interpretation of the evidence to the officer in charge of the incident.

Recording the Scene

1. Record time, date, and location of the scene.
2. Make a thorough and accurate record of the scene.

Exhibit Collection

1. Collect and package exhibits in a manner, which will prevent contamination.
2. Ensure exhibits are identified by appropriate labeling.
3. Establish a record of exhibits collected.

Case Management

1. Ensure continuity and security of exhibits, items, and records.
2. Maintain liaison with the officer in charge of the case and other specialists.
3. Prepare relevant statements, reports, and other documentation.

Competency and Proficiency Testing Crime-Scene Investigators

The emphasis inherent in internal and external proficiency tests is one of continual improvement. Proficiency testing is an integral part of an effective quality assurance program, to monitor performance and to identify areas where improvement may be needed. Hence a critical element in NATA's forensic science accreditation program has been the development of proficiency tests for crime-scene investigation.

Internal Competency and Proficiency Test Instrument

A proficiency-testing program is an essential criterion for accreditation of a facility. Both the internal and external proficiency tests measure the capability of a facility's investigators, thus ensuring their competency and therefore the reliability of any results produced. Each crime-scene investigator must complete an internal proficiency test instrument and each facility must complete an external proficiency test using CD-ROM as a medium annually.

The instrument for internal competency and proficiency testing replicates what is required from a crime-scene investigator undertaking the external (CD-ROM) proficiency test.

See **Figure 2** for an example of the competency and internal proficiency test instrument.

Crime-scene investigation, because of its subjective nature, presented a definite challenge in developing the concept of how to test crime-scene investigators. The initial committee of crime-scene investigators (CSAC), after considerable thought and discussion, came up with strategies in dealing with external proficiency tests for crime-scene investigators covering:

- concept
- platform
- management
- development
- delivery.

The conceptual stage of developing external proficiency tests was a challenge for CSAC and it was decided to produce the first proficiency test using video (analog) format and at the same time task a media development company to develop the concept of CD-ROM (digital). It was also decided to set up an independent committee, the Crime Scene Proficiency Advisory Committee (CSPAC), which was tasked with managing the external proficiency testing program, leaving the marketing and distribution to NIFS, and the work of shooting the actual mock crime-scene scenarios to a subgroup of CSPAC entitled the Proficiency Test Working Party (PTWP). Since its inception, CSPAC has become a standing committee of NIFS and is an accredited NATA proficiency test provider.

This involves assessment at an actual crime scene.

A. INITIAL ASSESSMENT OF THE SCENE

The crime scene investigator should establish if the crime scene guard at the scene has:

DESCRIPTION	Achieved	Not Achieved	Not Applicable	Comment
1. Assessed hazards, physical, electrical, gas, chemical, and biological				
2. Supplied first aid or medical attention as required				
3. Determined nature and size of the scene				
4. Determined entry and exit points that may have been used by suspect/s				
5. Removed all persons from the scene and recorded details of anyone who may have unintentionally or deliberately contaminated the scene				
6. Called for assistance (if required) to coordinate the scene				
7. Called any other experts (e.g., fingerprints, police surgeon, forensic pathologist, and plain clothes investigators) if required				
8. Defined the scene boundary with tape and guards				
9. Protected any endangered physical evidence				
10. Recorded details of all actions in an official notebook and maintained a log of persons who entered and left the scene				

Has the crime scene investigator:

DESCRIPTION	Achieved	Not Achieved	Not Applicable	Comment
1. Ascertained the circumstances of the incident				
2. Re-assessed scene boundary and protection				
3. Re-assessed health and safety risks				
4. Taken adequate safety precautions, additional checks, and protective clothing				
5. Determined if anyone else may have entered or left the scene (e.g. ambulance officers, witnesses, other victims or suspects)				

B. CONTROL OF THE SCENE

Has the crime scene investigator:

DESCRIPTION	Achieved	Not Achieved	Not Applicable	Comment
1. Identified an appropriate entry point to the crime scene				
2. Monitored cordon(s)				
3. Ensured a log is maintained				
4. Arranged to obtain a copy of log of events recorded by the first officer				

Figure 2 Competency and proficiency test crime scene investigation. Reproduced with permission from Horswell J (ed.) (2004) *The Practice of Crime Scene Investigation*. Boca Roton, FL: CRC Press.

DESCRIPTION				
5. Adopted appropriate procedures to prevent contamination and loss of evidence				
6. Ensured that the scene is adequately guarded				
7. Determined an entry and exit path for the investigator to commence examinations whilst minimizing loss of evidence				

C. EXAMINATION OF THE SCENE

Did the crime scene investigator:

DESCRIPTION	Achieved	Not Achieved	Not Applicable	Comment
1. Demonstrate an appropriate search pattern such as lane, grid, zone, or spiral NB: At least one of these techniques must be demonstrated				
2. Make detailed observations of the scene				
3. Consider and assess trace evidence during the search				
4. Consider possible contamination of evidence during the search				
5. Make arrangements to later search victims and/or suspects for evidence (if applicable)				
6. Assess the need for:				
a. Fingerprinting				
b. Forensic ballistics				
c. Forensic pathologist/police surgeon				
d. Video				
e. Photogrammetry/plan drawing				
f. Other experts or assistance				

D. INTERPRETATION OF THE EVIDENCE AT THE SCENE

Has the crime scene investigator:

DESCRIPTION	Achieved	Not Achieved	Not Applicable	Comment
1. Assessed the significance of evidence at the scene				
2. Considered possible sequences of events				
3. Determined the most probable scenario				

E. RECORDING THE SCENE
Photography

Has the crime scene investigator:

DESCRIPTION	Achieved	Not Achieved	Not Applicable	Comment
1. Taken adequate photographs:				
a. General				
b. Mid-range				
c. Close-up				
d. Technical				

Figure 2   Continued.

2. Taken adequate notes regarding:				
a. Times, dates, locations				
b. Description of scene				
c. Location of items				
d. Persons in attendance				
e. Lighting conditions				
f. Condition of locks, windows, doors				
g. Condition of items and objects				
h. Any other relevant details				

Plan

Has the crime scene investigator:

DESCRIPTION	Achieved	Not Achieved	Not Applicable	Comment
1. Arranged for appropriate plans: a. Completed a sketch plan which is a reasonable representation of the scene				
b. Taken adequate measurements for CAD/sketch plan				

F. EXHIBIT COLLECTION

Has the crime scene investigator:

DESCRIPTION	Achieved	Not Achieved	Not Applicable	Comment
1. Collected all relevant exhibits				
2. Packaged all items according to procedures				
3. Labeled all items collected in accordance with procedures				
4. Maintained a log of all items collected				

G. CASE MANAGEMENT

Scene Aspects

Has the crime scene investigator:

DESCRIPTION	Achieved	Not Achieved	Not Applicable	Comment
1. Maintained close liaison with first officer and investigator so as to process the scene effectively				
2. Maintained control				
3. Organized and planned the scene examination				
4. Evaluated options available				

Post Scene

Has the crime scene investigator:

DESCRIPTION	Achieved	Not Achieved	Not Applicable	Comment
1. Entered details of examination in the case management system				
2. Entered collected items in relevant recording system/s				
3. Obtained any other relevant paperwork for inclusion in the case folder				

Figure 2 Continued.

4. Examined items for evidence potential in an appropriate manner to avoid contamination and/or cross contamination				
5. Assessed items for further laboratory examination including possible options				
6. Completed all relevant forms and reports for items requiring further examination and forwarded them to the appropriate laboratory				
7. Secured exhibits for further examination				
8. Attended at case conference				
9. Ensured continuity is maintained for all exhibits				
10. Ensured appropriate quality assurance procedures have been adopted				
11. Prepared relevant statements and other documentation covering the following:				
a. Included an opening paragraph stating relevant qualifications and experience				
b. Presented the evidence in chronological order				
c. Explained the nature and extent of the examination				
d. Provided a detailed description of the scene				
e. Described details before presenting photographs in series				
f. Presented the information in a way that can be understood				
g. Labeled/captioned photographs appropriately				
h. Introduced exhibits appropriately				
i. Produced any charts, plans, etc. of scene				
j. Presented opinion evidence appropriately				

ADDITIONAL COMMENTS SECTION

Any other matters arising from this assessment which should be considered in the final assessment:

_____

_____

_____

_____

_____

_____

_____

_____

_____

_____

_____

_____

_____

_____

_____

Figure 2 Continued.

Has the crime scene investigator carried out additional specific procedures?

DESCRIPTION	Achieved	Not Achieved	Not Applicable	Comment
1.				
2.				
3.				
4.				
5.				
6.				
7.				
8.				
9.				
10.				
11.				
12.				
13.				
14.				
15.				

Crime Scene Investigator being assessed: ....
(name)

Assessor: ....
(name)

.... **Date:** ....
(signature)

Figure 2 Continued.

Crime-Scene Proficiency Advisory Committee

This committee was formed under the auspices of NIFS and initially comprised five senior crime-scene investigators from jurisdictions throughout Australia. CSPAC is responsible for the development of all external proficiency tests relating to crime-scene investigation.

Crime-Scene Proficiency Test

CSPAC develops one external proficiency test annually, which covers any or all of the following performance criteria:

- initial assessment of the crime scene
- control of the crime scene
- examination of the crime scene
- interpretation of evidence at the crime scene
- recording of the crime scene and evidence
- evidence collection
- case management.

The scenarios conceptualized by the Committee are representative of those encountered in normal crime-scene operations and reflect any jurisdictional-specific roles of crime-scene investigators throughout Australia.

The scenarios are mock crime scenes, which allow crime-scene investigators to carry out normal procedures as near to the real thing as possible. These crime scenes are fabricated by PTWP and photographed using still photography. The photographs are sequenced and overlapped using a special photographic camera mount on a tripod. They are then entered into the program by stitching the images together to provide a panorama of the scene, with the ability to move from one point in the scene to another, allowing zoom ability for close-up views of evidential material which has been seeded within the mock scene by PTWP. The resulting interactive CD-ROM program is known as "After the Fact." The concept of interactive CD-ROM technology is not new, as it has been available in animated games for some time. The application, for this purpose, is a first anywhere in the world, which has been followed by others in Australia in relation to the recording of actual crime scenes for replication as virtual reality used during investigations and court-room presentations. The concept has also surfaced in North America in relation to testing fire investigators.

After several draft versions, the first CD-ROM external proficiency test was distributed to 110 facilities throughout Australia in August 1999.

There are three aspects to the crime-scene proficiency test:

1. the crime scene
2. the investigation tools
3. the written test.

Each aspect is fully explained in detail on the program and it is important that all investigators representing the participating facility equate themselves fully with the functions of the program before attempting the assessment phase.

"After the Fact" allows the investigator to "walk through" a virtual crime scene and provides for realistic scene processing, including the following:

● photography
● notes
● collection and packaging of evidence.

Questions, predeveloped by the Committee and relevant to that particular scene, are presented to the investigator in accordance with the seven key performance criteria of crime-scene investigation.

Crime-Scene Investigation

The identification, recording, and retrieval of potential evidentiary material is practiced worldwide by individuals from a variety of backgrounds who possess a variety of qualifications and who have undertaken a variety of education and training programs.

Some countries employ bench scientists as crime-scene examiners, some countries employ uniformed or plain-clothed police, who have very little training as crime-scene examiners, and some countries employ professional scientists as crime-scene investigators.

Some jurisdictions have recently embarked on employing graduate scientists who are then trained as crime-scene investigators. The author has been a strong advocate in the past for the provision of scientific and forensic education and training to police officers who carry out the functions of crime-scene investigators. This has had varying degrees of success in Australia; however, it has worked particularly well in the author's own jurisdiction. What one

needs to avoid is a bench scientist undertaking crime-scene investigation duties in addition to his/her bench duties – these are two very distinct vocational activities, laboratory science and field science. Like all specialties, those who practice within a given specialty must practice their discipline to maintain current competencies and be in a position to provide evidence to a court of law that they have the expertise required to present evidence of "interpretation" or what is known in scientific circles as "hypothesis testing." It is only by carrying out many and varied crime-scene investigations that a crime-scene investigator will remain current and be in the position alluded to above. However, there are instances when laboratory scientists should be called to scenes to assist their field scientist colleagues. This would normally relate to the way in which the laboratory scientist would want the item or sample collected and handled given a particular set of circumstances. There is always room for other specialists to assist at the scene, such as fingerprint and forensic ballistics examiners. To take away the "interpretation" aspect of a crime-scene investigator's duties is to demean the practice of crime-scene investigation and those dedicated individuals who practice in the discipline.

The value of accreditation in crime-scene investigation cannot be understated. The old adage "rubbish in, rubbish out" applies when there is not an appropriately educated, trained, and equipped crime-scene investigator undertaking crime-scene investigation duties. There is another universally held view: "it does not matter how well equipped or qualified the staff are at the forensic science laboratory, if the material they are asked to analyze or examine is not relevant to the case, was not appropriately collected or packaged, or, indeed was not collected at all, then the forensic science laboratory will not be able to 'make it right' and provide useful information as the evidential value of such material is lost forever."

It is only by routine quality systems auditing and proficiency testing the individual crime-scene investigator and the system that the crime-scene investigation facility will be able not only to say that they are delivering a quality product, but be able to prove it.

A crime-scene investigation facility must be staffed with appropriately educated and trained scientists, who carry out their field science discipline, by not only attending the very complex crime scene, but also by attending the everyday routine crime scene. The crime-scene investigation facility should also possess quality systems forensic science accreditation which will indicate to their client, the courts, and hence the public, that the product they produce is a "quality" product that is backed up by a rigorously tested "quality system."

The addition of crime-scene investigation to the Australian forensic science accreditation program is an international achievement that has only come about through a persistent team effort.

One last closing comment: third-party quality systems accreditation, even though it is administratively hard work, is good management practice.

See Also

Accreditation: Forensic Specialties Accreditation Board

Further Reading

American Society of Crime Laboratory Directors, Laboratory Accreditation Board (ASCLD-LAB) (2000) *Laboratory Accreditation Manual*. Garner, NC: American Society of Crime Laboratory Directors.

Ashley W (2000) *Interactive CD-ROM Training and Proficiency Testing – Learning from Experience*.

Aumeer D, Shaheen B (2004) Quality in Australian forensic science, National Association of Testing Authorities. *Australia News* 111: 4–10.

Australian Federal Police (2002) *Quality Management System Forms, Forensic Services*. Canberra: Australian Federal Police Forensic Services.

Crime Scene Proficiency Advisory Committee (CSPAC) (1999) *Standard Operating Procedures*. Melbourne: National Institute of Forensic Science.

Gidley D (1992) Accreditation will enhance confidence, National Association of Testing Authorities. *Australia News* 65: 7.

Horswell J, Edwards M (1997) Development of quality systems accreditation for crime scene investigators in Australia. *Science and Justice* 37: 3–8.

Morling TR (1987) *Royal Commission of Inquiry into the Chamberlain Convictions, Report of the Commissioner*. Darwin, Australia: Northern Territory Government.

National Association of Testing Authorities, Australia (2000) *ISO/IEC 17025 Application Document – Supplementary Requirements for Accreditation in the Field of Forensic Science*. Sydney, Australia: National Association of Testing Authorities.

National Institute of Forensic Science (1993) *Corporate Plan 1993–1995*. Canberra: Australian Government.

Standards Australia (1999) *Australian Standard – General Requirements for the Competence of Testing and Calibration Laboratories AS ISO/IEC 17025*. Sydney: Standards Australia.

Tilstone WJ, Siegel JA, Saukko PJ, *et al.* (2000) Quality assurance. In: Siegel JA, *et al.* (eds.) *Encyclopedia of Forensic Sciences*. London: Academic Press.

Wright MJ (1994) *Crime Scene Investigation*. Proceedings of the 12th International Symposium on the Forensic Sciences, 21 to 25 November 1994. Auckland: Australian and New Zealand Forensic Science Society.

Toxicology

G R Jones, Office of the Chief Medical Examiner, Edmonton, AB, Canada

Introduction

When the results of analysis by a forensic laboratory are reported or presented in court, there is an obvious expectation that the testing was performed by a competent laboratory and that the results are reliable and accurate. At one time, there was an assumption that testing performed by a police or government laboratory was necessarily accurate. However, unreliable testing in several high-profile cases throughout the world has shown that government or police laboratories are just as capable of using "bad science" as any other laboratory (Dingo Baby case (Australia), Birmingham Six bombers (UK), Guy Paul Morin (Canada), FBI whistleblower Whitehurst (USA)). So, how do the courts know whether any laboratory is competent enough to get "the right answer"? The short answer is, there is no way to guarantee any laboratory will perform flawlessly. However, accreditation of the laboratory following administrative review and on-site inspection is a major step toward ensuring reliability and setting minimum standards.

Why are there Several Accreditation Programs?

There are several subdisciplines within forensic toxicology, some of which overlap, and some of which have their own distinct accreditation programs. The subdisciplines include postmortem forensic toxicology (medical examiner/coroner deaths), impaired driving cases (so-called driving under the influence (DUI)), drug-facilitated sexual assault cases, alleged attempted poisonings, so-called workplace-related drug testing (employment or preemployment testing for drugs of abuse in urine, hair, or saliva), methadone treatment-related testing, court-mandated forensic testing such as in child custody cases, and sports-related testing for both amateur and professional athletes. The design and focus of an accreditation program will depend partly on the specific area of forensic toxicology; the scope of testing may vary considerably and the standards applied may be different for the subdisciplines. For example, while fairly strict standards can be applied to the analysis of a small number of drugs of abuse in a simple and relatively consistent specimen like urine, it is not practical to apply exactly the same standards to a diverse range of postmortem specimens such as blood and tissues, some of which may be in a state of decomposition.

What do Most Accreditation Programs Have in Common?

By their nature, all accreditation programs have written standards with which the laboratory must comply in order to become accredited and remain so. The process starts with a comprehensive application that will assess whether the laboratory appears to meet at least the basic requirements. If that review is satisfactory, the laboratory must submit to an on-site inspection of its facilities, procedures, and personnel records by volunteer or paid personnel who have no connection with the laboratory. This process is usually aided by use of a comprehensive checklist that reflects the standards set by the accrediting organization. If the minimum standards are met, the laboratory will be awarded accreditation for a finite period of time (usually no more than 5 years), after which the laboratory must be reassessed by at least an on-site inspection. Many accreditation programs will also monitor laboratory performance between on-site inspections by review of proficiency test results and/or by requiring a documented internal audit of the laboratory's operations using its own staff.

What do Accreditation Programs Assess?

The specific nature of the different programs varies significantly, particularly between the USA and Europe, Canada, and Australia. However, they all generally assess the administrative operation of the laboratory, qualifications of personnel and adequacy of their training, existence and adequacy of standard operating procedures, adequacy of the chain of custody, review of the analytical procedures used, quality assurance (including quality control), reporting procedures, and safety. Individual programs differ in their approach and focus.

How do Accreditation Programs Differ?

Most of the forensic accreditation programs in Europe, Canada, and Australia are based on International Organization for Standardization (ISO) standards, primarily ISO 17025, usually supplemented by additional peer-written standards or guidelines. ISO standards are internationally accepted, at least by the very large number of signatory countries, and therefore have wide acceptance. They include widely accepted principles and standards of analytical laboratory practice, quality assurance, and quality control.

Examples of ISO 17025-based programs include that of the National Accreditation of Measurement and Sampling (NAMAS) in the UK, the National Association of Testing Authorities (NATA) in Australia, and the Forensic Science Accreditation program of the Standards Council of Canada. The disadvantage of the existing ISO-based programs is that specific standards for forensic toxicology are lacking or limited. ISO-based programs are very dependent on the existence of a fundamental infrastructure, the cornerstone of which is a strong quality-assurance program. The vast majority of these programs cover forensic science "in general" and are not focused toward forensic toxicology. Specifically for forensic toxicology, especially postmortem and some other areas, the disadvantage is that the nonroutine nature of such testing is sometimes difficult to fit into the "ISO mold." For example, ongoing quality monitoring is difficult for a drug assay that may only be performed once or twice a year. However, forensic toxicology laboratories in Canada, Australia, and the UK, and at least one in the USA have been accredited under ISO 17025 with appendices that include standards for the forensic sciences.

While at least one forensic science accreditation program in the USA is performed according to ISO standards, most forensic laboratories in the USA are based on peer-developed standards, although they invariably encompass many of the principles contained in the ISO standards. One advantage of the programs developed within the discipline is that they necessarily address some of the unique problems of that discipline.

Specific Accreditation Programs Covering Forensic Toxicology

There are five nationally available accreditation programs currently in the USA, only three of which are specific for forensic toxicology. Two of those programs are specific for so-called forensic urine drug testing (FUDT).

National Laboratory Certification Program (NLCP)

The NLCP is perhaps the most prominent program, mandated by the US Substance Abuse and Mental Health Services Administration under contract to Research Triangle Institute in North Carolina. The program stemmed from the "mandatory guidelines" published in the Federal Register in 1987, and subsequent revisions. However, this regulatory "certification" program has a very narrow focus, dealing with only five drug groups in urine (covering only eight drugs), in addition to integrity testing (to determine whether a urine sample has been adulterated or substituted); it does not cover the broader aspects of forensic toxicology. There have been discussions to include oral fluids and hair testing, although there are no plans to expand the list of drugs covered. This regulatory program covers the mandated testing of specific federal government employees and testing mandated by the US Department of Transportation. Laboratories must maintain a satisfactory score in quarterly proficiency tests and satisfactory performance in on-site inspections held every 6 months.

College of American Pathologists (CAP)

The CAP offers several accreditation programs in the clinical area, although only one is specific for forensic toxicology – specific for FUDT. It is broader than the NLCP program in that it covers a larger range of drugs of abuse in urine. Unlike the NLCP program, the CAP FUDT program is voluntary, unless mandated by local or state authorities. Satisfactory performance in the CAP FUDT proficiency test program, plus on-site inspections every 2 years, is required. (CAP also has a more general clinical chemistry accreditation program that covers clinical toxicology, including testing such as emergency drug screening and therapeutic drug monitoring. A broader range of drugs is covered than for FUDT, as is analysis in serum or plasma, in addition to urine. However, forensic toxicology is not specifically covered.)

While some aspects of each program are applicable to the broader aspects of forensic toxicology, these programs are otherwise inadequate for, for example, postmortem toxicology. Two other US programs are offered by the American Society of Crime Laboratory Directors Laboratory Accreditation Board (ASCLD/LAB) and the American Board of Forensic Toxicology (ABFT).

American Society of Crime Laboratory Director/ Laboratory Accreditation Board

The ASCLD/LAB program has currently accredited over 250 forensic laboratories of various sizes. Some are limited in scope, but many are broad-based forensic science laboratories that include forensic toxicology laboratories. The ASCLD/LAB program covers most of the conventional forensic science disciplines, of which forensic toxicology is one. The program checklist focuses on management of the laboratory, supervision, training, and quality assurance. However, very few questions in the ASCLD/LAB program checklist are specific to forensic toxicology. The program relies heavily on the judgment of individual on-site inspectors. The ASCLD/LAB program cycle is currently 5 years. However, laboratories are required to conduct periodic self-audits and maintain

satisfactory performance in a designated twice-yearly forensic toxicology proficiency test.

American Board of Forensic Toxicology

The ABFT laboratory accreditation program is designed specifically for medical examiner, coroner, police, private, and other laboratories performing postmortem toxicology and so-called human-performance toxicology. (Human-performance toxicology encompasses areas such as the detection and measurement of drug in drivers and other vehicle operators, as well as drug-facilitated sexual assault and similar testing.) It is the only program that was peer-designed and run specifically for laboratories performing broad-based forensic toxicology and is based on the *Forensic Toxicology Laboratory Guidelines*, first jointly published in 1991 by the Society of Forensic Toxicologists (SOFT) and the Toxicology Section of the American Academy of Forensic Sciences (AAFS). Those guidelines have subsequently been revised on at least three occasions; the latest version is available on the SOFT website. The ABFT program was first offered in 1996 and has slowly grown since that time, with a total of 16 laboratories accredited at the time this article was written. In order to maintain accreditation, laboratories must submit to an on-site inspection every 2 years and provide copies of all relevant proficiency test results annually. The 160-question checklist has sections covering laboratory administration, personnel, chain of custody and security, standard operating procedures, quality assurance and quality control, reporting, and safety, in addition to specific sections on all of the major analytical techniques. All questions are categorized as "essential," "important," or "desirable." Currently, laboratories must meet 100% of essential questions, at least 80% of important questions, and at least 50% of desirable questions.

Voluntary versus Regulatory or Mandatory Accreditation

For the most part, forensic toxicology testing is unregulated throughout the world, although there are some notable exceptions. The NLCP program for specific US federal employees and US Department of Transportation-regulated individuals has already been mentioned. However, for more general forensic testing, the state of New York passed legislation in 1996 requiring all public-sector forensic laboratories to be accredited. The ASCLD/LAB and ABFT programs are recognized for that purpose. Following some high-publicity failures in forensic testing, two other states, Texas and Oklahoma, have recently passed legislation requiring all forensic laboratories to become accredited; undoubtedly other states will follow. (It should be noted that many states and local authorities have regulatory programs for breath alcohol and the determination of blood alcohol, and even sometimes for laboratories performing urine drug testing (e.g., so-called workplace drug testing), but very few have legislation or regulations that cover the broader aspects of forensic testing and forensic toxicology specifically.)

The main advantage of mandatory accreditation is that it forces laboratories to upgrade their methods, procedures, and all aspects of laboratory operation. Even a conscientious laboratory director may delay these tasks if not forced to as a result of accreditation inspections, if there is a large and un-relenting backlog of casework. The secondary benefit of mandatory accreditation is that usually the state or local authority is forced to provide the necessary resources to allow facilities and equipment to be upgraded to the minimum standards required by the accrediting body. (A frequent excuse of laboratory directors for not pursuing voluntary accreditation is that they do not have the resources or time, because they are overworked and underfunded.) A local benefit is that preparing for initial accreditation and maintaining it can serve as a common goal for the entire staff of the laboratory, as well as instilling a sense of professional pride and accomplishment once accreditation is awarded.

Does Accreditation Ensure Acceptable, Error-Free Testing?

The short answer to this question is "no." The nature of any accreditation program is that it takes a "snap-shot" of a laboratory's operations at a specific point in time. It cannot guarantee that the quality of work produced by the laboratory will continue at the same level (it may stay the same, deteriorate, or improve). Staff may change between on-site accreditation visits. Accreditation certainly cannot guarantee that mistakes won't happen and bad practice won't creep in. However, accreditation, especially over a period of several cycles, should ensure that a minimum standard of practice is established, and that methods are properly documented, properly performed, and reliably reported.

See Also

Accreditation: Forensic Specialties Accreditation Board

Further Reading

Accreditation and Quality Assurance. Available online at: http://www.springerlink.metapress.com/.

American Board of Forensic Toxicology. Laboratory Accreditation Program. Available online at: http://www.abft.org/LabAccreditation.asp.

American Society of Crime Laboratory Directors, Laboratory Accreditation Board. Available online at: http://www.ascld-lab.org/legacy/indexlegacy.html.

Burnett D (2002) *A Practical Guide to Accreditation in Laboratory Medicine.* London: ACB Venture.

College of American Pathologists. Accreditation Programs. Available online at: http://www.cap.org/apps/cap.portal?_nfpb = true&_pageLabel = lab_accred_book.

Evans C (2003) *A Question of Evidence: The Casebook of Great Forensic Controversies, from Napoleon to O. J.* Wiley.

Hogg R (1996) *Dingo Baby case.* http://law.anu.edu.au/highcourt_project/Chamberlain%20Case%20rtf.rtf.

International Federation for Clinical Chemistry and Laboratory Medicine (IFCC) *Principles of Clinical Laboratory Accreditation (Policy Statement).* Available online at: http://www.ifcc.org/documents/Accreditation.pdf.

Morin GP (1998) Report of the Kaufman Commission on Proceedings involving Guy Paul Morin. Available online at: http://www.attoneygeneral.jus.gov.on.ca/english/about/pubs/morin/.

SAMHSA National Laboratory Certification Program. Available online at: http://workplace.samhsa.gov/DrugTesting/NatlLabCertPgm/INDEX.html.

Society of Forensic Toxicologists. Forensic Laboratory Guidelines. Available online at: http://www.soft-tox.org/Guidelines/default.asp.

The "Birmingham Six." http://www.innocent.org.uk/cases/birmingham6/.

Whitehurst F (1997) *FBI "Whistleblower."* US Department of Justice, The FBI Laboratory: An Investigation into Laboratory Practices and Alleged Misconduct in Explosives-Related and other Cases (April 1997). Available online at: http://www.usdoj.gov/oig/special/9704b/.

Accreditation *See* **Death Investigation Systems:** China; Japan; Nordic Countries; Certification of Death and the United Kingdom System; United States of America; **Forensic Psychiatry and Forensic Psychology:** Forensic Psychology, Education, Training and Certification; Forensic Psychiatry, Education, Training and Certification

AGE ESTIMATION IN THE LIVING

L Martrille and E Baccino, Centre Hospitalier
Universitaire de Montpellier, Montpellier, France

Introduction

Determining the actual age of a living individual
has great forensic significance, especially in the light
of a renewed outbreak of sometimes unlawful adolescent populations (illegal immigration, young people
seeking refugee status) and the subsequent rise
of delinquency among youths lacking proof of national identity. This may be exacerbated in some
countries by a mounting rate of family abandonment
or parental death.

Much less frequently, the court may also issue
orders aimed at determining the age of adults who,
for the most part, are born outside the country and
have not been officially registered with the state.

Age Estimation among Children and Young Adults: Justice for those Under Age

Although legislation regulating judicial rules for under-
age individuals varies from country to country, every
judicial system has set up age limits in regard to penal
procedures, as well as for penalties applicable to minor
delinquents. Thus, the magistrate needs to know the
age of individuals involved in penal proceedings.

For example, in France, there are no penal sanctions before the age of 13 years, even when an offense
has been committed. Another important age is 16
years because, after this age, prison sentences are
more important. The last significant age is 18 years,
the age of legal majority.

Age Determination Methods

The estimation of chronological age is derived from
the clinical, odontological, and radiological examination findings. Great interindividual variation in all
criteria being analyzed commands utmost caution of
interpretation and reservations in the final report to
the authorities.

Clinical Examination

Anthropometric criteria   Anthropometric measurements (e.g., weight, stature) are so highly variable
between individuals that they are of little value. It is
necessary to rely on easily measurable and replicated
criteria such as those found in growth percentile
curves. However, such reference groups of boys and
girls may not represent all the potential within their
generation, and even less so in cases where children
are of unknown origin: these results are not then
norms, but references to be interpreted.

Sexual maturity criteria   Tanner most precisely
described normal puberty development in both sexes.

In girls   The onset of puberty occurs between the
ages of 8 and 13 years. The growth of pubic hair
or labia majora precedes puberty by a few months
(P2 on the Tanner scale, average $10\frac{1}{2}$ years of age);
puberty begins with the development of the nipples
(S2 on the Tanner scale, average 11 years). Axillary
hair appears during stages S3 and S4 of breast development, about 12–18 months after the appearance
of pubic hair (average: 12 years of age). Around 13,
menstruation begins, about 18–24 months after the
first signs of puberty. The transformation of external
genital organs can also be seen: the vulva becomes
more horizontal due to forward tilting of the pelvis,
and the labia minora develop. Internal organs (uterus,
ovaries) also evolve. Other somatic changes are also
noticeable: growth of stature, muscular development,
and fat deposit on hips and thighs.

In boys   Puberty begins between the ages of 9 and
14 years in boys. The onset of puberty begins with
modification of the scrotum and penis and enlargement of the testicles, followed by the growth of pubic
hair (12 years). In accordance with stages P3 and P4
on the Tanner scale, axillary hair begins to grow (12 –
13 years), later followed by the growth of facial hair
between 15 and 20 years. The voice changes around
13–14 years, at stages 4 and 5. Also noticeable are
increased growth, broadening of the shoulders
(biacromial diameter), and increase in muscular mass.

The evolution of maturity is greatly influenced by
genetic and environmental factors, acute diseases that
may slow down growth temporarily, and psychosocial
factors. Precocious or delayed puberty, whether pathological or not, are eventualities that cannot be excluded on the basis of examination alone. Caution is
further warranted since a single secondary sexual trait
may remain isolated for a long time without any other
sign of development of puberty, without any spurt in
stature increase or rate of ossification.

Odontological examination   Dental aging may be
the most precise method of age estimation, especially
before the age of 15 years.

Dental age may be estimated either from the chronology of eruption of the teeth on the gum or from the mineralization of crowns and roots.

A dental formula allows good estimation of age, but, in contrast to the progressive calcification of dental germs, tooth eruption is more influenced by exogenous factors (anatomical characteristics of the maxilla, precocious puberty, heredity, and nutrition).

Chronological age estimation is relatively reliable during childhood, especially with regard to the second molar or "12-year-old tooth" which erupts between 12 and 13 years of age. Eruptions of the deciduous and permanent teeth have a well-known chronology before 15 years of age.

The level of development of crowns and roots is measured from dental X-rays and there are tables that correlate chronological age with the stages of development of crowns and roots. For better results these tables should be adjusted to correlate with ethnic and socioeconomic origins. These methods are more accurate than emergence because they take into account all teeth, even those that are yet to erupt. However the X-ray methods require substantial training and experience to be efficient.

After the age of 15, age estimation is based on the study of the third molar. Odontological methods are still very useful, although the relationship between third molar development and chronological age has been shown to be quite variable. In compensation, age could be estimated until the early 20s. The root begins to develop around the age of 15 and is complete around 21 years, with an average standard deviation of about 2 years. The third molar develops earlier in males than in females, and in mandibular than in maxillary arch. In forensic practice, if the third molar is totally erupted, or the root apices are completely closed, and the periodontal membrane has a uniform width around the tooth, there is a high probability that the chronological age is more than 18.

Alternatively, the third molar may be nonexistent, malformed, impacted, or extracted among young adults. Dental X-rays are very useful in such cases to make a differential diagnosis.

Several methods using computerized images of third molar root growth have been tested but are not currently used.

Bone Age

The evaluation of bone growth is based on the sequence of development of epiphyseal and round bone points of ossification, their growth rate, and the disappearance of cartilage in relation to established reference points.

It is critical to note that the goal of these methods was never to determine chronological age, but rather to evaluate bone development and evolution through time among children presenting with growth defects, to predict adult stature, or to check on the outcome of endocrine treatment.

Bone growth increases during puberty, a period when these tests are most reliable.

Methods   There are several methods of determining bone age:

- Quantitative methods require X-rays of half of the skeleton, are very penetrating, and are not often used.
- Qualitative methods are based on morphological variation of centers of ossification for a given articulation, and comparison to pictures of atlas of reference. The Greulich and Pyle atlas is the best known.
- Index methods: a numerical score is attributed to each step of ossification. For each given segment scores are added up to a total number which determines level of ossification.

Greulich and Pyle method   This method is based on frontal left-hand wrist and palm X-rays.

The purpose is to identify the carpal bones and the phalangeal epiphyses stage of ossification and compare them to those from the atlas of that particular sex. For both sexes there are reference sources for every 6 months or 1 year, depending on the age. Ossification-based aging is determined by comparing the subject X-ray to the atlas X-ray picture that best approximates it.

The Greulich and Pyle atlas was compiled in 1957 from a population of North American children, born between 1931 and 1942, and in a high socioeconomic stratum.

Bones displayed on each page of the atlas are of the same skeletal age. However, it was demonstrated that, barring any pathology, there could be a time lag between the stage of ossification of the carpal bones and the phalanges of 20 months for boys and 10 months for girls. The differential development of various bones may complicate the selection of atlas X-ray of reference. It is therefore recommended that primacy be given to the fingers.

Studies show that, if the average ossification age is close to the chronological age, standard deviation increases with age (it varies between 4, 7, and 13 months among boys over 17 depending on the study). For European children, the differences found between skeletal ages and chronological ages seem not to differ from the normal variations in skeletal maturation found initially by Greulich.

With this method, it is commonly accepted that, in order to obtain a reasonable bone age estimation, the result should be presented as an age range which takes into account the atlas pictures before (lower limit) and after (upper limit) the selected one.

A recent study concludes that the Greulich and Pyle method can be used for various ethnic groups. Low socioeconomic status may lead to age underestimation.

Taner and Whitehouse method This method is based on frontal left-hand wrist and palm X-rays.

This is a method based on a specific study of each bone to evaluate the development of certain hand and wrist bones. The first method studies 20 bones (radius, ulna, carpal bones (except the pisiform), and first, third, and fifth finger metacarpal and phalanges). The second method studies 13 bones, RUS (radius, ulna, short bones). Depending on developmental growth, each bone is divided into eight or nine stages. Each stage, documented by picture and diagram, is given a numerical score. The sum of the scores results in a score of skeletal maturation. Numerical results may be combined to obtain three types of skeletal development score: the carpal (TW3) score, the 20-bone (TW3) score, and the RUS (TW3) score. RUS provides the best age correlation, hence should be given priority in calculation.

It is imperative then to relate the chosen skeletal development age score to tables and curves of references to determine the age of ossification.

This method was devised from a population study of Scottish children born in the 1950s from rather low socioeconomic status.

For any given visualization, the difference between the most and the least advanced bone can generate an age difference of 3 months to 1 year. At best, the estimation then gives a variation of ±6 months.

Differences between various ethnic groups have been observed when age determination is based on the TW2 method. Several methods have generated conversion scales in order to adapt this method to local populations. A more recent atlas is now also available.

An advantage of this "bone-by-bone" method is that the examiner is not influenced by the stages of development of other hand bones.

Other methods The Sauvegrain and Nahum method is based on scoring elbow bones from frontal and profile X-rays. This method is valuable in populations of 11–15-year-old boys and 9–13-year-old girls, and can be a useful complement in forensics when the age is projected to be within this range.

The Risser test is based on a study of the development of the iliac crest points of ossification from a frontal view of the pelvis. The first ossification point appears around 13–14 years in females and 15–16 years in males. Ossification and complete fusion are generally completed in 3 years. Given significant variation in the development of ossification points of the iliac crests and strong potential for irradiation, this test is not systematically performed.

A scan test of the proximal end of the clavicle allows for the determination of four stages approximately separated by 2 years. This method could be used to estimate chronological age up to 29 years, and could be a useful complement to the TW3 and Greulich and Pyle methods.

Computer-enhanced methods Several such methods have been tested, one by Tanner himself: computer-enhanced methods allow for much more rapid analysis. Interobserver and intraobserver variability are greatly reduced. However, the quality of the radiography is critical to avoid important errors. In addition, underexposed or overexposed images that are poorly analyzed by the human eye are not so by the computer. Satisfactory image resolution is necessary, hence the fact that such methods are performed more to estimate bone age after the age of 10.

Computer-enhanced methods assisted by complex mathematical calculation methods called "neural network" have been proposed. Due to the greater precisions of such methods, results have been encouraging so far. Such technology, apparently in the process of being improved, is not currently in application, and these methods are not used in daily practice.

Other Factors

No method truly meets forensic needs.

There are essentially three sources of discrepancy between bone or dental age and chronological age: (1) inter- and intraindividual variability of growth; (2) systematic errors linked to the method itself; and (3) inter- and intraindividual variation among observers. For individuals in good health, skeletal age can be more than 1 year higher or younger than chronological age.

The rate of skeletal growth varies between various ethnic groups and between individuals residing in different countries, but it is the socioeconomic level that seems to play the most important role. Less favorable environments generate growth retardation. Overall, bones mature faster today than in the past. The application of the methods to subjects of unknown origin warrants extreme caution, especially given the fact that the patient's X-rays are never compared to his/her population of reference. National standards should be established and regularly updated.

If the Greulich and Pyle method is more rapid (and often the only one mastered) and more often used (1.5 mm per picture) than the TW2 (8 mm per picture), studies have shown that it is TW2 that retains the best correlation to chronological age and that offers better reproducibility.

The Greulich and Pyle atlas is the most widely used and has been recommended in practical situations. However, the authors themselves recognize the greater accuracy and reproducibility of the Tanner and Whitehouse method.

Epiphyseal fusion is more subject to population variability and puberty timing than dental development. Thus, dental age will often be closer to chronological age than bone age. Dental age is a more accurate index for age estimation for the early teens. Later in adolescence, only the third molar continues to form. The development of the third molar is quite variable, but allows estimation until the early 20s, whereas bone age, except the clavicle, allows estimation until 18 years of age.

No methods exist to estimate the age of living adults.

In Practice

Chronological age estimation begins with a clinical examination (anthropometric criteria, signs of sexual maturation) followed by odontological examination in order to determine dental status. If all teeth are erupted, including the third molar, it is not necessary to perform radiographs such as orthopantograms. If not, dental radiographs must be performed and interpreted by a forensic odontologist.

Any developmental disorders that may affect normal development should be taken in account.

Radiological bone examination should follow but be limited to a frontal X-ray of the left hand and wrist on the same picture (± the elbow if the age appears to be clinically less than 15 years).

The optimal course of action should aim at evaluating bone age from two methods, Tanner and Whitehouse and Greulich and Pyle. In our opinion, the Risser test should no longer be performed. Most often however, one must rely on the Greulich and Pyle atlas, since few trained teams will be able to master the TW3 method.

It is advisable to have a radiologist interpret the X-rays. It is the task of the medical examiner then to synthesize the clinical and radiological results.

In all cases, age estimation will and must be given as an estimation between two value points of discrepancy and should be discussed case by case. The expert must remain wary of puberty retardation and precocity, diseases, and socioeconomic factors that may affect the development of the individual examined.

Conclusion

Age determination is an important and frequent forensic act. The selected method should as far as possible be the most accurate, the most reproducible, and the least irradiating.

The tools at our disposal today can only indicate an age bracket, whereas the court would like to see age determination to the day. Chronological age can only be concluded to a certain degree of likelihood from the biological age, but not definitely determined.

It is necessary for medical examiners to devise new standards and/or to update them on a regular basis, so as to incorporate ethnic, geographic, and socioeconomic differences.

Beyond these requirements, computer-enhanced imaging should take the lead in the future.

See Also

Anthropology: Morphological Age Estimation

Further Reading

Bull RK, Edwards PD, Kemp PM, Hughes IA (1999) Bone age assesment: a large comparison of the Greulich and Pyle, and Tanner and Whitehouse (TW2) methods. *Archives of Diseases in Childhood* 81: 172–173.

Dermirjian A, Goldstein H (1976) New system for dental maturity based on seven and four teeth. *Annals of Human Biology* 3: 411–421.

Frisch H, Riedl S, Waldhör T (1996) Computer-aided estimation of skeletal age and comparison with bone age evaluations by the method of Greulich–Pyle and Tanner–Whitehouse. *Pediatric Radiology* 26: 226–231.

Greulich WW, Pyle SI (1959) *Radiographic Atlas of Skeletal Development of the Hand and Wrist,* 2nd edn. Stanford, CA: Stanford University Press.

Groell R, Lindbichler F, Riepl T, *et al.* (1999) The reliability of bone age determination in central European children using the Greulich and Pyle method. *British Journal of Radiology* 72: 461–464.

Gross GW, Boone JM, Bishop DM (1995) Pediatric skeletal age: determination with neural networks. *Radiology* 195: 689–695.

Kullman I (1995) Computerized measurements of the lower third molar related to chronologic age in young adults. *Acta Odontologica Scandinavica* 53: 211–216.

Marshall WA, Tanner JM (1969) Variations in the pattern of pubertal changes in girls. *Archives of Diseases in Childhood* 44: 291–303.

Marshall WA, Tanner JM (1970) Variations in the pattern of pubertal changes in boys. *Archives of Diseases in Childhood* 45: 13–23.

Mincer HH, Harris EF, Berryman HE (1993) The ABFO study of the third molar development and its use as an estimator of chronological age. *Journal of Forensic Sciences* 2: 379–390.

Pietka BE, Pospiech S, Gertych A, *et al.* (2001) Computer automated approach to the extraction of epiphyseal regions in hand radiographs. *Journal of Digital Imaging* 14: 165–172.

Schmeling A, Reisinger W, Loreck D, *et al.* (2000) Effect of ethnicity on skeletal maturation: consequences for forensic age estimation. *International Journal of Legal Medicine* 113: 253–258.

Tanner JM, Gibbons RD (1994) A computerized image analysis system for estimating Tanner–Whitehouse 2 bone age. *Hormone Research* 42: 282–287.

Tanner JM, Healy JR, Goldstein H, Cameron N (2001) *Assesment of Skeletal Maturity and Prediction of Adult Height (TW3 Method)*, 3rd edn. London: Saunders.

Ubelaker DK (1999) *Human Skeletal Remains, Excavation, Analysis, Interpretation*, 3rd edn. Washington, DC: Taraxacum.

ALCOHOL

Contents

Breath Alcohol Analysis

R G Gullberg, Washington State Patrol, Seattle, WA, USA

Introduction

As early as 1904, alcohol was recognized as a significant contributor to the risk of having an automobile accident. Since then, abundant epidemiological evidence supports the causal association between alcohol concentration in drivers (usually measured in the breath) and the risk of automobile accidents. Alcohol remains a major threat to traffic safety and is the drug most commonly encountered by forensic toxicologists. In order to address these concerns efficiently, breath alcohol measurement has emerged as the predominant method employed in "driving under the influence" (DUI) enforcement throughout North America, Europe, Australia, and other western nations. Programs have been established that integrate analytical methods, protocols, and trained personnel, all within a sound legal framework. Despite significant advancements in technology and legal structure, many challenges remain. The term alcohol will refer to ethyl alcohol, the organic compound found in alcoholic beverages.

Relevance to Traffic Safety

The role of alcohol in traffic safety has been the focus of enormous research effort. The vast majority of this work has relied on breath alcohol data when assessing accident risk. Breath alcohol analysis has also become widely employed in other transportation, research, public safety, and workplace contexts.

Several reasons exist for the widespread forensic application of breath alcohol measurement. These include: (1) minimal training and ease of analysis; (2) instrument portability; (3) immediate results; (4) computerized instrumentation; (5) noninvasive sample collection; (6) analytical reliability and robustness; and (7) widespread legal acceptability. Many jurisdictions, therefore, have enacted laws prohibiting specific breath alcohol concentrations (BrAC) and requiring subjects to provide breath samples under implied consent. Implied consent describes legislation where, by the operation of a motor vehicle, an individual has implied to have given his/her consent to submit to a breath alcohol test if requested by a law enforcement officer. Failing to do so results in driver's license revocation. A long history of case law exists for these issues. The measurement of breath alcohol, therefore, has substantial scientific and legal foundation.

Biological Considerations

Alcohol is consumed orally in most cases of forensic interest. Ethyl alcohol is a small (atomic mass unit $= 46$), polar organic molecule that is rapidly absorbed into the blood by simple diffusion across the mucosa lining the stomach and small intestine. Absorption from the stomach can be highly variable, depending on food content, alcohol concentration of the beverage, general gastric motility, and pyloric response. Approximately 25% of the ingested alcohol will be absorbed from the stomach while the remaining is rapidly absorbed in the upper portion of the small intestine. Upon entering the portal circulation, alcohol is transported to the liver where metabolism, predominantly via the alcohol dehydrogenase (ADH) pathway, occurs. The blood will distribute the alcohol to all parts of the body according to water concentration. Approximately 95% of the ingested alcohol is metabolized by enzymatic pathways in the liver with the remaining fraction being lost through sweat, urine, and exhaled breath. Alcohol pharmacokinetics generally follows a Michaelis–Menten model with linear (zero-order) elimination throughout most of the forensically relevant concentrations. Linear elimination has become an important assumption in cases requiring retrograde extrapolation.

The delivery of alcohol to the pulmonary circulation allows its measurement within the exhaled breath. The lungs of a healthy adult contain over 300 million alveoli and provide a surface area of $60 \, m^2$. The alveolar–capillary interface allows for the exchange of volatile gases, including alcohol. In accordance with Henry's law, alcohol will partition itself between the capillary blood and the alveolar breath as a function of temperature. At $37 \, ^\circ C$ this partition coefficient ($K_{blood/air}$) is approximately 1780:1. Following exhalation and airway interaction, the alcohol concentration in the breath sample is significantly reduced. Measurement ratios determined from venous blood alcohol concentration (BAC) and end-expiratory BrAC are generally closer to 2300:1. Because early breath alcohol instruments were developed as surrogates for BAC and statutes prohibited specific BAC levels, BAC/BrAC ratios have been the focus of much research and litigation. Position statements by the National Safety Council's Committee on Alcohol and Other Drugs in the early 1950s agreed that "Available information indicates that this alveolar air–blood ratio is approximately 1:2100." In 1972 this ratio was reaffirmed by the Committee. From these and other position statements has emerged the practice in North America of reporting BrAC as grams per 210 liters. The assumed ratio of 2100:1 has resulted in many legal challenges owing to the many analytical and biological factors influencing it. This highly variable relationship between the within-subject BAC and BrAC is illustrated in **Figure 1**, which plots both the BAC and BrAC for the same subject over time along with the corresponding BAC/BrAC ratio. The ratio is clearly not constant, even within the same subject. Issues and challenges regarding the uncertainty of this ratio, therefore, have prompted many jurisdictions to adopt statutory

language prohibiting specific BrAC (e.g., 0.08 g per 210 l) and BAC (e.g., 0.08 g per 100 ml) results separately. Moreover, one must use caution when reading and comparing the scientific literature regarding alcohol measurement since jurisdictions use a variety of different units. The measurement units used within each jurisdiction usually have a substantial procedural and legal history.

Differing within-subject pharmacokinetic models of BAC and BrAC have forensic significance. Since breath alcohol actually arises from arterial blood, it may differ in concentration from that of venous blood collected simultaneously. These arteriovenous differences are greatest during the absorption phase where BrAC (g per 210 l) frequently exceeds venous BAC (g per 100 ml). Following the peak (probably describing most subjects arrested for drunk driving), BrAC will generally be less than that of venous BAC, as illustrated in **Figure 1**.

Sampling is another very important consideration in measuring breath alcohol. While being voluntarily provided by an intoxicated individual, there can be significant variability in breath measurement results. Unlike blood, the subject is significantly involved in the breath-sampling process. Measurement results, therefore, are influenced by length of exhalation, preexhalation breathing pattern (e.g., hyper- or hypoventilation), breath temperature, preexhalation inhalation volume, and the alveolar composition of the sample. Modern instrumentation is designed to obtain representative and repeatable breath samples by employing several sampling criteria. **Figure 2** illustrates two separate breath alcohol expirograms from the same individual collected within minutes of each other. The reported results (those obtained at the end of exhalation) show typical variation observed in forensic practice.

The variability observed in forensic breath alcohol measurement has two components – the analytical

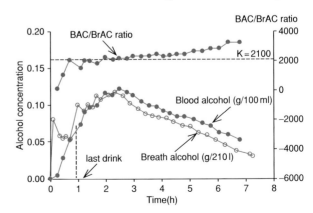

Figure 1 Corresponding blood (BAC) and breath alcohol concentration (BrAC)–time curves for the same individual along with the computed BAC/BrAC measurement ratio.

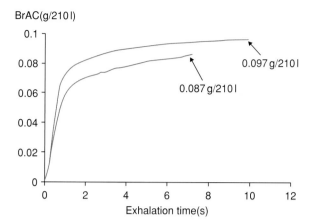

Figure 2 Two breath alcohol exhalation curves (expirograms) collected a few minutes apart from the same subject following two separate continuous exhalations into a computerized breath alcohol instrument. The large variability between samples is clearly illustrated.

and biological (sampling). If we consider these components as independent contributors to total variance, we can employ the equation:

$$S_T^2 = S_A^2 + S_B^2 \qquad [1]$$

where S_T^2 = total variance, S_A^2 = analytical variance, and S_B^2 = biological (sampling) variance. Consider as an estimate of the analytical component of variance an instrument that obtains a standard deviation of 0.0026 g per 210 l to 0.0009 g per 210 l on $n = 10$ sequential simulator standard results measured over 16 days near the concentration of 0.08 g per 210 l. The total variance, determined from an estimated standard deviation of 0.0033 g per 210 l, is obtained from evaluating duplicates on a large number of subjects also having concentrations near 0.08 g per 210 l. Employing these estimates in eqn [1] we determine that the biological (sampling) component contributes only 92% to the total measurement variance. This information can assist in identifying where efforts should be focused for minimizing the total variance. Sampling parameters based on exhalation time, volume, and flow rates can be developed within the analytical software that will require near-equivalent samples each time. These parameters must not be so strict, however, so that a large proportion of individuals are unable to comply. Similarly, features associated with the analytical, environmental, and simulator device can also be evaluated to minimize the analytical source of variance.

Analytical Methods

Work with animals in 1910 began to establish much of the physiological foundation for measuring alcohol

in breath. Further work with humans in 1927 showed that breath was a suitable surrogate for blood alcohol. The work of Rolla Harger in 1931 led to the development of the Drunkometer – the first commercially available breath alcohol instrument. The analytical method was the oxidation of ethanol in a solution of potassium permanganate within which a color change was measured. Harger also recognized the importance of obtaining an end-expiratory sample and incorporated the measurement of carbon dioxide to estimate alveolar breath. The Drunkometer began to be used by law enforcement agencies during the late 1930s. Finally, the Breathalyzer, developed by Robert Borkenstein in 1954, became the most widely used evidential instrument for breath alcohol determination. The Breathalyzer also employed a colorimetric method using potassium dichromate in a sulfuric acid solution and was designed to collect only the last fraction (52.5 ml) of breath from a prolonged exhalation. The Breathalyzer continues to be used by several law enforcement agencies today.

Modern Instrumentation

Computerized instruments employing infrared absorption and electrochemical technologies have now become state of the art. Employing computerized technology, manufacturers have developed highly automated instruments that ensure end-expiratory samples, provide printout results, transfer data to a host computer, monitor system performance, reject defective test results, and provide several other "intelligent" features capable of monitoring and controlling the analytical process. These modern instruments are also capable of performing automatic internal and external (simulator or gas) standard measurements along with barometric pressure monitoring when employing gas standards.

A large number of instruments are available for use by law enforcement agencies today. The National Highway Traffic Safety Administration (NHTSA), an agency within the US Department of Transportation, has published a conforming products list containing over 75 different instruments produced by 20 different manufacturers. Only a brief description of a few of the more widely used instruments for forensic purposes will be presented. Since every jurisdiction purchasing modern instruments requests different features, the ones discussed here are only representative of the features as employed within specified jurisdictions. All of these features can be altered or employed by all of the manufacturers, owing to the flexibility offered by computerized technology. Moreover, where predetermined criteria are not met, all of the instruments can be programmed to abort tests, require additional samples, and display and preserve message codes. Many of the analytical features of each instrument, therefore, are largely determined by the customized requests of end users.

The BAC Datamaster (National Patent Analytical Systems, Mansfield, OH) is widely used throughout North America and Europe. The instrument (**Figure 3**) employs infrared absorption to quantify the alcohol concentration in accordance with Beer's law.

The instrument employs two or more wavelengths (i.e., 3.37 and 3.44 μm) to distinguish between ethanol and one or more interfering substances (typically acetone). A basic condition of Beer's law requires that the same number of frequencies be employed as compounds to be distinguished. In addition, filters of these frequencies must be sufficiently separated to avoid overlap and of sufficient quality to approximate monochromatic light. These basic principles are appropriately applied in all modern infrared breath alcohol instruments discussed here. The BAC Datamaster is computerized with an attached keyboard. Customized software allows flexibility for a variety of analytical and data collection features. Breath-sampling parameters generally include: (1) minimum of 5 s of exhalation; (2) maximum slope for the breath alcohol expirogram; (3) minimum flow rate of approximately 4 l min^{-1}; and (4) a minimum breath volume of 1.5 l. The instrument also monitors several of its analytical systems including: (1) blank tests; (2) sample chamber purging; (3) internal standard; (4) external control standards; (5) sample chamber temperature; (6) duplicate breath test agreement; (7) pump operation; (8) software integrity; (9) presence of "mouth alcohol." Failing to comply with predetermined standards results in an aborted test.

The Intoximeter EC/IR (Intoximeters, St. Louis, MO) is another computerized instrument (**Figure 4**) employing electrochemical (fuel-cell) technology to quantify the breath alcohol. Infrared is also employed for the purpose of detecting "mouth alcohol" by monitoring the expirogram slope over time.

The instrument has a keyboard allowing for data collection. The breath-sampling parameters generally include: (1) minimum flow rate of 0.2 l s^{-1}; and (2) a minimum breath volume of 1.5 l. Several system parameters are also monitored, including: (1) blank tests; (2) fuel-cell solenoid operation; (3) diagnostic checks; (4) fuel-cell integrity; and (5) presence of "mouth alcohol." When failing to comply, status codes are preserved in memory for subsequent evaluation. The risk of acetone interference is further minimized by the fuel-cell characteristics and associated algorithms since the time for acetone reaction on the cell surface is largely different than that of ethanol.

The Intoxilyzer 5000 (CMI, Owensboro, KY) represents another widely used computerized instrument. This instrument (**Figure 5**) also quantifies the

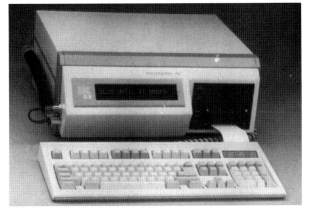

Figure 4 The Intoximeter EC/IR breath-testing instrument. Reproduced with permission from Intoximeters, Inc., St. Louis, MO.

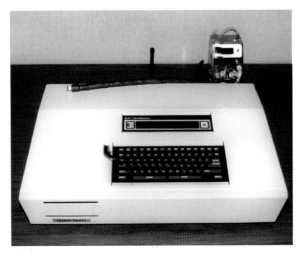

Figure 3 The BAC Datamaster breath-testing instrument showing a wet-bath control simulator standard device attached.

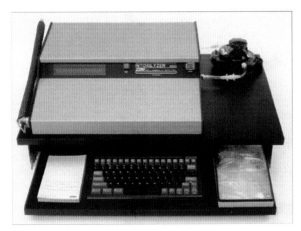

Figure 5 The Intoxilyzer 5000 breath-testing instrument. Reproduced with permission of CMI, Inc.

alcohol by means of infrared absorption. Multiple filters can be employed (depending on customer request) to distinguish between ethanol and several other potential interfering substances. The instrument also has a keyboard allowing data collection and printout capabilities. Self-diagnostics are also performed. Breath-sampling parameters generally include: (1) minimum flow rate of $0.151s^{-1}$; (2) minimum exhalation time of 2 s; (3) minimum volume of 1.1 l; and (4) a maximum slope of 7% for the expirogram (**Figure 2**).

The Intoxilyzer 8000 represents one of the newest computerized evidential instruments offered by CMI. This instrument is smaller than the Intoxilyzer 5000 and, with 12 V power capability, can be employed in either a stationary or mobile environment. The instrument employs infrared absorption technology with frequencies at both 3.5 and $9\,\mu m$, thereby improving the specificity for ethanol. The sample chamber volume is 30 ml with an infrared path length of 25 cm (10 in.). A unique feature offered with this instrument is the attachment of either a magnetic strip or bar code reader for the acquisition of driver's license information. Software is encoded within flash read-only memory (ROM) devices with the capability of being remotely revised or updated. The instrument also contains an ethernet port for those requesting that capability. The capability of data collection, printouts, and the attachment of external standards is also included.

A newer evidential instrument is the Drager 7110 (National Drager, Durango, CO). This instrument (**Figure 6**) employs dual technology (infrared and fuel-cell) to quantify the alcohol and thereby improve specificity. The typical agreement required between the two analytical methods is 0.008 g per 210 l or within 10% of the infrared result, whichever is greater. Differences exceeding these limits are assumed to be the result of an interfering substance.

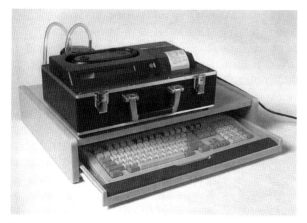

Figure 6 The Drager 7110 breath-testing instrument. Reproduced with permission from Intoximeters, Inc., St. Louis, MO.

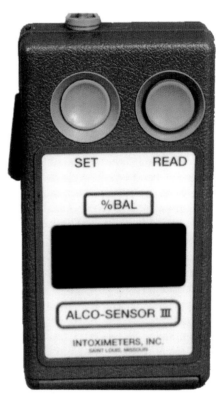

Figure 7 The Alco-Sensor III handheld breath-testing instrument. Reproduced with permission from Intoximeters, Inc., St. Louis, MO.

Moreover, the infrared frequency is near $9\,\mu m$, thereby avoiding the many organic compounds with the carbon–hydrogen stretch near $3\,\mu m$. The instrument is also computerized, offering data collection, printout of results, and system diagnostics.

Several handheld instruments designed for portable screening tests at the roadside are also available. Many of these models also appear on the NHTSA conforming products list. One such instrument (**Figure 7**) is the Alco-Sensor III (Intoximeters, St. Louis, MO). Like most handheld models, this instrument employs electrochemical (fuel-cell) technology.

Some handheld units also offer an attachable printer, data collection, error detection features, and breath-sampling parameters. These handheld devices are largely employed for prearrest purposes to establish probable cause. Indeed, these handheld devices also find wide application in the workplace, schools, hospitals, alcohol treatment facilities, and jails because of their simple and inexpensive operation, immediate results, portability, and robustness.

Measurement Protocols and Quality Control

The serious consequences of a DUI conviction require both adequate instrumentation and sound measurement protocols. Indeed, professional forensic practice should pursue the most reliable and confident analytical results possible. Results that are fit-for-purpose require a total program approach, including: (1) appropriate instrumentation; (2) sound testing protocol; (3) trained personnel; (4) initial and periodic evaluation of equipment; (5) sound administrative rules; (6) careful record-keeping; and (7) full disclosure.

Fitness-for-purpose is the assurance that appropriate confidence can be attached to measurement results sufficient for their intended application. All measurements possess error, resulting in uncertainty. A sound protocol will minimize both systematic and random errors to acceptable levels and identify cases where they are exceeded. Moreover, standards for acceptable results should be sufficiently strict so that not every subject tested will comply. An acceptable level of test rejection (i.e., 5%) will ensure that sufficiently rigorous forensic standards are being employed. There will not be admissible forensic breath alcohol evidence in those cases failing to comply with the predetermined criteria and other evidence (i.e., driving, field sobriety tests, etc.) must be relied upon.

The evidentiary weight assigned to breath test evidence is largely determined by the quality of the program/protocol producing them. At a minimum, the following should be considered in the program/protocol design: (1) specific language of the DUI statute; (2) critical concentrations prohibited by statute; (3) instruments employed and their capability; (4) training required; (5) printout results (information and format); (6) accuracy and precision requirements; (7) interpretability of results; (8) data collection capabilities; (9) unique legal challenges; and (10) program funding and control. Moreover, key individuals should be consulted regarding program/protocol development, including: (1) prosecutors; (2) law enforcement agencies; (3) judges; (4) traffic safety organizations; (5) forensic scientists; and (6) legislators. All of these have relevant interests and contributions regarding forensic breath alcohol measurement.

Quality control is largely determined by the careful integration of instrumentation and measurement protocol. Important considerations will include: (1) using preapproved instrumentation; (2) operation by qualified personnel; (3) preexhalation observation period (i.e., 15 min); (4) internal standard verification; (5) duplicate breath samples; (6) external control standard; (7) purging between all analyses; (8) error detection capability; and (9) printout of results. Preexhalation observation ensures that a recently consumed alcoholic beverage will not bias the result due to "mouth alcohol." The external standard is

preferred over simply an internal standard check because it measures the analyte of interest. The internal standard is simply an optical or electronic signal generator that is useful but limited. The external standard may consist of a wet-bath simulator device heating an alcohol/water solution to 34 °C to provide a headspace vapor alcohol sample of known concentration. Although any constant simulator temperature could be employed, 34 °C has been selected by most manufacturers because of its proximity to end-expiratory human breath temperature. The external standard may also consist of a compressed gas standard of known alcohol concentration. Gas standards, however, need to account for atmospheric pressure and the absence of water vapor. Although the measurement correspondence required for external standards varies between jurisdictions, typical values are from 5% to 10%. Duplicate breath samples agreeing within predetermined standards (i.e., within 0.02 g per 210 l or ±10% of their mean) are important to ensure precision and account for the largest source of total variance (the biological/sampling component). Purging between all sample analyses to predetermined levels (i.e., ≤0.003 g per 210 l) is also important to preclude a carryover effect. Although the third decimal place is informative for measuring precision, many jurisdictions prefer to report results truncated to the second decimal place as further forensic precaution. A carefully designed printout document showing all critical results and analytical units will further enhance interpretation. Finally, although not forensically necessary, data collection by a host computer can enhance program and instrument evaluation.

Legal Foundation and Challenges

There exists a long history of legal construction and case law regarding breath alcohol testing in both North America and Europe. The statutory framework generally consists of: (1) statutes prohibiting specified BrAC; (2) implied-consent statutes; and (3) statutes authorizing specified equipment, procedures, and personnel. Most jurisdictions possess *per se* legislation that prohibits motor vehicle operation while having specified BrACs. There will generally be coexisting legislation prohibiting the operation of a motor vehicle while "under the influence" of alcohol – accommodating the absence of a breath test. While simplifying the case by linking the offense to a measured result, *per se* statutes have also generated increasingly technical defense challenges regarding the analytical procedure. Challenges are particularly acute when results are near the prohibited limits. Nevertheless, jurisdictions continue to enact *per se* legislation while appellate courts continue to uphold their constitutionality. Implied-consent legislation continues to provide the foundational leverage for obtaining breath alcohol evidence.

The statutory foundation for program implementation is also necessary. Program details are generally found within administrative rules authorizing all aspects of the program, including instrumentation, protocols, and personnel. Careful consideration must be given to the drafting of these rules. They should not be overly detailed, thereby interfering with legal interpretation and admissibility. Program details are best left to policy manuals that are easily amended and available to responsible personnel. There also exists a great deal of appellate case law proceeding from US v. *Frye* (1925) and *Daubert* v. *Merrill Dow Pharmaceuticals* (1993) supporting the analytical methodology.

Recent incentives from the US federal government have encouraged states to adopt legislation prohibiting alcohol concentrations of 0.08 g per 210 l or more while driving. Many political, economic, and public health and safety interests have motivated these efforts. Many jurisdictions have also increased the penalties associated with DUI conviction, including: jail time, license revocation, increased financial penalties, eliminating deferred prosecutions, and enhanced penalties at higher concentrations. Statutes also emphasize different groups, including: (1) 0.02 g per 210 l limit for minors (i.e., zero-tolerance); (2) 0.04 g per 210 l for commercial vehicle operators; (3) 0.08 g per 210 l for drivers in general; and (4) enhanced penalties for 0.15 g per 210 l or more. Moreover, some jurisdictions prohibit specified concentrations depending on the number of previous convictions. These efforts to link the offense or penalties to specific concentrations have important implications for breath alcohol analysis. Low concentration statutes, for example, must consider the limit-of-detection (LOD) capabilities. Similarly, estimating the uncertainty must consider the concentration, of which the variance is a function. Indeed, all of these analytically dependent issues fuel the continuing debate in DUI litigation.

Many legal challenges are raised by the defense regarding the admissibility of breath alcohol evidence in DUI litigation. Several of these are general and occur in most jurisdictions. Others are specific to a particular jurisdiction due to unique statutory language, nature of the offense, and its consequences, specific administrative rules, unique analytical/protocol features, previous case law, and unique rules of evidence. In many jurisdictions the defense effort is directed towards having the evidence suppressed in pretrial hearings, realizing the persuasive nature before a jury. Where suppression is not possible, the attempt is to minimize the weight of the evidence. Several common defense challenges and possible prosecution responses include:

1. Uncertainty in measurement results: this is often an issue for results near critical *per se* levels. The forensic scientist must be prepared to compute and discuss the quantitative uncertainty employing appropriate variance estimates.
2. Breath alcohol is not determined at time of driving: this often leads to performing some retrograde extrapolation, which is fraught with uncertainties. Many jurisdictions have enacted laws prohibiting specified BrACs within a specified time (i.e., 2 h) of driving.
3. Technical details regarding administrative rules: all technical aspects of the administrative rules become elements for challenge. If, for example, the temperature of simulator thermometers is specified, their accuracy, certifying records, and traceability all become an issue. These technical details are best left to policy manuals.
4. Instrument repair history: sound breath-test programs will maintain careful records documenting the certification and maintenance history on all instruments. The reliability of an instrument with a large set of maintenance records is often questioned by the defense. Prosecutors should focus on the protocol and safeguards under which the defendant's test was performed. A proper and complete record for the defendant's results in which all criteria were satisfied should be interpreted as independent of prior instrument problems. Moreover, modern instruments are designed to abort a test if any of the critical analytical criteria fail to be met.
5. The potential for interfering substances: historically, acetone has been considered the only organic compound remotely possible of interfering with forensic breath-testing. In recent years, other volatile organic compounds, primarily from occupational exposure, have also been suggested as potential biases. Instrument manufacturers have addressed these concerns through: (1) employing additional filters in the infrared region; (2) use of fuel-cell technology; (3) employing other less susceptible frequencies in the infrared region (i.e., 9 μm); or (4) use of dual technology. Significant literature exists documenting the minimal risk of interference in a properly performed forensic breath alcohol test.
6. Use of database records to discredit test results: instruments with a large number of "error" records may also be challenged. The prosecution should argue that the defendant's test is

independent of previous results. In addition, administrative rules can be framed so the loss of database records does not preclude the admissibility of test results.

7. Linearity cannot be inferred outside concentrations tested: for results greater than the limits tested by the instrument, the defense might argue that the same accuracy and precision cannot be inferred. Although technically correct, prosecutors should argue that the offense is exceeding a specific concentration, not that the measured result has a specified accuracy or precision.

8. Challenges based on biological considerations: the defense might argue that the longer the person exhales, the higher will be the result. **Figure 2**, however, reveals the small increase in BrAC over exhalation time. This issue is addressed by carefully defining in the administrative rules the sample and measurement objective. For example, the sampling objective might be defined as obtaining an end-expiratory breath sample following a full single exhalation.

9. Software reliability: the defense will often argue the instrument software is either inadequate or not properly evaluated. Fitness-for-purpose should be emphasized by the prosecution. Agencies purchasing instruments should ensure the manufacturer has appropriately tested and documented the software for the forensic context of breath alcohol testing.

10. Traceability of measurement results: traceability of breath alcohol results to some national authority (e.g., National Institute of Standards and Technology, International Organization for Standardization (ISO), OIML (International Organization for Legal Metrology)) may be challenged by the defense. Documentation showing traceability through control standards (simulator or gas) to the national authority should be maintained and provided.

Obviously, these reflect only a small number of the many challenges proffered by the defense regarding breath test evidence. Each jurisdiction will face many challenges unique to its programs. Forensic scientists must work closely with local prosecutors and law enforcement agencies to ensure a cooperative effort in order to address the many defense challenges they will face. Oftentimes, changes are necessary in analytical or procedural elements to achieve legal admissibility and confidence in court.

The Future

Breath alcohol analysis has become firmly established within the analytical, legal, and traffic safety communities as an important tool facilitating the apprehension and prosecution of the alcohol-impaired driver. Nevertheless, improvements can be made in many areas. Indeed, there remain many areas to be explored, amenable to creative research.

Improving quality control remains a priority as the seriousness of drunk driving convictions continues to escalate in most jurisdictions. Breath alcohol evidence, employed in over 90% of DUI cases in North America, must be obtained and presented in a manner that maximizes its informative and evidentiary value. Measurement protocols should include at a minimum those elements discussed earlier. In addition, measurement results should ideally be presented along with an assessment of their uncertainty. Many European jurisdictions accommodate this by including correction factors. Further work is also needed regarding the performance of wet-bath simulator versus dry-gas standards. Finally, the computerized features of instruments should be enhanced to allow monitoring of instrument performance over time.

Further research is needed regarding the potential risk of interfering substances. Unanswered questions remain regarding which volatile organic compounds and what exposure, biological or analytical conditions pose a measurable risk for undetected interference. Moreover, the optimal combination of analytical and procedural features to address the interference problem has yet to be defined.

"Intelligent measurement" and expert systems need further investigation to identify relevant applications for forensic breath alcohol measurement. Techniques may be available to make simulator devices more reflective of the dynamics and variability of human breath exhalation. Many "intelligent" features exist for enhancing system performance and measurement confidence.

Improving the communication and interpretation of analytical results for the court also presents an important challenge. Optimal analytical results are of no value if the court is left confused regarding the information. Improving this communication process may include some combination of: (1) clear and professional oral presentation; (2) use of visual aids; (3) printout document appearance and informative value; (4) use of analogies to explain technical detail; (5) providing estimates of uncertainty; and (6) full disclosure. Disclosure of material to the legal community, for example, can be enhanced through internet accessibility. Many areas capable of improving the communication and informative value of breath alcohol measurement have yet to be explored.

Many areas of program administration deserve further research. Such areas include: (1) records to be retained; (2) optimal instrument certification schedules; (3) levels of personnel responsibility; (4) level of technical training for personnel; (5) instrument evaluation and approval process; (6) criteria used for field assignment of instruments; (7) advantages of employing a single instrument type; (8) internet provision of documentation; (9) computerized training of personnel; and (10) data collection and/or remote monitoring of instruments. Indeed, successful programs will involve thoughtful design, contributions from many different people, and the appropriate integration of instrumentation, protocols, and personnel.

Conclusions

Forensic breath alcohol measurement remains a prominent tool for confronting the problem of the alcohol-impaired driver. The biological understanding and analytical methodology are well established. The legal foundation is firm. Many challenges and opportunities, however, still remain. Quality control can still be improved while data collection and analysis need further application. The primary forensic objective remains, however, to provide the court with relevant and material evidence of the highest possible integrity.

Further Reading

Borkenstein RF (1960) The evolution of modern instruments for breath alcohol analysis. *Journal of Forensic Sciences* 5: 395–407.

Borkenstein RF, Crowther RF, Shumate RP, Ziel WB, Zylman R (1974) The role of the drinking driver in traffic accidents (the Grand Rapids study). *Blutalkohol* 11: 1–131.

Council on Scientific Affairs (1986) Alcohol and the driver. *Journal of the American Medical Association* 255: 522–527.

Dubowski KM (1970) Measurement of ethyl alcohol in breath. In: Sunderman FW, Sunderman FW Jr (eds.) *Laboratory Diagnosis of Diseases Caused by Toxic Agents*, pp. 316–342. St. Louis, MI: Warren H. Green.

Dubowski KM (1992) *The Technology of Breath-Alcohol Analysis*. DHHS publication no. *ADM 92-1728. Washington, DC: US Department of Health and Human Services, National Institute on Alcohol Abuse and Alcoholism.

Dubowski KM (1994) Quality assurance in breath-alcohol analysis. *Journal of Analytical Toxicology* 18: 306–311.

Dubowski KM, Essary NA (1984) Response of breath-alcohol analyzers to acetone: further studies. *Journal of Analytical Toxicology* 8: 205–208.

Emerson VJ, Holleyhead R, Isaacs MDJ, Fuller NA, Hunt DJ (1980) The measurement of breath alcohol: the laboratory evaluation of substantive breath test

equipment and the report of an operational police trail. *Journal of the Forensic Science Society* 20: 3–70.

Jones AW (1982) How breathing technique can influence the results of breath-alcohol analysis. *Medicine Science and the Law* 22: 275–280.

Jones AW (1992) Blood and breath alcohol concentrations. *British Medical Journal* 305: 955.

Jones AW (1996) Measuring alcohol in blood and breath for forensic purposes – a historical review. *Forensic Science Review* 8: 1–32.

Jones AW, Andersson L, Berglund K (1996) Interfering substances identified in the breath of drinking drivers with intoxilyzer 5000S. *Journal of Analytical Toxicology* 20: 522–527.

Lowry W, Garriott J (1979) *Forensic Toxicology: Controlled Substances and Dangerous Drugs*. New York: Plenum.

Mason MF, Dubowski KM (1976) Breath-alcohol analysis: uses, methods and some forensic problems – review and opinion. *Journal of Forensic Science* 21: 9–41.

National Highway Traffic Safety Administration (1999) Highway safety programs; model specifications for devices to measure breath alcohol. *Federal Register* 64: 30097–30100.

Philipps KA (1977) The "nuts and bolts" of testifying as a forensic scientist. *Journal of Forensic Science* 22: 457–463.

Wilson HK (1986) Breath analysis: physiological basis and sampling techniques. *Scandinavian Journal of Work and Environmental Health* 12: 174–192.

Blood and Body Fluid Analysis

D M Hunsaker, University of Louisville School of Medicine, Louisville, KY, USA
J C Hunsaker III, University of Kentucky College of Medicine, Frankfort, KY, USA

Introduction

Ethyl alcohol (EA), the psychoactive ingredient in alcoholic beverages, is universally available. Indiscriminate consumption is commonly associated with violence and disease. The most frequently detected drug by both clinical and forensic toxicology laboratories, EA is the leading cause of or contributor to drug-associated death, and constitutes the major catalyst in nonfatal trauma. For these reasons it has come to be regarded as unique, both historically and in current practice, and therefore is commonly discussed separately from other licit or illicit drugs of abuse.

In these contexts the task of the forensic pathologist or other forensic expert, as interpretive toxicologist, is to decide whether EA affected the subject's antemortem psychological, behavioral, and physiological function (**Table 1**). In official medicolegal death investigation additional issues arise regarding the role of EA in the demise of the individual (**Table 2**).

Assessment of the effects of EA necessarily relies on properly collected, stored, transported, analyzed, and reported specimens from the subject. In order to reach scientifically sound conclusions on the range of effects and mode of action of EA, the medicolegal official must be familiar with the fate and disposition of consumed EA in the body. This intellectual, correlative process in turn rests upon a thorough understanding of the interplay between quantitated results from blood or other fluid matrices. Significantly coupled with the breadth of analytical results is a sound understanding of individual tolerance to EA. When these interconnected factors are mastered, the expert is judicially qualified to offer evidence-based opinions in medicolegal settings (**Table 3**).

Table 1 Primary role of medicolegal expert assessing effects of ethyl alcohol on the living

Determination of impact on physiological function
Evaluation of effect on behavior in multitask activities
 Operation of motor vehicle (DUI or DWI)
 Skill at control of machinery
 Workplace-related activity
Assessment of influence on social behaviors

DUI, driving under the influence; DWI, driving while intoxicated.

Table 2 Questions by expert adjudging role of ethyl alcohol (EA) in medicolegal death investigation

Was EA solely causative in death?
Did EA act as a synergist to other toxins, causing death when no toxin alone is responsible for the fatality?
How did the BAC, quantitated postmortem, affect behavior shortly before death?
What was the BAC at the time of injury in cases of delayed death?

BAC, blood alcohol concentration.

Table 3 Responsibilities of the expert evaluating ethyl alcohol in blood and body fluids

Function as interpretive toxicologist
Master the state-of-the-art science on the fate and disposition of alcohol in the body
Understand the physiological, behavioral, and psychological effects of alcohol on humans
Oversee appropriate collection and analysis of fluid specimens
Maintain or confirm chain of custody for transport of specimens
Recognize the interrelationships between alcohol concentrations in blood and body fluids
Correlate laboratory findings with autopsy and the background of either death or event
Provide scientifically sound expert opinions on the effects of quantitated alcohol

Analytical toxicologists have reliably identified and quantified EA in virtually all body tissues, fluids, and secretions (**Table 4**). In the clinical setting the desired sample is venous blood appropriately collected via venepuncture, from which serum is typically segregated and analyzed enzymatically. Breath, saliva, and, with qualification, urine, serve as substitutes or complements when phlebotomy is legally or practically contraindicated.

The gold standard in testing postmortem fluid EA levels for medicolegal purposes is whole blood by headspace gas chromatography (HS-GC). In regard to the short postmortem interval prior to the onset of decomposition, countless studies have established the comparative ratio of postmortem whole-blood EA concentration (blood alcohol concentration or BAC) to other matrices (**Table 5**). Postmortem decomposition spuriously increases BAC due to endogenous production by overgrowth of normal, fermentative flora in the gut, with substantial ($>0.20\%$) artifactual elevations reported in some cases. Vitreous humor is a reliable comparison medium to differentiate antemortem consumption from postmortem production. Intravascular fluids from embalmed bodies may be utilized selectively to estimate the antemortem BAC by comparison with constitutive volatiles in embalming fluid.

EA is the most frequently analyzed drug by the toxicologist in consultation with coroners, medical examiners, physicians in emergency departments, directors of poison control centers, and police. Optimal specimens are required for accurate analysis by the laboratory technician as practitioner of analytical toxicology, as well as for evaluation of the analytical results by the expert as interpretive toxicologist.

The BAC, which distinctively rests upon collection and analysis of the specimen obtained at a discrete time, is dependent above all on the individual's

Table 4 Body fluids suitable for analysis of ethyl alcohol in medicolegal investigation

Blood (whole blood, plasma, serum)[a]	Gastric and proximal small-bowel contents
Urine[a]	Bone marrow
Vitreous humor	"Decompositional" fluid
Cerebrospinal fluid[a]	Fluid from embalmed bodies
Saliva[a]	Sequestered intracranial hematomas
Bile	Sweat[a]
Synovial fluid	Amniotic fluid[a]
Pericardial fluid	Maternal breast milk[a]
Dialysis fluid[a]	Lavage fluid[a]
"Cavity blood"	Aspirated vomitus[a]
Tears[a]	Pleural fluid

[a]Samples not limited to autopsy; they may be collected during life from hospitals or clinics.

Table 5 Summarized ratios: body fluid to whole blood alcohol concentration

Specimen	Average ratio or range
Serum or plasma	1.0–1.15
Vitreous humor	1.05–1.34
Urine	1.17–1.5
Bile	1.03–1.10
Cerebrospinal fluid	1.1
Saliva	1.08–1.12
Pericardial fluid	Variable
Synovial fluid	1.01–1.32
Tear fluid	1.08–1.20
Amniotic fluid	0.5
Bone marrow	0.34–0.53
Gastric contents	Variable
Pleural fluid	Variable
Solid organs not addressed in discussion	
Brain	0.65–0.96 (site-dependent)
Liver	0.6
Kidney	0.7
Skeletal muscle	0.89–0.91
Spleen	Variable
Testicle	"High correlation"

unique tolerance to and absorption, distribution, and metabolism of the drug. Correlation of the BAC to the level detected in a particular body fluid from one or more other body compartments is particularly important in death investigations for several reasons: (1) support of reliability of the blood level in evaluating the degree of intoxication; (2) resort to other body fluids when a satisfactory blood sample is unavailable or contaminated; and (3) quality assurance and proficiency of testing. Such correlative analysis requires the establishment of relative distribution ratios and standard deviations from the mean. Ideally, each investigatory agency should establish its own experience-based parameters. Experts may also refer to many studies establishing comparative ratios (with standard deviations and ranges) between whole-blood EA levels and other biologic fluids and tissues (**Table 5**).

Analytical Methodology

Specific analytical methods are necessary for the analysis of EA because of potential interference by a variety of volatile substances in postmortem specimens. Laboratory methods for the analysis of EA in biological specimens are classified as chemical, biochemical, and instrumental. Wet chemical analyses include distillation or microdiffusion utilizing the inherent volatility characteristics of alcohol, which allows for separation, oxidation, and subsequent detection. A well-known example of this chemical methodology is the Breathalyzer developed by Borkenstein

in 1954. Biochemical methods utilize the enzyme alcohol dehydrogenase (ADH). Physiochemical methods include gas chromatography (GC), high-performance liquid chromatography (HPLC), and gas chromatography–mass spectrometry (GC-MS).

Gas Chromatography

GC is the most common methodology for the measurement of EA in postmortem biological specimens, owing to its specificity, sensitivity, and reproducibility. EA has been measured by several GC methods, including solvent-based extraction, protein precipitation, and distillation techniques, direct injection, or headspace analyses. Headspace analysis and direct injection techniques are current applications of choice. Direct injection techniques generally require injection of a liquid sample into the gas chromatograph equipped with a flame ionization detector (FID). The specimen may be an undiluted sample, a protein precipitated sample, or a diluted sample of the specimen with an aqueous solution of an internal standard (commonly, 1-propanol and *t*-butanol).

Dual-column HS-GC is nearly completely specific for EA. It is a proven test method acceptable in most courts of law affording admissibility of analytical results on which to base expert testimony. HS-GC with FID precisely detects EA at concentrations as low as $0.01\,\mathrm{g\,dl^{-1}}$. It also distinguishes EA from other alcohols, aldehydes, ketones, and other analytes in the mixture. Headspace analysis techniques physically rely on Henry's law wherein the ratio of a dissolved substance in solution is dependent on temperature, pressure, and concentration of the fluid medium. The measurable amount of volatile in the headspace above the liquid medium is proportional to the volatile liquid concentration in solution. The headspace procedure employs diluted blood samples of aqueous solution with internal standards, which are placed in small, capped bottles. After incubation produces the vaporized mixture, which includes an inert carrier gas, the headspace (gas phase) is injected into a closed system via the single injection port. The injection splits into two attached capillary columns (stationary phase(s)), variably coated to interact predictably with analytes of interest. EA is initially separated, based on the appropriately calibrated GC parameters and columns, and subsequently quantified using computer-aided techniques. Separation of the volatile compounds, as the vapor phase is carried through the column, depends on the relative differential affinity of each analyte for the stationary phase. A detector at the end of the column, which is designed for FID, creates over time electrical signals that are converted to quantitative results. In addition to temperature, optimal analysis also depends on the condition at which the vapor is at equilibrium with the liquid specimen, flow rate of the carrier gas, material packing the column, column length, and the kind of detector. In sum, the discrete, absolute, or relative retention times (min) depicted on the gas chromatogram provide qualitative analysis, while the peak height or area for each analyte affords quantitative analysis (**Figure 1**). Although GC-MS techniques are the most definitive assay for EA analysis, these tests are not widely employed in forensic laboratories because they require considerable expertise and are more expensive.

Biochemical Methods – Immunoassays

Hospital and clinical laboratories commonly apply enzymatic methods, utilizing ADH, to determine EA in blood and urine because gas chromatographs are often unavailable. The instrument-based biochemical reaction is similar to *in vivo* enzymatic reactions controlling EA metabolism. The coenzyme, nicotinamide adenine dinucleotide (NAD), is reduced as a byproduct of the oxidation reaction of EA to acetaldehyde. Various trapping reagents, e.g., hydrazine or semicarbazide, trap acetaldehyde and drive the

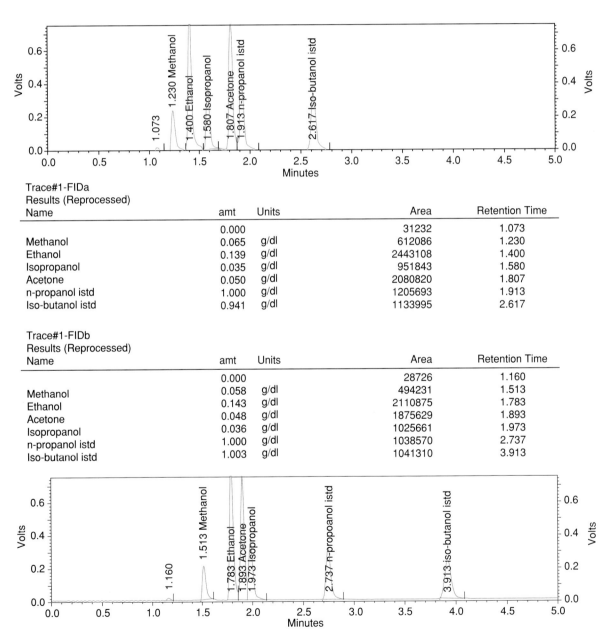

Trace#1-FIDa
Results (Reprocessed)

Name	amt	Units	Area	Retention Time
	0.000		31232	1.073
Methanol	0.065	g/dl	612086	1.230
Ethanol	0.139	g/dl	2443108	1.400
Isopropanol	0.035	g/dl	951843	1.580
Acetone	0.050	g/dl	2080820	1.807
n-propanol istd	1.000	g/dl	1205693	1.913
Iso-butanol istd	0.941	g/dl	1133995	2.617

Trace#1-FIDb
Results (Reprocessed)

Name	amt	Units	Area	Retention Time
	0.000		28726	1.160
Methanol	0.058	g/dl	494231	1.513
Ethanol	0.143	g/dl	2110875	1.783
Acetone	0.048	g/dl	1875629	1.893
Isopropanol	0.036	g/dl	1025661	1.973
n-propanol istd	1.000	g/dl	1038570	2.737
Iso-butanol istd	1.003	g/dl	1041310	3.913

Figure 1   Gas chromatogram (dual-column headspace gas chromatography with flame ionization detector (HS-GC-FID)) with both columns depicting retention times and levels of methanol, ethanol, isopropanol, and acetone with internal standards, *n*-propanol and isobutanol.

oxidative metabolism of EA to the right. The reaction produces the reduced form of NAD, NADH, which can be measured spectrophotometrically at 340 nm. Radiative energy attenuation is a modified enzymatic method utilizing the NADH produced by an ADH-catalyzed ethanol/NAD reaction. The NADH product combines with a thiazole blue dye to form a chromogen. Measured fluorescence quantifies the EA in the liquid specimen.

The automated enzymatic method is a quick and easy way to detect EA. However, it lacks the specificity of HS-GC because the presence of other alcohols such as isopropanol may interfere chemically and yield an inconclusive, false-positive result. Unlike HS-GC, antigen–antibody reactions are subject to cross-reaction with other substances within the blood and for that reason are not regarded as a reliable method for testing BAC in a medicolegal or juridical context.

Specimen Selection and Collection in Living Subjects

Currently accepted venepuncture consists of cutaneous application of a nonalcoholic antiseptic (e.g., povidone iodine) and withdrawal of a sufficient aliquot of cubital venous or fingertip capillary whole blood by a sterile needle to a sealed sterile vial. Anticoagulants and microorganism-inhibiting chemicals are typically added. Importantly, venous blood does not precisely reflect the cerebral BAC, which ultimately defines the biochemical effects of EA, unless absorption and distribution of EA are complete at collection (Table 6).

Table 6 Accepted collection, transport, and storage of blood from living persons

Cutaneous application of nonvolatile antiseptic
Percutaneous venepuncture of cubital vein or fingertip capillary
Withdrawal of sample by sterile needle to sterile container
Vacuum glass collection tubes are acceptable legally
Filling container sufficiently to avoid evaporation
Use of clean container without anticoagulant allowing blood to clot (for serum)
Use of preservatives/anticoagulants (for whole blood and plasma):
  1–2% sodium fluoride
  EDTA or potassium oxalate
Proper labeling, laboratory request form, and chain of custody on or with container
Refrigeration (4 °C) or prompt delivery to analytical laboratory
Recording receipt and disposition of specimen by receiving analyst
Analysis or storage (refrigeration or frozen: −20 °C) of specimen

EDTA, ethylenediaminetetraacetic acid.

Randomly collected, first-voided urine is generally valuable only in confirming the presence of EA, because the urine alcohol concentration (UAC) is subject to multiple uncontrolled variables. Since the 1990s saliva, or oral fluid, has gained acceptance as a satisfactory matrix for on-the-spot testing for EA, both qualitative and semiquantitative, applicable to workplace or clinical settings such as emergency departments.

Specimen Selection and Collection – Postmortem

If possible, recovery of available antemortem or perimortem blood, blood components, or other body fluids (Table 4) from the victim, collected by investigators or medical personnel, is a recommended practice after declaration of death. The earliest collected sample frequently provides more accurate information about the question of antemortem intoxication by EA than do samples from autopsy, particularly when treatment over variable periods of time includes fluid resuscitation. This applies particularly in cases of traumatic exsanguination, urgent operative procedures, and prolonged hospitalization before death. For both living and deceased subjects, it is necessary to consider potential antemortem dilution from therapeutic administration of blood and other fluids.

In most postmortem cases, there is undoubtedly greater opportunity – in contrast to limitations within the clinical arena – to collect a variety of biologic specimens for laboratory analysis (Table 7). Under optimal circumstances, utilizing multiple specimens at autopsy from various compartments and subcompartments of the body helps to support the accuracy of a given quantitative result and thereby facilitates optimal interpretation.

The most critical, vigorously debated issue with regard to blood sample collection before putrefaction in contemporary postmortem medicolegal practice is the phenomenon of site-to-site differences in BAC, both within-case and between-case. Traditionally, "heart blood" or "central blood" (blood aspirated from either the intact cardiac chambers, the intrapericardial great vessels arising from and exiting the heart, or a mixture from these sites) has been routinely collected for EA analysis. This practice has been justified in view of various studies finding no statistical significance between heart blood and femoral blood ("peripheral blood") EA content. More recent controlled experiments addressing this issue were designed to collect fluid from multiple sites (pericardial fluid, left pulmonary vein, aorta, left heart, pulmonary artery, superior vena cava, inferior vena

Table 7   Accepted collection of routine samples for ethyl alcohol analysis after death

Intravascular blood (central and peripheral), as available:
  $\geq$50 ml, as available, from each site via clean wide-bore needle and syringe
  Commercially available gray-top Vacutainer or
  30 ml glass container with 250 mg NaF ($=$ 1–2% NaF) or
  Polypropylene test tubes with Teflon-lined screw caps
  Aspirate from heart chambers, supravalvular aorta, pulmonary artery, vena cava
  Percutaneous or direct phlebotomy from femoral (or subclavian) vein
  Refrigerate/freeze (4–20 °C) promptly before delivery to analytical laboratory
Intravesical urine
  $\geq$250 ml, as available
  Aspirate with needle to syringe through dome of distended urinary bladder
  Aspirate directly after superior cystotomy of collapsed urinary bladder
  Preserve in clean container, preferably with NaF
  Refrigerate/freeze till timely analysis
Ocular vitreous humor
  $\geq$4–6 ml, as available, from both globes
  Ophthalmocentesis with clean needle and 5 or 10-ml syringe
  Avoid forceful aspiration to prevent retinal detachment
  Preserve in clean container with NaF
  Refrigerate/freeze till timely analysis
Cerebrospinal fluid
  $\geq$2–6 ml, as available
  Preferred: aspiration via clean needle/syringe directly from cerebral cisterns or proximal cervical canal after opening skull
  Avoid "blind" percutaneous suboccipital or lumbar puncture owing to potential contamination to analyte and paraspinal soft tissue
  Preserve in clean container, NaF optional
  Refrigerate/freeze till timely analysis
Synovial fluid
  $\geq$2–4 ml, as available
  Percutaneous arthrocentesis (knee joint) via clean needle/syringe
  Preserve in clean container with NaF
  Refrigerate/freeze till timely analysis
Gastric/small-bowel contents
  Following removal of block of esophagus, stomach, duodenum, pancreas:
  Place all contents into clean volumetric container
    via compression of stomach, forcing contents out of esophageal segment or
    through gastrotomy in relatively avascular region
  Quantitate and characterize contents (food, liquid, slurry, foreign bodies)
  Preserve 50 ml uniform sample in clean container
  Preserve 100 ml nonuniform sample (liquid/solid/semisolid) in clean container
  Refrigerate/freeze till analysis
Bile
  Collect and quantitate all liquid contents ($<$0.5–65 ml)
  Choledochocystocentesis via clean needle/syringe before hepatic evisceration
  Preserve contents in clean container
  Refrigerate/freeze till analysis
Sequestered intracranial (epidural, subdural) hematomas
  Quantitate and remove maximal amount of fluid and clot on opening skull
  Preserve in clean container
  Refrigerate/freeze till analysis

NaF, sodium fluoride.

cava, right heart, right pulmonary vein, femoral vein, and stomach), either simultaneously or at defined intervals, and at different environmental temperatures. Such experiments have demonstrated the chaotic, site-dependent unpredictability of BAC at autopsy in some cases, an artifact attributed to simple diffusion of EA from the stomach or esophagus to adjacent regions and to the circulation.

Blood and its Constituents

In postmortem sampling, available "whole blood" remains the most desirable specimen for analysis. In light of contemporary evidence, some recommend autopsy collection of at least two samples of blood, one peripheral and one complementary central sample, if case specifics permit. In order to avoid artifacts and difficulties with postmortem redistribution, it is strongly recommended that the medicolegal investigator collect peripheral blood as the optimal sample, drawn by a wide-bore, clean needle with new syringe preferentially from the femoral vein and, when such a sample is not collectable, secondarily from external iliac vein or subclavian vein. It is necessary to avoid "milking" the vein to prevent admixing the blood with tissue fluid.

Specifically designed clean containers are utilized for specimen collection. Depending on the design and specimen type, these rubber-stoppered, glass collection tubes may contain sodium fluoride, heparin, potassium oxalate, EDTA, or no additives at all. The anticoagulant and bacteriostatic actions of sodium fluoride are optimal for preserving and storing whole blood drawn at autopsy. If blood is analyzed by GC, plastic containers are the most optimal receptacles. For analysis of volatiles, some sample should be retained in a Teflon-lined screw top to prevent diffusion.

In addition to potential postmortem artifactual site-to-site alterations, the BAC from various regions of the intact circulation and EA concentration in other body compartments vary during the absorption phase of EA metabolism. Therefore, it is necessary to specify unequivocally the source of the sample or the site of collection of whole blood. Arterial BAC may be at least 40% higher than venous BAC in the absorptive phase. It is equally important that the blood specimen should not be mixed from various sources, such as intermingled central and peripheral blood.

Pooled blood from the pericardial sac and bloody fluid recovered from extravascular body cavities (which are not blood!), especially in trauma, are less reliable toxicological specimens to quantitate EA, but may be used if these are the only blood-related source. The pooled or bloody fluid may have either a higher or lower level of EA than that in intravascular blood *per se* (central or peripheral), and accordingly may make meaningful interpretation of the reported "BAC" virtually impossible. If such samples are the only ones obtainable, antemortem BAC is merely an estimate. Bloody fluid from body surfaces or from the relevant scene are unreliable, inappropriate sources for toxicology evaluation.

In collecting blood samples at autopsy there are factors influencing the concentration of EA that are not pertinent to antemortem techniques. Diffusion of significant amounts of EA from the esophagus or stomach into the adjacent pericardial cavity and heart is likely to occur, and becomes increasingly significant as the postmortem interval increases. Yet, if there is a short period of time, measured in hours, between the last drink and death, diffusion of EA from the gut to the "heart blood" will not be substantial. Under circumstances where the autopsy is performed within 48 h of death, diffusion of alcohol from the gut to the heart is relatively insignificant. As noted, femoral or subclavian venous (peripheral) blood sites are preferable to central blood. These samples may be difficult to obtain secondary to insufficient volume and in cases of traumatic hypovolemia ("empty-heart sign"). As EA distributes to total body water, it is important prior to the onset of putrefaction to consider the water content of the blood sample in interpreting BAC. For example, the sample with a low hematocrit (volume of red cells to total blood volume) yields a higher level of EA due to the greater water volume. In cases of significant hypovolemia, sampling other compartments is necessary. When the remains are incinerated, the vascular compartment may contain only uniformly coagulated or anhydrous, "baked" clot. Such a sample should be collected even though the EA level has little meaning without correlating EA concentration in other available matrices.

Withdrawing a "blind" postmortem sample via precordial percutaneous pericardiocentesis to collect blood is indisputably flawed and to be avoided. Central blood specimens contain blood that is drawn by direct observation from the heart or the great vessels. In summary, external "blind" chest puncture is not considered an acceptable procedure for the collection of a blood sample for subsequent EA analysis. False elevations of EA in bloody fluid collected by external chest puncture can be confirmed by analysis of postmortem vitreous humor or urine. Without autopsy, it is recommended to collect peripheral blood.

In contrast to the practices of clinical laboratories, most forensic toxicology laboratories analyzing postmortem samples report BAC from whole blood preserved in sodium fluoride. Yet, as most forensic experts are frequently called upon either to interpret results from or analyze antemortem serum or plasma samples, it is incumbent on the expert to appreciate different results from various specimens. Researchers conclude that using serum, plasma, or whole blood for EA analysis produces essentially equivalent results for clinical and forensic purposes, as long as the final report clearly specifies the specimen (serum, plasma, whole blood). Under most physiological conditions, serum or plasma contains about 10–20% more water than an equal volume of whole blood. EA levels are correspondingly, but only slightly, higher in these samples. The average EA ratio of whole blood to serum or plasma is approximately 1:1.15.

Vitreous Humor

As a quality control measure, concomitant comparative quantitation of EA in the postmortem vitreous humor (VAC; vitreous alcohol concentration) is an excellent means of interpreting the reported BAC, whether central or peripheral. Because the intact, relatively avascular intraorbital globe is anatomically isolated from other tissues or fluid, it serves as an excellent compartment to obtain unadulterated, typically sterile vitreous humor for quantitation. Characteristically, VAC lags approximately 1–2 h behind BAC at metabolic equilibrium. Therefore, BAC in the absorptive phase is higher than VAC. At the plateau or equilibrium phase, the reported average ratio of BAC:VAC is 1:1.05–1.34 by virtue of the differential water content of these matrices. In the postabsorptive or elimination phase, VAC is higher than the BAC. Such comparative analysis is helpful in establishing whether the deceased was in the absorptive or elimination phase at death. Given the well-documented BAC:VAC ratios, reference to the VAC is also very useful in inferring the probable BAC at death when intravascular blood or other body fluids are not readily available.

As in all extrapolations based upon EA levels in extravascular matrices, a conservative approach is always prudent in estimating the BAC from the VAC at autopsy. The EA distribution ratio (VAC:BAC) (femoral blood) may exhibit wide variation in light of recent research. Investigators recommend a conservative approach by dividing the postmortem VAC by 2.0 to arrive at an estimate of the equivalent (femoral) BAC, which, although lower than the "true value," may then be offered with a higher degree of confidence in the medicolegal arena.

Other Body Fluids

When blood or vitreous humor is not available, such as in decomposition, trauma, or contamination, other aqueous body tissues may be used to quantitate EA, which is readily miscible in water. Ideally, because the level of alcohol in the central nervous system directly affects behavior and activity, the best sample for measurement of EA concentration is brain. Obviously, this is not feasible for living individuals. Although brain is usually readily available at autopsy, it is not the specimen of choice for several reasons:

1. Blood from the vascular compartment is usually easier to obtain and process.
2. The appropriately determined BAC adequately reflects the effect of EA on the brain.
3. Simultaneous sampling of various brain regions yields significant differences in the EA concentration.

4. It is more practical, technically efficient, and economically sound to analyze blood regularly when such high-caseload volumes are involved.

Other tissues and samples used for blood alternatives are urine, gastric contents, bone marrow, bile, intracerebral and paradural hematomas, synovial fluid, cerebrospinal fluid (CSF), and others catalogued in **Table 4** (in addition to solid organs, e.g., liver, kidney, brain, spleen and lung, cardiac, smooth or skeletal muscle, a topic not relevant to this discussion). Many researchers have reported an established range and ratio of EA in these various body fluids to BAC (**Table 5**). Limited research suggests that synovial fluid from intact joints serves as a readily obtainable, adequate substitute for vitreous humor in estimating perimortem BAC. These tabulations are valuable and afford reasonable inferences with respect to BAC when intravascular blood is unavailable. BAC estimations must be expressed conservatively within a wide range when they are derived from extravascular biological fluids (or tissues). If biological fluids other than peripheral blood specimens are collected, the EA concentration derived from stomach or gastric contents (gastric alcohol content: GAC) may be referenced to improve the accuracy of the estimated BAC. One study of 60 autopsy cases suggested that a GAC $>0.5 \, g \, dl^{-1}$ at death likely indicated "recent" ingestion and that the subject was in the preabsorptive phase; and, further, that a subject with a GAC $<0.5 \, g \, dl^{-1}$ may be considered in the postabsorptive state. With the realization that the removal of EA from the stomach, especially in real-life drinking circumstances, is subject to multiple variables regarding end of drinking and time to peak BAC, this comparison may improve – in the absence of a reliable history – the estimation of the pharmacokinetic state of the individual at the time of death.

CSF can be used for EA analysis; however, use of CSF EA levels is of limited value in light of studies indicating that EA does not reach the CSF in maximum concentration until 3 h after the end of drinking and also exhibits delay in distribution equilibrium. If the posttraumatic survival of an individual is prolonged, the postmortem analysis of EA from sequestered intracerebral or paradural hematomas may be of value in estimating retrospectively the BAC at the time of injury.

Urine

With qualification, urine is potentially an acceptable medium to estimate BAC and to determine the pharmacokinetic phase of the subject at the time of collection. The preferred sample is ureteral urine. Excreted

EA from the renal circulation as a glomerular filtrate prior to mixing with water in the tubules is virtually identical to that in the water content of blood in that vascular compartment. Clinically or at autopsy, collection of ureteral urine is not practical. The urinary bladder is a storage container for eliminated urine until voiding. In the absence of pathological or drug-related conditions affecting urine production, urine continuously enters and collects in the bladder. It contains variable time-and-volume-dependent concentrations of EA.

Confounding factors in collection are inherent in the measurement of UAC. In living subjects, the stored urine must be voided and a subsequent urine specimen collected over time (30–60 min) with no EA consumption or postvoiding alteration. If, for example, after arrest for presumptive driving under the influence (DUI), a first void is followed promptly (≤30 min) by withdrawal of a venous blood sample and then a second void (60 min (range 30–130)), reference limits for UAC/BAC have been established to estimate the subject's venous BAC. Once-voided urine should only be used as a qualitative test for EA. Toxicological urinalysis, though often based on one void in practice, is generally of little or no value *per se* to estimate an individual's BAC at a given time.

At autopsy, UAC represents the cumulative or integrated sum of different BACs *intra vitam* over time, encompassing various phases of EA metabolism. Pooled urine merely estimates an average urine concentration over the collection time. The quantitated UAC may be used for rough estimates of BAC in that timeframe. The reported average UAC:BAC ratio is 1:1.33, but the experimentally determined range is great, reportedly from 1:0.21 to 1:2.17–2.44. UAC:BAC comparisons may also be used to delineate the stage of metabolism the individual is in at the time of specimen collection: absorptive phase UAC:BAC <1.0; postabsorptive phase UAC:BAC >1.3.

Decomposed or Embalmed Specimens

Thorough intravascular embalming renders blood a medium unavailable for determining preembalming BAC. Vitreous humor may serve as a suitable substitute. In such cases the toxicologist must analyze a sample of the embalming fluid to compare with the VAC. In general, many embalming fluids, usually composed of formaldehyde, either do not contain EA or have relatively low levels compared to other volatiles. In commercially manufactured embalming fluid, other volatiles may include acetone, methanol, isopropanol, and occasionally EA. Typical formulas

distinguishing the volatiles in embalming products are readily available. Another technical difficulty in analysis of EA in cases of exhumation–embalming arises when dehydration of tissue or postmortem synthesis of alcohol is present after prolonged burial. EA may be elevated in bodies that have not been embalmed in a timely manner. The BAC is therefore likely due to postmortem production of EA.

Postmortem decomposition, even at an early stage, falsely elevates BAC and complicates the task of the interpretative toxicologist. Fermentative flora, primarily bacteria, fungi, and yeast, enter the vascular compartment postmortem, metabolize glucose or protein, and produce endogenous EA chemically identical to that in alcoholic beverages. Because of relative isolation from the putrefactive processes, urine from the bladder and vitreous humor, which reside in relatively sterile compartments, are sometimes spared of this phenomenon.

Investigators report postmortem BAC as high as 0.22% attributable to endogenous production. In moderate-to-severe decomposition, simultaneous analysis of either vitreous humor or urine devoid of EA supports the conclusion that the postmortem BAC is due to endogenous fermentation by microorganisms. Bodies that have been stored in cold environments generally will have minimal endogenous alcohol production. Endogenous fermentation also applies to victims of drowning, who frequently undergo severe decompositional change even in temperate climates. Moreover, dilutional factors may occur, especially in fresh-water drowning. Therefore, the BAC quantified from postmortem samples may actually be lower than the true level. Specific variations are not known at this time due to the lack of research in this area.

The endogenous generation of EA by microorganisms is not unique to the postmortem period. Such considerations are also relevant to the living, particularly exemplified by subjects with metabolic complications of diabetes mellitus with urinary tract infections, or sepsis. In diabetics, discrepancies between BAC and UAC, where the latter demonstrates abnormally elevated amounts of EA, may be attributable to urinary retention and incontinence. As a result of this phenomenon, postmortem UAC in diabetics is unreliable.

Summary

In evaluation of the behavioral or lethal effects of EA, appropriately collected and handled specimens are required for both the analytical and the interpretative toxicologist. Currently there is near universal consensus that the preferred antemortem and postmortem specimen is peripheral whole blood. A confounding factor affecting interpretation of the BAC in the early postmortem period is the occasional site-to-site difference in EA levels. For optimal evaluation and if resources permit, simultaneous collection of peripheral whole blood and a complementary, backup central sample is desirable. Other extravascular fluids or analytes with comparative ratios of EA to whole blood may be utilized as a gauge of its effects on the brain. Vitreous humor is a satisfactory complement to peripheral BAC and should be collected routinely for EA analysis. Several critical factors influence the distribution ratio and must be considered. Foremost among these is the stage of alcohol distribution at collection. The optimal specimen is collected at maximum BAC plateau or during the elimination phase. In spite of detailed historical investigation and thorough postmortem sampling, the medicolegal investigator may not be able at autopsy to pinpoint the pharmacokinetic phase of the individual at the time of death. If, for example, the specimen is collected during the absorption stage, then total body distribution has not been achieved. Evaluation of the reported BAC from that sample requires recognition of this limitation. Cautiously interpreted comparative ratios of whole-blood BAC to extravascular matrices are of value in making reasonable estimates of the BAC at death when a suitable blood sample is unavailable. With decomposition or embalming, interpretation of the BAC is fraught with difficulty even when other matrices are analyzed.

In living subjects plasma or serum is an acceptable body fluid for interpretation when designated as such. Properly collected urine samples may be used cautiously to estimate the BAC when blood is unavailable. Saliva has gained acceptance as a body fluid suitable for analysis of EA and monitoring intoxication in a variety of clinical settings.

See Also

Alcohol: Breath Alcohol Analysis; **Autopsy, Findings:** Postmortem Drug Measurements, Interpretation of; Postmortem Drug Sampling and Redistribution; **Crime-scene Investigation and Examination:** Collection and Chain of Evidence; **Toxicology:** Methods of Analysis, Antemortem; Methods of Analysis, Postmortem

Further Reading

Backer RC, Pisano RV, Sopher IM (1980) The comparison of alcohol concentrations in postmortem fluids and tissues. *Journal of Forensic Sciences* 25: 327–331.

Baselt RC (2004) Ethanol. In: Baselt RC (ed.) *Disposition of Toxic Drugs and Chemicals in Man*, 7th edn., pp. 411–414. Foster City, CA: Biomedical.

DiMaio VJ, DiMaio D (2001) Interpretive toxicology: drug abuse and drug deaths. In: DiMaio VJ, DiMaio D (eds.) *Forensic Pathology*, 2nd edn., pp. 507–545. Boca Raton, FL: CRC Press LLC.

Ellenhorn MJ, Schonwald S, Ordog G, Wasserberger J (1997) Alcohols and glycols. In: *Ellenhorn's Medical Toxicology Diagnosis and Treatment of Human Poisoning*, 2nd edn., pp. 1127–1165. Baltimore, MD: Williams and Wilkins.

Felby S, Nielsen E (1994) The postmortem blood alcohol concentration and the water content. *Blutalkohol* 31: 24–32.

Freimuth HC (rev. by Spitz WU) (1993) Forensic aspects of alcohol. In: Spitz WU (ed.) *Spitz and Fisher's Medicolegal Investigation of Death Guidelines for the Application of Pathology to Crime Investigation*, 3rd edn., pp. 767–775. Springfield, IL: Charles C Thomas.

Garriott JC (ed.) (2003) *Medical–Legal Aspects of Alcohol*, 4th edn. Tucson, AZ: Lawyers & Judges.

Huckenbeck W, Bonte W (2004) Alkoholie. In: Madea B, Brinkmann (eds.) *Handbuch gerichtliche Medizin*, Bd 2, pp. 379–518. Berlin, Heidelberg, New York: Springer Verlag.

Houts M, Baselt RC, Cravey RH (2003) Ethanol. In: Houts M, Baselt RC, Cravey RH (eds.) *Courtroom Toxicology*, vol. 4, pp. Etha-1–Etha-30. New York: LexisNexis Matthew Bender.

Jones AW (2002) Reference limits for urine/blood ratios of ethanol in two successive voids from drinking drivers. *Journal of Analytical Toxicology* 26: 333–339.

Jones AW, Holmgren P (2001) Uncertainty in estimating blood ethanol concentrations by analysis of vitreous humor. *Journal of Clinical Pathology* 56: 699–702.

Ludwig J (ed.) (2002) *Handbook of Autopsy Practice*, 3rd edn. Totowa, NJ: Humana Press.

Pounder DJ, Smith DRW (1995) Postmortem diffusion of alcohol from the stomach. *American Journal of Forensic Medicine and Pathology* 16: 89–96.

Saukko P, Knight B (2004) Forensic aspects of alcohol. In: Saukko P, Knight B (eds.) *Knight's Forensic Pathology*, 3rd edn., pp. 552–559. London: Arnold.

Scheinin LA (1999) Forensic aspects of alcohol intoxication. In: *American Society for Clinical Pathology Check Sample, Forensic Pathology No. 99-9 (FP-250)*, p. 127. Chicago, IL: American Society for Clinical Pathology.

Williams RH, Leikin JB (1999) Medicolegal issues and specimen collection for ethanol testing. *Laboratory Medicine* 30: 530–537.

Winek CL, Esposito FM (2003) Antemortem and postmortem alcohol determinations. In: Wecht CH (ed.) *Forensic Sciences*, vol. 2, pp. 31B-1–31B-75. New York: LexisNexis Matthew Bender.

Zumwalt RE, Bost RO, Sunshine I (1982) Evaluation of ethanol concentrations in decomposed bodies. *Journal of Forensic Sciences* 27: 549–554.

Acute and Chronic Use, Postmortem Findings

A W Jones, University Hospital, Linköping, Sweden

Introduction

Mention the word alcohol to a chemist and this conjures up a family of organic compounds with broadly similar chemical properties and with each molecule containing one or more hydroxyl (-OH) groups. Alcohol is a generic name for a large group of organic chemical substances derived from hydrocarbons by replacing one or more of the hydrogen atoms with hydroxyl groups. Examples of alcohols commonly encountered in forensic medicine and toxicology are methanol, ethanol, isopropanol, *n*-propanol, and ethylene glycol. The basic properties of these primary alcohols (methanol, ethanol, and *n*-propanol), secondary alcohol (isopropanol), and the dihydroxy alcohol (ethylene glycol) are summarized in **Table 1**. The alcohol of prime concern in this review is ethanol or ethylalcohol, which is the ubiquitous psychoactive substance in alcoholic beverages (beers, wines, and distilled spirits).

Alcohol is a legal drug and, although most people drink in moderation, many progress to become heavy drinkers and sometimes become alcohol-dependent; in short they are addicted to alcohol and can be diagnosed clinically as alcoholics. People drink alcohol for different reasons. The first experience of this social drug often occurs during adolescence when teenagers and young adults perhaps out of curiosity or peer pressure make their drinking début. Some will then stop or curb their drinking owing to the nausea they experienced, whereas others continue to drink alcohol throughout adult life. Excessive drinking and abuse of alcohol lead to problems within the family, with the police, and at the workplace.

Alcohol has been referred to as the Jekyll and Hyde of the drug world because moderate drinking has a number of beneficial effects on a person's health and gives feelings of well-being. Drinking small amounts of alcohol tends to relax people by lowering their inhibitions and encouraging social interaction. Recent research has shown that 1–2 drinks per day, especially in the form of red wine, is an effective prophylactic treatment for cardiovascular diseases such as stroke. However, for about 10–15% of the population who choose to drink alcohol, particularly men, initial moderate consumption escalates into abuse, which wrecks lives and causes considerable morbidity and mortality. Alternatively, the production, advertisement, and sale of alcoholic beverages represent a major source of government income via taxation, making this legal drug a double-edged sword.

In most countries alcohol-related injuries constitute a major public health problem with enormous costs for society both directly owing to the medical intervention necessary for alcohol-related diseases and also indirectly through alcohol-related accidents. Impairment of body function and diminished performance after heavy drinking are responsible for 30–40% of traffic fatalities in most countries, these being caused by drunk drivers. In addition, many problems in the workplace and in the home, including domestic violence, are another consequence of heavy drinking. Besides driving under the influence, overconsumption of alcohol and drunkenness are underlying factors in many criminal offenses including murder, sexual assaults, and rape as well as the aggressive behavior of drunken hooligans. Autopsy reports show that people committing suicide as well as those who die by drowning have high blood alcohol concentration (BAC). The analysis of alcohol in biological specimens therefore represents the most commonly requested service from forensic science and toxicology laboratories.

An overview of the forensic science aspects of alcohol is presented, particularly acute and chronic effects on the individual, and issues of importance and concern in relation to postmortem toxicology of alcohol, including a correct interpretation of the results.

Reporting Blood Alcohol Concentrations

Because of the well-established relationship between the concentration of alcohol in a person's blood or breath and the risk of causing a traffic accident, most countries have established threshold limits of alcohol concentration above which it is an offense to drive a motor vehicle. However, these punishable limits differ between countries owing to tradition, lifestyle, and not least various political forces and public opinion. In most European countries a BAC limit of 50 mg per 100 ml is enforced, whereas Norway and Sweden have adopted a threshold of 20 mg per 100 g blood (21 mg per 100 ml). The UK, Ireland, and most US states as well as the provinces of Canada are more tolerant to driving after drinking: the legal blood alcohol limit is 80 mg per 100 ml. In a few remaining US states the threshold alcohol limit for driving is set at 100 mg per 100 ml (**Table 2**).

The concentration units used to report the results of forensic alcohol analysis depend in part on the kind of biological fluid analyzed, whether blood, breath, or urine. Moreover, some countries use mass/mass units (Germany and the Nordic countries) although

Table 1   Characteristic features of various alcohols commonly encountered in forensic toxicology and legal medicine

Property	Methanol	Ethanol	n-propanol	Isopropanol	Ethylene glycol
CAS number	65-46-1	64-17-5	71-23-8	67-63-0	107-21-1
Molecular weight	32.04	46.07	60.09	60.09	62.07
Molecular formula	C_2H_4O	C_2H_6O	C_3H_8O	C_3H_8O	$C_2H_6O_2$
Chemical formula	CH_3OH	CH_3CH_2OH	$CH_3CH_2CH_2OH$	$(CH_3)_2CHOH$	$(CH_2OH)_2$
Structure	Primary aliphatic alcohol	Primary aliphatic alcohol	Primary aliphatic alcohol	Secondary aliphatic alcohol	Dihydroxy aliphatic alcohol (diol)
Structural formula					
Common name	Wood alcohol	Beverage or grain alcohol	Propyl alcohol	Rubbing alcohol	Antifreeze
Boiling point	64.7 °C	78.5 °C	82.6 °C	82.5 °C	197 °C
Melting point	−95.8 °C	−114.1 °C	−126.5 °C	−88.5 °C	−13 °C
Density	0.791 at 20 °C	0.789 at 20 °C	0.805 at 20 °C	0.785 at 20 °C	1.11 at 20 °C
Water solubility	Mixes completely	Mixes completely	Mixes completely	Mixes completely	Mixes completely
Main metabolites	Formaldehyde and formic acid	Acetaldehyde and acetic acid	Propionaldehyde and propionic acid	Acetone	Glycolic, glyoxylic, and oxalic acid

CAS, Chemical Abstract Service Registry Number.

Table 2   Threshold concentration limits of alcohol in whole blood and breath for operating a motor vehicle in various countries and the blood:breath ratios of alcohol used to establish the breath alcohol limits

Country	Blood alcohol concentration	Breath alcohol concentration	Blood:breath ratio of alcohol
Most European countries	0.50 mg ml^{-1}	0.25 mg l^{-1}	2000:1
The Netherlands	0.50 mg ml^{-1}	220 μg l^{-1}	2300:1
Norway, Sweden[a]	0.20 mg g^{-1}	0.10 mg l^{-1}	2100:1
Finland	0.50 mg g^{-1}	0.21 mg l^{-1}	2400:1
USA	0.08 or 0.10 g per 100 ml	0.08 or 0.10 g per 210 l	2100:1
UK and Ireland[b]	80 mg per 100 ml	35 μg per 100 ml	2300:1
Canada	0.08 g per 100 ml	0.08 g per 210 l	2100:1

[a]Because a blood alcohol concentration of 0.20 mg g^{-1} is equivalent to 0.21 mg ml^{-1}, the actual blood:breath ratio operating is 2100:1.
[b]If urine is the specimen collected and submitted for analysis, the threshold concentration of alcohol is 107 mg per 100 ml.

most use mass/volume units. Because the specific gravity of whole blood is 1.055 on average, 100 mg per 100 ml blood is close to 95 mg per 100 g blood (**Table 2**). When the analysis of alcohol is done at hospital or clinical laboratories the specimens used are plasma or serum and these contain more water and therefore more alcohol than an equal volume of whole blood. In addition, the unit of concentration used to report results is mmol l^{-1}, where 21.7 mmol l^{-1} = 100 mg per 100 ml. The average plasma-to-whole-blood ratio of alcohol determined empirically is 1.15:1, which leads to a 15% higher concentration of alcohol in the plasma after the red cells are removed by centrifugation.

Most countries now use breath alcohol instruments in traffic-law enforcement to establish whether a person has consumed too much alcohol for driving. This has necessitated creating threshold breath alcohol concentration (BrAC) limits and thus avoiding the need to translate results into the equivalent BAC in every case. The critical BrAC limits were derived from the preexisting BAC limits by assuming a population average blood:breath ratio of alcohol (BAC:BrAC). Unfortunately, different countries opted for different BAC:BrAC ratios when their threshold BrAC limits were being set. Moreover, the units of concentration used to report blood and breath alcohol measurements differ between countries;

Table 3 Interrelationships between the concentration units used to measure and report blood alcohol concentrations for clinical and legal purposes

UK and Ireland (mg per 100 ml (mg%))	USA and Canada (g per 100 ml (g%))	Most European countries (g l^{-1})	Nordic countries and Germany (mg g^{-1} or g kg^{-1})^a
50	0.05	0.50	0.47
80	0.08	0.80	0.76
100	0.10	1.00	0.95
150	0.15	1.50	1.42
200	0.20	2.00	1.89

^{a}The specific gravity of whole blood is taken as 1.055, whence density is 1.055 g ml^{-1}.

examples of the current BAC and BrAC limits and the blood:breath ratios used in different countries are shown in (**Table 3**).

In connection with alcohol use in the workplace, especially by those engaged in safety-sensitive work, a BAC of 40 mg per 100 ml is enforced throughout the USA. Furthermore, for people below 21 years a zero-tolerance policy has been instituted for driving, which in practice means a legal blood alcohol limit of 20 mg per 100 ml. This is motivated by the fact that young people are overrepresented in alcohol-related road traffic crashes, which emphasizes the need for stricter control of their drinking habits. The legal drinking age in the USA is 21 years, although teenage drinking is a fact of life and is virtually impossible to control. Nevertheless, establishing a minimum legal drinking age (21 years) and a low BAC (<20 mg per 100 ml) for driving has resulted in a decline in alcohol-related highway deaths among young people.

Alcoholic Beverages

The concentration of alcohol in alcoholic beverages is expressed as percent by volume (% v/v), namely ml alcohol per 100 ml beverage. When required to calculate the amount of alcohol ingested from a given number of drinks these v/v percentages need to be converted to weight percent (% w/v) or g per 100 ml, which is done by multiplying v/v with the specific gravity of alcohol (0.79), leading to the equivalent w/v concentrations shown below.

- Beers 2.5–6.0% v/v – 2.0–4.7% w/v (g per 100 ml)
- Table wines 8–12% v/v – 6.3–9.5% w/v (g per 100 ml)
- Sherry/port 16–20% v/v – 12.6–15.8% w/v (g per 100 ml)
- Spirits 35–50% v/v – 27.6–39.4% w/v (g per 100 ml)

Besides the problem posed by different alcohol concentrations in similar drinks, the situation is further complicated because different volumes are dispensed as a standard measure depending on country and establishment where the alcoholic beverages are served. In the USA, the alcohol equivalent of a standard drink corresponds to a 12 oz (approximately 360 ml) bottle or can of beer, a 5 oz (approximately 150 ml) glass of wine, or a $1\frac{1}{2}$ oz (approximately 45 ml) serving of distilled spirits. Assuming that beer is 5 vol%, wine 12 vol%, and spirits 40 vol%, a standard drink thus corresponds to 14 g pure ethanol or an amount that requires 2 h to become eliminated from the body by metabolism in the liver. Obviously, the exact quantity of ethanol depends on the alcoholic strength of the beverage, which can vary widely for beers (2–10% v/v).

In the UK, a standard drink is referred to as a unit of alcohol and this corresponds to 8 g ethanol, and is considered broadly equivalent to half a pint of beer, a small glass of table wine, or a single measure of distilled spirits. The current recommendation for sensible drinking without risk of damaging health is 1–2 units per day. For men, risky drinking implies consumption of 8 units of alcohol daily (64 g) over a long period of time, which will eventually lead to alcohol-related health problems. For women, the amount of alcohol considered harmful is 6 units of alcohol or 48 g per day. The smaller size and lower body weight in women mean less body water to dilute the alcohol and therefore a higher BAC for the same dose ingested compared with men. In addition, hormonal differences might make the female gender more vulnerable to the untoward effects of alcohol and its metabolites.

Methods of Measuring Alcohol in Body Fluids

The methods used to measure alcohol in body fluids are the same regardless of whether the specimens are taken from the living or dead. However, differences exist depending on whether alcohol is measured in breath as opposed to liquid specimens like blood, urine, or saliva. Over the years, the methods for measuring alcohol in body fluids have undergone radical changes. Between 1900 and 1950 nonspecific wet-chemical oxidation methods dominated. In the early 1950s more selective enzymatic procedures appeared using the enzyme alcohol dehydrogenase (ADH) extracted from horse liver and/or yeast. Today highly selective physicochemical methods are used for analysis of alcohol in body fluids such as gas–liquid chromatography and mass spectrometry.

The first methods of breath alcohol analysis used the principles of chemical oxidation with dichromate and photometric detection of the endpoint as with the famous Borkenstein Breathalyzer® instrument, which was widely used by police forces in the USA, Canada, and Australia. More modern instruments for breath alcohol analysis rely on infrared (IR) spectrometry for quantitative analysis of ethanol or electrochemical (EC) oxidation, which is the basis of the so-called fuel-cell instruments. Some breath alcohol instruments make use of both analytical principles (IR and EC), thus furnishing an enhanced selectivity for the analysis and identification of ethanol. Breath alcohol testing is noninvasive and therefore ideal for conducting on-the-spot tests in drivers. Several kinds of handheld devices are available for testing motorists at the roadside. Such breath alcohol screening tests are also being used in accident and emergency departments to test for alcohol intoxication in casualty patients.

Point-of-care testing is currently in vogue and minimally invasive procedures such as the analysis of exhaled air have many advantages over blood sampling. Another noninvasive approach uses saliva (oral fluid) as a biological specimen for analysis of alcohol and a number of enzymatic test kits are available for this purpose.

The principles and basic features of the various methods used to analyze ethanol in blood and breath are summarized in **Table 4**. The current method of choice in forensic science and toxicology laboratories is headspace gas–liquid chromatography (HS-GC), which first appeared in the early 1970s. Besides the determination of ethanol, the same HS-GC technique can be applied to analyze a wide range of low-molecular-weight volatile substances that might be present in the biological specimens, such as methanol, acetone, isopropanol, and toluene. In brief, the HS-GC method entails sampling the air or vapor phase, called the headspace, above the liquid specimen (e.g., blood or urine) contained in an airtight glass vial kept at a constant temperature of 50 or 60 °C. After air–liquid equilibrium is established, an aliquot of the vapor phase is removed either using a gas-tight syringe or with some automated system and transferred into the HS-GC column for gas chromatographic analysis.

Table 4   Summary of the analytical methods used to determine ethanol in body fluids

Method of analysis	Basic principle of the analytical method
Chemical oxidation	The ethanol is first separated from the biological matrix by distillation, diffusion, aeration, or protein precipitation. The resulting aqueous ethanol is then oxidized, usually with a mixture of potassium dichromate and sulfuric acid, and the reaction endpoint is determined by volumetric titration or by spectrophotometry
Enzymatic oxidation	Ethanol is first separated from the biological matrix as above; the pH of the aqueous distillate is adjusted to between 8 and 9 with semicarbizide buffer, and the coenzyme (NAD^+) is added. Oxidation of ethanol is achieved by adding the enzyme alcohol dehydrogenase derived from yeast and the reaction is monitored by formation of the reduced coenzyme (NADH) at 340 nm by ultraviolet spectrometry
Gas chromatography using liquid injection	An aliquot of blood or other body fluid is diluted 1:5 or 1:10 with an aqueous solution of internal standard (either n-propanol or t-butanol). About 1–5 μl of the diluted specimen is injected into the gas chromatograph fitted with a polar stationary phase (e.g., polyethylene glycol) and a flame ionization detector is used for quantitation
Gas chromatography using headspace analysis	An aliquot of blood or other body fluid is diluted 1:5 or 1:10 with an aqueous internal standard as above. The diluted specimen is allowed to equilibrate in an airtight glass vial for 20 min before an aliquot of the vapor phase (called the headspace) is removed with a gastight syringe or other means (instruments fitted with automated injectors are common) and transferred into a gas chromatograph for analysis
Infrared spectrometry	Ethanol in the vapor phase (e.g., breath) is quantitatively determined by infrared spectrometry according to the Lambert–Beer law. Ethanol absorbs infrared radiation at wavelengths of 3.4 μm corresponding to the C-H stretch and at 9.5 μm corresponding to the C-O stretch
Electrochemical oxidation	Ethanol in the vapor phase (e.g., breath) is quantitatively determined by electrochemical oxidation with a platinum black catalyst and an acid electrolyte mounted with electrical connections to form a fuel cell. The ethanol molecules enter one side of the cell and are oxidized via acetaldehyde to acetic acid; the current produced is proportional to the concentration of ethanol in the sample

A recommended practice in forensic science is to make all determinations of BAC in duplicate. To enhance the selectivity of the assay the chromatographic conditions should differ for each aliquot of the duplicate and this requires the use of two different stationary phases that give unique retention times (RTs) for ethanol. The RT is defined as the time in minutes measured from the point of injection to the appearance of the apex of the peak on the chromatogram. RT is characteristic of the substance analyzed and is used for qualitative analysis or identification by comparison with pure known compounds. In practice it is rare that different substances have the same RT under the same chromatographic conditions and even rarer if two different GC systems are used for the analysis. Quantitative analysis is achieved by measuring the height or area under the GC peak response and for many volatile compounds a flame ionization detector (FID) is the universally accepted method. The detector response from the FID is remarkably linear over a wide range of concentrations encountered in forensic toxicology from 0 to 600 mg per 100 ml and higher.

Alcohol in the Body

Alcohol is a small polar molecule (molecular weight 46.07) and mixes with water in all proportions. Alcohol is easily absorbed from the stomach and small intestine by passive diffusion according to the concentration gradient existing. Drinking alcohol in the form of whisky (40% v/v), wine (10% v/v), or beer (5% v/v) will be expected to show different rates of absorption. The alcohol from the stronger drink is likely to become absorbed faster and give higher peak BACs for the same dose. Some basic characteristics of ethanol in the body and body fluids are summarized in **Table 5**.

Trace amounts of alcohol are produced naturally in the body mainly through the action of microorganisms and yeasts in the jejunum and colon that utilize dietary carbohydrates as substrates for biosynthesis of alcohol. However, the concentration of endogenous ethanol reaching the peripheral venous blood remains very low (<0.1 mg per 100 ml) as determined by highly sensitive and specific methods. Indeed, if any alcohol is produced in the gut it first has to enter the portal venous blood and pass through the liver before reaching the peripheral circulation. The alcohol-metabolizing enzymes located in the liver can effectively metabolize low concentrations of endogenously produced alcohol and only trace amounts are detectable in the peripheral circulation. Endogenous ethanol production therefore lacks any clinical or forensic significance.

Absorption of Alcohol

After drinking beer, wine, or spirits, the alcohol (ethanol) present in these beverages mixes with the total body water without binding to plasma proteins and the solubility of ethanol in fat and bone is negligible. How fast alcohol enters the blood stream depends on many variable factors, particularly the amount ingested, the rate of drinking, and especially the speed of gastric emptying. Alcohol can be absorbed

Table 5 Characteristic features of ethanol and its distribution in body fluids

Property	Value
Molecular weight	46.07
Density	0.79 g ml^{-1}
Critical diameter	4.4 Å
Dielectric constant	26
Energy value	$\sim$7.1 kcal g^{-1}
Spirits 40 vol%	31.6 g per 100 ml
Wine 12 vol%	9.5 g per 100 ml
Beer 5 vol%	4.0 g per 100 ml
SI units 21.7 mmol l^{-1}	100 mg per 100 ml
Standard drink contains	8–10 g ethanol
Plasma:whole blood distribution ratio	1.15:1 (wide range)[a]
Urine:whole blood distribution ratio	1.30:1 (wide range)[b]
Distribution volume	0.6 l kg^{-1} (women) 0.7 l kg^{-1} (men)
Proportion metabolized and excreted	95% and 5%
Elimination rate from blood (range)	10–25 mg per 100 ml per h[c]
Elimination rate from body (range)	6–18 g ethanol per h[c]

[a]The values in any individual case depend on the water content of the specimen, which in turn depends on blood hematocrit.
[b]The urine:blood alcohol concentration ratio is lower on the ascending limb compared with the descending limb of the blood alcohol curve and increases as blood alcohol concentration decreases.
[c]Values apply to the vast majority of people.

through the stomach and also from the small intestine (duodenum and jejunum) where the rate of absorption is faster owing to the larger internal surface area provided by the villi. The alcohol contained in beer and wine tends to be absorbed more slowly than alcohol from whisky and vodka, not only because of the lower concentrations present but also because malt beverages and wines contain sugars as well as other constituents that tend to delay gastric emptying owing to an altered gastric pH caused by the buffer capacity of the drink.

Eating a meal during or before drinking alcohol diminishes the rate of alcohol absorption into the blood because the food tends to delay stomach emptying. The resulting peak BAC is lowered after food and the time that alcohol remains in the body is shorter under these conditions compared with taking the same amount on an empty stomach. This is illustrated in **Figure 1**, which shows mean concentration–time profiles of ethanol derived from analysis of whole blood from 10 subjects who drank 0.3 g ethanol per kg either after an overnight fast (empty stomach) or after eating a standardized breakfast (after food).

Another factor influencing the absorption rate of alcohol is a person's blood sugar level. It seems that hyperglycemia slows and hypoglycemia accelerates gastric emptying, which means that the time of day when drinks are consumed and other determinants of blood sugar, e.g., eating low-carbohydrate diets, pregnancy, and diabetes, are important to consider. Hormonal changes depending on age, menstrual cycle, and menopause in women might account for gender differences in gastric motility and rate of alcohol absorption. Some commonly used medications

(aspirin, cimetidine, ranitidine) can alter gastrointestinal motility and this is reflected in drug-induced changes in ethanol absorption rate. Smoking cigarettes is known to delay the opening of the pyloric sphincter, thereby slowing the absorption of alcohol into the portal venous blood. It seems that a host of environmental and possibly gender-related differences exist that modulate gastric emptying and alter the peak BAC and the acute impairment effects seen after a given dose of alcohol.

Distribution of Alcohol

A person's BAC depends not only on the dose and the rate of absorption of alcohol from the gut but also on the body weight and particularly the amount of muscle and fatty tissues in the body. Having a high proportion of fat instead of lean tissue means a higher BAC for a given dose of alcohol because leaner individuals have more body water into which the alcohol ingested becomes diluted. Since women tend to be smaller than men and also have more fatty tissue per kg body weight and therefore less body water, a given amount of alcohol in a female drinker is expected to produce a higher BAC and therefore a greater intoxicating effect. This makes women more susceptible to the health hazards of prolonged heavy drinking.

All body fluids and tissues take up alcohol in proportion to their water content and the ratio of blood flow to tissue mass determines the speed of equilibration into the various body compartments. Most of the body water resides in the skeletal muscles so only a part of the ingested alcohol is circulating in the blood stream. The ratio of blood flow to tissue mass is high for organs such as the lung, the brain, and the kidney, which rapidly equilibrate with the absorbed alcohol. However, for the resting skeletal muscles in the arms and legs the ratio of blood flow to tissue mass is considerably less and a longer time is necessary to attain equilibrium with the concentration of alcohol in the arterial blood. This leads to arterial–venous difference in ethanol concentration, which are particularly marked during the absorption and distribution stages of ethanol metabolism. By 60–120 min postingestion, the arterial–venous differences are abolished and for the remainder of the time alcohol is present in the body, providing no further drinks are taken, the concentration in the venous blood is slightly higher than in the arterial blood.

The relationship between a person's BAC and the amount of alcohol absorbed and distributed in all body fluids and tissues is given by the following simple equation:

$$A = \text{BAC} \times V_\text{d} \times \text{body weight} \qquad [1]$$

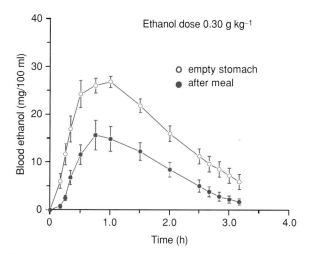

Figure 1 Comparison of the concentration–time profiles of ethanol in blood after drinking a moderate dose of alcohol (0.3 g kg^{-1}) on an empty stomach (10-h fast) or after eating a meal.

Table 6   Relationship between blood alcohol concentration (mg per 100 ml) and the amount of alcohol (g) absorbed and distributed in all body fluids at time of sampling. Values are shown for the average nonobese healthy adult person with body weights (kg) ranging from 50 to 90 kg

Blood alcohol (mg per 100 ml)	Subject[a]	50 kg[b]	60 kg	70 kg	80 kg	90 kg
20	Male	7.0	8.4	9.8	11.2	12.6
	Female	6.0	7.2	8.4	9.6	10.8
50	Male	17.5	21.0	24.5	28.0	31.5
	Female	15.0	18.0	21.0	24.0	27.0
80	Male	28.0	33.6	39.2	44.8	50.4
	Female	24.0	28.8	33.6	39.4	43.2
100	Male	35.0	42.0	49.0	56.0	63.0
	Female	30.0	36.0	42.0	48.0	54.0
150	Male	52.5	63.0	73.5	84.0	94.5
	Female	45.0	54.0	63.0	72.0	81.0
200	Male	70.0	84.0	98.0	112.0	126.0
	Female	60.0	72.0	84.0	96.0	107.9

[a]The volumes of distribution of ethanol were assumed to be 0.7 l kg^{-1} for men and 0.6 l kg^{-1} for women.
[b]Conversion factor: 1 kg = 2.2 lb and therefore 50 kg is 110 lb.

where A is the amount of alcohol in grams absorbed and distributed in all body fluids at the time of sampling blood, BAC is the person's BAC in units of g l^{-1} (not mg per 100 ml), body weight in kilograms, and V_d is the volume of distribution of alcohol expressed as liters per kilogram (l kg^{-1}) body weight. The average V_d parameter for healthy nonobese males is 0.7 l kg^{-1} and for healthy nonobese females 0.6 l kg^{-1}. By rearranging the above equation it becomes obvious that V_d corresponds to the ratio of the concentration of alcohol in the whole body (dose $= A$/kg) to the concentration of alcohol in the blood (BAC). Since alcohol only distributes into the total body water, the ratio of alcohol in the body to alcohol in the blood is the same as the ratio of percent water in the body to percent water in the blood.

Assuming a total body water of 60% for men and 53% for women and a blood water of 82% w/v for men and 86% w/v for women (because of their lower hematocrit) predicts a V_d of 0.73 l kg^{-1} for men and 0.62 kg^{-1} for women. Obviously there are appreciable inter- and intraindividual variations in the actual values depending on the person's age, gender, and the amount of adipose tissue in the body, as indicated by studies of body composition and body mass index (BMI). The magnitude of variation in V_d is about ± 20% within the same gender. **Table 6** was constructed using the above equation to give the amounts of alcohol in grams absorbed and distributed in all body fluids for healthy men and women with body weights ranging from 50 to 90 kg. The calculations were based on measured blood ethanol concentrations from 20 to 200 mg per 100 ml.

Metabolism and Elimination of Alcohol

Once absorbed from the gut, the alcohol molecules are transported to the liver by the portal venous blood where hepatic enzymes begin to clear the drug from the blood stream. The principal alcohol-metabolizing enzyme is ADH, which converts ethanol into its primary toxic metabolite acetaldehyde (**Figure 2**) which fortunately is swiftly transformed into acetate by another hepatic enzyme called aldehyde dehydrogenase (ALDH).

The same enzymes are also involved in the metabolism of methanol, as illustrated in **Figure 2**. Indeed, the classic treatment for patients poisoned with methanol is to administer ethanol intravenously to achieve an initial BAC of 100–150 mg per 100 ml and keep this constant by administering more ethanol at a constant rate of 7–10 g h^{-1}. This treatment prevents the oxidation of methanol into its toxic metabolites formaldehyde and formic acid, and any unmetabolized methanol can be removed from the blood stream by dialysis. Bicarbonate is also given to the patient to counteract acidosis caused by excess formic acid in the blood. Another more modern antidote for methanol poisoning is the drug fomepizole (4-methylpyrazole), which is a competitive inhibitor of ADH.

The catalytic activities of both ADH and ALDH display racial and genetic variations including polymorphism and isoenzymes exist with different characteristics including specificity for substrates and k_m and V_{max} values (**Figure 2**). Many people of Asian descent (40–50%) have an inherent low tolerance to alcohol and experience nausea even after a couple of drinks because they inherit a defective form of the ALDH enzyme. The enzyme is less capable of

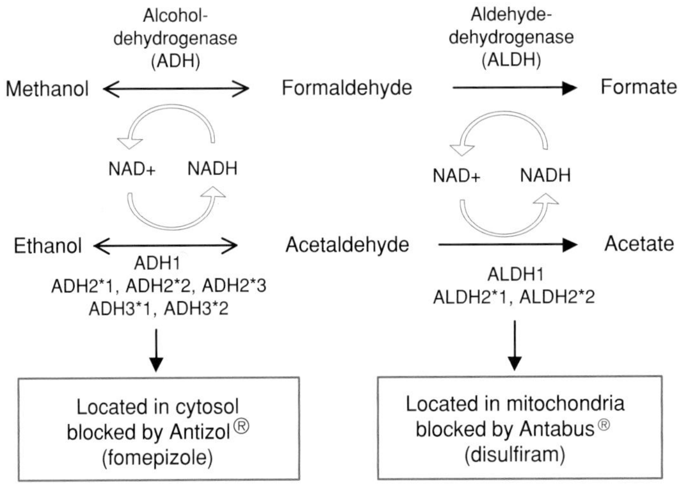

Figure 2 Scheme showing the enzymatic oxidation of ethanol and methanol via alcohol dehydrogenase (ADH) and aldehyde dehydrogenase (ALDH) and the various isozymes involved and examples of drugs that inhibit ADH (fomepizole or 4-methylpyrazole) and ALDH (disulfiram).

effectively metabolizing the acetaldehyde produced during the oxidation of ethanol and abnormally high concentration of acetaldehyde appear in peripheral blood. The high blood acetaldehyde triggers a range of unpleasant effects including facial flushing, nausea, tachycardia, and breathing difficulties, and this deters people from continuing to drink. These individuals are afforded a protection from becoming heavy drinkers and alcoholics owing to their inability to metabolize acetaldehyde effectively. The same effect can be achieved by giving Antabuse® (disulfiram), a drug treatment known as aversion therapy for alcoholics (**Figure 2**). This medication works by blocking the action of ALDH so if a treated person drinks alcohol he/she suffers the consequences caused by the high concentration of blood acetaldehyde.

Oxidative Metabolism

The bulk of the dose of alcohol ingested (93–95%) undergoes oxidative metabolism. This process occurs primarily in the liver, whereby ethanol is converted enzymatically first to acetaldehyde and then to acetate by the action of ADH and ALDH, respectively. These enzymes are located in the cytosol fraction of the liver (ADH) and mitochondria (ALDH) (**Figure 2**). Only small amounts of ethanol (5–7%) are excreted unchanged in breath, sweat, and urine, which means that drinking water to increase production of urine or hyperventilating the lungs or exercising to increase the formation of sweat are not effective ways of lowering the BAC to sober up quicker. There is an abundance of ADH in the liver so even people with serious liver dysfunction, such as hepatocellular carcinoma or cirrhosis, are capable of metabolizing ethanol, albeit at a slightly slower rate.

Another enzyme system engaged in the metabolism of ethanol is known as cytochrome P4502E1 (CYP2E1), which is located in a subcellular component of the hepatocyte know as smooth endoplasmic reticulum, particularly the microsomal fraction. The CYP2E1 as well as many other microsomal enzymes (e.g., CYP2D6, CYP2C9, CYP2C19) are important for the metabolism of endogenous substances as well as drugs and xenobiotics taken into the body. The CYP2E1 enzyme has a higher k_m for oxidation of ethanol (40–60 mg per 100 ml) and therefore comes into play when BAC reaches higher concentrations, as in heavy drinkers and alcoholics. Moreover, the CYP2E1 enzyme is inducible after a period of binge drinking so that alcoholics and others with very high BAC can clear ethanol more effectively from the blood stream. This accounts for the faster rates of disappearance of ethanol from blood reported during detoxification of alcoholics (30–35 mg per 100 ml per h). Many adverse drug–alcohol interactions are caused by the CYP2E1 enzyme, which is also involved in metabolism of the over-the-counter medication acetaminophen (paracetamol). Hyperactive CYP2E1, caused by heavy drinking, can result in liver damage and cell death owing to a toxic metabolite of acetaminophen. Furthermore, many dangerous environmental chemicals (e.g., chlorcarbons and hydrocarbons) are substrates for CYP2E1 and these can also be converted into toxic metabolites. The fate of ethanol in the body and the proportions metabolized and excreted are illustrated in **Figure 3**.

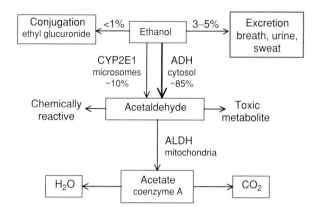

Figure 3 Scheme showing the fate of ethanol in the body, the relative amounts oxidized via alcohol dehydrogenase (ADH) and cytochrome P450 (CYP2E1), and conjugation and excretion in breath, sweat, and urine.

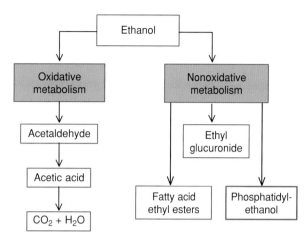

Figure 4 Comparison of the metabolites of ethanol produced by oxidative and nonoxidative metabolic pathways.

Gastric Metabolism of Ethanol

Although ethanol is primarily metabolized in the liver where most of the enzymes are located, studies have shown that ADH also occurs in the lung, kidney, and gastric mucosa. Great interest was aroused some years ago when investigators claimed that a considerable fraction of the dose of ethanol consumed was already eliminated in the stomach by class IV isozymes of ADH in the gastric mucosa. Interestingly, the activity of gastric ADH was found to be lower in women than in men and also less in alcoholics compared with moderate drinkers. It was argued that women and problem drinkers were more vulnerable to the ill-effects of ethanol and reached higher BAC for the same pattern of drinking because they lacked the capacity for ethanol metabolism in the stomach. This would mean an enhanced systemic availability of ethanol and a greater risk of organ and tissue damage as well as more pronounced acute effects on the person's performance and behavior. The magnitude of gastric first-pass metabolism was found to be greater during repetitive drinking, which is more in keeping with daily life, as compared with ingesting a bolus dose.

In another series of publications, it was shown that gastric ADH was rendered less effective when certain medication, such as aspirin, Tagamet®, and Zantac®, had been taken before drinking. This was explained by drug-induced inhibition of the gastric ADH enzyme so people who combined alcohol with this medication were more liable to reach a higher BAC because less was metabolized presystemically in the stomach. However, the significance of gastric ADH as a protective barrier against alcohol's effects is still a matter of conjecture and debate. It was found that the difference in BAC curves with and without the drug was highly dependent on the dose of alcohol ingested and the fed/fasted state of the individual. Whether the liver or the gut is the primary site for first-pass oxidation of ethanol is therefore still unresolved.

Nonoxidative Metabolism

It has been known for many years that a very small fraction (<1%) of the dose of ethanol consumed undergoes a phase II conjugation reaction with glucuronic acid to produce ethyl glucuronide (EtG), which is then excreted in the urine. Recent studies have shown that EtG has a much longer elimination half-life than ethanol itself and can therefore be detected in blood and urine long after ethanol is no longer measurable. This means that analysis of EtG in blood or urine could serve as a marker to detect recent consumption of alcohol. This would be useful when monitoring outpatient alcoholics and others in rehabilitation programs who are required to refrain from drinking.

Other examples of nonoxidative pathways of ethanol metabolism are the synthesis of fatty acid ethylesters (FAEE) and phosphatidylethanol (PEth) products formed during enzymatic reactions between ethanol and various free fatty acids (esterification) and phospholipid adducts, respectively. Both FAEE and PEth are being actively researched as markers of excessive drinking and also as possible explanations for ethanol toxicity to body organs and tissues. The oxidative and nonoxidative metabolites of ethanol are compared in **Figure 4**.

Rate of Alcohol Disappearance from Blood

The speed at which alcohol disappears from the blood stream is often discussed in forensic and legal medicine because this information is needed when retrograde estimations of a person's BAC are required, such as in drink driving cases. It sometimes happens that the BAC at the time of driving or involvement in a traffic accident needs to be estimated from the BAC measured several hours later at a time when the blood was drawn. In properly conducted experiments the rate of ethanol disappearance from the blood, which is commonly referred to as the β-slope or burn-off rate, usually ranges from 10 to 25 mg per 100 ml h^{-1} in the vast majority of people. These rates were obtained from controlled drinking experiments and tracing the concentration–time profiles of ethanol. Only those blood samples on the postabsorptive elimination phase of the BAC profile can be used to calculate the disappearance rate of ethanol from blood (**Figure 5**). This rate is given by the slope of the line (β-slope) or the ratio C_o/min_o in units of mg per 100 ml h^{-1}. The volume of distribution of alcohol is derived from the ratio dose (g kg^{-1})/C_o and takes the units l kg^{-1}.

In healthy people with moderate drinking habits a disappearance rate of 15 mg per 100 ml h^{-1} is considered a good average value, although in heavy drinkers, including many apprehended drunk drivers, higher mean rates are found, such as 19 mg per 100 ml h^{-1}. Alcohol starts to become metabolized from the moment it enters the body and this process continues at a constant rate per unit time (zero-order kinetics). When a measured BAC needs to be converted into the amount of alcohol a person has consumed, the amount lost through metabolism since beginning to drink must be considered. This can be done by using eqn 2, where ($\beta \times t$) is the amount of alcohol eliminated since the start of drinking, that is 0.15 mg per 100 ml h^{-1} multiplied by the number of hours elapsed.

$$A = [BAC + \beta \times t] \times V_d \times body\ weight \qquad [2]$$

To obtain an estimate of the rate of elimination of alcohol from the whole body one needs to consider the volume of distribution of alcohol, which depends on, among other things, the size of the individual and the total body water. The amount of alcohol eliminated from the body is given by the product of β and V_d and has units of g kg^{-1} h^{-1}. As a rule of thumb, a human being can eliminate 0.1 g 100% ethanol per kilogram body weight per hour regardless of gender, so a man or woman of 80 kg body weight eliminates 8 g ethanol per hour or approximately one unit of alcohol.

Table 7 shows likely rates of alcohol elimination from the blood stream (β-slope) and the body as a whole and also the conditions under which these values might be observed in practice.

Distribution of Alcohol into Body Fluids

Many different body fluids and tissues have been used for the determination of ethanol in clinical and forensic medicine and the choice depends on whether samples are taken from living or dead bodies. The specimens most commonly obtained are listed in **Table 8**, although it should be noted that the concentration of alcohol is not the same in the various fluids or tissues listed. The main reason for this is the different amounts of water and the time after end of drinking when the samples are obtained or how long after drinking death occurred in the cause of forensic autopsy work.

Urine

Much has been written about the relationship between alcohol in blood and urine in both living

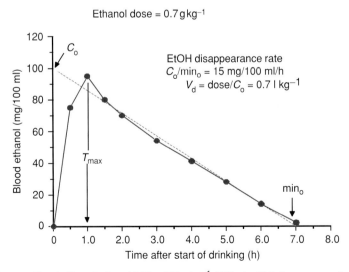

Figure 5 Concentration–time profile of ethanol after drinking 0.7 g kg^{-1} (160 ml whisky) on an empty stomach and the method of calculating disappearance rate from blood (β-slope) and the volume of distribution (V_d).

Table 7 Expected elimination rate of alcohol from blood and the whole body under different treatments or conditions

Elimination rate from blood (mg per 100 ml per h)	Elimination rate from whole body (g h^{-1})^a	Conditions/treatment necessary
8–10	4–5	People with liver dysfunction (e.g., owing to cirrhosis or carcinoma) or those who are malnourished or eat low-protein diets. Treatment with the drug fomepizole (4-methylpyrazole) will also slow elimination of ethanol
10–12	5–6	Healthy individuals who drink moderate amounts of alcohol after an overnight (10-h) fast
12–16	6–8	After ingestion of a moderate dose of ethanol under nonfasting conditions
16–25	8–12	Healthy individuals who reach appreciably high blood alcohol concentration (>120 mg per 100 ml) such as drunk drivers
25–35	12–17	Alcoholics or very heavy drinkers immediately after a drinking spree (e.g., during detoxification). Even heavy drinking for several days might show enhanced rates. Treatment with protein-rich diets or conditions that cause hypermetabolic conditions (e.g., burn trauma, hyperthyroidism)

^{a}The above values apply to a healthy nonobese individual with a body weight of 70 kg and an ethanol volume of distribution of 0.7 l kg^{-1}.

Table 8 Examples of biological specimens used for determination of alcohol in forensic casework when dealing with living and dead subjects

Living subjects	Deceased subjects (postmortem)
Whole blood	Whole blood
Cubital vein^a	Cubital or jugular vein
Radial artery	Femoral vein^a
Capillary or fingertip sample	Cardiac (heart) blood
Plasma or serum^a	Stomach contents
Freshly voided urine^a	Bladder urine^a
Tears	Vitreous humor^a
Cerebrospinal fluid	Cerebrospinal fluid
Saliva	Bile
Sweat	Bone marrow or synovial fluid
Breath	Various tissues
Free-expired	Brain
End-expired^a	Muscle
Rebreathed	Liver

^{a}Recommended specimens if available.

subjects and also in cadavers. Indeed, in postmortem toxicology urine is an important biological specimen for the analysis of alcohol and comparing the concentration in urine and blood can help to resolve whether postmortem synthesis might have occurred. Except in conditions like diabetes or other disturbances in carbohydrate metabolism, bladder urine does not normally contain sugar, which is the usual substrate for microbial synthesis of ethanol. This means that the risk of postmortem synthesis of ethanol is seemingly less in bladder urine compared with blood specimens.

In healthy people, urine is produced in the kidneys and enters the bladder at a rate of about 1 ml min^{-1} or 60 ml h^{-1}, although this production might increase 10-fold during a period of alcohol-induced diuresis close to the peak BAC. Drinking water will not dilute the concentration of ethanol in the urine because this depends on the concentration of ethanol in renal

artery plasma, which cannot be lowered by drinking liquids. Urine is therefore an excellent body fluid to verify that a person has used a particular drug, including alcohol, and urine drug testing is a large commercial enterprise in most countries. However, interpreting the concentrations of ethanol determined in urine and blood taken at autopsy is not always easy because urine tends to pool in the bladder, during which time the blood ethanol concentrations might have changed considerably, especially during the absorption phase. Urine is secreted in batches so the ethanol concentration in a voided sample will not reflect the concentration of ethanol in renal artery blood at the time of voiding. Much depends on the particular stage of alcohol pharmacokinetics and how long the person might have survived after drinking alcohol before death occurred. But also in living subjects the relationship between urine and blood

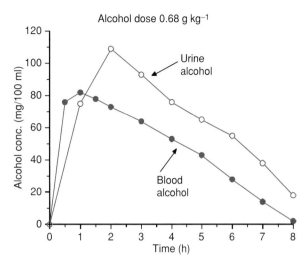

Figure 6   Concentration–time profiles of ethanol in blood and urine after drinking a moderate amount of alcohol ($0.68\,\mathrm{g\,kg^{-1}}$) in 20 min on an empty stomach. Alcohol was in the form of neat whisky and the bladder was emptied before the start of drinking.

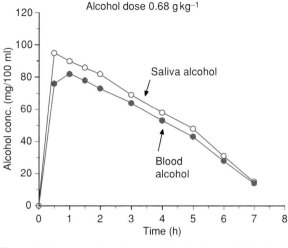

Figure 7   Concentration–time profiles of ethanol in blood and saliva after drinking a moderate amount of alcohol ($0.68\,\mathrm{g\,kg^{-1}}$) in 20 min on an empty stomach. Alcohol was in the form of neat whisky.

alcohol can differ widely depending on the position of the blood alcohol curve and the storage time in the bladder before voiding (**Figure 6**).

The magnitude of variation in urine vs blood alcohol concentration ratios is an important consideration whenever attempts are made to estimate BAC indirectly from the concentration determination in urine. Although the average urine:blood ratio of ethanol in the postabsorptive phase is about 1.3:1, the values vary widely in any individual case depending on many factors. A conservative estimate of BAC from UAC can be obtained by using a considerably higher UAC:BAC ratio such as 1.5:1 or higher, depending on legal requirements, such as beyond a reasonable doubt or more likely than not. **Figure 6** shows the relationship between alcohol in blood and bladder urine in one subject who consumed 0.68 g ethanol per kg body weight on an empty stomach in 20 min. Note that the bladder was emptied before drinking started and then every hour for up to 7 h.

Saliva

Saliva is a watery fluid produced by the parotid, the submaxillary, and the sublingual glands, although the mixed oral fluid collected for determination of drugs also contains mucous secretions from the mouth. The use of saliva as a body fluid for analysis of alcohol and other drugs has expanded greatly over the past decade. A number of methods have been developed for sampling saliva such as by chewing on cotton wool or parafilm to stimulate production of an appropriate specimen. For drugs like ethanol, which enter the saliva by simple diffusion from the arterial

blood supply to the salivary glands, the time lag between alcohol entering the blood stream and appearing in the saliva is very short. Only the nonprotein-bound fraction of a drug enters the saliva, which makes alcohol an ideal candidate for oral fluid analysis because of its negligible binding to albumin and other plasma proteins. Accordingly, the concentration of alcohol in saliva should be the same as that in the water fraction of the blood. Studies have found that the mean saliva:blood alcohol ratio is about 1.08:1 and this was remarkably constant during absorption, distribution, and elimination of alcohol in the body. The main disadvantage of saliva as a biofluid for drug analysis is the small volume available and the fact that some people, owing to a dry mouth, will not be able to produce the required sample on demand.

Figure 7 shows an example of the pharmacokinetic profiles of ethanol in saliva and blood in one subject who drank 0.68 g ethanol per kg body weight on an empty stomach in 20 min. Note that the saliva profile is closer to the blood alcohol profile than the urine alcohol profile (**Figure 6**) owing to a shorter time lag for alcohol to enter the oral fluids compared with the urine in the bladder, which is stored until voided.

Breath

A small fraction (1–2%) of all the alcohol ingested is exhaled in the breath. Alcohol diffuses from the pulmonary capillary blood across the alveolar–capillary membrane into the alveolar spaces and into the respiratory passages. The amount of ethanol leaving the body via the lungs depends primarily on the blood/air partition coefficient for alcohol, which is about 2000:1 at body temperature (37 °C). With a BAC of 100 mg per 100 ml the concentration of ethanol in alveolar air is only 0.05 mg per 100 ml (100/0.05 = 2000). If ventilation of the lungs is $41\,min^{-1}$ or $2401\,h^{-1}$, only 120 mg of ethanol (0.12 g) leaves the body with the exhaled air every hour. This amount is negligible compared with the amount lost by hepatic metabolism, which corresponds to 6–8 g of ethanol per hour.

The analysis of alcohol in breath has found many applications in both clinical and forensic medicine as a rapid noninvasive test for alcohol consumption and if necessary as a way to estimate the amount of alcohol in the body. A wide variety of breath alcohol analyzers have been developed and used for both roadside screening of drivers and also for evidential purposes, as discussed elsewhere in this encyclopedia.

Figure 8 compares venous blood ethanol and breath ethanol concentrations in one subject tested with an infrared breath alcohol analyzer (Intoxilyzer 5000). Note the slightly higher breath readings at the first sampling point just 15 min after drinking ended

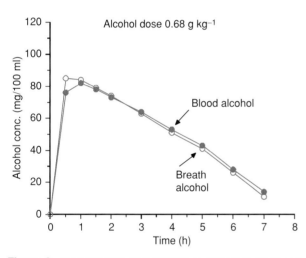

Figure 8 Concentration–time profiles of ethanol in blood and breath after drinking a moderate amount of alcohol $(0.68\,g\,kg^{-1})$ in 20 min on an empty stomach. Alcohol was in the form of neat whisky and the breath alcohol analyzer was Intoxilyzer 5000 based on infrared analysis.

and the lower results at all later times, which can be explained by arterial–venous differences in blood ethanol concentration. The alveolar and end-exhaled concentration of alcohol is closer to arterial BAC and not venous BAC.

Vitreous Humor

The vitreous humor (VH) of the eye is a clear fluid widely used in postmortem toxicology not only for determination of ethanol but also for measuring glucose, potassium, chloride, and lactate as well as certain drugs of abuse. VH is particularly useful when bodies are badly damaged or when putrefaction has occurred. VH specimens are easy to obtain using syringe and needle and this procedure can be done even before a complete autopsy is performed. The remoteness of the eye from the gut where bacteria start to spread makes VH less prone to artifacts caused by contamination with microbes and postmortem diffusion of alcohol from the stomach and chest cavity. Indeed, VH can sometimes be used as a specimen for alcohol analysis in embalmed bodies. The concentration of alcohol in VH helps to verify the BAC at autopsy and if necessary BAC can be estimated from VH concentration, albeit with large uncertainty.

Table 9 shows ethanol distribution ratios of VH/blood and urine/blood from a large autopsy material.

Effects of Alcohol on the Body

The effects of alcohol on human performance have been investigated extensively and the cardinal signs and symptoms of drunkenness are common knowledge – lack of judgment and restraint, slurred speech, unsteady gait. The effects of alcohol depend not only on the amounts consumed (the dose) but also on the speed of drinking: larger doses and faster drinking times lead to a more pronounced effect on the person's performance and behavior. An unusually rapid absorption of alcohol such that BAC passes 120–150 mg per 100 ml within 30 min after the end of drinking often results in nausea and vomiting caused by an action of alcohol triggering a vomit reflex in the brain.

Table 9 Mean distribution ratios of ethanol for urine/blood and vitreous humor/blood in specimens taken at autopsy. The vitreous data represent all causes of death but the urine data were alcohol-related deaths only (alcoholism or acute alcohol poisoning)

Body fluids	n	Mean blood alcohol concentration (median)	Mean vitreous humor concentration or urine alcohol concentration (median)	Mean ratio[a] (median)	95% range
Vitreous humor/blood	505	170 (150)	199 (180)	1.17 (1.18)	0.63–1.45
Urine/blood	1118	309 (320)	372 (380)	1.25 (1.21)	0.85–2.0

[a]Calculated for cases with blood alcohol concentration exceeding 50 mg per 100 ml because ratios increase sharply as blood alcohol concentration decreases.

Table 10 Typical signs and symptoms of acute alcohol influence as a function of a person's blood alcohol concentration when observations were made close to the maximum value after a single oral dose

Blood-alcohol (mg per 100 ml)	Signs and symptoms of alcohol influence[a]
<20	No untoward effects or outward signs
30–50	Mild euphoria and impairment of certain skilled tasks that require divided attention
50–100	Reduced inhibitions, increased talkativeness, sensory and motor disturbances, slower reaction time, especially in choice situations
100–150	Lack of coordination, unsteady gait, slurred speech, prolonged reaction to sights and sounds
150–200	Obvious drunkenness, significantly slower reaction time even for simple tasks, nausea and vomiting in some people, ataxia, aggressiveness
200–300	Inability to stand upright and walk without support, incoherent speech, motor areas of the brain severely depressed with distorted perception and judgment
300–400	Confusion, stupor, or coma with shallow breathing and risk of death
>400	Heightened risk of death through respiratory paralysis and cardiopulmonary arrest

[a]Large intersubject variations exist within each blood-alcohol concentration range owing to different drinking patterns and the development of tolerance to alcohol, and individuals may exhibit very different effects.

Table 10 lists some of the typical signs and symptoms of alcohol influence at various BAC intervals, although it is important to note that wide variations exist both between and within individuals from occasion to occasion. Much depends on the person's age and experience with drinking alcohol and particularly the speed of intake, beverage type and whether food was eaten, and not least the development of acute and chronic tolerance. Impairment is more pronounced on the rising part of the blood–alcohol curve compared with the declining phase several hours after end of drinking, and this is known as the Mellanby effect.

Acute Intoxication

Drinking alcohol interferes with many bodily functions including reaction time and the ability to perform skilled tasks, especially those that require divided attention. Cognitive functions are initially influenced (e.g., impairment of thinking, learning, memory) followed by motor skills and vision, all of which increases the likelihood of an accident, especially when skilled tasks like driving are performed. Alcohol reaches the brain almost immediately after drinking starts and the initial effects are felt after just one drink. There is a strong dose–effect relationship between the BAC and degree of inebriation, especially when the BAC curve is in the ascending phase, that is, during absorption of alcohol into the blood stream as it crosses the blood–brain barrier to influence brain functions. After the peak BAC or BrAC is reached in the descending phase of the curve, a marked recovery in both objective and subjective feelings of intoxication is evident. Seemingly the brain adapts to the alcohol environment and several hours after the

maximum BAC is reached, highly sensitive tests are needed to detect any residual alcohol impairment.

Alcohol exerts its effects on the brain by interfering with the normal functioning of nerve cells and chemical messengers (neurotransmitters). The wide spectrum of ethanol's effects, progressing from euphoria and excitement to muscle relaxation and ataxia, sedation, and stupor, and ending in coma and respiratory failure (**Table 10**), suggest the involvement of several different receptor systems including dopamine, gamma-aminobutyric acid (GABA$_A$), glutamate (*N*-methyl-D-aspartate receptor), and serotonin as well as others.

Tolerance

People react to drugs in different ways and accordingly they display wide intersubject variation in how much alcohol is required to elicit a certain effect or cause a change in behavior. Some people tolerate alcohol better than others, especially after a long period of continual drinking. Intake of the same dose of alcohol to reach the same BAC causes less effect in a tolerant person as evidenced by both performance tasks and objective ratings. Alternatively, an increasing amount of drug is necessary to produce the same effect and this as illustrated in **Figure 9**, is demonstrated by a shift in the concentration–effect curve to the right.

There are several different kinds of tolerance to alcohol:

• Acute tolerance can be defined as an adaptation to the effects of alcohol within a single drinking session in a person hitherto alcohol-free. Measures of alcohol-induced motor impairment at a given BAC on the rising limb of the curve are more pronounced than at the same BAC on the descending limb after the absorption and distribution terminates. Acute tolerance is particularly marked for subjective feelings of intoxication recorded at various times after drinking. The development and recording of acute tolerance in humans and dogs were first noted about 100 years ago by the British pharmacologist Sir Edward Mellanby.

- Metabolic or dispositional tolerance develops after a period of continuous heavy drinking and this is reflected in a more rapid rate of elimination of alcohol from the blood compared with after drinking a single dose. The mechanism of metabolic tolerance has been traced to a specific group of enzymes located in the microsomal fraction of the liver cell denoted CYP2E1. These enzymes are activated during chronic drinking and "learn" to dispose of alcohol more effectively. This form of enzyme induction is associated with an increased rate of alcohol degradation with less time being needed to clear alcohol from the body, thereby reducing the duration of alcohol's effects on performance and behavior.

- Chronic tolerance is represented by a progressive change brought about by continuous heavy drinking and this tends to develop over months or years of alcohol exposure. A given BAC produces less of an effect on the individual for measurements made at the same time after end of drinking, thus eliminating the confounding influence of acute tolerance. The effect–concentration relationship is shifted to the right in an alcohol-tolerant subject (**Figure 9**). One consequence of chronic tolerance after prolonged heavy drinking is the emergence of physical dependence. This means that when drinking stops abruptly the tolerant person experiences abstinence, which is associated with a range of unpleasant and often life-threatening effects including anxiety, restlessness, convulsions, delirium tremens, and hallucinations, and many have died after abrupt withdrawal of alcohol.

Depressant drugs used to treat abstinence symptoms include barbiturates and, more recently, benzodiazepines such as diazepam and lorazepam, all of which are agonists for the $GABA_A$-receptor complex. Despite long interest in the phenomenon of acute and chronic alcohol tolerance and dependence, the exact cellular mechanisms involved are obscure, although several neurochemical synapses and receptors are probably involved (mainly $GABA_A$ and glutamate).

The phenomenon of acute alcohol tolerance is well illustrated in **Figure 10**, where it can be seen that after drinking neat spirits on an empty stomach, the

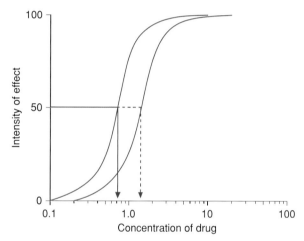

Figure 9 Illustration of the development of chronic tolerance with a parallel shift in the effect–concentration curve to the right.

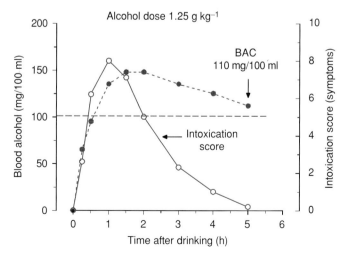

Figure 10 Relationship between blood-alcohol concentration and the well-known signs and symptoms of alcohol intoxication at various times after drinking alcohol as a bolus dose ($1.36\,g\,kg^{-1}$) as neat spirits in 15 min and on an empty stomach.

symptoms of alcohol influence were no longer measurable by 6 h postdrinking, although the mean BAC was still relatively high, being close to 110 mg per 100 ml.

The temporal variations in signs and symptoms of alcohol influence, depending on the rising or falling phase of the BAC curve, are shown by the data in **Table 11**, which come from a Finnish study by Alha. The data show that symptoms of intoxication are more prevalent at lower BACs on the absorption phase compared with the postpeak period several hours postdosing. In most subjects the signs and symptoms of being under the influence of alcohol were no longer evident by 2–2½ h postpeak. This provides experimental verification of what has become known as the Mellanby effect or acute tolerance to alcohol.

Metabolic Effects of Alcohol

Ethanol is unique among drugs of abuse in that it exerts two completely different actions: one of these is nutritional, providing energy (7.1 kcal g^{-1}) and another is impairment of the central nervous system and disruption of intermediary metabolism. During the hepatic oxidation of ethanol (**Figures 2** and **3**) there is a marked change in the redox state of the liver and the coenzyme NAD$^+$ is reduced to NADH, which offsets other NAD-dependent metabolic reactions. Among other things, pyruvate is reduced to lactate, causing varying degrees of lactic acidosis, which in turn inhibits the renal excretion of uric acid, which accumulates in joints and precipitates attacks of gout. The ethanol-induced increase in NADH/NAD$^+$ ratio also explains the characteristic fatty liver seen in heavy drinkers and alcoholics.

In some individuals who drink excessively over many years, fatty liver progresses to hepatitis and eventually liver cirrhosis and death. The change in redox state in the hepatocyte leads to inhibition of fatty acid oxidation, which in turn increases the synthesis of triglycerides. The excess NADH also hampers hepatic gluconeogenesis so if glycogen stores are deleted, as often happens in heavy drinkers who neglect to eat properly, this leads to an alcohol-induced hypoglycemia.

Acetaldehyde, the toxic metabolite of ethanol by all known oxidative pathways (**Figure 3**), has been incriminated in many of the untoward effects of heavy drinking, including hepatotoxicity, cancer, and cell death and also addiction and dependence.

Identifying Problem Drinkers

Judging whether a person drinks too much alcohol is not always easy because some alcoholics furiously deny their actual pattern of consumption. Obtaining an accurate drinking history by self-reports, clinical interviews, and questionnaires is notoriously difficult. Accordingly, more objective ways to identify heavy drinkers are needed for use in preventive medicine and clinical practice to validate self-reported alcohol consumption. Biochemical markers such as altered urinary metabolites or the activity of certain serum enzymes or an abnormal blood chemistry after a period of continuous heavy drinking have attracted much attention. Laboratory testing for hazardous drinking has become an important area of addiction medicine and in rehabilitation programs, such as in drunk drivers who reapply for a driving permit.

Well-controlled population surveys have shown that only about half of the known total consumption of alcohol in a country can be accounted for by results from questionnaire surveys. Accordingly, various laboratory tests have been developed to aid in the diagnosis of hazardous or harmful drinking. Among others, carbohydrate-deficient transferrin (CDT) and γ-glutamyltransferase (GGT) are well-known

Table 11 Percentage of individuals (healthy men) diagnosed as being under the influence at various times after they drank neat spirits on an empty stomach. Comparisons were made on the rising (absorption) phase and declining phase of the blood-alcohol curves 1–1½ and 2–2½ h postpeak

Blood alcohol concentration (mg per 100 g)	Percentage under the influence on rising (absorption) phase	Percentage under influence 1–1½ h postpeak	Percentage under influence 2–2½ h postpeak
12–50	50% (40/80)^a	#	0% (0/4)
51–80	57% (47/83)	5% (1/18)	0% (0/28)
81–100	66% (33/49)	4% (1/23)	4% (1/24)
101–120	77% (40/52)	36% (8/22)	21% (4/19)
121–140	69% (29/42)	38% (8/21)	15% (3/20)
141–160	91% (30/33)	#	#

^{a}Proportion of individuals under the influence of alcohol.
#, None with these blood-alcohol ranges.

Table 12 Biochemical markers or indicators of acute and chronic intake of alcohol

Biochemical marker	Specimen for analysis	Comments
Ethanol (EtOH)	Blood, breath, saliva, urine	Highly specific and useful to prove acute alcohol intake; sensitivity depends on amount of alcohol consumed
Ethyl glucuronide (EtG)	Blood or urine	More sensitive than analysis of ethanol, this metabolite is a useful marker for recent drinking up to 24 h after a drinking spree
5-hydroxytryptophol (5-HTOL)	Urine	The predominant urinary metabolite of serotonin is 5-hydroxyindoleacetic acid (5-HIAA), although this shifts towards 5-HTOL during catabolism of alcohol. This leads to an increased ratio of 5-HTOL:5-HIAA, which remains elevated for 10–20 h after end of drinking
γ-glutamyl transferase (GGT)	Serum	This serum marker is elevated after chronic drinking and although fairly sensitive it lacks specificity because other factors can elevate the readings and cause positive results (e.g., various drugs, other liver diseases)
Carbohydrate-deficient transferrin (CDT)	Serum	A widely used marker with good specificity for detecting long-standing heavy drinking
Mean corpuscular volume (MCV)	Red blood cells	Routine clinical laboratory test
Transaminases (AST, ALT)	Serum	Routine clinical laboratory tests, although not very sensitive or specific for alcohol abuse

examples of biochemical tests that can signify prolonged heavy drinking and early damage to organs and tissue. Some markers (EtOH, EtG, and 5HTOL/5HIAA: see **Table 12** for abbreviations) are useful to detect relapse to drinking in connection with rehabilitation of alcoholics or drug abusers. This places high demands on the sensitivity of the test, which is reflected in a high percentage of true-positive results. If tests are used for medico-legal purposes the results should have high specificity, that is, a small likelihood of obtaining a false-positive result.

The ideal marker should exhibit 100% sensitivity and 100% specificity, but this is never achieved in practice because reference ranges for normal and abnormal values tend to overlap. Nevertheless, the use of biochemical tests for monitoring a person's drinking habits is increasing and is now used in connection with granting life insurance policies and sometimes in connection with job applications.

The main features of some widely used alcohol markers are summarized in **Table 12**.

Toxicity of Alcohol

The toxicity of alcohol is low compared with many other drugs and toxins when one considers that tens of grams (25 g and more) are necessary to bring about a pharmacological effect compared with milligram amounts of other drugs (e.g., 5–10 mg diazepam, 10 mg morphine, 100 mg codeine) in first-time users. However, the ratio of effective dose to lethal dose for ethanol is fairly narrow, being only about 8:1, considering that a BAC of 50 mg per 100 ml causes euphoria whereas 400 mg per 100 ml causes

Table 13 Postmortem blood-alcohol concentration in men and women when death was attributed to acute alcohol poisoning and when alcohol was the only drug present

Gender	n	Age ± SD (years)	Blood alcohol concentration (mean ± SD) (mg per 100 ml)
Men	529	54 ± 11	355 ± 87
Women	164	53 ± 12	373 ± 83
Both	693	54 ± 11	360 ± 86

death. Alcohol can kill in various ways besides sudden deaths associated with acute alcohol poisoning and chronic alcoholism. In deaths on the roads and in the workplace as well as in suicides and other kinds of trauma, alcohol intoxication and drunkenness are overrepresented.

Deaths ascribed to acute alcohol intoxication are often the result of asphyxia caused by a depression of the respiratory center in the lower brainstem (medulla oblongata). This usually occurs when BAC is between 300 and 500 mg per 100 ml depending on tolerance. Another mechanism of death is suffocation by inhalation of vomit because a deeply comatose person might lack a gag reflex or die through positional asphyxia when lying face-down or in some other compromising position. Deaths resulting from inhalation of vomit need to be verified by histological examination of the lungs.

The BACs measured in femoral venous blood at autopsy when death was ascribed to acute alcohol intoxication are given in **Table 13** for a large case series of postmortem examinations. The age of the men and women was about the same; being in their mid-50s, but the women had a somewhat higher mean BAC of 373 versus 355 mg per 100 ml compared with the men. However, the BAC at autopsy is probably an underestimation of the highest BAC reached, owing to the metabolism (breakdown) of alcohol that takes place up to the time of death.

If nothing remarkable is found at autopsy apart from a fatty liver, then death may have resulted from severe metabolic disturbances after binge drinking combined with food deprivation or malnutrition. A metabolic acidosis may be caused by an accumulation of ketone bodies in the blood (ketoacidosis) as well as excess lactic acid, both of which are common in alcoholics since normal metabolic processes are disrupted during ethanol metabolism.

Postmortem Aspects

The quantitative and qualitative analysis of ethanol in postmortem specimens is a relatively simple task and the methods available are no different from those applied to specimens from living subjects. However, interpreting the results of alcohol analysis in postmortem specimens requires care owing to numerous analytical and physiological artifacts. The recommended blood-sampling site for toxicological specimens is a femoral vein after cross-clamping the femoral artery and transection of the vein before draining the femoral venous blood. Taking blood from the heart or pleural cavity is not recommended because of the risk of contamination with alcohol possibly remaining in the stomach if there was drinking just before death. How the body was handled and transported from the place of death to the postmortem examination and whether some agonal event might have caused stomach contents to enter the lungs heightens the risk of a postmortem artifact occurring.

In bodies without signs of putrefaction and when the specimens are preserved in a refrigerator at $+4\,^{\circ}C$ there is little risk of alcohol being produced or destroyed through the action of bacteria and yeasts. Moreover, if the sampling and analysis of ethanol are done the same day as the autopsy then chemical preservatives are not necessary. For longer delays such as when specimens are transported or sent by mail to another laboratory it is imperative to include sodium or potassium fluoride as a preservative to give a final concentration of 1–2%. The fluoride ion functions as an enzyme inhibitor and prevents the production of ethanol by microbial and fermentation processes.

Results of postmortem blood alcohol analysis are strengthened if additional body fluids are submitted for toxicological analysis, particularly bladder urine, VH, and cerebrospinal fluid (CSF). These liquids, which are almost 100% water, are obtained from the urinary bladder, the eye, and the base of the neck (cisternal fluid), and are expected to contain more ethanol than an equal volume of blood, which is only 80% w/w water. Besides different water content, however, there are also temporal variations in the concentrations reaching body fluids and cavities. The urine:blood, VH:blood, and CSF:blood ratios of alcohol change as a function of time after drinking.

During drinking and on the ascending limb of the BAC profile when the alcohol is being absorbed into the blood stream, the concentrations of ethanol in urine, VH, and CSF are lower than or about the same as in venous blood. On the descending limb of the BAC profile, corresponding to the postabsorptive phase, the concentration of ethanol in urine, VH, and CSF are always higher than in the blood. Indeed, alcohol might still be measurable in these alternative specimens even though BAC is reported as negative. In autopsy work a blood ethanol concentration below 10 mg per 100 ml is usually reported as being negative.

Many alcohol-related fatalities involve traumatic events, resulting in open wounds and massive blood loss, which increase the risk of bacteria entering the body and postmortem synthesis of ethanol occurring. These risks are heightened at elevated environmental temperatures (summer months) and when a long time is needed to recover the bodies, e.g., after air disasters or drowning. Although a fluoride preservative is routinely added to blood specimens taken at autopsy it should not be overlooked that some alcohol might have been synthesized in body cavities between the time of death and autopsy.

Obtaining blood for alcohol analysis from a subdural hematoma or clot in the brain can sometimes furnish useful information because of the reduced or nonexistent blood circulation to the clot. The person's BAC at the time of sustaining the injury and formation of the clot decreases owing to hepatic metabolism but the poor circulation in the clot means that alcohol concentrations remain elevated. The concentration of ethanol in the sequestered hematoma gives an indication of the person's BAC several hours earlier, e.g., at a time when the trauma occurred. For example, if a drunken person suffers a blow to the head but survives, albeit being unconscious for several hours prior to death, the subdural or epidural hematoma might contain an appreciable concentration of alcohol. With a survival period of say 10 h and a rate of alcohol elimination corresponding to 15 mg per 100 ml h^{-1}, a person's BAC decreases by 150 mg per 100 ml from the time of the trauma until the time of death. At autopsy, the concentration of ethanol in the blood clot is expected to be considerably higher than in a femoral venous blood sample. In practice, the rate of formation of the clot and other factors need to be considered.

Conclusion

Knowledge about the disposition and fate of alcohol in the body, including the relative amounts metabolized and excreted and the rates of distribution into various body fluids and tissues, has not changed much since the 1950s. However, much has been learnt about the biochemistry of alcohol and the effects on various metabolic pathways, particularly those related to liver pathology after chronic drinking. The mechanism of action of alcohol in the brain and effects on other body organs (e.g., pancreas) has also advanced considerably since the 1950s.

Ethanol can now be determined in body fluids and tissues with a high degree of precision, accuracy, and specificity and on-the-spot methods using the analysis of saliva and breath are currently available. The limited selectivity of older wet-chemical methods of analysis had always posed a problem in postmortem toxicology because of the risk of cross-reaction with other organic volatiles possibly present in body fluids, such as the products of putrefaction. Although carbon monoxide poisoning was once the major cause of death, especially in suicides, it seems that acute alcohol intoxication, alcohol-related disease, road traffic fatalities, and drowning now dominate among out-of-hospital deaths. Because alcohol is a legal drug its negative impact fails to receive the same publicity and media attention as illicit drugs like heroin, cocaine, and cannabis.

Gender and genetic differences in the metabolism of alcohol continue to be a popular research field and subtle differences have been noted, especially between different racial groups. A smaller volume of distribution for ethanol in women, a faster and more variable absorption from the gut, a lower activity of gastric ADH enzyme, a swifter hepatic clearance, and a higher concentration of acetaldehyde are physiological factors that make females more sensitive to alcohol than males. Although a person's drinking habits depend on a complex interaction between social, cultural, and genetic factors, there is a host of nutritional, biochemical, and hormonal influences that seem to make some people more vulnerable than others to the untoward effects of alcohol consumption.

Alcohol intoxication not only figures in a large proportion of unnatural and suspicious deaths but also in natural deaths, and some feel that blood alcohol analysis is needed in all out-of-hospital deaths. The concentration of ethanol in a specimen taken from a single sampling site is virtually impossible to interpret without additional information such as reliable case history and circumstances surrounding the death as well as measuring alcohol concentration in other biofluids (urine, VH, CSF). Great care is needed when interpreting the results of analyzed postmortem blood specimens and when a statement is made for legal purposes about the person's state of inebriation at the time of death.

Alcohol has always been and probably will remain the number-one drug of abuse in modern society and requests to measure alcohol in body fluids and to interpret the results for legal purposes will remain the most commonly requested service from forensic science and toxicology laboratories.

See Also

Alcohol: Breath Alcohol Analysis; Blood and Body Fluid Analysis; **Forensic Psychiatry and Forensic Psychology:** Drug and Alcohol Addiction

Further Reading

Agarwal DP, Seitz HK (eds.) (2001) *Alcohol in Health and Disease.* New York: Marcel Dekker.

Alha AR (1951) Blood alcohol and clinical inebriation in Finnish men: a medicolegal study. *Annals Academiae Scientiarum Fennicae, Series A* 26: 1–92.

Gibbons B (1992) Alcohol – the legal drug. *National Geographic* 181: 3–35.

Jaffe JH (ed.) (1995) *Encyclopedia of Drugs and Alcohol.* New York: Macmillan Library Reference, Simon and Schuster and Prentice-Hall International.

Jones AW (1991) Forensic aspects of alcohol metabolism. In: Mahley A, Williams RL (eds.) *Forensic Science Progress*, vol. 5, pp. 33–90. Berlin: Springer-Verlag.

Jones AW (2000) Alcohol; post-mortem. In: Siegel JA, Saukko PJ, Knupfer GC (eds.) *Encyclopedia of Forensic Sciences*, pp. 112–126. London: Academic Press.

Jones AW (2003) Disposition and fate of ethanol in the body. In: Garriott JC (ed.) *Medical-Legal Aspects of Alcohol*, 4th edn., pp. 47–112. Tuscon, AZ: Lawyers and Judges.

Jones AW (2003) Biochemistry and physiology of alcohol: applications to forensic science and toxicology. In: Garriott JC (ed.) *Medical-Legal Aspects of Alcohol*, 4th edn., pp. 113–148. Tuscon, AZ: Lawyers and Judges.

Jones AW, Pounder DJ (1998) Measuring blood alcohol concentration for clinical and forensic purposes. In: Karch SB (ed.) *Drug Abuse Handbook*, pp. 327–356. Boca Raton, FL: CRC Press.

Karch SB (ed.) (1998) *Drug Abuse Handbook.* Boca Raton, FL: CRC Press.

Klatsky AL (2003) Drink to your health. *Scientific American* 288: 62–69.

Lieber CS (1982) *Medical Disorder of Alcoholism.* Philadelphia, PA: WB Saunders.

O'Neal CL, Poklis A (1996) Postmortem production of ethanol and factors that influence interpretation: a critical review. *American Journal of Forensic Medicine and Pathology* 17: 8–20.

Pounder DJ, Jones AW (1998) Measuring alcohol post-mortem. In: Karch S (ed.) *Drug Abuse Handbook,* pp. 356–374. Boca Raton, FL: CRC Press.

Wallgren H, Barry H III (1970) *Actions of Alcohol.* Amsterdam: Elsevier.

Walls HJ, Brownlie AR (1985) *Drink, Drugs and Driving,* 2nd edn. London: Sweet and Maxwell.

Alcohol Back-tracking Calculations *See* Back-tracking Calculations

---

ALLERGIES

A Aggrawal, Maulana Azad Medical College, New Delhi, India

Introduction

The term allergy was first used in 1906 by an Austrian child specialist, Clemens von Pirquet (1874–1929) to denote exaggerated sensitivity of certain persons to innocuous exogenous particles such as animal dander, pollen, milk, jewelry, or washing powder. About 20% of all people, on coming into contact with such particles, exhibit symptoms like severe breathing difficulties, rashes, urticaria, or stomach upsets. von Pirquet coined this word from the Greek *allo,* meaning different, and *ergon,* meaning work. Literally, therefore, an allergy is something that "works differently" from the normal. Substances such as pollen or chemicals in washing powder, which elicit such abnormal responses, are called allergens. Allergens can enter the body in four principal ways: (1) ingestion (milk, peanuts); (2) inhalation (pollen, hay); (3) injection (bee stings, venoms); and (4) contact (washing powder, cosmetics). Allergic reactions would usually give rise to symptoms related to the exposed organ system. Thus ingested allergens may cause nausea, vomiting, and abdominal distress; inhaled allergens, bronchial asthma and respiratory distress; injected allergens, local redness and swelling; and contact allergens, dermatitis. All allergens can cause generalized life-threatening symptomatology, such as hypotension and shock.

A secondary allergen is an agent that induces allergic symptoms because of cross-reactivity with an allergen to which the individual is sensitive.

Allergoids are formaldehyde-modified allergens in order to favor the induction of immunoglobulin G (IgG: blocking antibodies) rather than IgE (antibodies causing most allergic reactions). These are analogous to toxoids prepared from bacterial exotoxins.

Allergen Nomenclature

In the initial days of allergy research, allergens were being discovered so rapidly that their nomenclature had become confusing, haphazard, and parochial. To bring a uniformity to its nomenclature, the Subcommittee for Allergen Nomenclature of the International Union of Immunological Societies (IUIS) recommended that all biologically derived allergens be designated by the first three letters of the genus (italicized), followed by a space; the first letter of the species name (again italicized), followed by a space; and a Roman numeral indicating the order of discovery of that antigen in that species. Thus, the allergen *Amb a* II indicates that it is the second antigen isolated from the ragweed *Ambrosia artemisiifolia.* Other common allergens are *Lol p* I to *Lol p* IV from perennial ryegrass pollen *Lolium perenne, Fel d* I from the domestic cat *Felis domesticus, Rat n* I from the rat *Rattus norvegicus, Equ c* I to *Equ c* III from the horse *Equus caballus, Der p* I and *Der f* I from two house dust mites *Dermatophagoides pteronyssinus* and *D. farinae* respectively, *Alt a* I from the fungus

Alternaria alternata, and *Gad c* I from the codfish *Gadus callarias*.

Classification of Allergies

The term allergy is quite commonly used interchangeably with hypersensitivity. A number of hypersensitive or immune disorders are known to clinicians. These can be classified in four principal ways. One of the simplest is to classify the reactions by source of antigen (**Table 1**). Levine in 1966 proposed a classification based on the time of onset of allergic symptoms (**Table 2**).

A third classification is according to their predominant clinical manifestations (**Table 3**).

Gell and Coombs in 1975 classified allergic reactions according to the immune mechanism involved (**Table 4**). This classification is most widely used by clinicians today.

Type I reactions are mediated by IgE, type II and III by IgG, and type IV by antigen-specific effector T cells. IgG are by far the most abundant immunoglobulins in the serum, and IgE the least. The levels of variousimmunoglobulins in human serum are: IgG $600–1400 \, mg \, dl^{-1}$, IgA $60–380 \, mg \, dl^{-1}$, IgM $40–345 \, mg \, dl^{-1}$, IgD $3 \, mg \, dl^{-1}$, and IgE $5 \times 10^{-3} \, mg \, dl^{-1}$.

Each of the above classifications helps us to understand and gain useful insights into the nature and diversity of allergic reactions.

It is important to appreciate that the term allergy has been used by various authorities in a variety of ways. Different authors mean different things when they use the term allergy. It has been noted above that the term allergy is used as a synonym of hypersensitivity by several authorities. This implies an adverse and idiosyncratic reaction to a substance – mostly foreign, but in some cases the body's own constituent too. Most pathologists however use the term allergy to describe only the IgE-mediated mast cell degranulation and corresponding clinical disorders. In this usage allergy is synonymous with immediate hypersensitivity.

In a medicolegal context, however, allergy should be used in the former sense, i.e., any adverse and idiosyncratic reactions to a substance, since all four categories (mentioned in **Table 4**) can have medicolegal implications. Examples include anaphylactic shock following drug injections such as penicillin (type I), mismatched blood transfusions and drug-induced lesions (type II), serum sickness (type III), and transplant rejection (type IV). It is in this sense that the term allergy will be used in this article. In addition, we would also include anaphylactoid reactions, which include non-IgE-mediated mast cell degranulation, such as those caused by neuromuscular

Table 1 Allergic reactions classified by the source of antigen

Source of antigen	Typical examples
Exogenous	Reactions to plant pollens, milk, animal dander
Homologous	Reactions to isoantigens such as transfusion reactions
Autologous	Autoimmune disorders such as systemic lupus erythematosus, rheumatoid arthritis, etc.

Table 2 Allergic reactions based on their time of onset

Reaction type	Time of onset	Clinical presentation (allergic symptoms)
Immediate	0–1 h	Anaphylaxis, laryngeal edema, fall in blood pressure, urticaria/angioedema, wheezing
Accelerated	1–72 h	Urticaria/angioedema, laryngeal edema, wheezing
Late	>72 h	Hemolytic anemia, serum sickness, drug fever, exfoliative dermatitis, Stevens–Johnson syndrome, interstitial nephritis

Table 3 Allergic reactions classified according to their predominant clinical manifestations

Allergic reaction	Predominant clinical manifestation
Anaphylaxis	Bronchospasm, laryngeal edema, hypotension
Cutaneous reactions	Vasculitis, pruritus, maculopapular rash (also known as morbilliform rash), photosensitivity reactions, exfoliative dermatitis
Destruction of blood elements	Hemolytic anemia, neutropenia, thrombocytopenia
Pulmonary reactions	Interstitial/alveolar pneumonitis, fibrosis
Renal reactions	Nephrotic syndrome, glomerulonephritis, interstitial nephritis
Hepatic reactions	Hepatocellular damage, cholestatic reaction
Serum sickness	
Drug fever	
Lymphadenopathy	
Systemic vasculitis	

blocking agents, opiates, radiocontrast media, dextrans, and a myriad of other low-molecular-weight chemicals, since these are also important from a medicolegal point of view. These agents do not cause a true IgE-mediated anaphylactic reaction. Instead, they act directly on the mast cells and basophils, causing degranulation, and all associated signs and symptoms.

Table 4 Allergic reactions classified by mechanism involved

Type	Typical example	Immune mechanism involved
Type I Anaphylactic type	Anaphylaxis, atopy such as allergic conjunctivitis, rhinitis, some forms of asthma, urticaria, angioedema	Immunoglobulin E-mediated disorder. Release of vasoactive amines from mast cells
Type II Cytotoxic type	Transfusion reactions, erythroblastosis fetalis, myasthenia gravis, drug-induced lesions such as anemia caused by alpha-methyldopa and sedormid purpura	IgG and/or IgM bind to cell surface, causing lysis or phagocytosis
Type III Immune complex type	Serum sickness, Arthus reaction, rheumatoid arthritis	Antigen–antigen complexes bind to tissues and activate complement system. Tissue destruction occurs
Type IV Cell-mediated (delayed) hypersensitivity	Tuberculosis, transplant rejection	T lymphocytes are sensitized on a previous exposure and release lymphokines, causing tissue destruction

Tests for Allergy

A number of tests are available for allergy. They are broadly classified as *in vivo* and *in vitro* tests. Common forms of *in vivo* tests include immediate skin tests, delayed skin tests, patch skin tests, conjunctival challenge, oral challenge, and bronchial challenge. Among the *in vitro* tests, one of the most common and frequently performed tests is the radioallergosorbent test (RAST).

RAST

First introduced in 1967, RAST measures circulating allergen-specific IgE antibody. The term allergosorbent means that the allergen of interest (say, penicillin, insulin, or latex) is bound to a solid support, forming an allergosorbent. This solid support could be a carbohydrate particle, paper disk, a cotton thread, plastic ball, synthetic membranes, or even the wall of polystyrene testtubes or plastic microtiter wells.

If the allergist wants to diagnose a patient's allergy to, say, penicillin, he/she would use an allergosorbent containing the antigen of interest – in this case, penicillin. The allergosorbent is then exposed to the patient's serum. If the serum contains antibodies (IgE) against penicillin, they would bind to the allergosorbent. Excess serum is washed away. The allergosorbent is then reacted with a radiolabeled, highly specific antihuman IgE antibody. The amount of anti-IgE binding to the allergosorbent is proportional to the amount of IgE bound to the allergosorbent. Thus, by measuring the radioactivity levels, true levels of IgE against penicillin can be found. Currently RAST is available for a number of allergens, among them penicillin, insulin, chymopapain, muscle relaxants, thiopental, protamine, trimethoprim, and latex (**Figure 1**).

The radio label (in the radiolabeled, antihuman IgE antibody) is usually ^{125}I. More recently, enzymatic labels have become increasingly popular, producing enzyme-linked immunosorbent assay (ELISA). If an enzyme is used to label the anti-IgE, one more step is used, in which a proper substrate, which changes color in the presence of enzyme, is added. The intensity of color would then indicate the levels of IgE present in the blood.

Improper Use of RAST and its Attendant Medicolegal Implications

Increasing allergy litigations against doctors have seen increased use of RAST in recent times. It has led to commercialization and subsequent abuse of RAST. Companies have been selling RAST kits for drugs and chemicals which do cause anaphylactoid reactions, but have not been demonstrated to cause true IgE-mediated anaphylactic reactions (such as radiocontrast media). Performance of RAST in such cases is not only superfluous, but misleading. Increasing reliance of doctors on RAST in such cases would not prevent anaphylactoid reactions, and can invite unnecessary litigation.

Medicolegal Considerations in Allergy

Allergic disorders have a wide variety of inherent medicolegal implications, which are of relevance to forensic and legal personnel. Examples illustrating the different phenomena are given below.

Allergic Asthma

One of the most common conditions seen by doctors is allergic asthma. Generally, physicians rely on their clinical judgment to gauge the severity of their symptoms and the effectiveness of medications. In 1991, however, the US National Institute of Health

I

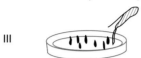

Allergen molecules (say penicillin)
bound to cellulose disk (allergosorbent)

II

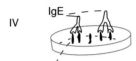

Serum of the patient to be tested for
allergy to penicillin. If he is allergic, it
would contain penicillin-specific IgE molecules

III

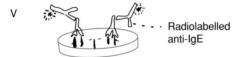

Patient's serum is mixed with allergosorbent

IV

IgE

Penicillin molecules
After washing IgE molecules remain sticking to allergosorbent.
The next stage is to mix radio labeled anti-IgE

V

Radiolabelled
anti-IgE

Radiolabeled anti-IgE sticks to IgE molecules. The amount
of radioactivity measured gives the levels of IgE in patient's blood

Figure 1 Principle of radioallergosorbent test (RAST).

published *Guidelines for the Diagnosis and Management of Asthma* and mailed it to 150 000 pediatricians, internists, pulmonologists, family practitioners, and allergists. These guidelines prescribed a set of recommendations which seem to set a standard of care for doctors. For instance, it is recommended that office spirometry be conducted in the initial assessment of all patients, and periodically thereafter, as appropriate. It was also recommended that clinicians consider using peak expiratory flow rate (PEFR) as measured by peak flow meters at home to monitor patients over 5 years old with moderate to severe asthma. The recommendations also said that peak flow measurements provided a simple, quantitative, reproducible measure of airway obstruction that can be obtained using inexpensive, portable peak flow meters. They correlate well with forced expiratory volume in 1 s (FEV$_1$) and provide an objective measurement. These measurements were considered akin to measuring glucose levels in a diabetic, or blood pressures in a hypertensive patient.

It was noted that neither patients' reporting of severity of symptoms nor physicians' clinical judgment were the true indicator of the severity of disease. The only objective criteria were the pulmonary function tests as noted above. Patients' responses to medication were also to be assessed by these tests.

A case is on record where a young asthmatic woman in her 20s died of an exceptionally severe attack. It was later discovered that her physician and the emergency medicine doctors had failed to conduct the objective pulmonary function tests outlined above in the report. Had they done the tests, they may have probably discovered that the patient was not responding well to treatment, and may have considered hospitalization, which could have saved her life. The woman's relatives sued the doctors, and the case was settled for a substantial sum.

Occupational Allergies and Compensation

Most countries now have laws regarding general aspects of health and safety at work. Employers are required by law to look after the health of their employees. In the event of an employee becoming ill in the workplace, the employer will be responsible and liable for compensation, especially if negligence on the employer's part is proved. Some important acts catering to workers' safety are Health and Safety at Work Act 1974 and Control of Substances Hazardous to Health Regulations 1988 in the UK, Health and Safety at Work Act 1977 in Sweden, Worker Health and Environment Act 1977 in Norway, and The Workmen's Compensation Act 1923, and The Factories Act 1948 in India.

Allergic manifestations occurring in work environments may attract various medicolegal provisions of the above acts, relating to compensation, relocation, or premature retirement. Examples are given below.

Hypersensitivity pneumonitis Hypersensitivity pneumonitis is a lung inflammation induced by antibodies specific for substances that have been inhaled. If these inhaled substances are related to work, and/or are present in the work environment, they would attract relevant legal provisions relating to compensation.

Bagassosis The fungi *Thermoactinomyces saccharic* and *T. vulgaris* thrive in pressings from saccharis. Subjects working in sugarcane mills may inhale dust from molding hot sugarcane bagasse and develop type III (Arthus reaction) hypersensitivity. The condition is expressed as a hypersensitivity pneumonitis.

Farmer's lung This is another instance of hypersensitivity pneumonitis. Farmer's lung is caused by *Actinomycetes* (or other organic dusts), which thrive in moldy hay. Subjects working in such environments may develop antibodies to the mold spores. Subsequent inhalation of dust containing spores may induce hypersensitivity pneumonitis characterized by nausea, chills, fever, coughing, tachycardia, dyspnea, and cyanosis. Treatment would include standard antiallergic regimens such as those consisting of cromolyn sodium and corticosteroids.

Humidifier lung This condition, also known as air-conditioner lung, is common among workers involved with refrigeration and air-conditioning equipment. The hypersensitivity is due to the various species of the fungi *Micropolyspora* and *Thermoactinomyces*. Symptoms of the acute form consist of chills, cough, fever, dyspnea, anorexia, nausea, and vomiting. The chronic form of the disease is characterized by fatigue, chronic cough, dyspnea on exercise, and weight loss.

Bird fancier's lung Known variously as bird breeder's lung, pigeon breeder's lung, or hen worker's lung, this form of hypersensitivity pneumonitis is due to antigens in bird droppings.

Tables 5 and 6 list these and some other cases of hypersensitivity pneumonitis, along with the antigen involved. In all these cases, the subject experiences flu-like symptoms, with productive cough and weight loss. Specific precipitating antibodies can be demonstrated in some cases. Pulmonary function tests show a restrictive defect in early disease and a restrictive, obstructive, or mixed defect in late disease. Chest X-rays would show signs of pneumonitis. If the disease is recognized early, the employee may be relocated in service or considered for premature retirement. If the disease is not recognized, it may progress to interstitial fibrosis, which could invite heavy compensation.

Employers in these professions must conduct a regular check-up of all their prospective employees, including chest X-rays, complete blood profile, and pulmonary function tests before inducting them in work. Once an employee is inducted, the same tests must be conducted at regular intervals, perhaps every 6 months. As seen above, if pulmonary function tests are not conducted regularly, and occupational hypersensitivity pneumonitis develops, it may be difficult to convince the jury that the employer was not negligent with regard to employees' health.

Finally, it may be added that certain forms of hypersensitivity pneumonitis may not necessarily be associated with a particular profession. The most recent example is the so-called "hot tub lung" caused by *Mycobacterium avium* complex (MAC), which thrives in hot tubs. Hot tubs provide an excellent growth environment for MAC; the warm temperature promotes growth. The steam and bubbles generated efficiently vaporize the organism, facilitating easy inhalation.

It has recently been recommended that physicians maintain a high index of suspicion for hot tub lung and include questions about hot tub use in their routine review of symptoms in patients with respiratory problems. Not doing so may invite charges of medical negligence.

Allergy to laboratory animals (ALA) ALA is a well-known occupational disease in subjects working with these animals. The most common animals to which personnel are allergic include mice, rats, guinea pigs, rabbits, hamsters, dogs, cats, and monkeys. About 20% of all workers exposed to animals display allergies. The most common clinical manifestation is rhinoconjunctivitis which comprises sneezing, nasal

Table 5 Some common instances of hypersensitivity pneumonitis (HP) due to biologically derived antigens, which may attract medicolegal provisions

Disease name	Antigens	Exposure
Antigens originating from bacteria and fungi		
Bagassosis	Thermophilic actinomycetes	Moldy bagasse (pressed sugarcane)
Cheese-washer's lung	Fungus (*Pencillium casei* or *P. roqueforti*)	Cheese casings
Compost lung	Fungus (*Aspergillus*)	Compost
Farmer's lung	Thermophilic actinomycetes fungus (*Aspergillus* spp.)	Moldy hay
Humidifier (air-conditioner) lung	Bacteria (*Bacillus subtilis, B. cereus, Klebsiella oxytoca*), fungus (*Aureobasidium pullulans*), amebae (*Naegleria gruberi, Acanthamoeba polyhaga, A. castellani*)	Mists from standing water
Japanese summer-type HP	Fungus (*Trichosporon cutaneum*)	Damp wood and mats
Malt worker's lung	Fungus (*Aspergillus clavatus*)	Moldy barley
Maple bark-stripper's lung	Fungus (*Cryptostroma corticale*)	Moldy wood bark
Metal-working fluids HP	*Mycobacterium chelonae*, fungi	Microbially contaminated, water-based metal-working fluids
Mushroom worker's lung	Thermophilic actinomycetes	Mushroom compost
Sequoiosis	Fungi (*Graphium* spp., *Pullularia* spp.)	Moldy wood dust
Suberosis	Fungus (*Penicillum frequentans*)	Moldy cork dust
Wood pulp worker's lung	Fungus (*Alternaria* spp.)	Moldy wood pulp
Wood trimmer's disease	Fungus (*Rhizopus* spp.)	Moldy wood trimmings
Antigens comprising proteins other than from bacteria and fungi		
Mollusc shell HP	Aquatic animal proteins	Mollusc shell dust
Bird breeder's lung	Avian proteins	Bird droppings and feathers

Table 6 Some common instances of hypersensitivity pneumonitis (HP) due to chemicals acting as antigens, which may attract medicolegal provisions

Disease name	Antigens (chemical involved)	Exposure
Isocyanate HP	• Toluene diisocyanate (TDI): most dangerous • Hexamethylene diisocyanate (HDI): less dangerous than TDI • Methylene bisphenyl diisocyanate (MDI): least dangerous and the preferred substitute for TDI and MDI	Paints, resins, polyurethane foams
TMA HP	Trimellitic anhydride (TMA)	Plastics, resins, paints

congestion, and itchy, watery eyes. It occurs in up to 80% of symptomatic workers. Dermatologic symptoms, including contact urticaria (hives) itchy maculopapular eruption, occur in up to 40% of symptomatic workers. About 20–30% of the symptomatic workers suffer from respiratory symptoms, including asthma, wheezing, cough, and chest tightness. Asthma is the most serious symptom and may not be reversible after removal from exposure.

Symptoms usually start within 1 year of the beginning of exposure (in one-third of all cases). Most who develop allergies will do so within 3 years of employment (up to 70%).

In the case of allergy to mouse (*Mus musculus*), the most common allergen involved is *Mus m* I, found primarily in mouse urine, but also in dander and hair, and *Mus m* II, found mostly in hair and dander. In the case of guinea pig, the allergens are *Cav p* I and *Cav p* II, found in hair, dander, and urine; in the case of rabbit, *Ory c* I, found in hair, dander, and saliva, and *Ory c* II, found in hair, dander, and urine; in the case of cat, *Fel d* I, found in hair, dander, and saliva; and in the case of dog, *Can f* I, found in hair, dander, and saliva.

It is important to remember that most animal allergens are only a few microns in size (between 1 and 20 µm) and, as such, can remain airborne for hours. Removal of animals from the work environment therefore may not bring immediate relief.

It is recommended that there should be a preemployment medical examination of all prospective employees. Very few laboratories are currently doing these examinations. Even those which are conducting such examinations are found lacking in conducting specialized tests for animal allergies. For instance, in one study it was found that less than 5% of preemployment examinations included skin testing for hypersensitivity. The tests should be thorough, including lung function tests, blood profile (for increased IgE levels), and skin tests. In addition job applicants must be required to furnish information regarding personal history of allergy, asthma, and, most importantly, allergy to animals. A history of allergy to animals must be an immediate disqualifier.

If an employee develops ALA despite all screening tests, immediate steps must be taken to limit the exposure. The steps may include limiting the hours of exposure, withdrawing the individual from those procedures most likely to put him/her at risk, use of respiratory protection and other personal equipment, use of a safety cabinet where possible, increased periodic monitoring, and monitoring the progress of disease. If possible, shifting the employee to administration may be considered.

It is important to realize that if an employee develops an allergic disease to a laboratory animal, in several countries it may be required by law to report this to the proper authorities. For instance, in the UK occupational asthma resulting from working with laboratory animals must be notified to the Health and Safety Executive under the Reporting of Injuries, Diseases and Dangerous Occurrences Regulations of 1985. Occupational asthma (such as that developing from exposure to laboratory animals) is a prescribed occupational disease in most countries and qualifies for disability benefit.

Latex allergy   Natural latex is the sap of the tropical rubber tree *Hevea brasiliensis*. It is a colloidal dispersion of rubber particles (*cis*-1,4-polyisoprene) in water, and contains a complex mixture of organic substances including many proteins. Allergy to natural rubber latex (NRL) proteins (latex allergy) was first reported to cause glove-related contact urticaria in 1979. Later there were several reports of fatal reactions to latex enema tips. The incidence of latex allergy in recent years seems to have increased due to increased condom and glove use (both latex products) in the wake of acquired immunodeficiency syndrome (AIDS) and hepatitis epidemics. In high-quality, costlier latex gloves, leachable chemicals and water-soluble proteins are removed with a costly process. Poorly manufactured gloves may have a higher protein content, causing more reactions.

Latex allergy can be detrimental to both healthcare workers (doctors, surgeons, nurses) and their patients. Patients with spina bifida are 500 times more prone to latex allergy than the general population.

This could be due to their repeated exposure to latex. The incidence in the general population is less than 1%.

The most common symptoms of latex allergy are localized contact urticaria, pruritus, erythema, and urticarial wheals. Cornstarch used as glove powder adsorbs NRL allergens, rendering them airborne, and this can cause an acute attack of asthma in susceptible persons. The UK Medical Devices Agency has advised against its use. It is further recommended that sensitized individuals should use NRL gloves with a low extractable protein content ($<50\,\mu g\,g^{-1}$), or gloves made from alternative material such as neoprene (polychloroprene) or elastyrene (styrene butadiene). However these have financial implications, as they could be more expensive.

If a doctor finds that a patient is allergic to latex, he/she should immediately inform the patient about this. The patient should also be told to wear a Medic-Alert bracelet stating "allergy to latex." Hospitals should make sure that staff are not allergic to latex. If an employee is found to be allergic, gloves made of alternative material should be provided.

Recently a nurse from South Wales, UK, successfully sued her employers because she was allergic to latex. Interestingly the hospital had provided her with vinyl gloves, but contact with colleagues wearing latex or with latex-contaminated dust was enough to trigger an allergic reaction in her. The appellate court held that in such cases the employer held a strict liability.

Drug Allergy and Anaphylaxis

Allergy to drugs is a very important issue from a medicolegal standpoint. A number of medical negligence suits have been filed against doctors who failed to conduct sensitivity tests before injecting, say, penicillin. A number of other drugs can cause allergy, and the practicing physician would do well to keep them in mind.

Type I hypersensitivity reactions (anaphylaxis)   These are the most serious and dramatic allergic reactions to drugs such as penicillin, cephalosporins, allergenic extracts, and insulin. Anaphylactoid reactions can be caused by radiocontrast media and aspirin. It is vital for radiologists to take an informed consent from the patient before administering radiocontrast media. Two types of radiocontrast media are currently available. One is the conventional high-osmolar radiocontrast media (HORCM). Their osmolality is seven times that of plasma. Anaphylactoid reactions to HORCM (urticaria, wheezing, dyspnea, hypotension, death) occur in 2–3% of individuals receiving intravenous or intraarterial injections. If there is a previous history of reactions to HORCM, the chances of having a repeat reaction on reexposure are as high as 33%. Death occurs in about 1:50 000 intravenous procedures. It is hypothesized that the high osmolality of HORCM may cause direct degranulation of mast cells.

It might be prudent for radiologists to use low-osmolality radiocontrast media (LORCM), which is a relative new entrant in the field. The osmolality of these agents is only twice that of plasma. The incidence of a repeat reaction with LORCM is just about 2.7%, even in patients who have shown a previous reaction to HORCM. However, their cost is 20 times that of HORCM.

Type II hypersensitivity reactions Certain drugs, such as penicillin, quinidine, and methyldopa, can cause type II hypersensitivity reactions causing antibody-mediated destruction of red blood cells (hemolytic anemia) or platelets (thrombocytopenia). The drug binds to the cell surface and serves as a target for antidrug IgG antibodies, causing destruction of the cell. Penicillin is known to cause all four types of hypersensitivity reaction.

Allergy to antisnake venom (type I, type III hypersensitivity) Antisnake venom is prepared by hyperimmunizing horses against snake venom. The sera from these horses are then used to manufacture antisnake venom. Since it contains foreign proteins, it can induce violent anaphylaxis (type I hypersensitivity) or serum sickness (type III hypersensitivity). Adequate testing must be done before injecting antisnake venom. This includes injecting 0.1 ml of the antisnake venom intradermally. A wheal of 1 cm surrounded by erythema of about the same width developing in 5–20 min would indicate that the subject is allergic.

If the subject is found to be allergic, antisnake venom must be given with great caution. Medications for anaphylaxis must be available.

Most snakes are nonpoisonous and giving generalized polyvalent antisnake venom in every instance of a snakebite may not be very good practice. If the relatives and friends have killed the snake, and have brought it with them, it must be identified. A good emergency physician must know the basic differences between a poisonous and a nonpoisonous snake for this reason. Doing so may avoid unnecessary medicolegal complications.

Herxheimer reaction (type III hypersensitivity) This is a form of serum sickness (type III form of hypersensitivity), which occurs following the successful treatment of certain infections such as syphilis, trypanosomiasis and brucellosis. During infection antibodies are formed against these organisms. A successful drug therapy will cause lysis of these organisms, releasing into the circulation a significant amount of their antigens. This may cause a violent antigen–antibody reaction, which may have medicolegal connotations. Before starting treatment in such cases, it is always advisable to inform the patient of the possibility of these reactions. Furthermore, it is advisable for the physician to obtain a written signed consent form from these patients.

Allergy to Human Seminal Plasma

This bizarre condition, first described in 1958 by Specken, has led to successful divorce suits. The female is allergic to her partner's seminal plasma. This causes a stinging, burning, or itching sensation in the vagina immediately after intercourse, with pain in some cases. Local redness, swelling, severe vulvovaginitis, rhinitis, dyspnea, wheezing, and even life-threatening asthma after intercourse have been reported. Many women experience the symptoms for the first time during their honeymoon. These symptoms have also been reported following intrauterine insemination.

In an interesting case, a concurrent allergy to human seminal plasma and latex in a woman has been described. Though the condition is rare, its existence could lead to successful divorce suits. The condition effectively means that a woman cannot have sex. She would experience allergic symptoms after sexual intercourse irrespective of whether the partner used a condom or not. If a condom was used, latex allergy would be the culprit, and if not, it would be the seminal allergy.

Bestiality and Allergy to Animal Sperm

In an extremely unusual case, allergy to dog sperm has been reported. In October 1971, a 42-year-old divorced woman, who had four children and who was pregnant for the fifth time by her boyfriend, reported dizziness and syncope. Her attending physician found her to be hypotensive. She admitted to having had sexual contact with her German Shepherd dog 20 min before her arrival. A scratch test with dog sperm was found to be positive.

Peanut Allergy

Peanut allergy is a known phenomenon, and has invited several successful litigations against doctors. The allergy is due to proteins found in peanuts. These proteins are not destroyed by cooking, so fresh, cooked, and roasted peanuts can cause an allergic reaction. About 1% of all people could be allergic to peanuts.

It is the doctor's duty to inform the parents of children with serious food allergies that their condition is potentially life-threatening. They should also be taught how to use epinephrine (adrenaline) in cases of emergency. On January 24, 2002, a jury ordered two US Middlesex County physicians to pay $10 million to a 13-year-old boy Ray Varghese, who had suffered brain damage after eating peanut candy on Christmas day 1996, because they had failed to inform his parents of the severity of his allergy to peanuts. The parents of Ray Varghese successfully alleged in court that they were not prescribed an EpiPen (epinephrine) that could have prevented their son's brain damage.

Allergy and Sudden Infant Death Syndrome (SIDS)

A M Barrett, a pathologist at the University of Cambridge, UK, was the first to suggest, in 1954, that the cause of enigmatic SIDS could be hypersensitivity to milk. Six years later he, together with two of his colleagues, W E Parish and R R A Coombs (of Gell and Coombs classification fame), conducted a few ingenious experiments to show that milk allergy could indeed be the cause of SIDS. They showed that instillation of a very small amount of milk – too little to cause choking (say, about 0.25 ml) – over the glottis into the larynx of unsensitized conscious guinea pigs was without clinical effect. However, the same procedure repeated over guinea pigs sensitized to milk could result in characteristic anaphylactic reaction, often leading to death. The postmortem findings in such animals did not resemble those found in typical cot-death cases.

If, however, the guinea pigs were lightly anesthetized – an experimental condition used to simulate the condition of the sleeping child – milk introduced into the larynx had quite a different effect. In the unsensitized animal there was no effect, as before. In the sensitized animal, on the other hand, there was a complete lack of the anaphylactic reaction that was seen in the conscious animals. The animal stopped breathing after some time without any sign of struggle. Death sometimes occurred immediately, but the majority died within an hour. The pathological findings in these animals resembled those found in SIDS.

This definitely seemed to indicate that allergy to milk could be a causative factor in SIDS. Later, in November 1960, Parish, Barrett, and Coombs along with two more colleagues, Gunther and Francis E Camps, published a paper outlining their experiments to provide more experimental evidence in favor of their theory. They examined sera from actual cases of cot deaths for their level of milk antibodies. Instead of using milk, they used recovered stomach contents from actual cases of SIDS and used it for instillation in guinea pigs. They conducted experiments to see if individual milk proteins casein, α-lactalbumin, and β-lactoglobulin could produce a lethal effect. And finally, they compared the pathological findings in guinea pigs killed in this way with those found in human cot death.

They found that anesthetized guinea pigs sensitized to cow's milk died rapidly and without struggling when a small quantity (about 0.25 ml) of either cow's milk or stomach contents recovered from cases of SIDS was instilled over their larynx. A 1% solution of casein or a 1% solution of β-lactoglobulin introduced in the same way also produced death. The histopathological changes in the lungs of experimental animals resembled those found in cases of cot deaths. This seemed to prove quite conclusively that milk allergy was indeed the cause of SIDS.

Many workers in later years seemed to corroborate the allergy theory, but suggested different causative allergens. Some workers found increased levels of serum IgE antibodies to dust mite and *Aspergillus*, suggesting that these could be the possible offending allergens. Elevated serum tryptase levels were also found in many cases of SIDS, which seemed to indicate mast cell degranulation just before death, which in turn seemed to corroborate the allergy theory.

But several other workers produced evidence that allergy may not be the causative mechanism in SIDS at all. Elevated serum tryptase levels were explained by stating that it could be caused by a hypoxic stimulus due to the prone position of the child, or it could be due to terminal respiratory failure which would occur in all cases of death. It was suggested that elevated tryptase levels could also be due to passive diffusion from the lung after death, and could just be a postmortem artifact.

The allergy and SIDS controversy is still ongoing, and unresolved, with workers producing evidence for and against the allergy theory at regular intervals.

Exercise and Allergy

Allergy to exercise is a known condition, and may invite medicolegal considerations, especially in army personnel, sports coaches, and trainers, and other persons involved in strenuous work. Exercise in susceptible people causes massive release of histamine in the body. Sometimes only exercise is needed, while at other times the person has to eat something before exercise. Occasionally the person has to eat a particular food before exercise to trigger the allergy.

Allergy to exercise can take very bizarre forms. A German group has recently reported a man who got this allergy every Friday while gardening, but not while gardening on other days. This was because he treated himself to a slice of poppyseed cake every Friday before his garden work. Allergy to poppy seeds was proved with tests, but it needed the extra trigger of exercise to accentuate the allergic manifestations.

Postmortem Examination in Allergic Deaths

Quite frequently, a forensic pathologist is faced with an anaphylactic death. Undoubtedly this is one of the most difficult situations to handle; an inexperienced pathologist can easily ruin the autopsy if he/she does not take some basic precautions.

Precautions

It is important to remember in such cases that the autopsy should be conducted as soon as possible after death, because the findings, especially those in the larynx, may recede rapidly after death. Medicolegal formalities may tend to take time, but the earlier they are completed, the better it is for the pathologist. If the body has to be embalmed, the neck organs should be removed before. A detailed history is very helpful, since it would determine proper sampling procedures. Most common allergic deaths encountered are deaths due to drug anaphylaxis (e.g., penicillin), anaphylactoid reactions (e.g., radiocontrast media), exposure to certain plants, and stings due to bees, wasps, and fire ants.

It is useful to take a chest X-ray before starting an autopsy. In fact, the clinician would do well to take it immediately after pronouncing death in such cases; a delay can often cause remission of findings. Pulmonary edema and congestion in chest X-rays may indicate a possible anaphylactic reaction.

External Examination

On external examination, one must search for injection sites or sting marks. Time spent on this simple procedure is well worth it, and may save a lot of embarrassment to the pathologist later. Concentrate on areas like the cubital fossa, front of forearms, back of the hand, both gluteal regions, and areas which are swollen. These are the areas where an injection is likely to be given. Stings are more likely to be on the face and neck, although they can be on any exposed part. Such lesions on covered areas generally rule out insect stings, and indicate injections. If such lesions are found, they must be photographed and excised with a minimum 5 cm margin. The excised tissue should immediately be frozen at $-70\,°C$, and submitted for antigen–antibody reactions. Observe for foam around the mouth and nostrils.

Internal Examination

Neck organs must be removed and a photograph of the rima of glottis taken from above, together with the epiglottis. This photographic record may prove very valuable in a court of law. This would also be useful in cases where a second autopsy may be ordered, which is not entirely unusual, given the raised suspicion levels of distressed relatives regarding medical negligence in such cases. Finally these photographs may be useful given the fact that laryngeal edema may subside very rapidly. By the time the pathologist has returned to the neck organs after dissecting the rest of the organs, he/she may find that laryngeal edema has subsided considerably. For histologic study, larynx and epiglottis must be fixed in Zenker's or Bouin's solution.

A detailed examination of the tracheobronchial tree and lungs may prove very rewarding. It is not unusual to find foamy edema in the trachea and bronchi. Lungs may show pulmonary edema and congestion. There may be diffuse or focal pulmonary distension alternating with collapse. A microscopic examination may reveal eosinophilic leukocytes. Just as in the case of trachea and larynx, it is useful to take photographs of the lungs for similar reasons. Weights of lungs must also be recorded; grossly overweight lungs point to pulmonary edema. Lungs should not be perfused with fixative as it may cause artificial distension.

A microscopic examination of the spleen may show eosinophilic leukocytes in red pulp.

Special Investigations

A sample of blood must be submitted for drug levels (or sting antigens) alleged to have been injected. Samples must also be frozen and submitted for IgE against the suspected drug/antigen.

See Also

Autopsy: Procedures and Standards; **Autopsy, Findings:** Sudden Infant Death Syndrome; **Drug-Induced Injury, Accidental and Iatrogenic; Drugs, Prescribed:** Product Liability; Testamentary Capacity; **Sudden Infant Death Syndrome, Etiology and Epidemiology**

Further Reading

Aggrawal A (1993) Allergies. In: Aggrawal A (ed.) *Some Common Ailments*, pp. 1–8. India: National Book Trust.

Buckley MG, Variend S, Walls AF (2001) Elevated serum concentrations of β-tryptase, but not α-tryptase, in sudden infant death syndrome (SIDS). An investigation of anaphylactic mechanisms. *Clinical and Experimental Allergy* 31: 1696–1704.

Galiher GO, DeRobertis LR (1999) The legal aspects of the latex protein allergy epidemic. *Hawaii Medical Journal* 58: 160, 167.

Gibofsky A (1996) Legal issues in allergy and clinical immunology. *Journal of Allergy and Clinical Immunology* 98: S334–S338.

Giroux-Slavas J (1999) Latex allergy: a potential liability issue. *Pennsylvania Dental Journal (Harrisburg)* 66: 14–17.

Guidelines for the Diagnosis and Management of Asthma (1991) *National Asthma Education Program Expert Panel Report.* Publication NIH 91-3042. Bethesda, MD: Department of Health and Human Services.

Holden TE, Sherline DM (1973) Bestiality, with sensitization and anaphylactic reaction. *Obstetric Gynecology* 42: 138–140.

Hunskaar S, Fosse RT (1993) Allergy to laboratory mice and rats: a review of its prevention, management and treatment. *Laboratory Animals* 27: 206–221.

Kohn P (1999) The legal implications of latex allergy. *Registered Nurse* 62: 63–65. Erratum in *Registered Nurse* 1999; 62: 9.

Parish WE, Barrett AM, Coombs RRA, Gunther M, Camps FE (1960) Hypersensitivity to milk and sudden death in infancy. *Lancet* ii: 1106–1110.

Rice B (2002) A $10 million allergy case. Could it happen to you? *Medical Economics* 79: 36–38.

Rubsamen DS (1993) The doctor, the asthmatic patient, and the law. *Annals of Allergy* 71: 493–494.

Schappi GF, Konrad V, Imhof D, Etter R, Wuthrich B (2001) Hidden peanut allergens detected in various foods: findings and legal measures. *Allergy* 56: 1216–1220.

Wakelin SH, White IR (1999) Natural rubber latex allergy. *Clinical and Experimental Dermatology* 24: 245–248.

Zemenick RB (1994) Medicolegal implications of pulmonary function testing. *Annals of Allergy* 73: 275–276.

ANIMAL ATTACKS AND INJURIES

Contents

Fatal and Nonfatal

A W Fegan-Earl, Forensic Pathology Services, London, UK

Introduction

Since the evolution of humans, there has been interaction between human beings and animals for a whole host of different reasons, either through human control and mastery of animals, such as the keeping of food animals and agriculture and companion animals, or more simply, with human beings as part of the food chain as an example of prey for an animal.

As a result of the diversity of animals within different continents and countries, detailed local knowledge of the fauna may assist in the interpretation of injuries that are perceived to have been caused by animals. However, as the world grows smaller and nonindigenous animals are kept, this geographical specificity ever diminishes. This also applies to increasing tourism.

As in all ecosystems, there exist complex relationships between all animals, including humans, although to some extent we have removed ourselves from some of these natural interactions.

When an individual dies without immediate intervention from authorities, such as in an isolated dwelling or a remote region, he/she simply becomes part of the ecological cycles relevant to that region. In this context companion animals dependent upon their keeper for care and food may simply view the body now as a source of nutrition, leading to postmortem depredation. Such depredation may present a series of bizarre changes to law authorities that may be perceived as suspicious or even thought of as homicide.

Knowledge of the local ecology, of which the fauna is but one part, may assist in the interpretation of a crime scene. Hence the natural processes of decomposition with the well-documented entomological successions that visit a corpse may be of great value in estimation of the time of death. Similarly, the finding of a specific animal species, or marks left by such a species, may aid in consideration of the locus of a crime or of sites of body storage.

Injuries caused by animals may be virtually pathognomic of that animal or nonspecific, and it is here that local knowledge of the fauna may be of value. A limited survey of some of the injuries will now be undertaken, passing through various orders of animals.

Mammals

Mammals include some of the largest carnivores on the planet, including the felids (cats) and canids (dogs), together with bears. Such animals are well equipped to prey on a range of animals, including human beings, with powerful jaws and claws and shearing teeth. The sheer size and speed of many of these animals are relevant to the rapid overpowering of an individual. The victim of such an attack will have invariably suffered multiple and severe injuries as a result, and it may be that identification of the deceased presents a problem owing to the extent of the injuries and the secondary depredation that may occur. Indeed, the level of secondary scavenging may make the task of identifying original injuries difficult, if not impossible, in areas that are well populated by such animals. Injuries observed will represent a mixture of laceration from claws, and the parallel nature of such injuries may give an assessment of the size of animal involved, together with bite marks. Such marks, if in isolation, may present a clean appearance suitable for appropriate photography and odontological interpretation. Distances between certain teeth may assist in the assessment of animal size. Defense injuries may be seen upon the body, but overpowering by large animals may preclude identification of such changes. Certain animals such as bears may show a predilection for the face. Underlying tissues and organs will be crushed and lacerated, and possibly absent either from direct ingestion by the animal or secondary scavenging.

It is of course not only the carnivores from higher animal orders that present a danger to humans. The large herbivores present a risk, either from accidental injuries as a result of size, or from defense of territory or their young. Within agriculture, many of the beasts of burden present such a size that if an individual becomes interposed between the animal and another firm surface, crushing may become a distinct possibility. Death may then result from traumatic asphyxia, or from multiple crushing injuries to the chest, abdomen, and head. Usually the history and setting should readily explain the situation. Aggressive behavior from bovines may result in goring by the horns, with major internal injury and hemorrhage. Similarly, trampling from stampede may cause multiple blunt injuries, with occasional recognizable patterns. Specifically, horseshoes may leave a patterned mark upon the body, following kicks or stampedes from equids. In more tropical climes, animals such as the hippopotamus, rhinoceros, and elephant are well known for the danger that they present to human life, causing more fatalities than more expected animals such as predatory carnivores.

Odontological assessment may assist in defining the species of animal. Furthermore, recovery of hairs from the body may allow comparison with animal hair collections.

Most fatal animal attacks are caused by large animals where the size and power of that animal simply overpower the individual. However, as in many aspects of forensic medicine, the young, old, or infirm may be particularly at risk from attacks from smaller animals that in other circumstances would be relatively innocuous. In addition, lack of experience in handling an animal may result in provocation of that animal and resultant aggressive and dangerous behavior. The author has seen an example of a baby killed by three ferrets that had escaped their cage: death occurred through shock and blood loss as a result of multiple bites.

Dog attacks may be encountered now that ownership is so widespread. Studies have shown that the majority of attacks occur on the owner's property, with a quarter caused by dogs on the loose. There are many complex factors that relate to dog attack; particularly relevant is their pack animal hierarchy, with animals sometimes testing the victims of attack in terms of dominance. Individual animals may be responding to cruel treatment or as a response to pain. They may be unfamiliar with a victim and see him/her as a threat. Children are most at risk from dog attack, with those aged between 1 and 4 years sustaining the most serious injuries. Dog breed is relevant, with Pit Bull Terriers, German Shepherds, and Rottweilers most commonly associated with attacks, both fatal and nonfatal. These are inherently aggressive and powerful dogs so perhaps these findings are not surprising. Such attacks may result in multiple and severe bites, with powerful jaws capable of severely lacerating tissues and injuring underlying muscle and even bone. Peripheries may be at risk, as when an individual attempts to defend him/herself. The author has recently seen a case where a dog attacked an individual who was suffering a seizure. In this attack the larynx was severely crushed, with compromise of the airways.

Attacks from packs may result in considerable mutilation of the body. In the peri- and postmortem period, a dog may cause injuries. Dogs may paw at their owners if in a collapsed state, leaving parallel abrasions and lacerations. Once dead, depredation may occur, especially if the animal is locked within the dwelling. This is a simple reaction for the search for food. It has been recorded that animals have absorbed drugs from the bodies of their owners following such depredation. The extent of such depredation may be extensive, with exposed parts of the body reduced to skeleton in a short time. Injuries may be difficult to distinguish from true marks of violence, and in this case examination of the dog for tissue around the mouth or even the stomach contents may be of value. A further case is quoted whereby two individuals were noted to be engaged in a severe altercation: one of the pair was found dead a short time later. The ears were missing and parallel lacerations were found, causing obvious concern to the police. The deceased had died of a coronary thrombosis, and collapsed. In the perimortem period his five dogs had become excited and frightened, leading to this perimortem attack.

In the living, bite marks may be examined and considered by a dental specialist to consider the size of the dog that caused the injury. The prominent canid canine teeth produce characteristic bite marks. Extensive surgery may be required following an attack and the chance of infection, both local and systemic, from the bacterial flora of the dog's mouth, should not be overlooked.

Birds

The majority of birds will not present a risk to humans. Their usual interaction will be through depredation of the dead (or nearly dead) body. One possible exception is the large flightless birds, such as the emu, rhea, ostrich, and cassowary. As a result of their flightless condition they have powerful muscular legs, equipping them for rapid transit over the ground. Attacks have been recorded where severe penetrating lacerations have been sustained by individuals when the bird was approached, leading to torrential hemorrhage and disemboweling.

Reptiles and Amphibians

One of the first animals to come to mind will be the crocodilians. Noted for their hunting skills, the larger species such as the Nile crocodile, *Crocodylus niloticus,* give rise to fatalities. Their habit of sudden explosive ejection from the water to grasp the prey, followed by rolling underwater, is a devastatingly successful method of attack. Few animals are so readily able to disarticulate a limb, demonstrating the animal's power. Death is usually due to drowning. The teeth marks may give a clue as to the nature of the attacking animal, as the arcade of puncture wounds may be highlighted by the position of the fourth premaxillary tooth, that may be seen in the animal with the jaws opposed. Frequently bodies may be decomposed and significantly scavenged as a result of the crocodilian habit of storing corpses underwater to allow softening and easier removal of tissues.

The Komodo dragon may give rise to fatalities. Its mouth flora is populated by pathogenic bacteria that give rise to septicemia. In its small natural environment, such a mechanism guarantees food in spite of the animal's relative lack of agility. If threatened, the Gila monster may inject venom that is capable of causing death through severe cardiac compromise.

Of course, snakes are a group that gives rise to many injuries or deaths. Venomous snakes may cause death following envenomation either by neurotoxic or hematotoxic methods. The former may rapidly cause death as a result of respiratory paralysis. Hematotoxins cause progressive hemorrhage and disseminated intravascular coagulation and run a more protracted course. Neurotoxic snakes often leave inconspicuous bites whereas hematotoxic snakes leave bites that swell and bleed. Identification is paramount and local casualty departments often have an identification guide to facilitate administration of the correct antivenom. Laboratory tests may also be employed.

Constricting snakes may cause death from crush asphyxia. Frail and small individuals are more at risk, especially babies and small children. Fatal snake attacks are now encountered more frequently in nonindigenous areas due to the keeping of exotic species.

The highly colored arrow frogs from the Amazon are well known for their secretion of toxins upon the skin. Although used by native Indians on their arrows to kill small monkeys, fatalities do not usually occur in humans.

Fish

Death may occur as a result of interaction with fish and other marine life. The most obvious example is the shark: a large number of species are capable of attacking and causing significant injuries to human beings. Limbs may be grasped first, leaving curved bite marks representing the dental arcade of the animal. The power of the animal is reflected in the incision through different layers of tissues, including bone, in a similar way to crocodilians. Victims may be considerably disrupted following feeding of the sharks. Brushing of the rough shark skin against the individual may give rise to multiple dermal abrasions.

The piranha is always considered to be capable of stripping a body of flesh within minutes, although this has never been substantiated. Nonetheless, these fish have extremely powerful jaws and can produce multiple bites of about 3 cm diameter.

Some fish are capable of producing an electric shock, such as the electric eel, the electric catfish, and the electric ray. The charge is rarely of sufficient strength to kill.

A variety of fish are capable of envenomation by means of defensive spine, but these rarely cause death; rather there is more pain at the site of the sting.

Lower Marine Creatures

Many smaller creatures are capable of inflicting significant stings that on rare occasions cause death. The jellyfish can cause widespread stings, particularly the larger species with long tentacles, such as the Portuguese man o' war. They give rise to acutely painful erythematous and edematous lesions in the shape of the touching tentacle.

Cone shells use a very sharp poisonous barb to hunt, and may cause injury if accidentally stepped on, leaving a single penetrating injury at the site of injury.

Arthropods

This vast and diverse group includes insects, spiders, and scorpions, and centipedes, all of which have members dangerous to humans. In terms of injuries, often a small and inconspicuous sting injury is present, accompanied by varying degrees of edema and erythema.

Wasp and bee stings are common. They may prove fatal when large numbers of stings are sustained, such as in swarm situations. Individual stings may prove fatal when the subject is allergic, and develops fatal anaphylaxis.

Flies, particularly blowflies, may be of value in entomological consideration of a body or scene. Some researchers have investigated the uptake of drugs from a dead body upon which they are feeding for a qualitative assessment – this is called forensic entomotoxicology.

Ants, particularly in tropical climes, may sting causing painful but local reactions. They may be a common visitor to the corpse, and can produce curious serpiginous lesions that may be mistaken for marks of violence. Marks at the limits of clothing, e.g., at the collar, may cause artifact such as apparent ligature marks.

Spiders and scorpions are generally less dangerous than is popularly believed. Nevertheless, several powerful toxins are produced by species such as *Latrodectus*, the black widow, to name but one. With spiders a paired set of puncture wounds may be seen, corresponding to the fangs.

Summary

This has been a brief summary of the injuries, fatal, and nonfatal, that may be encountered following human interaction with animals. As in all aspects of forensic medicine, the history and setting are of vital importance, but as stated, with a smaller world and increased travel, pathologists may see exotic lesions not encountered before. It is worth noting the interaction of animals with the dead body, and the artifacts that can be produced.

See Also

Animal Attacks and Injuries: Predation; **Entomology**; **Odontology:** Bite Mark Analysis; **Venom**; **Veterinary Aspects of Forensic Medicine, Wild Animals**

Predation

R Rabinovich, The Hebrew University of Jerusalem, Jerusalem, Israel
T Kahana, Division of Identification and Forensic Science, Israel National Police, Israel

Introduction

Lethal injuries sustained from animal attacks are uncommon in most medicolegal practices; their frequency and nature vary among geographical regions of the world. Antemortem animal injuries can be the direct or indirect cause of death, especially in cases where the victim is very young or incapacitated by disease.

Taphonomic changes induced by animal activity are however very common; most forensic practitioners have encountered them in their daily practice. Bodies that have been left undisturbed for various lengths of time usually present some degree of animal disturbance; the assessment of the ante- and perimortem injuries in these cases can pose some difficulty.

Combination of perimortem and postmortem injuries is frequently encountered, especially where the fauna is abundant, i.e., rural areas. Moreover, as animals are driven out of their natural habitats more attacks are observed. Still, numerous attacks occur in known animal–human settings like zoos, circuses, and the private domain (house, garden, etc.).

The circumstances surrounding the incident are a necessary tool for treatment planning and future prevention of similar cases. When only "dry bones" survive, the identification of the manner and cause of death can only be achieved by taphonomical methods. Under such conditions the circumstances of death might be obliterated by postmortem processes; animal activity on cadavers plays a major destructive role due to animals' tendency to dismember the body as well as damage the tissues. Moreover, natural conditions such as water, vegetation, and sun exposure influence the final condition of the body.

A further phenomenon to be considered when conducting forensic examinations is the prevalence of zoonotic diseases that are transferred through contact between humans and animals. The prevalence of infectious diseases has increased considerably in the wake of animal domestication; increasing population morbidity is associated with sedentism and population density concomitant with agriculture and urban life.

Zooarcheologists, forensic pathologists, and anthropologists have developed differential diagnostic criteria to identify diverse predators and their remarkable patterned injuries on bones.

The pathognomonic and taphonomic findings associated with animal attacks can be described according to the taxonomic classification of the injuring agent.

Insects and Arachnids

Ticks are blood-feeding external parasites of mammals, birds, and reptiles throughout the world. Ticks can cause paralyses, toxicoses, and allergic reactions and are vectors of a broad range of viral, rickettsial, bacterial, and protozoan pathogens. There are hard ticks – Ixodidae – and soft ticks – Argasidae.

Approximately 12 argasid species (*Argas* and *Ornithodos*) are frequently found attached to humans who enter tick-infested caves and burrows. Hard ticks have three distinct life stages: larva, nymph, and adult; the completion time of the entire life cycle may vary from less than a year in tropical regions to over 3 years in cold climates, where certain stages may enter diapause of several years until hosts are again available.

Death caused by insects' stings is seldom due to envenomation but rather to some form of anaphylactic shock. Bees and wasps are the most commonly involved insects in these types of death. Most stings are evinced as a small red lesion surrounded by a pale rim and a pink flare. Occasionally, multiple and very closely grouped stings are the result of an attack of swarms of wasps or bees accidentally or intentionally disturbed.

During postmortem examination, insects may be observed within the clothing of the victim and the bee sting may be found embedded in the injury itself. Postmortem findings may include pathognomonic signs of hepatic and renal failure and rhabdomyolysis.

There are very few taphonomic changes associated with these insects although, since they are parasitic on the maggots of other insect species that colonize bodies and in a few instances on the decomposing body itself, they tend to affect the entomologic assessment of the postmortem interval.

Scorpions and spiders are responsible for very few deaths, although they are invariably poisonous. The general rule is that the danger of any given venom is inversely proportional to the weight of the victim; thus it follows that lethality is most commonly associated with children. The examination of the body discloses a relatively unremarkable local lesion, sometimes a closely spaced double injury, erythema, local pallor, and ulceration, depending on the species involved and on the survival period. Autopsy findings are nonspecific and include pulmonary and brain edema, local necrosis, disseminated intravascular coagulopathy, and myocardial damage.

Anthropophagic activity of various insects – such as ants, cockroaches, and beetles – can sometimes simulate antemortem trauma; these are mostly superficial skin defects, arranged in linear or circular formations (**Figure 1**).

In all cases of suspected insect and arthropod attack an enzyme-linked immunosorbent assay (ELISA) test should be used for the identification of the specific immunoglobulin E, complemented by serum assay for tryptase. Recent investigation on the postmortem detection of anaphylaxis suggests that the assay of serum tryptase by itself should not be relied upon, especially in the latter postmortem stages.

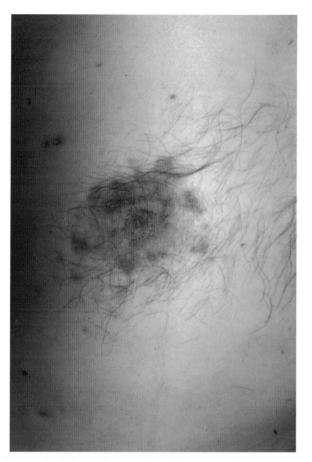

Figure 1 Anthropophagic activity of insects causing superficial skin defects, arranged in linear or circular formations.

Marine Animals

Death by marine animals is mostly associated with attacks of large fish – such as sharks, barracudas, and moray eels – and with poisoning by venomous fish and to a lesser extent by soft-bodied animals like hydroids. While attacks of marine fauna can cause intense pain from envenomation, death is unlikely to occur from the sting itself unless the victim is allergic to the venom; however, the intense symptoms caused by the envenomation may lead to drowning due to collapse.

Death due to direct trauma from schools of small fish such as the South American piranha fall mostly in the realm of folklore; similarly, some species of eel that produce an electric jolt of up to 500 V are unlikely to cause death. Nevertheless, these types of attack can render the victim at risk of death by drowning.

The postmortem changes associated with the anthropophagous behavior of small fish are notorious; these creatures feed on easily accessible soft tissue such as eyes, lips, and digits (**Figure 2**) and have been known to gnaw on bone. The telltale marks of their teeth can be seen on the margins of the wound as a row of connected small semicircles, the size of the fish's teeth. Similarly, small crustaceans that adhere to most surfaces slowly destroy the cortical surface of the bone.

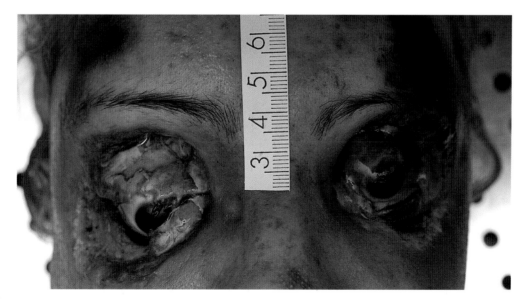

Figure 2 Postmortem changes associated with small fish that feed on soft tissue like eyes, lips, and fingers and gnaw the bone.

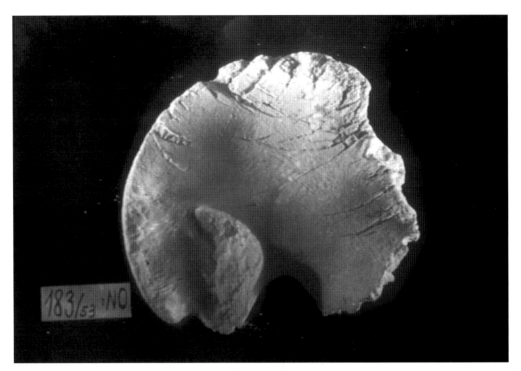

Figure 3 Telltale marks of shark teeth on a human os coxa. Note the distance between the scratches on the bone that fit the shape of the shark teeth.

The majority of marine fauna lethal attacks are associated with sharks: there are about 50 reported attacks annually, of which approximately 7% are lethal. Sharks attack in both shallow and deeper water. The types of injury are related to the type of attack and to the size and species of the shark. While feeding, their serrated sharp teeth that are set in consecutive rows leave pathognomonic signs, i.e., gouges, deep cuts, and avulsion of soft tissue. Being unable to chew their prey they strip it, thus they tend to attack the extremities from the thigh down (**Figure 3**). When bumped into at a high speed, shark's skin causes long deep regular abrasions in the victim's skin and its underlying tissue.

Rodents

Deadly attacks by rodents are extremely rare; they are usually associated with small children of low socio-economic background or debilitated persons. In these cases death, commonly caused by large species of rats, is due to blood loss resulting from multiple rat bites; subcutaneous bleeding around the wounds is the main indication that the injuries were inflicted while the victim was still alive. Autopsy findings often reveal signs of hypovolemic shock.

Postmortem scavenging is common among wild and domestic rodents; they are well known to alter or destroy the indicators of the cause of death and preclude the visual identification of the victim. Rodents tend to gnaw on bone, to wear down on their incisors, leaving telltale sets of parallel striations on the osseous cortex. Postmortem rodent-caused injuries are usually wedged, paired, clean, small incisions without subcutaneous bleeding (**Figure 4**).

Porcupines are known to collect and modify both dry and meaty bones. They leave a typical pattern of gnawed trails, thinning the bones in a fan-shaped pattern and creating "windows" in the shaft produced by heavy gnawing and scooping out material (**Figure 5**).

Birds

Serious injuries from birds resulting in death are very rare. The forensic literature mostly records postmortem stablike or puncture wounds caused by the hard bills of crows, owls, buzzards, or seagulls. Scavenging is a common feeding behavior of various species of birds, and remains are often completely defleshed in a matter of hours by these efficient foragers. Damage to bone occurs from the stripping

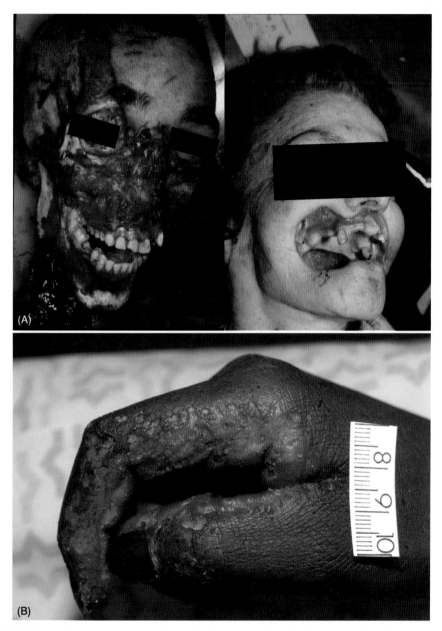

Figure 4   (A, B) Postmortem injuries made by rodents – paired incisions without subcutaneous bleeding.

and tearing action of the beaks and talons and small punctures and scratches on bone cortical surfaces are left.

Finally, there have been instances where small birds have utilized the thoracic cavity of a skeletonized individual for nesting.

Small Carnivores

"Man's best friend" – the domestic dog – accounts for the majority of deaths caused by animal attacks. Attacks occur most often in the household domain,

frequently against children and old adults. The majority of the lesions occur on the head, neck, and face, although they can be seen on the upper and lower extremities as well. The wounds are characterized by pairing of injuries resulting from the canine teeth, along linear parallel abrasions. Dogs can sometimes inflict blunt-force trauma by lifting their heads rapidly when excited, striking the victim in the throat area. Pets can sometimes paw their dead owners in an attempt to rouse them, inflicting groups of parallel abrasions that can be confused with injuries associated with assault.

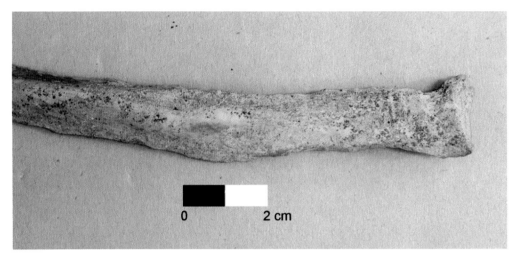

Figure 5   Bones with typical fan-shaped gnaw pattern consistent with porcupine behavior.

Canids leave typical postmortem damage patterns over the bones, characterized by rounded punctures, peglike penetrating injuries, and shallow scratches. Severe damage caused by gnawing of the softer bony parts (proximal epiphyses) is frequently detected.

Pack attacks by feral or wild dogs and wolves pose a greater danger of fatal injuries, similar to those produced by single animal attacks but often covering a larger area of the body. Not many reports have been related to deadly attacks of wolves on human; they are more often associated with attacks on flock animals. Overpopulation of foxes near or even in settled areas must be considered as dangerous. The scavenging behavior of packs of foxes can produce postmortem artifacts that can be easily misinterpreted as perimortem injuries.

Large Carnivores

Wild game attacks on humans occur mainly in rural areas, natural parks, zoos, and circuses. Large cats such as lions and tigers have been known to assault humans, although humans do not constitute their natural prey. The primary injuries sustained from these attacks are a series of parallel abrasions, multiple deep bite injuries, and lacerations with an abraded rim, consistent with the tapered claws of the animal. Punctured wounds similar in shape to those inflicted by smaller carnivores are often observed in the neck area of the victim. Shaking the victim by the neck is not uncommon, resulting in hypertension injuries. Furthermore, feeding on carcasses results in eventration, loss of tissue, and extensive bone injury.

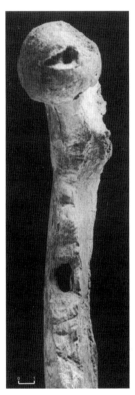

Figure 6   Human modified bones from a Chalcolithic mortuary site at Kissufim Road, Israel. Carnivore modification on a right femur diaphysis, medial view. Reproduced from Le Mort F, Rabinovich R (2002) The taphonomic and mortuary practices. In: Goren Y, Fabian P (eds.) *Kissufim Road: A Chalcolithic Mortuary Site Antiquities Authority*, pp. 66–81. IAA reports monograph series no. 4. Jerusalem, Israel.

Attacks by hyena are uncommon, though they have been reported from Ethiopian villagers. Hyenas are known to plunder graves, dispersing the remains and leaving a puzzling scene for the unsuspecting investigator (**Figure 6**). Many carnivores crack bones with their teeth – the propensity of hyenids to feed on large diameter bones is legendary. Both species, spotted hyena (*Crocuta crocuta*) and striped hyena (*Hyaena hyaena*), tend to take chunks of their prey to their den, breaking and damaging the bones. Unique morphological features of hyena teeth and skull are associated with bone cracking. In addition to the morphological adaptations to lifting and carrying large and heavy loads, their ability to remove and destroy carcasses is noteworthy; scratches, furrows, puncture marks, and gnawed areas are typical of bone damage by hyena (**Figures 7** and **8**).

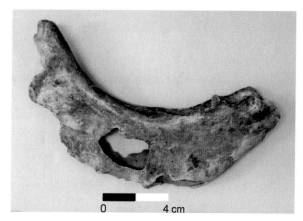

Figure 7 Hyena gnawing marks on a camel mandible. Note the amount of severe gnawing and of missing bone.

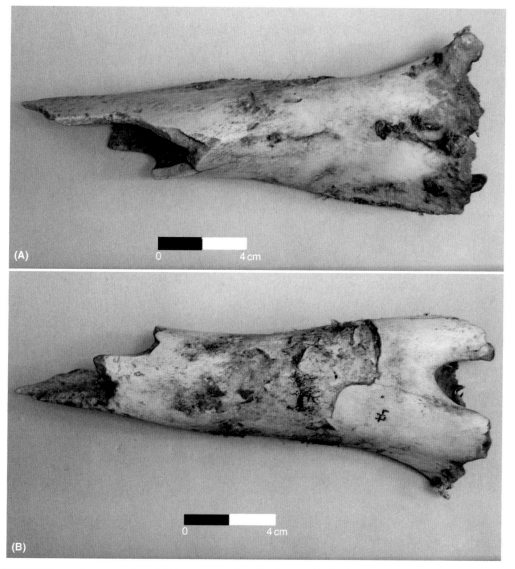

Figure 8 Typical gnaw marks on a donkey right humerus produced by hyenas. Notice (A) the missing epiphyses and (B) the typical pit and scratch marks.

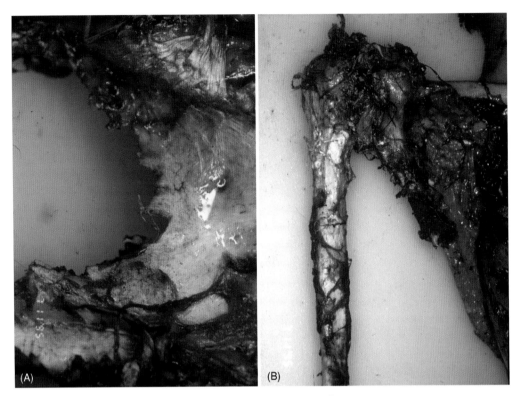

Figure 9 Taphonomic changes on cadaveric remains produced by wild pig feeding.

Human–bear conflict resulting in attacks has become less rare as bear populations have increased. Bears tend to bite, puncture soft tissues (i.e., abdomen), scratch the neck, thighs, and hips, and leave tracks at the crime scene. Cases of injuries or lethal attacks are known to be caused by the grizzly bear (*Ursus arctos horribilus*), black bear (*U. americanus*), and brown bear (*U. arctos*).

Large Herbivores

Farm animals such as cows, bulls, and horses tend to produce blunt-force and crushing injuries. The majority are nonspecific injuries produced by the weight of the animal pressing the victim against a wall or a fence. Notwithstanding, specific injuries often produced by kicking and trampling are consistent with the shape of the hoofs, while bull-goring wounds vary between clean lacerations produced by the tip of the horns to large irregular penetrating injuries.

Crushing and trampling are common features caused by the largest herbivores, i.e., elephants, rhinoceros, and hippopotamus. Their attacks are a known cause of death in rural Africa as well as of handlers in zoos. The injuries encountered at autopsy may include piercing by tusks and crushing injuries as

the result of being trapped in a confined space by the bulk of the animal.

There are no reports of postmortem injuries produced by farm herbivores, although omnivores like domestic pigs have been known to feed on cadavers (**Figure 9**).

Reptiles

Snake attacks are not very common; most bites are what experts call "dry bites," in which no venom is released. A majority of those bitten are snake handlers or individuals who have snakes as pets. Though snake bites are rarely fatal, when left untreated they can result in severe tissue damage or loss of fingers, toes, or limbs. Typically, poisonous snake bites cause intense pain and swelling at the site of the injury. Tingling around the lips and tongue, abnormal bleeding, and muscle weakness may also occur. Traumatic asphyxia due to the tendency of some species of snake to squeeze the victim has been known to occur. Teeth marks can be seen on the victim in the form of small puncture marks.

Crocodiles and alligators are widespread all over the world. Most attacks are known from Australia, Tanzania, and Florida. People tend to be attacked near water, or while swimming, and quite often the victim is pulled into the water. The powerful jaws of these reptiles are known to cause severe injuries, tearing and dismembering body parts. Injuries may vary from minor lacerations and puncture wounds to major abdominal chest and limb trauma. Fatal victims are often found dismembered and decapitated.

Summary

At first glance, animal attacks would appear to be easily identified and the classification of the wounding agent a straightforward endeavor. In fact, a variety of animals can leave similar patterns of damage, and when other taphonomical processes are engaged, such as exposure to sun or water, the medicolegal investigation is further obscured.

The careful documentation of scat, hair, footprints, and claw marks can serve as auxiliary proxies for the exact identification of the animal responsible for the attack. The magnitude of the damage changes along the animal's guild, mainly by feeding behavior and size (i.e., carnivores versus herbivores, small or large), thus lion and fox are unlikely to leave similar damage patterns.

In theory the size of a wound serves as an indicative measure of the wounding animal, but it is not accurate enough to separate between animals of similar body and dental size. Thus, we can differentiate relatively easily the damage caused by a mouse and a wolf, but less so that caused by a tiger and a hyena. If severe damage to bones is involved, including cracked long bones, then we can safely assume that we are dealing with hyena postmortem activity.

The location of the damage along the body, its description, and the probability of a certain animal to be the cause of death should be taken into consideration while examining any case. Familiarity of the forensic practitioner with the local fauna and with the various aspects related to taphonomic changes of the cadaver is of paramount importance in the correct assessment of animal perimortem and postmortem attacks.

See Also

Animal Attacks and Injuries: Fatal and Nonfatal; Anthropology: Archeology, Excavation and Retrieval of Remains; Bone Pathology and Antemortem Trauma

Further Reading

Animal attack: www.igorilla.com/gorilla/animal/.

Baum J, Kahila Bar-Gal G (2003) The emergence and co-evolution of human pathogens. In: Greenblatt CL, Shpigelamn M (eds.) *Emerging Pathogen: Archaeology, Ecology and Evolution of Infectious Disease*, pp. 67–78. Oxford, UK: Oxford University Press.

Binford LR (1981) *Bones: Ancient Man and Modern Myths*. New York: Academic Press.

Brain CK (1981) *The Hunters or the Hunted? An Introduction to African Taphonomy*. Chicago, IL: University of Chicago Press.

Caldicott DGE, Mahajani R, Kuhn M (2001) The anatomy of a shark attack: a case report and review of the literature. *Injury, International Journal Care Injured* 32: 445–453.

Horn K, Halsey JF, Zumwalt E (2004) Utilization of serum tryptase and inmunoglobulin E assay in the postmortem diagnosis of anaphylaxis. *American Journal of Forensic Medicine and Pathology* 25: 37–43.

International Shark Attack File (ISAF) www.flmnh.ufl.edu/fish/Sharks.

Iscan MY, McCabe BQ (2000) Animal effects on human remains. In: Knupfer JC (ed.) *Anthropology, Encyclopedia of Forensic Sciences*, pp. 196–206. San Diego, CA: Academic Press.

Norwood S, McAuley C, Vallina Van L, *et al.* (2000) Mechanisms and patterns of injuries related to large animals. *Journal of Trauma: Injury, Infection and Critical Care* 48: 740–744.

Rothschild MA, Schneider V (1997) On the temporal onset of postmortem animal scavenging. "Motivation" of the animal. *Forensic Science International* 89: 57–64.

Tsokos M, Schulz F (1999) Indoor postmortem animal interference by carnivores and rodents: report of two cases and review of the literature. *International Journal of Legal Medicine* 112: 115–119.

ANTHROPOLOGY

Contents

Overview

T Kahana, Division of Identification and Forensic Science, Israel National Police, Israel

Introduction

Anthropology (*anthropos* – human, *logos* – science) is the study of the biological and cultural aspects of humans. The field encompasses a wide scope of specialized knowledge from social behavior, language, kinship, and religion to body build, ancestry, and evolution. There are two main divisions within the science of anthropology: cultural and physical anthropology.

Cultural anthropology is the subdivision of the field that deals with behavior and beliefs organized into an integrated system that is learned and shared by specific human groups. Traditionally, cultural anthropologists have studied the cultures of existing, nonliterate, less technologically complex societies, although the research techniques developed in studying these groups have been transferred to the study of all societies. Similarly, ethnologists study both the culture of living people and cultures no longer in existence but for which there are written records, while social anthropology is usually restricted to the analysis of social organization of modern societies. There is a great overlap in the various cultural and sociological aspects studied by anthropology; interdisciplinary investigations encompassing ethnological, sociological, economical, psychological, and religious aspects of society are very common, effectively blurring the limits between these fields.

Linguistics, the scientific study of languages, is another subdiscipline of cultural anthropology. Languages – being the main tool by which humans communicate, organize themselves, and transmit their culture from one generation to the next – are an essential key to the understanding of culture in its integrity.

Archeologists are concerned with the reconstruction of cultural history and daily life of ancient cultures. In a sense, archeology is the sociocultural anthropology of extinct civilizations. By means of highly developed technologies of excavation and observation of remains, the archeologist is able to reconstruct past cultures and to study their changes, movement, contacts, and influences on each other.

Physical anthropology is the branch of anthropology concerned with the study of the biological aspects of humans; the field encompasses two basic areas: human evolution and human variation. Further subdivision within physical anthropology includes: paleoanthropology, the study of human fossils; osteology, the study of bones; primatology, the study of nonhuman primates; paleopathology, the study of ancient disease; and forensic anthropology, the application of physical anthropology techniques in questions of law.

The understanding of the morphology of the skeleton and the techniques implemented to reconstruct life histories of humans has led to the development of forensic anthropology, i.e., the identification of human remains within the medicolegal domain.

The origins of forensic anthropology can be traced to the end of the nineteenth century when the French criminologist Alphonse Bertillon devised the first classification and identification system to identify criminals based on anthropometry. During the twentieth century the discipline became well established, with forensic anthropologists all over the world collaborating in almost all stages of forensic investigations associated to, but not solely with, personal identification of human remains.

Given the fact that bones and teeth survive much longer than soft tissue, many physical anthropologists specialize in the detailed study of skeletal and dental functional anatomy, physiology, and pathology, their expertise being of substantial value in forensic casework. In addition to providing clues as to the personal identity of a deceased, anthropologists assist in sorting human from nonhuman remains, diagnose skeletal trauma, and estimate the mechanism that produced the injuries. Comparing antemortem and postmortem radiographs, examining photographs of living individuals to determine the identity of the persons depicted and establishing the biological age of living individuals are some of the tasks of the anthropologist. Finally, this discipline has been essential in the investigation of mass graves and identification of victims of mass disasters.

Scope of the Field

The first query addressed by anthropologists when law enforcement agencies or members of the medicolegal community request their services is related to the nature of the remains. Many an embarrassment could have been avoided if the anthropologist was involved from the early stages of the investigation: for example the remains submitted for examination as human are nothing but polymer-resin models of bone, the refuse of a picnic, or just a hoax (**Figure 1**).

Once the remains have been established as human, it is important to determine their provenance. Usually skeletal material is considered of medicolegal

significance if the time of death can be estimated to be within the last 50–70 years, although this judgment is not always easy.

The state of preservation of the remains is one of the main aspects that distinguish the contemporary from the noncontemporary remains. Taphonomy, the study of postmortem processes which affect the condition of dead organisms, such as the effects of scavenging, natural dispersion, and the physicochemical influence of the environment on bones, has been extensively studied by forensic anthropologists. Examples of these would include interference by carnivores, both large and small, the effect of insect infestation, weather conditions, and other postmortem events, which alter the remains. Although highly dependent on environmental conditions, the principal indications of the state of preservation of osseous remains include the presence of soft tissue on them, their color, texture, amount of hydration, fragility, and mass.

The presence of body modifications is another important clue in the determination of the postmortem interval, certain common forms of modifications typical of ancient people, i.e., cradle-boarding, and alterations in the shape of the teeth that, when observed, easily exclude the remains from being of forensic interest. Conversely, the presence of remnants of medical interventions like dental restorations, prosthetic devices, and surgical reduction of fractures or discolorations related to antibiotic treatment is a clear indication of a modern provenance of the remains.

Personal belongings associated with the skeletal remains and the conditions of interment also provide excellent clues to their source. Bodies recovered from coffins, embalmed, or in association with grave

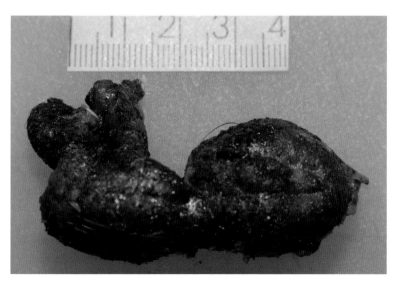

Figure 1 A rubber "fetus" found in a stairwell and submitted for anthropological examination as a suspected stillbirth or a case of infanticide.

goods, are usually of no forensic concern, while those found in shallow graves, covered by a blanket or within a plastic bag are unlikely to be archeological. Furthermore, the presence of hinges, small springs, and perforations in articulations indicate that the bones are an anatomical specimen (**Figure 2**).

Determining the minimal number of individuals present within the remains is of great importance not only in mass disaster situations, but also in common graves and criminal investigations, as well as in civil claims. The possibility of commingling should be considered whenever parts of a skeleton are collected from scattered areas, or when cremated remains are being studied. Anatomical examination and the discovery of duplicated parts can achieve separation of commingled remains into discrete individuals. These can be sorted according to age, sex, stature, general morphologic characteristics, ancestry, and the probability of articulation of the various segments.

Forensic anthropologists are often called upon to assist in the exhumation of human remains, either from clandestine shallow graves or from cemeteries. The exhumation process, which is carried out with techniques similar to those of an archeological

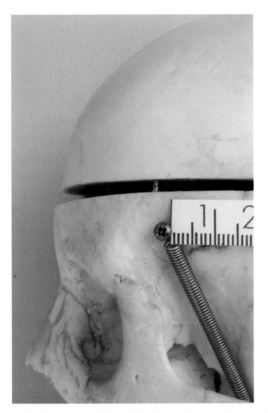

Figure 2 Human skull found in the cupboard of a recently deceased dental surgeon. The presence of springs, screws, and pins in the skull indicate that this is an anatomical specimen of no forensic interest.

excavation, is usually carried out in collaboration with forensic archeologists. The presence of the anthropologist at the excavation site is instrumental in determining the minimal number of individuals as well as distinguishing natural taphonomic processes such as fauna damage to the bones, discarding non-human remains, and recording all human elements present in the grave. Although most of the anthropological analysis of exhumed remains is carried out in the laboratory, proficiency in field techniques is vital to ensure meticulous removal of small and fragile items such as teeth, bullets, and personal effects, that are often critical in the identification of the deceased and determination of cause and manner of death.

The investigation of attempted genocide often includes locating and opening mass graves. This task is invariably undertaken by multidisciplinary teams including forensic pathologists, archeologists, and anthropologists who work in close collaboration to obtain accurate and unbiased information regarding the fate of the victims thus interred. Frequently, the permission to investigate mass graves is granted after a protracted period of time and the cadavers are partially or completely skeletonized. In these cases the skills of the forensic anthropologist, especially in osteology, are helpful in sorting through the commingled remains in a systematic manner, thus maximizing the preservation of evidence.

Anthropological Profile

Perhaps the most important step in the identification of unknown human remains is the creation of a biological profile of the individual studied. Describing the remains in such a way as to permit law enforcement and other investigating agencies to narrow the range of possible identities is crucial; it is here that the knowledge of human variation and the application of physical anthropology techniques play a key role in individualizing the deceased.

Developing an anthropological profile entails estimating the age, sex, ancestry, and stature of the particular individual through the interpretation of skeletal shape and size of the remains. Furthermore, unique characteristics such as congenital or acquired malformations of the individual that could have been known to the relatives or friends of the missing person are recorded. Positive identification based on an anthropological profile can be achieved only if specific individualizing features like signs of medical intervention previously recorded or unique anatomic characteristics are found. Nevertheless, exclusion of identity can be easily accomplished if the antemortem information is contradicted by the profile of the remains.

Age Estimation

The estimation of age at death of an individual is based on biological changes that take place throughout life. There is a high statistical correlation between the chronological age of a person and the biological stage of growth and development; the assessment of biological age is usually most accurate in the early phases of development and decreases as the individual gets older.

The life history of an individual can be subdivided into four phases based on the developmental and degenerative changes that characterize them: prenatal, childhood, juvenile, and adulthood. The estimation of age at death in each of these phases relies on the inspection of the various sets of events that take place during the specific phase.

The pace of growth and development differs between the sexes and between various biological groups and the onset of the diverse age indicators is affected by genetic and environmental factors. Thus they should be taken into consideration whenever the sex or the ancestry of the individual is known either by the presence of remnants of internal or external sex organs, or because there is a presumed identity.

Skeletal maturation proceeds from the formation of cartilage models through the ossification of bony centers to the complete formation of the bone itself. Ossification begins by the sixth fetal month and proceeds at a bone-specific, regular rate. Age estimation during the fetal period relies on length-for-age standards of the long bones, the progressive ossification of the cranium, and the size and closure of the fontanelles.

During the fetal and neonatal periods, age estimation is based mainly on the degree of calcification of the deciduous teeth, which can be evaluated by radiographic means. The ossification standards are sometimes difficult to apply in a forensic setting, depending on the conditions of the remains. Not all bones may be present, and their absence can be misinterpreted as lack of development instead of the result of taphonomic processes (**Figure 3**).

In childhood, the successive development of the temporal, occipital, and sphenoid bones, the closure of the fontanelles, the rate of dental development, and the sequence of appearance of the secondary centers of ossification are useful age indicators.

The most accurate source of information for age estimation during the juvenile phase is the sequence of fusion of epiphyses and the unification of the three bones of the os coxa. The standard deviation of the estimate in this stage is greater than the assessment based on the appearance of the centers of ossification during childhood and oscillates between 2 and 4 years depending on the sex and ancestry of the individual.

The onset of puberty differs between populations; thus, extreme caution should be exercised when establishing age during the juvenile period. Forensic anthropologists generally implement dental standards when analyzing subadult remains. However, it is important to evaluate all the skeletal age indicators rather than depending on one to avoid exclusion of possible matches.

Once the individual has reached the final stages of growth and development, the estimation of age at death becomes less accurate since it depends chiefly on subtle and highly variable degenerative changes in the skeletal tissue. Postmaturity age changes involve mainly the remodeling of bony and cartilaginous structures, which are very sensitive to internal and

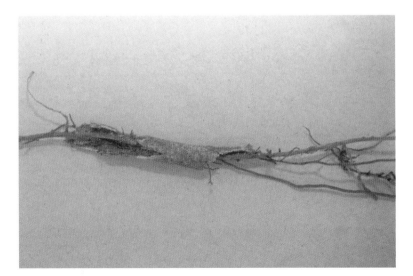

Figure 3 Long bone shaft of a newborn skeleton exhumed *circa* 50 years after death. The absence of epiphyses is the result of taphonomic processes.

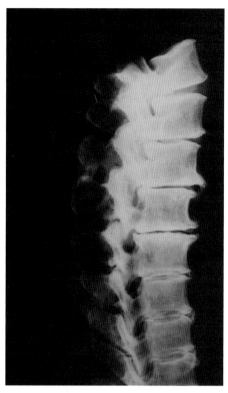

Figure 4 Radiograph of the thoracic and lumbar spine of a 73-year-old man, found in an advanced stage of decomposition. Note the collapsed vertebral bodies, lipping and osteophytes concomitant with age-related degenerative changes.

external factors, including the health status, lifestyle, and genetic makeup of the individual.

Adult age estimation is based on degenerative skeletal changes best observed in the various articulations. Pubic symphysis morphology is considered one of the most reliable indicators of adult age. This method is especially useful in the estimation of the age of individuals from late teens until the fifth decade of life. The mineralization of the costal cartilage of the ribs is also a valuable age indicator in adults. The gradual closure of the cranial sutures during adulthood is an unreliable procedure when used in itself but helpful when considered together with other age indicators (**Figure 4**).

Microscopic changes in the cortical bone and dental structure can be correlated with biological age, although these histological techniques require the sacrifice of the specimens, which later on can be detrimental for comparison with antemortem records. In addition, biochemical aging techniques and age estimation from radiographic assessment of the trabecular bone are also used when studying skeletal remains; their accuracy is somewhat contestable in the forensic realm.

A variety of aging techniques are recommended in the literature, and the choice should be based on the preservation of the skeletal remains and on the accuracy of the method. Most authors recommend that, when possible, a battery of aging techniques should be applied to enhance the accuracy of the estimation.

Sexual Dimorphism

The attribution of biological sex of the remains investigated is a critical stage, as it excludes 50% of individuals within the population to be considered. Furthermore, the estimation of biological age and stature depends on the correct determination of sex, since the standards for doing so are gender-specific.

The correct determination of sex is limited to adolescent and adult individuals. Although sex differences have been quantified in fetal and child skeletons, they are subtle and highly variable until the secondary sex characteristics develop during the juvenile period. Attempts at establishing sex in prepubescent bones utilizing measurements of growth-based differences between males and females are far from definitive. Nevertheless, some traits, such as the morphological differences in the ventral aspects of the pubic bone which can be detected in individuals as young as 14 years old, have been reported in literature.

As a rule, male skeletons are larger and have more rugged areas for muscle attachment, while females tend to be more gracile and maintain a child-like morphology. Nevertheless, most methods of sex determination are limited by some degree of morphological overlap and individual deviation from the central tendencies. Moreover, since certain populations differ in skeletal size and robustness, the researcher must be able to identify the population from which the remains come when determining the sex.

In the adult, the rate of accuracy of sex attribution in most populations is about 90%. Sexual dimorphism is most reliably diagnosed in the pelvic girdle and the skull, although most areas of the skeleton display some form of dimorphism.

In general the articulated female pelvis presents a wide outlet compared to that of the male and the subpubic angle appears noticeably wider in the female. These and other morphological differences are the result of the evolutionary adaptation that enables the relatively large-brained human infant to pass through the birth canal (**Figures 5** and **6**).

Aside from the pelvic girdle, the skull contains most of the morphologic characteristics that enable the anthropologist to determine biological sex. The female skull retains a "child-like" (pedomorphic) shape throughout life, while the typical male skull

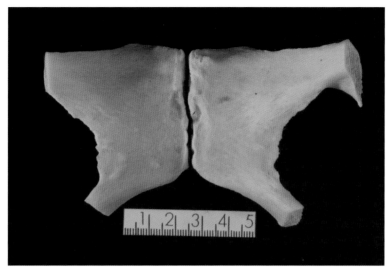

Figure 5 Dorsal aspect of a female pubic bone showing scars of parturition.

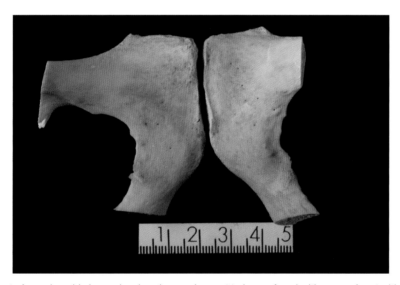

Figure 6 Dorsal aspect of a male pubic bone showing rim erosion, not to be confused with scars of parturition.

tends to be larger and more robust. This is best reflected in areas of muscle attachment and bio-mechanical stress, such as brow ridges and mandible.

Quantification of sexual dimorphism is especially effective in the postcranial skeleton. The size of joint surfaces, particularly in the humeral and femoral head areas, the body-to-manubrium rate, and the diameter of long bones are some of the sex-related metric traits available to the investigator. There is, however, some overlap in the cut-off points of sexual-ly dimorphic traits across biological groups. The ma-jority of the discriminant function formulae devised to determine biological sex are highly population-specific, thus they should be applied with prudence.

The best approach to ascertain sex with the highest degree of accuracy is to assess the entire skeletal pattern of the remains. Sex adjudication of very fragmented or charred skeletal remains should be cautiously undertaken; this can be better accom-plished by genetic analysis to avoid misclassification of the remains, precluding the possibility of a later positive identification.

Ancestry

There is an ongoing debate among physical anthro-pologists concerning the subdivision of humans into distinct racial groups. The basis for this contro-versy stems from the natural repugnance of enlightened scientists to the atrocities perpetrated throughout history in the name of racial cleansing. Notwithstanding, physical differences in populations are an important contribution to the process of records screening and personal identification in forensic anthropology.

The division of the populations of any species into biological races tends to be arbitrary to some degree, but when it comes to human races, the attribution of an individual to a certain population is often impossible due to the complexity of human mating and migration patterns. Racial attribution to a set of human remains may be hindered by the very wide range of variation within each racial group and the considerable overlap between members of different races; moreover many individuals bear the genes of two or more racial groups. Finally, the attribution of population membership is often socially constructed and rather arbitrary; oftentimes it reflects social group membership, which can be a matter of personal choice or happenstance.

The races of the world have been divided in different ways; most but not all anthropologists identify five basic biological groups based on morphological characteristics: (1) Mongoloids (Japanese, Chinese, and Amerindians); (2) Negroids (African and American Blacks); (3) Caucasoids (Europeans, West Asians, Asian Indians, and some American people); (4) Australoids (Australian and Melanesian Aborigines); and (5) Polynesians.

The designation of an individual to a particular biological ancestry group should always be based on the entire complex of traits associated with race. The level of experience of the forensic anthropologist with the populations that inhabit the area where the remains are found is critical.

The craniofacial skeleton holds the majority of morphometric traits useful in race determination. In Negroid individuals the lower face projects forward (facial prognathism), the skull is long and narrow, the nasal aperture is wide, and the nasal sill is guttered. Mongoloid individuals show in the malar and midnasal area an anterior projection, giving the appearance of a somewhat flatter facial skeleton than that of the Caucasoids. The white-caucasian skull tends to be high, rounder, and with an almost completely straight lower face (orthognathism); the nasal aperture is narrow and the nasal sill very sharp-edged. In Polynesians the facial and alveolar prognathism is moderate.

Other facial features helpful in race assignation include the palate, the zygomaticomaxillary suture, the visibility of the oval window through the external auditory meatus, and the morphology of the mandible. Dental morphological traits differ in their frequency among various biological groups, and their presence can be used as an indicator of race in conjunction with other skeletal traits.

In the postcranial skeleton there are few reliable criteria for race determination. Intermembral indices, such as the ratio of tibia-to-femur length and the radius-to-humerus length along with the anterior curvature of the femoral shaft and the intercondylar angle, have been suggested as good indicators for racial affinity.

Stature Estimation

Establishing the living height of an individual from skeletal remains is a routine and straightforward practice in forensic anthropology. Nevertheless, the assessed value may be deficient in the identification process, not only because of the normal changes in an individual's stature during the day and throughout life, but also because of the lack of accuracy in most antemortem records regarding reported stature. As a rule, there is a difference in the way individuals perceive their own stature from actual height; men tend to report in their driver's license that they are as much as 5 cm taller than they really are.

Stature estimation from skeletal remains can be obtained by either anatomical or mathematical methods. The anatomical technique requires the measurement of the height of the cranium and of each vertebra from C2 to S1, the physiological lengths of the femur and tibia, and the articulated height of the talus and calcaneum.

The mathematical method for stature estimation is based on the correlation between discrete bones and body parts and stature. Regression formulae based on measurements of single bones and combination of various bones specific for sex and population are implemented.

The best bones from which to reconstruct living stature are the long bones of the lower limb, since they are the most important components of height. Likewise, vertebral segments have been found to be useful in stature estimation, especially in mutilated human remains. When the preferred skeletal element is not present within the remains, stature may be estimated from other bones, but the accuracy of the estimate will be dramatically low.

When the skeletal remains are incomplete, stature reconstruction can be achieved from various segments of long bones. The application of these formulae requires some experience in osteology to be able to identify the correct landmarks in long bone fragments.

Finally, although the body build or robustness of an individual can be reconstructed from the prominence of the muscle attachments and the diameter of the long bones relative to their total length, the weight of an individual cannot be ascertained from the skeleton.

Habitus

Some occupations and activities, which involve heavy labor or repetitive actions, may leave an imprint on the bones. Enlarged areas of muscle attachments in certain bones (hypertrophy) can be indicators of specific activities, i.e., the presence of sharp tubercles in the mandibular condyles is often associated with playing woodwind instruments. Similarly, spurs or ridges of bone, facets, and grooves in areas that are normally smooth, and bone deformations can be the result of a specific occupation or habit. Since these types of markers can have a genetic as well as an age component, the investigator should be extremely cautious when stating a specific occupation as part of the anthropological profile.

Assessing the handedness of unidentified individuals would be highly desirable as approximately 95% of humans are right-side-dominant, thus determining that the remains are those of a left-handed person would significantly narrow down the search for possible identification. Unfortunately, there are several problems in the assessment of handedness and an error could impede reaching the correct antemortem records.

Individualizing Characteristics

Personal identification of human remains is accomplished when specific features of the skeleton can be equated to data recorded in medical and radiological records during the life of the individual.

Congenital and acquired pathologies, the presence of healed fractures, and specific degenerative changes are excellent markers for positive identification of human remains. Furthermore old surgical and prosthetic devices that might be evident within the remains are invaluable to the investigator, once the anthropological profile has limited the search to a few records. Likewise, anatomic variation of osseous features – such as the spinous processes, the outline of the frontal sinuses, the unique pattern of the trabecular bone, and various abnormalities in bone fusion – can be utilized to achieve positive identification (**Figure 7**).

Imaging techniques, such as skull-photo-superimposition and facial reconstruction, have been used to achieve personal identification when no other techniques are accessible; the scientific value of these methods is a constant subject of debate among forensic scientists, although their value for ruling out possible identifications is universally agreed.

Skeletal Trauma

Analyzing signs of trauma on bone, i.e., patterned wounds, gunshot wounds, sharp wounds, and the

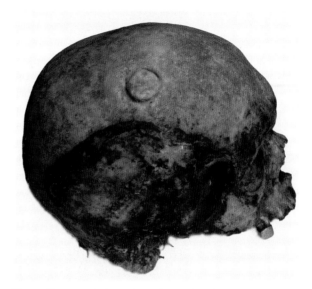

Figure 7 Lateral view of a male cranium found in the woods. Observe the circular healed defect on the right parietal compatible with a surgical procedure. The identification of the victim was possible after the anthropological profile narrowed the search to a missing individual suffering from Parkinson's disease who had undergone a craniotomy 15 years earlier.

presence of healed and unhealed fractures, falls within the realm of forensic anthropology. Understanding both normal anatomy and possible pathologic or anomalous variations can greatly increase the accuracy of the diagnosis of trauma by ruling out natural phenomena (**Figure 8**).

Usually, the remains analyzed have an extended postmortem interval and are either decomposed or skeletonized. Taphonomic processes, such as carnivore activity or geological processes, should be distinguished from perimortem trauma; however, it is not always possible to determine the age of a bone injury since detectable vital reaction takes several days.

The Role of Forensic Anthropology in Mass Casualty

The accumulated knowledge and experience of forensic investigators over the years has led to the development of standard procedures for processing and identifying victims of mass disasters and multiple death scenes. Forensic anthropologists, pathologists, biologists, and odontologists play key roles that complement each other in the medicolegal investigation of these events.

During the search and recovery phases on the site of the incident, anthropologists not only devise search criteria based on the scope and nature of the event, but organize grid systems for retrieval of human

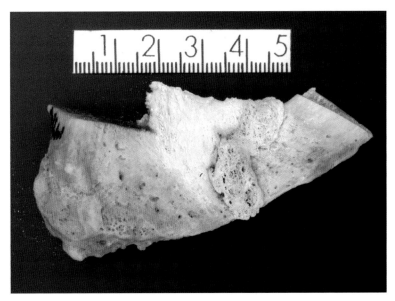

Figure 8   Osseous callus on a pubic bone, detected after thermochemical preparation of the specimen. This finding, the result of a motor vehicular accident, was paramount in narrowing down the search within the missing persons files.

remains and associated personal effects similar to the techniques implemented in archeological digs.

At the time of initial processing of the cadavers in the designated work area, forensic anthropologists are instrumental in identifying and reassociating fragmentary bodies. On the ensuing stages of the investigation, their lore is applied to creating anthropological profiles of the victims and collaborating in the positive identification endeavor.

The prominent role of the anthropologists in the efficient resolution of incidents that require a vast number of identifications is recognized worldwide. In fact, most emergency forensic organizations and international teams investigating mass graves from war crimes include forensic anthropologists in their organic makeup.

Summary

Forensic anthropology has been defined as the application of the science of physical anthropology to the legal process. The anthropologist's skills in osteology are instrumental, not only in generating anthropological profiles and establishing the positive identity of unidentified human remains, but also in contributing data on skeletal trauma and pathology.

The academic training of forensic anthropologists worldwide includes a vast knowledge not only of osteology but also of anatomy, growth, and development, and genetics as well. Most forensic anthropologists from North and South America undergo thorough studies in all fields of anthropology including archeology, thus are well versed in field techniques. In the rest of the world, physical anthropology is mostly taught in medical and odontology faculties, being better versed in radiography, odontology, and pathology. Nevertheless, all practicing forensic anthropologists acquire the required skills as they work in close collaboration with other experts.

The techniques implemented to achieve positive identification of human remains are common to odontologists, radiologists, and pathologists. However, by virtue of the broadness of the field of physical anthropology, i.e., skeletal biology, dental anthropology, paleopathology, and human evolution, the competence of the anthropologists often provides a more comprehensive analysis of unidentified human remains.

See Also

Anthropology: Archeology, Excavation and Retrieval of Remains; Stature Estimation from the Skeleton; Bone Pathology and Antemortem Trauma; Pediatric and Juvenile; Sex Determination; Determination of Racial Affinity; Handedness; Role of DNA; **War Crimes:** Pathological Investigation

Further Reading

Byers ST (2001) *Introduction to Forensic Anthropology. A Textbook*. Boston, MA: Allyn and Bacon.
Cox M, Mays S (eds.) (2000) *Human Osteology in Archaeology and Forensic Science*. London: Greenwich Medical Media.

Haglund WD, Sorg MH (eds.) (1997) *Forensic Taphonomy – The Postmortem Fate of Human Remains.* Boca Raton, FL: CRC Press.

Kahana T, Hiss J (1997) Identification of human remains: forensic radiology. *Journal of Clinical Forensic Medicine* 4: 7–15.

Scheuer L (2002) Application of osteology in forensic medicine. *Clinical Anatomy* 15: 297–312.

Reichs KJ (ed.) (1998) *Forensic Osteology,* 2nd edn. Springfield, IL: Charles C Thomas.

Archeology, Excavation and Retrieval of Remains

W D Haglund, International Forensic Program, Physicians for Human Rights, Shoreline, WA, USA
T Simmons, University of Central Lancashire, Preston, UK

Introduction

The basic role of the forensic anthropologist is to determine the identity of human remains. This is traditionally accomplished by first estimating the biological profile (age, race, sex, and stature) of an individual and then assessing any unique identifying biological characteristics, such as antemortem pathology or trauma. The forensic anthropologist is also trained to interpret both peri- and postmortem trauma, i.e., those injuries sustained around the time of death (with the understanding that they may have contributed to the cause of death) and any damage sustained to the skeleton after death that may aid in understanding the history of the remains before they were deposited in the position in which they were located and from which they were retrieved.

The forensic archeologist interprets both the artifacts found and the context in which they were found in order to reconstruct the history of the scene. When combined, the evidence of forensic archeologists and forensic anthropologists can provide a very precise picture of the events leading to the death and the subsequent disposal of the individuals found at the crime scene.

Contributions of Anthropologists and Archeologists to the Excavation and Recovery of Human Remains

The fundamental challenge to forensic death investigators is to maximize the recovery of human remains and evidence. Human remains, any portion of a human body in any condition, especially those that are skeletonized, burned, buried, or disarticulated and scattered, may render them difficult to recognize and complicated to recover. Common outdoor scene issues are to: (1) locate remains; (2) maximize as complete a recovery as possible; (3) differentiate ante-, peri-, and postmortem trauma or other modification of remains; and (4) resolve taphonomic issues from the scene and its context that shed light on the relationships among the events of death and subsequent fate of the remains (**Table 1**).

In the forensic context, taphonomy includes the decomposition of remains, their skeletonization, dispersal, modification, or destruction. Overcoming these challenges necessitates successful search strategies, use of special techniques to maximize recovery and documentation of remains and evidence, and utilizing taphonomic data to unravel postmortem events that may involve movement, modification, or destruction of human remains. Such information, based upon the scene context, can be utilized to make supportable inferences regarding the postmortem fate of human remains. The participation of forensic archeologists and anthropologists in the excavation and retrieval of remains can provide a basis for improving the quality of the analysis of the case in later stages of an investigation.

Locating Human Remains and Graves

Contributions of forensic anthropologists and archeologists to the retrieval of human remains are summarized in **Table 1**. The following discussion will elaborate on search strategies for locating human remains both on the surface of the ground and buried.

Surface Remains

In the domestic context, the initial discovery of surface remains is often by chance, e.g., a dog brings home a human bone from the woods nearby; a hiker or hunter stumbles across human remains in a remote area, or a driver stops the car on the shoulder of the

Table 1 Major contributions of forensic archeologists and anthropologists in the field

Rapid field assessment
Distinguish human from nonhuman bones
Determine search strategy for surface remains and graves
Recovery of surface remains
Excavation of graves
Exposure, documentation, and recovery of remains
Provide skeletal inventories
Determine presence of multiple remains
Minimize commingling when multiple individuals are involved
Resolve taphonomic issues such as types of bone modification and periods in which they may have occurred

highway to relieve himself and in the process discovers human bones. In international investigations (e.g., former Yugoslavia), witnesses, even individuals who actually escaped death, may lead investigators to sites of ambushes or extrajudicial killings.

Upon discovery of human remains, the first question to be addressed is: are the remains human or nonhuman? The second question is: are they of forensic significance? It is generally considered that deaths that occurred over 50–75 years prior to when the remains are located are unlikely to generate a prosecution.

When surface human remains, especially those partially or fully skeletonized, are discovered, often only a portion of the skeleton is initially found because body parts or bones have often been overlain by seasonal debris, dispersed, or even destroyed, commonly by animals. To complicate matters, initial responding investigators, who are inadequately trained in the recognition of human skeletal remains, may attempt to recover these remains without expert advice or assistance. When this happens, often subsequent scene visits are necessary to address questions that arise with regard to: (1) incomplete recovery of remains; (2) detailed searches not being conducted in trajectory paths between scattered clusters of remains; or (3) documentation and/or mapping at the scene not being sufficient to respond to questions that arise about the scene.

As with all crime scenes, organized search strategies must be carried out. The strategy employed depends on the size of the area to be searched as well as the terrain. Participants in searches must be trained in the recognition of isolated skeletal elements and have qualified forensic anthropologists available to confirm their findings.

Standard grid searches may be warranted once the remains have been discovered and confined to a relatively small area. In locating scattered skeletal remains, line searches are most useful for large areas and often used with care in wooded areas as well. In conducting a line search, the spacing between participants must be adjusted to allow a complete view of the surface space between them. If any evidence is encountered along this path, it should not be moved until fully evaluated by the appropriate investigators, and a marker, such as easily visible flags, is used to mark the position. The flags are left in place until the search is concluded. This allows for the large-scale (or even aerial) photography of the area in order to document the distribution of evidence locations within the scene. Once this is completed, additional grid searches can be employed, encompassing the area where the remains are concentrated.

Under certain circumstances a radial search pattern is also useful. This is primarily when the remains are located at a focal point, such as under a tree on the top of a hill, and/or when there are a limited number of search participants. In a radial search, one investigator begins at the focal point (the tree) and slowly walks an expanding spiral out from this point. The radial search works best if supplemented by secondary searches conducted on straight lines, or spokes radiating from the focal point; these intersect the spiral at several points and may be useful in locating additional remains. As in the line search, evidence should be flagged, but not collected, when initially encountered.

Several questions need to be addressed when processing scenes involving scattered skeletal remains. From what location(s) were the remains scattered? Often movement will occur from the original location where the individual died or where the body was originally deposited. This is usually the primary site of decomposition, except in cases of subadults (children) or major portions of adults, which can be moved by canids. Larger carnivores are capable of moving adult bodies. Movement of incompletely decomposed body components to another area results in secondary sites of decomposition. The significance of sites of decomposition is that these are the most likely areas where not only parts of remains but artifacts (portable objects such as cartridges, bullets, ligatures, blindfolds, medical appliances such as joint prostheses, clothing, and/or personal effects) may be shed. Decomposition sites may be marked by odorous, discolored staining caused by decomposition fluids soaking into the ground. The presence of insect puparium or yellowish discoloration of low overhanging deciduous foliage may also provide visual clues to where a body decomposed. Knowledge of the process of soft-tissue deterioration and the relative sequence in which bones or body parts become separated aids in distinguishing primary versus secondary decomposition sites.

What is the composition of the primary and secondary clusters of remains? It is crucial, when processing scenes of scattered remains, that not only the relative position of artifacts and human remains is mapped, but also a detailed inventory of the bones or artifacts contained in each location needs to be made. Understanding whether or not bones in separate locations represent anatomically related units helps to determine in what stage of the decomposition process scattering took place. For example, if bones of a closely grouped cluster represent bones of the same anatomical region, for example a lower leg and foot, they were more than likely removed from the remains as an articulated body unit.

A following question is: what were the most likely trajectories of dispersion? Knowledge of the decomposition site(s) and scatter pattern can often allow deduction of the most likely dispersal trajectories. It is along these trajectory paths between larger bone finds that small pieces of bone or teeth, often crucial in identification of the deceased, are found. Special circumstances that may affect dissociation and scatter are preexisting trauma, terrain, or purposeful dismemberment.

Locating Graves

Although chance discovery of buried remains may occur in the course of digging activity, such as preparation for construction, it is most common that a general area is suspected of containing a grave and it is the localization of the actual gravesite that is problematic. A variety of methods has been applied to finding buried remains and not all methods are amenable to particular environments. With all approaches to locate graves, with the exception of trenching, findings must be confirmed by actual digging.

Witness Statements

Accurate witness statements are the most reliable method of locating a grave. Unfortunately, it is not uncommon for witnesses to indicate the general area where a grave is supposed to be located, but not be able to pinpoint the exact position, even when he/she was present at the time of burial. Clandestine disposal of remains may take place under hurried or stressful circumstances, for example, at night or under other conditions of subterfuge. Over time, familiar landmarks in the landscape may change through human development or natural processes. Vegetation grows, dies, or changes in makeup. Memories of witnesses dim or fail. When relying on witness testimony, it is preferable to obtain information from more than one source if possible. Even then, disagreements may abound.

Visual Clues

Clues to the location of a grave include changes in the ground surface contours, vegetation death and subsequent regrowth, and damage to nearby trees and shrubs, as well as surface scatters of artifacts relating to the grave (e.g., cartridge casings, shreds of clothing, displaced skeletal elements). Soil removed in digging a grave is placed adjacent to the hole being dug and then used to fill the grave once the body is in place, leaving disturbance vegetation near the grave and a heap of dirt at its surface. Surrounding vegetation may be killed during the process. New plant growth will emerge, at times quite luxuriant

as it is well-fertilized by the organic products of decomposition and the bioturbation of the soil from the disturbance by organisms, e.g., mixing, trampling, and plant and root penetration. Thus, to the trained botanical eye, the plant community of the grave may look quite different from that of the surrounding area. As the process of decomposition continues and soft tissue is destroyed, the soil filling the grave sinks, ultimately leaving a shallow depression. Frequently, graves are dug shallowly, in haste, too small to contain the remains and parts of the body or skeleton will stick out of the newly sunken earth.

Aerial Imagery

Aerial imagery takes advantage of an elevated point of view and relies upon the fact that surface indications of signs of digging activity or potential graves stand out from their general background. Historically, aerial photography has been the most utilized aerial imagery. An extraordinary example of the use of satellite photographs was those that demonstrated actual digging of graves and subsequent disturbance of the graves for the 7000 Bosnian victims of the Srebrenica massacre of 1995.

Probes

A simple probe can be made from a stainless steel rod approximately 1 cm in diameter with a T-shaped handle (**Figure 1**). Two types of probe have been utilized to explore subsurface areas suspected to hold graves: (1) a probe consisting of a solid metal rod; or (2) a core sampling probe. The utility of probing is to detect differential soil compaction and the presence of decomposing materials. Thinner probes are used when detecting remains, because the core types may cause significant damage to buried remains. Careful insertion of the thinner, solid probe allows detection of relative differences in subsurface compaction. In places where decomposition fluids have permeated the area, simply smelling the tip of the withdrawn probe will indicate the presence of decomposing materials. Use of a probe that provides a sample core can indicate subsurface strata and potentially disturbed areas can be compared with control cores from adjacent undisturbed areas. When decomposing carcasses are encountered, the odor of the probe shaft is the "tipoff." A drawback to probing is that one cannot determine the difference between the odor of decomposing human and nonhuman carcasses. When the probe is employed in areas of high water tables, localization of the grave may be problematic due to contamination by mobilized fluid components of decomposition to the general area surrounding the origin of decomposition.

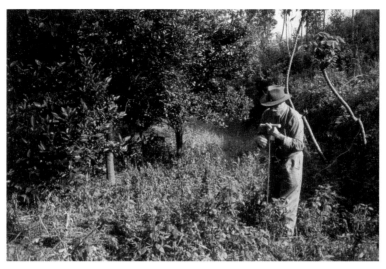

Figure 1 Use of a probe, to locate graves in Rwanda 1996.

Skimming, "Peeling" off to Subsurface Levels

Skimming or shaving thin layers of surface materials and soil, a routine technique of archeologists detecting subsurface features, is also quite effective for localizing disturbances indicative of potential graves. This can be done by small hand tools as well as by utilizing machinery when dealing with large areas (**Figure 2**).

The mixing of soil horizons that occurs when a hole is dug frequently leaves a darker soil in the grave compared to the undisturbed subsoil around it. This soil change can often be clearly seen once the excavation is below the topsoil and the pit outline may be clearly visible as the profile is revealed in the trench. The information revealed in the profile can also help to demonstrate if the grave was reopened after the initial bodies were deposited, either to add or to remove material.

Trenching

Trenching simply involves excavating parallel trenches through an area suspected to contain buried remains until they are encountered. Trenches must be close enough together to insure that potential remains between them will not be missed. A case demonstrating the use of trenching was the 1995 search for two individuals who had been buried 12 years previously near the Honduran village of El Magular. At the time of their original discovery, their decomposed bodies were found by locals off to the side of a road at the edge of a banana grove. As is customary, the regional medical authority conducted a brief exam and the bodies were buried in the area where they had been discovered. Through the intervening years, the

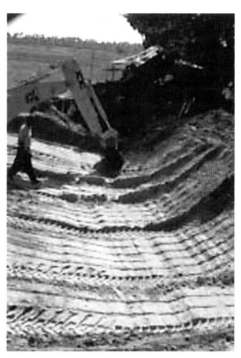

Figure 2 Heavy machinery can be used to "skim" the superficial layers of soil in order to locate graves when large areas are involved, Sri Lanka, Acheh Peninsula, 1999.

banana grove had been eradicated, and the road had been widened with its route now encroaching on to part of the old banana grove. As surface features had been drastically altered, test trenches were dug at three different areas pointed out by witnesses. Even though all three witnesses had been involved in burying the bodies, they could not agree on the location. As the work progressed, more witnesses, claiming to know where the bodies were buried, came forward with opinions as to why their memory of events was the correct one.

It was decided to extend the trenching over the whole area, first placing priority on the most reasonable scenarios. With labor provided by nearly 40 volunteers, digging work progressed for 5 days and resulted in 250 linear meters of 1.5-m-deep trenches until the remains were finally encountered.

Remote Sensing

Recent innovations in efforts to locate graves have utilized geophysical prospecting techniques routinely used in civil-engineering projects. Methods that have shown the most promise are side-scanning sonar, ground-penetrating radar, proton magnetometer, and electrical resistivity. The basis of these techniques is their ability to discern subsurface anomalies, but unfortunately not to discriminate human remains from other anomalies.

Exhumation of Buried Remains

Prior to discussing exhumation of buried remains it is necessary to address the different uses of the terms exhumation and excavation. In the USA, excavation implies only digging, not the surface recoveries or exhumations of human remains. Exhumation implies specifically the recovery of human remains from a buried context. In the UK, the term excavation may be used in lieu of exhumation to describe an organized dig (or surface recovery) of artifacts and/or remains using archeological methods and techniques.

Prior to excavation, once a grave has been located, surface features and evidence are documented. Potential evidence is then mapped and collected. The grave's boundary is then determined and a strategy for its excavation planned. Sometimes a test trench is dug across the grave and into undisturbed soil to determine the depth of the grave, its extent and condition and the disposition of remains, and the configuration of the natural stratigraphic sequence of the undisturbed area adjacent to the grave. The natural stratigraphic sequence of the subsurface can also be determined by digging a control trench away from the immediate area of the grave. Test trenching allows determination of the logistical needs of the excavation and necessary specialists for it and the subsequent examination of remains.

The grave fill on top of the remains is then removed in a layered sequence, preferably leaving as much of the grave walls intact as possible. The grave wall will have tool marks of the hand tools or machines used to dig the grave. For large mass graves, working trenches will be needed to provide drainage, sumps, or a convenient location to place removed overburden for later removal. Once remains are exposed they need to be mapped and photographed prior to removal. In dealing with mass graves it may be necessary to expose the surface of several remains in order to determine which remains should be removed first. Once the grave is emptied, a metal detector can be passed over the grave floor in order to detect metal objects, such as bullets, which may have penetrated it. Impressions of tread or track marks from digging machines or footprints should be documented. Finally, the grave should be refilled, not left as a hazard.

The Forensic Paradigm Shift

As with any discipline when applied to the forensic arena, experts must be aware of the special requirements of working in the medical–legal context. Unlike working in some areas of academia, where opinions, often based on tantalizing observations, thrive, yielding papers and theories, in forensics they may literally prove fatal. Several lessons need to be learned.

One lesson deals with legal issues crucial to the handling and documentation of evidence. Admissibility of evidence and even complete investigations may be compromised for lack of proper collection, documentation, and storage of evidence. Chain of custody, the accountability for evidence, must be maintained and documented from the time of its discovery to the time of its presentation in court. Such documentation includes a trail of where, when, why, and in whose possession evidence has been kept. Unless otherwise directed, strict discretion must be maintained as far as the investigation and its findings are concerned.

For those not experienced in dealing with death investigations, as happens increasingly, added stresses are present when working in the arena of international investigations involved with war crimes, genocide, and crimes against humanity. Experts may not be accustomed to working out of their own countries. Meeting the everyday needs of food, lodging, travel, and logistics may be daunting. Availability of potable water and electricity, security issues such as mines, and other unexploded devices create added burdens to the work. Unfamiliar circumstances such as checkpoints and the presence of military personnel and weapons may prove stressful.

For those traditional archeologists and anthropologists who deal with human remains, skeletal remains are the norm. There is a relatively safe psychological distance when working with bones and/or historic and prehistoric human remains that is not present when one deals with recently dead human remains. Instead of simple skeletal remains, the dead may be fleshed and/or decomposed. Clothing may not be unlike that worn by workers. Materials such as currency, watches, jewelry, and combs may be similar to those the workers carry with them everyday. Highly personal photographs and documents, such as letters, may reveal intimate details of the victim's life. The truth of human inhumanity to others is demonstrated by evidence of the circumstance and causes of death. For many experts, meeting surviving families is not a routine experience and may cause extreme discomfort. These are but a few of the psychological ramifications of forensic work. All of these factors tend to foreshorten empathetic distance between workers and the remains.

See Also

Anthropology: Overview; Taphonomy; Bone Pathology and Antemortem Trauma; Cremated Bones; Sex Determination; Role of DNA; **Autopsy:** Procedures and Standards; **Deaths:** Trauma, Musculo-skeletal System; **Death Investigation Systems:** United States of America; **Odontology:** Overview; **Postmortem Changes:** Overview; **War Crimes:** Site Investigation; Pathological Investigation

Further Reading

Burns KR (1999) *Forensic Anthropology Training Manual.* London: Prentice Hall.

Haglund WD (1998) The scene and context: contributions of the forensic anthropologist. In: Reichs K (ed.) *Forensic Osteology II,* pp. 4–62. Springfield, IL: Charles C Thomas.

Haglund WD, Sorg MH (eds.) (1997) *Forensic Taphonomy: The Postmortem Fate of Human Remains.* Boca Raton, FL: CRC Press.

Haglund WD, Sorg MH (eds.) (2001) *Advances in Forensic Taphonomy: Methods, Theory, and Archeological Perspectives.* Boca Raton, FL: CRC Press.

Hunter J, Roberts C, Martin A (1996) *Studies in Crime: An Introduction to Forensic Archeology.* London: BT Bastford.

Killim EW (1990) *The Detection of Human Remains.* Springfield, IL: Charles C. Thomas.

Reichs KJ (1986) *Forensic Osteology: Advances in the Identification of Human Remains.* Springfield, IL: Charles C. Thomas.

Steadman DW (2003) *Hard Evidence: Case Studies in Forensic Anthropology.* Upper Saddle River, NJ: Prentice Hall.

The Society for Historical Archeology (2001) *Archeologists as Forensic Investigators: Defining the Role. Historical Archeology* (35) 1. Uniontown, PA: The Society for Historical Archeology.

Taphonomy

W D Haglund, International Forensic Program, Physicians for Human Rights, Shoreline, WA, USA
M H Sorg, University of Maine, Orono, ME, USA

Taphonomy: The Scientific Study of Postmortem Processes in Context

Forensic taphonomy is the interdisciplinary study and interpretation of postmortem processes of human remains in their depositional context, i.e., the history of a body following death. Taphonomic details are critically important for estimating time since death and differentiating injuries from postmortem changes. A careful taphonomic assessment can provide valuable information about the death event, transport of the victim's body by a perpetrator or by natural forces, and the timing and nature of events after death. Taphonomy attempts to provide an organized approach to data collection during the recovery of remains, as well as the understanding of postmortem environments and their interaction with the human body.

Historical Background

The term taphonomy was created in 1940 by combining the Greek terms for burial or grave (*taphos*) and laws (*nomos*), meaning literally the laws of burial. First applied in paleontology, taphonomy developed into a structured approach to explain the history of a set of remains, termed the "death assemblage," from the time of death until its discovery, with a focus on reconstructing ancient ecological communities. Archeologists and paleoanthropologists adopted and enhanced taphonomic methods during the 1970s with the goal of better interpreting human biology and behavior in the archeological context. For example, they studied bone modification by scavenger species, and butchering modification by modern hunter–gatherer people in order to differentiate the taphonomic signatures of nonhuman scavengers from that of human cultural food preparation. They developed models of bone weathering and devised experiments to simulate rivers and their effects on the transport of particular types of bones. Some scientists did naturalistic observation of particular species or environmental processes as they occur in nature. Others performed actualistic or experimental research. These efforts produced models that could be applied to archeological data.

In 1985 forensic anthropologists began applying taphonomic models and techniques to the understanding of forensic cases, coining the term forensic taphonomy. Early applications focused on the effects and processes of scavenger modification, primarily by wolves and dogs, as well as the effects of transport of human remains in river currents or ocean environments. At about the same time, entomologists, botanists, and other natural scientists were becoming more involved in forensic cases. They utilized plants and animals associated with bodies as biological clocks to estimate the postmortem interval, or to document the changes in the body which could have been moved, wounded, or otherwise modified. Forensic taphonomy is best accomplished using an interdisciplinary approach, to the extent possible depending on resources allocated to death investigation within a particular jurisdiction, nation, or culture.

Taphonomic Information in the Forensic Context

In many instances, the modifications to the remains that result from taphonomic processes, the taphonomic overprint, must be figuratively stripped away in order to discern information about the death event. This may involve, for example, differentiating skeletal injuries at the time of death – perimortem trauma – from postmortem artifacts.

Alternatively, postmortem sequences and processes may themselves produce forensic evidence of, for instance, transport or modification of the remains after death by the perpetrator. In both cases, the forensic taphonomy approach focuses on the condition of the remains within the context of their deposition and/or discovery. This often involves multiple disciplines such as anthropology, entomology, botany, or marine biology, thus utilizing expertise across the natural sciences to reconstruct and interpret particular aspects of the postmortem environment.

Primary Postmortem Processes

Taphonomic processes begin at the point of death, as the body begins a series of chemical and physical processes termed decomposition. Autolysis involves the dynamic chemical breakdown of cellular functions and structures due to the absence of oxygen and loss of thermoregulatory capacity. The concomitant process of putrefaction includes the action of internal and external bacteria and fungi, which utilize the body's nutrients to fuel their own physiology and reproduction. Both autolysis and putrefaction are facilitated by heat; freezing slows or stops decomposition, although it may itself produce cellular damage and breakdown. Dry heat removes the moisture essential for decomposition and creates mummification, a drying and hardening of tissues. The presence of excess moisture facilitates saponification and the generation of adipocere, a variable waxy solidification of tissues that occurs with the build-up of fatty acids and a byproduct of autolysis.

As soft tissue decomposes and is lost into the environment, the body will skeletonize, exposing cartilage and bone tissue. The subsequent loss of organic substances within the bone has a much longer time frame, on average, than soft-tissue loss. Bone in the living organism, composed of both organic and inorganic substances, tends to retain its shape after death due to the underlying inorganic or mineral matrix, unless the environment is acidic. Minerals in the bones may be replaced chemically by minerals in the sediments, while maintaining the original shape of the bones, a process termed diagenesis. This occurs over long time periods and leads to fossilization.

The processes of decomposition in both soft and hard tissues are variable in their intensity, location, and range. These processes may vary at different locations within the same body, even within the same bone element, or among multiple bodies in the same depositional context. For example, soft tissue on extremities such as hands and feet may mummify, while the torso, having more soft tissue and moisture, skeletonizes. Similarly, bodies in a mass grave, with the same postmortem intervals, may vary greatly in decomposition depending on their position in the body mass, whether more exposed to environmental factors on the periphery, or more protected by other bodies within the core of the body mass. It is important to appreciate, record, and interpret accurately such microenvironmental variation.

The Context: Ecological Perspectives

Introduction of a dead organism into an environment creates a cascade of ecological events as scavengers and processes of decomposition interact with physical and chemical factors to assimilate and recycle the remains. These processes are dynamic, as the microenvironment changes with each succession of organisms attracted by the body, or, secondarily, attracted by the presence of the scavengers of the remains.

In some cases remains may be preserved from consumption and certain forms of decomposition by body covering, burial, or somewhat extreme environmental conditions, such as freezing temperatures, excessive dryness, extremes of pH, or other shielding from scavengers. In these cases destruction of soft and/or hard tissues may be delayed considerably, for example by mummification. In the most extreme cases, such organic remains may ultimately become mineralized or fossilized.

Thus, the taphonomic history of a dead organism is the result of a complex and dynamic interplay between environmental factors that promote or delay decay and preservation. Although it is possible to understand scientifically and generally predict individual processes affecting taphonomic changes, for example, the impact of freezing on decomposition, the interaction of multiple processes and sequences associated with a particular case creates a unique history requiring interpretive judgment, combined with scientific data. For example, estimating the postmortem interval based on generic, regional models of decomposition would be complicated in a case that underwent partial decomposition indoors, after which the body was moved outside by a perpetrator, followed by bear scavenging and transport of body parts.

Forensic taphonomy has focused research on individual processes and taphonomic agents, such as observing decomposition rates in a controlled microenvironment. Research has also been done on a series of actual forensic cases in which taphonomic details are known, observations have been calibrated and documented, and a model has been produced, such as canid scavenging stages in a particular region. Taphonomic agents, including temperature, moisture, chemicals, plants, animals, sediment, and water, can theoretically be identified by a particular signature. In some cases the signatures are not unique and additional data may be needed about the context, for example, to differentiate overlapping patterns.

The Structure of Forensic Taphonomy Inquiry

Forensic taphonomy seeks to answer questions regarding time of death, location of body deposition and decomposition, sequences of events at and after the time of death, and interpretation of injury. The bulk of taphonomic research has focused on four major categories: (1) decomposition; (2) transport; (3) scavenging; and (4) associated organisms. Both terrestrial and aquatic environments have been the subject of taphonomic study for decades.

Postmortem Interval and Condition of Remains

Forensic taphonomists have utilized case series of human deaths in which postmortem interval is known to build regionally specific models of terrestrial and aquatic decomposition, most of which are based in North America. Each model, in which the condition of remains is the dependent variable, typically includes several phases of soft-tissue decomposition and skeletonization, associated in a general way with the time since death. Differences between

models are due to relative amounts of atmospheric moisture and heat as well as potential for freezing, i.e., variables associated with climate. Burial and body covering alter these chronologies. Generally, a body that is not preserved by freezing can reach one of three endpoints: (1) skeletonization; (2) mummification; or (3) saponification. The more likely changes to take place are: (1) skeletonization in humid environments; (2) mummification in dry environments; and (3) saponification in wet environments.

Caution is needed in applying models to individual cases. Model case series tend to be small in size, the range of variation within phases is large, and unique microenvironmental contexts or circumstances may interfere with the usual taphonomic processes, for example, deposition in a cave or other protected area. The condition (and hence the decomposition phase) of different body parts, for example, the head versus the pelvic region, may differ within the same individual, due to the amount of associated soft tissue. Disarticulation, which refers to separation of bone elements at the joints by decomposition or scavenging animals, may hasten decomposition (i.e., appear to have a shorter postmortem interval) or hasten soft-tissue desiccation (i.e., appear to have a longer postmortem interval). Body coverings, such as heavy boots, can protect soft tissue for long periods of time, suggesting a very short postmortem interval.

The most accurate estimates of postmortem interval are produced using biological clocks, i.e., the association of the remains with organisms for which there are well-known metamorphic or developmental processes. When remains are exposed in natural settings, associated sarcosaprophagic insects (postmortem scavengers) go through a fairly well-timed metamorphosis specific to their species and region. Forensic entomologists may be able to reconstruct the postmortem interval fairly accurately within the first several weeks after death by identifying the insects and their metamorphic phases. Plant growth may also suggest general time periods. Phases of mammalian scavenger consumption and use are much less precise, but can suggest general time frames. Other organisms, such as barnacles attached to bones in marine contexts (**Figure 1**) can suggest a minimum elapsed time following exposure of the bone surface. Growth rates of associated plants can also suggest minimum postmortem intervals.

Most research by forensic taphonomists focuses on the loss of soft tissue to which they attach very broad time frames, usually weeks or months. Following the loss of soft tissue, bone may also decompose. Models associated with bone degradation, often referred to as weathering, tend to offer descriptive and qualitative phases without precise temporal referents (**Table 1**). For example, desiccation cracks are followed by

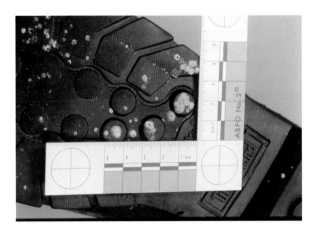

Figure 1 Barnacles on a boot sole. Marine biologists can use the total diameter of barnacles associated with human remains in some cases as an indicator of minimum postmortem interval. This requires knowledge about the specific species of barnacle in conjunction with information about the marine ecological context.

Table 1 Weathering stages in bone

Stage	Condition of bone
0	Soft tissue present; bone greasy
1	Bone surface exposed; thin cracks parallel to fiber structure of bone
2	Flaking of the outer surface, usually associated with cracks
3	Superficial bone surface has a rough texture, edges of cracks are rounded
4	Bone surface course, rough, and fibrous; cracks are open and invade deeper layers
5	Bone fragile and falling to pieces

Adapted from Behrensmeyer AK (1978) Taphonomic and ecologic information from bopne weathering. *Paleobiology* 4: 150–162.

exfoliation of bone cortex, but in between these phases timing is relative (**Figures 2** and **3**). Bone in both terrestrial and aquatic settings may break down due to abrasion, erosion, and dissolution, as well as from the actions of plants and animals (**Figures 4–7**).

Location of Sites of Deposition and Decomposition

A taphonomic approach is helpful in locating sites where the body may have been disposed and sites where the remains rested during the decomposition process. Tracking such sites allows the sequential movement of bodies and body parts to be determined and may prove invaluable in locating missing body parts, such as teeth, that may have been shed during the movement from one location to another.

Sites of decomposition are also of potential evidentiary significance. As soft tissue decomposes, items such as earrings, hair, clothing, and their contents are separated from the human remains. The context

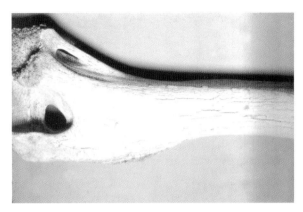

Figure 2 Bone weathering showing widening of linear cracks due to extreme drying.

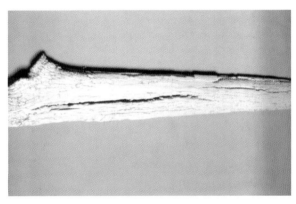

Figure 3 Bone weathering showing deep invading cracks and fragile condition with exfoliation of cortex.

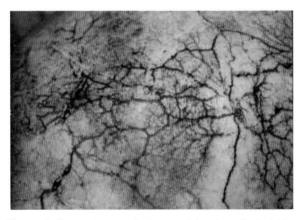

Figure 4 Root patterns etched on cranial surface. Such etching is caused by secretion of acidic products.

of the original deposition of the remains may also give clues to how the body arrived at the site.

Visual indicators may often be present at decomposition sites. Decomposition may initially depress, and then greatly enhance associated plant growth. The process of putrefaction and gas build-up can cause sediments overlying a buried body to bulge, then

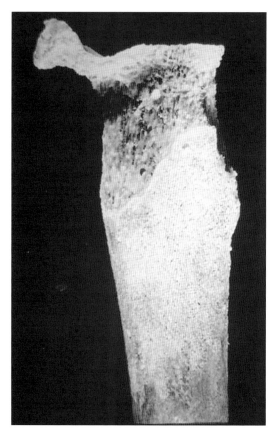

Figure 5 Sea snail modification of a distal tibia, producing a circumferential pedestal effect.

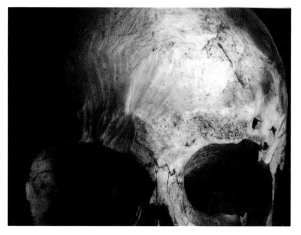

Figure 6 Rodents have modified this cranium, removing elevated brow ridges and exposing spongy bone below (above right orbit). Broad, parallel-scraping defects produced by rodent incisors can be seen above the left orbit. Courtesy of Emilee Mead.

collapse; putrefaction can also increase the chances for a body in water to float, or to resurface after first sinking.

Scavengers are attracted to bodies by scent. The dispersal of scent from a body can be modeled as a cone, with decreasing concentration and increasing

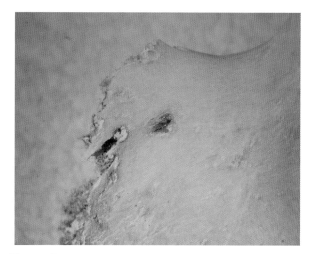

Figure 7 Canid modification of an innominate, including gnawed edge (left) and canine tooth punctures (center).

diameter further from the body or scent source. Animals use olfaction to detect scent cone directionality by sensing relative concentration of the odor. Cadaver air-scent dog search teams can benefit from an understanding of the principles of scent distribution in air, sediment, and water. Scent can be moved from its primary source by wind or water currents, and the scent cone can be interrupted or rearranged by changes in topography or vegetation. It is important for searchers to interpret these potential complexities correctly in terms of their effects on dog (or human) olfaction. In some cases dogs may alert in an area where no visible remains are present because scavengers have removed them, but where decomposition scent has penetrated the ground.

Consumption of dead organisms by scavengers results in a dispersal of a set of remains within an environment. For example, a scavenger's stomach or scat at some distance from the original body deposit may contain remains. Dogs and coyotes are known to transport portions of bodies as far as 1.5 km from the original source.

Birds, fish, mammals, and invertebrates may all participate in scavenging. Knowing the taphonomic signature of the particular animal and plant taxa is helpful in reconstructing the pattern and range of dispersal, as well as in interpreting bone modification.

Reconstructing Postmortem Sequences

The reconstruction of postmortem sequences requires consideration of variation in rates of certain processes as well as in the timing and order of modification by taphonomic agents. The potential permutations are extensive, requiring the investigator to merge theoretical understanding of taphonomic change with a historical approach that considers unique events and event sequences.

Table 2 General effects of moving water on bone

General patterns	Possible effects on crania
Bones may be moved	Facial bones are more easily damaged or destroyed
Movement affected by size, density, and shape of bone	Thin bone plates frequently become perforated
Fast currents more likely to move bone than slow currents	Exposed edges become abraded
Bone may become buried, later exposed and moved	Surface may become pitted, scratched, or gouged
Bones tend to orient with flow direction	Anterior tooth enamel may become chipped
Edge-rounding increases with transport distance	Bones may become disarticulated
Abrasion varies with riverbed type	Single-rooted teeth are more likely to be lost
Riverbed topography may affect bone movement	Algae may stain bone surfaces
	Staining tends to be circumferential
	Matrix tends to become packed into foramina

Adapted from Nawrocki SP, Pless JE, Hawley DA *et al.* (1997) Fluvial transport of human crania. In: Haglund WD and Sorg MH (eds.) *Forensic Taphonomy: The Postmortem Fate of Human Remains.* Boca Raton, FL: CRC Press.

Primary, secondary, and even tertiary taphonomic sequences may modify remains. Secondary and tertiary phases usually ensue if and when the remains change environments or locations. With longer postmortem intervals potential complexity increases, yet the available data may decrease. Evidence for the primary processes of decomposition and scavenger consumption may be superimposed by secondary processes of transport of the body or parts of the body, for example by riverine (**Table 2**) or flood waters. Tertiary sequences, such as associated root growth into bone that reaches a beach after floating, may overlie the signs of water transport.

Because the econiches of plant and animal taxa may be discontinuous and specific, the association of particular species with a set of remains may provide clues about movement of the remains. For this reason, plant and animal remains associated with the body or body part should be treated as potential trace evidence of prior locations.

Interpreting Injury to Bone

Taphonomic data are often critical for the correct interpretation of defects or modifications of bone. Blunt- and sharp-force defects may be related to perimortem trauma or due to postmortem artifact. The term perimortem, as used in forensic taphonomy, refers to the condition of skeletal remains at the time of the modification, rather than the physiological

moment of death. Bone that is fresh has not lost substantial moisture or fat; it will tend to fracture differently than a dry bone. Bone modifications that occurred when the bone was fresh are somewhat distinctive. Vital reaction in soft tissue is used by pathologists to identify changes before death. Vital reaction in bone consists of the build-up of bone tissue associated with healing. However, this is usually not macroscopically visible for up to a week after the injury. Thus, defects in bone, which appear to have occurred while the bone was chemically fresh, and which lack any signs of vital reaction or healing, are assumed to be perimortem, i.e., to have occurred at or around the time of death. Physiologically, the perimortem period can extend into the antemortem and postmortem time frames.

Some defects are difficult to interpret. Nonhuman taphonomic agents can mimic human modifications. (Modifications produced by humans, e.g., due to dismemberment, are also termed taphonomic if they occur after death.) Pseudo cutmarks have been created, for example, by animals that have fallen into natural trap caves, survived for some time, and scratched animal bones in the cave with their hooves. Similarly, large carnivores are able to break the relatively large shafts of human long bones with their jaws, creating perimortem modification that can resemble blunt trauma. In some cases it may not be possible to differentiate human from nonhuman agents for defects occurring in the perimortem period.

Attention to the taphonomic context can be very helpful in ruling out nonhuman taphonomic mimics. The assessment of taphonomic signatures in association with access to the death/deposition scene by particular taphonomic agents can be used to rule out some hypothetical causes of bone defects.

Theoretical and Methodological Issues in Forensic Taphonomy

The development of the theoretical and methodological basis of forensic taphonomy has emerged from research in paleoanthropology, archeology, and paleontology. However, the focus of forensic taphonomists differs. First, the emphasis on the early postmortem period requires that forensic taphonomists pay much more attention to the decomposition of soft tissue. Secondly, forensic taphonomy is an applied science. The primary data, coming from cases involving human death investigation, are often collected from within a sensitive and restricted context. Ethical and legal issues strictly limit research. Rather than experimental design, forensic taphonomy is more likely to utilize individual case studies and case series to develop models and generate hypotheses. Nonhuman animal models have generally been used in taphonomic experimentation. In rare instances, donated cadavers have provided research materials.

The interdisciplinary approach and need for data regarding the taphonomic context have influenced how body recoveries are done. More attention to careful data collection and archeological technique has raised the bar in death investigation. As this field develops, and specialties emerge, it will be critical to maintain interdisciplinary collaboration.

The scientific base for decisions and interpretations in forensic taphonomy will continue to be based on model building and qualitative assessment of probability and goodness of fit of individual cases in the courtroom. Appreciation and articulation of the range of variations is critical, with careful attention to the microenvironmental taphonomic context, comparison with documented taphonomic signatures, and a disciplined process of ruling out competing hypotheses.

Each death is a unique event. Our ability to understand and explain it based on science, i.e., through the application of principles and models, is partially limited by the chaos and random disorder of unique historical sequences. However, forensic judgments about the time and place of death, as well as perimortem injuries associated with the death, are nevertheless enhanced through a disciplined taphonomic approach to both the body recovery and examination.

See Also

Animal Attacks and Injuries: Fatal and Nonfatal; Predation; **Anthropology:** Overview; Archeology, Excavation and Retrieval of Remains; Stature Estimation from the Skeleton; Bone Pathology and Antemortem Trauma; Cremated Bones; Morphological Age Estimation; Pediatric and Juvenile; Sex Determination; Determination of Racial Affinity; Handedness; Role of DNA; **Autopsy:** Procedures and Standards; **Deaths:** Trauma, Musculo-skeletal System; **Death Investigation Systems:** United States of America; **Healing and Repair of Wounds and Bones**; **Injury, Fatal and Nonfatal:** Blunt Injury; **Odontology:** Overview; **Postmortem Changes:** Overview; **War Crimes:** Site Investigation; Pathological Investigation

Further Reading

Bonnichsen R, Sorg MH (eds.) (1987) *Bone Modification.* Orono, ME: Center for the Study of the First Americans.

Byrd JH, Castner JL (eds.) (2001) *Forensic Entomology: The Utility of Arthropods in Legal Investigations.* Boca Raton, FL: CRC Press.

Grauer A (ed.) (1994) *Bodies of Evidence: Reconstructing History Through Human Skeletal Remains.* New York: Wiley-Liss.

Haglund WD, Sorg MH (eds.) (1997) *Forensic Taphonomy: The Postmortem Fate of Human Remains.* Boca Raton, FL: CRC Press.

Haglund WD, Sorg MH (eds.) (2001) *Advances in Forensic Taphonomy: Methods, Theory, and Archeological Perspectives.* Boca Raton, FL: CRC Press.

Lyman RL (1994) *Vertebrate Taphonomy.* Cambridge, MA: Cambridge University Press.

Micozzi MS (1991) *Postmortem Change in Human and Animal Remains.* Springfield, IL: Charles C Thomas.

Morse D, Duncan J, Stoutamire J (1983) *Handbook of Forensic Archaeology and Anthropology.* Tallahassee, FL: Rose Printing.

White TD (1992) *Prehistoric Cannibalism at Mancos 5MTUMR-2346.* Princeton, NJ: Princeton University Press.

Stature Estimation from the Skeleton

T Sjøvold, Stockholm University, Stockholm, Sweden

Introduction

Stature is one of the characteristics that may be used to identify an individual. From birth to adulthood, stature increases until a maximum is reached. However, even during growth, stature is not a fixed measurement for any individual. It is known to decrease slightly during the day, and also with age, especially after about the age of ~30 years. Decrease in stature during the day is mostly caused by compression of the elastic vertebral disks because of the weight carried by the vertebral column. The thickness of the vertebral disks is regained during normal periods of sleep. Normally, the decrease is ~1 cm, but if, for instance, heavy loads are carried, the result may be a decrease of several centimeters. The most important factors causing decrease in stature due to age are the gradual loss of elasticity of the vertebral disks and the individual changes of posture due to aging processes in general.

Together with hair and eye color, stature is given in passports for identification purposes. Though the accuracy of individual stature given in passports has been challenged in forensic journals, such an information may still be regarded as a guideline in cases when stature estimates are being compared with passport information of missing persons. The stature given in the passport may, however, not always have been recorded in connection with issuing the passport. For instance, hearsay information may have been entered, or erroneous values may have been transferred from a previous passport. In addition, stature may have been measured according to different protocols, or at different times of the day. At any rate, however, a deviation of ~1 cm from the figure recorded may be considered as sufficiently accurate.

Estimates of the stature may be obtained from its relation to measurements of the bones of the skeleton. Methods or formulas for estimating the stature from the skeleton may be based on any measurement of any bone or part of bone. In general, the more information about the stature contained in the measurement or combination of measurements the more exact is the estimate obtained. More specifically, the higher the correlation between the body proportions expressed by each measurement and the stature, or the higher the multiple correlation between several measurements and stature, the better the result. However, since in all populations there are individuals with relatively long trunks and short extremities (and also the other way around), there is always a variation in body proportions for any given stature, and consequently, in all populations, for any given bone measurement there is a certain variation in stature. This explains why there is no guarantee that any stature estimate is exact. Every stature estimate has a certain error, which sometimes may be derived mathematically, sometimes empirically, and sometimes not known or mentioned at all.

In principle, any bone may be used, but measurements of one or more of the six long bones provide the most reliable estimates. Methods even exist for stature estimation based on incomplete bones. In general, such an approach starts with the reconstruction of a particular measurement of the complete bone according to mathematical principles. However, if a series of complete bones from some collection of skeletons is available, it is possible to compare an incomplete bone with the complete ones, and then measure the complete bone which matches the size fairly accurately, if such a bone is found.

Because the six long bones of the skeleton are paired, some methods based on these bones have been restricted to only one side. The argument in such cases is that the counterpart from the opposite side is almost equal in length. The bone from any side may therefore be used, but when the complete pair is available, the mean measurement of right and left bone should be inserted.

Methods for Estimating Stature from the Skeleton

The source materials for developing methods for stature estimation from the skeleton differ in character. They are of three basic types:

1. Collections of cadavers where cadaver lengths have been measured before and bone measurements taken after maceration. It had already been observed by the end of the nineteenth century that the length of the cadaver tended to be about 2.5 cm longer than the actual stature of the individual when living. This is explained by the relaxation of ligaments and vertebral disks as well as a flattening of the vertebral curvature after rigor mortis. This means that the bone measurements are exact, but stature has to be adjusted, both concerning the amount that has to be subtracted because of the extension of the corpse as well as corrections because of reduction due to age.
2. Collections of living individuals where stature is known but the bone lengths have to be estimated from corresponding somatometric measurements on the body. In this case, it is possible to select the material so that reduction of stature due to age is eliminated. Thus, in this case stature is known, but the bone lengths have to be estimated. The advantage of such a method is that large samples may be collected by measurement of individuals according to the same protocol, the disadvantage is the errors introduced when bone lengths are estimated.
3. Collections of individuals where both stature when living as well as bone lengths after death are known. These are considered ideal if it is not influenced by older individuals whose statures have been reduced due to age.

Four different principles have been applied for stature estimation from the skeleton. The apparently most simple is based on crude ratios between the stature and the skeletal measurements, because for every individual the stature may be expressed by the skeletal measurement multiplied by a certain factor. But within any collection of individuals, the different factors vary slightly from individual to individual. Attempts have been made to use factors based on the mean measurements of the bones, assuming more or less explicitly that the error made compared to the exact proportion between stature and bone length for a given individual is small. So far, however, the actual standard errors connected with the use of crude factors have not been calculated. The errors made therefore remain unknown, which is a disadvantage of the method.

The second principle is based upon regression equations, either as simple regression equations, when the stature is estimated from one bone measurement, or multiple regression equations, when the stature is estimated from several measurements simultaneously. Simple regression is a method in which the stature is calculated as a product of the bone measurement and a factor plus a constant term. Multiple regression involves differential weighting of the bone measurements used which means that the factors with which to multiply each of the bone measurements are differentiated according to the importance of the measurement. The stature is calculated as the sum of products of each measurement and individual factors plus a constant term. All factors and constant terms are mathematically determined from a source material where both stature and bone measurements are known according to one of three types of source materials. For this process least-squares linear regression is used. This is a mathematical method that minimizes the standard error of the stature estimate, and from that point of view this is the best choice for estimating stature. It should not be confused with an alternative solution by which stature is estimated from each bone measurement used by means of simple regression, and the mean of the estimates is regarded as the final stature estimate. The standard error of this method is, however, not simply the mean of the standard errors, because the bone measurements used are already correlated to some degree. Some of the information used is therefore common to each of the simple regression equations. Because of this, it is not advisable to use the mean value of several simple regression estimates, though it is frequently done. It is clear that the standard error of a mean value of simple regression estimates is larger than the standard error of a multiple regression estimate based on the same measurements, although how much larger has not been investigated for any of the methods published. Since multiple regression equations involve as many dimensions as the number of measurements involved, as well as the stature, such equations may be difficult to conceive, whereas simple regression equations are only bivariate and easy to understand. Since simple regression estimates of the stature based on different bone measurements generally differ, an estimate based on the mean value of the estimates may be felt to be more reliable than an estimate based on any particular simple regression estimate. Such an estimate is based on information from all bone measurements involved, though some of the information is duplicated because of the correlation between the measurements, in contrast to multiple regression where the duplicated information has been mathematically eliminated.

One negative property of least-squares regression that had been overlooked for a long time in stature estimation research was that, at least from a mathematical point of view, the tallest individuals tended to be underestimated and the shortest overestimated. The reason was that only the error between the actual and the estimated statures in the source materials was considered because the method aimed at minimizing the sum of squares of the errors.

The third principle aims at reproducing correctly the stature of the tallest and the shortest individuals, at the cost of a slightly higher standard error. This kind of method has, so far, only been developed for situations comparable to simple regression, estimates of stature based on the measurement of one bone at a time. It is related to least-squares regression. The method, known as the reduced major axis method, minimizes the sum of products of the deviation between actual and estimated stature and corresponding actual and estimated bone measurements in the source material. This kind of equation may also well be used in order to estimate the bone measurement from the stature, whereas this is not even possible for simple regression, because another regression equation is needed.

Another problem is that the regression line passes through the mean values of the bone measurements as well as the mean stature. The mean values as well as the correlation between the bone measurements and between the bone measurements and stature are used for the calculation of the different factors and constants used in the regression equations. Because every method is based on a given source material, the mean values and the correlations involved are estimates. If this is taken into account, the standard error is a minimum at the calculated mean values, but tends to broaden in a doubly hyperbolic fashion if the mean values are increased or decreased. The reason is that errors of the direction of the calculated regression line compared with that based on the parent population from which the sample is obtained are taken into account. However, although this problem in stature reconstruction from the skeleton is occasionally mentioned in the forensic literature, it is secondary when compared with the number of methods from which to choose in a given case.

The fourth principle is called the anatomical method. It is based on the sum of measurements of the skull height, the individual vertebrae of the vertebral column, the femur, tibia, and talus and calcaneus in articulated position, to which estimates of missing soft tissue are added, depending on the sum of the measurements.

Development and Use of Methods for Stature Estimation from the Skeleton

Developments before World War II

A large number of methods for estimating stature from long bones are still in use, though a small number dominates. The earliest attempt that has still some relevance today was published by Manouvrier in

France in 1893. The material used was taken from an earlier thesis in forensic medicine by Rollet who studied the relation between the long bones of the skeleton and the length of dissection-room cadavers. Following a long, theoretical discussion, Manouvrier provided a series of tables giving the estimated stature for each of the six long bones. These tables have been used and reprinted several times even after World War II.

Manouvrier's tables were empirical, and it seems that the values used in the tables have been smoothed. The range of variation of the stature and corresponding bone lengths was restricted, depending on the measurements available. For bone lengths outside the tabulated range, crude factors were given with which to multiply the bone length to estimate the stature. But if the values in the tables are plotted, it is seen that the proportion between stature and bone lengths changes along the tabulated range of variation, whereas it is fixed outside the tabulated range, a contradiction which Manouvrier did not realize. What was formally estimated, however, was the cadaver length, since a dissecting-room material was used, but it was already known that the length of the cadaver exceeded that of the stature of the individual when living by an amount of approximately 2.5 cm, which therefore had to be subtracted from the estimate.

In 1899 one of the most influential methodological papers on how to estimate stature from the skeleton was published by one of the world's greatest statisticians, Pearson, who introduced the principle of regression, which had been developed a little more than a decade earlier. Regression equations have been used for almost all subsequent methods for estimating stature. Pearson used the same material as Manouvrier, but provided a mathematical solution, in contrast to Manouvrier's empirical solution.

Pearson also turned to the problem of whether the formulas developed using a French sample might be applied to other populations and to prehistoric individuals. Pearson's test case was the Ainu from northern Japan, where a number of skeletons had been excavated. Since the statures of the individuals excavated were not known, it was assumed that their mean stature corresponded to the mean stature of the living Ainu, which in modern terms would imply that no secular changes were assumed to have occurred. The regression equations developed based on the French material seemed to fit well even to the Ainu.

Thirty years later, in 1929, the physician Stevenson working in Peiping published new formulas for Chinese individuals, based on a dissecting-room sample from northwestern China, in the journal *Biometrika* edited by Pearson. Contrary to Pearson's findings, he found that the proportions of the French material did not correspond with those of the Chinese sample, so that Pearson's regression equations should not be applied to Chinese, nor should the regression formulas developed by means of the Chinese sample be applied to the French or to the Ainu for that matter. Pearson added a lengthy editorial note to the paper, where he concluded that regional regression methods had to be developed, and also that regression equations had to be developed separately for each sex because of differences in body proportions.

Following Pearson's advice, a number of regression methods based on national criteria, i.e., from China, France, Finland, Germany, Greece, India, Japan, Portugal, and the USA have been published, and continued until the present century. The most comprehensive study before World War II was carried out by the German anthropologist Breitinger, who measured the stature of 2428 male athletes and their limb proportions as a starting point to estimate the corresponding long bone measurements. This is so far the largest study of measurements on living individuals used for estimates of stature from the skeleton.

Developments after World War II

A major breakthrough was made during the 1950s by the anthropologist Trotter and the statistician Gleser. They developed new regression equations based on measurements of long bones from World War II casualties, from the battlefields of the Pacific, in connection with a repatriation program after the war. The identity of each individual was known, as well as the stature when living. Thus both the actual stature and the bone lengths were known, a situation which was ideal. Since only males were included, regression equations for females were developed based on female skeletons from a dissecting-room collection. Prior to the calculation of the regression equations, another study based on dissecting-room skeletons had provided information about the actual decrease in stature due to age, so that age could be corrected for when necessary. A second, similar opportunity offered itself in connection with repatriation of US war casualties from the Korean war. This time regression equations were calculated for males only.

One particular result was that the regression equations from the Korean war differed slightly from those of the Pacific war. The reason was that the mean stature had increased slightly, affecting body proportions involving the long bones as well. Trotter and Gleser concluded that stature is in "a state of flux" and stressed not to use a regression equation for a different population than the one for which it had been developed.

The regression equations by Trotter and Gleser have been by far the best-known method during roughly the last half century. They have been and are still widely used, not only because they are based on a source material which is close to ideal from a methodological point of view, but also because formulas for groups of different ethnic affiliations had been developed, i.e. for Caucasian, Mongoloid, Mexican, and American Blacks. Since it is well known that secular changes of stature occur, however, and that people in virtually all countries have become taller during the last 100 years, the choice of which regression formula to use may be difficult when the mean stature of the background population of an individual is not known. This is particularly a problem in many forensic cases when a more-or-less complete skeleton of an unknown individual exists. The problem is even greater if the sex is also unknown.

Two different approaches have been made to overcome this problem. One approach by the anthropologist Sjøvold is based on an observation made by another anthropologist, Olivier, who in the early 1960s compared regression equations by Trotter and Gleser with regression equations based on a collection of identified skeletons from German concentration camps which had been measured in connection with a repatriation program after World War II. Olivier discovered that the simple regression lines were literally parallel, at a distance which roughly corresponded to the difference in the mean stature between the source materials. Supported by still more examples, it appeared that the stature/long-bone length proportion tended to be dependent on or to adapt itself to the stature.

The approach used was called "the line of organic correlation," a generalization of the reduced major axis method, and was used for Caucasian samples at first. This seemed to solve a forensic problem, that the nationality of a skeleton discovered did not seem to be necessary in order to estimate the stature. As for the need for different equations for males and females, it was discovered that much of the difference in body proportions could be explained by differences in stature, and it was therefore possible to make a synthesis of previous methods for stature estimation, valid for both sexes, based on mean values of stature and long-bone measurements. For dissection-room samples, which generally consist of old individuals, it was assumed that the postmortem extension of the corpse roughly amounted to the decrease in stature due to old age, as far as mean values were concerned. In forensic cases, the mean stature of the parent population of an individual is unknown. But it may be inferred that the most likely stature of that individual should be close to the mean value. Statistically speaking, the "expected" value of the stature is equal to the mean value of the parent population. The same arguments are applicable to the different ethnic groups, which led to a synthesis for worldwide populations.

Another argument for the use of a synthesis is that the different source materials used are ill defined from a genetical point of view. What is known is only that they were available, whereas the genetical relations between the individuals are unknown. It is even unlikely that all the individuals of a certain material originated from the area where they were studied. Strictly speaking, therefore, they just represent samples of "humans," characterized by certain mean statures and certain long-bone length proportions.

Another approach was based on the observation that the relationship between the mean stature and the mean length of the femur appears to be fairly stable around the world. Feldesman made a worldwide survey of similar samples for which the synthesis based on mean values was made. It may be inferred that similar assumptions have been made for use of the different types of source materials. This is an example of the use of a crude factor. Although the survey was based on the relation between the measurement of the femur and stature, the reverse relationship was used to estimate the stature from the length of the femur, based on the stature/femur relationship of 3.74. Although it may be shown empirically that this factor tends to overestimate tall and underestimate short individuals, one argument for its use is that every regression equation (or any mathematical formula for estimating stature from the skeleton) has a standard deviation, and tests showed the method to provide more exact results than those obtained by means of regression equations. Later tests, however, showed that a generic regression, quite similar to the weighted line of organic correlation, provided even more exact results. A standard deviation of the estimates based on the stature/femur relationship was not given, which means that only point estimates were used.

In late 1950s, the so-called "anatomical method" was developed by Fully. The source material was the identified skeletons which had been repatriated from the German concentration camps. This method consists of the sum of the basibregmatic height of the skull, the height of the vertebrae from "axis" through the first sacral vertebra, the bicondylar length of the femur, the physiological length of the tibia, and the articulated height of the talus and calcaneus. For skeletal heights between 153.5 and 165.5 cm, 10.5 cm was added to account for soft tissue, for skeletal heights above 165.5 cm, 11.5 cm should be added and 10.0 cm should be added for those below

153.5 cm. This method is independent of ethnic affiliation as well as of sex. The drawback is that it is very cumbersome to use, and requires a complete skeleton. The empirical error is the smallest among all methods for estimating stature, amounting to about 2.5 cm.

Recommendations

The more that is known about the individual such as sex and ethnic affiliation, the better. The method developed by Fully is, in principle, the best one to use, but it is very cumbersome and requires a complete skeleton. Use of regression equations based on regional samples is recommended if the mean stature fits the parent population from which the individual case derives. The methods by Trotter and Gleser are widely used, though based on a source material with a mean stature shorter than today, whereas Sjøvold's method circumvents the problem of the mean stature of the parent population. It should be recollected that all methods based on mathematical principles aim at an estimation of the maximum stature of an adult individual before decrease due to age. For older individuals, therefore, the correction derived by Trotter and Gleser should be used, subtracting 0.06 (age at death − 30) cm from the estimated stature for individuals older than 30 years.

See Also

Anthropology: Cremated Bones; Morphological Age Estimation; Determination of Racial Affinity

Further Reading

Fully G (1956) Une nouvelle méthode de détermination de la taille. *Annales de Médicine Légale* 36: 266–273.

Krogman WM, İşcan MY (1986) *The Human Skeleton in Forensic Medicine.* Springfield, IL: Charles C. Thomas.

Manouvrier L (1893) La détermination de la taille d'après les grands os des membres. *Mémoires de la Societé d'Anthropologie de Paris* 4: 347–402.

Olivier G, Aaron C, Fully G, Tissier G (1978) New estimation of stature and cranial capacity in modern man. *Journal of Human Evolution* 7: 513–518.

Pearson K (1899) On the reconstruction of stature of prehistoric races. *Transactions of the Royal Society, Series A* 19: 169–244.

Rösing FW (1988) Körperhöhenrekonstruktion aus Skelettmaßen. In: Martin R, Knußmann R (eds.) *Anthropologie: Handbuch der vergleichenden Biologie des Menschen. Begründet von Rudolf Martin,* vol. 1, pp. 586–600. Stuttgart: Fischer.

Sjøvold T (1990) Estimation of stature from long bones using the line of organic correlation. *Human Evolution* 5: 431–447.

Stevenson PH (1929) On racial differences in stature long bone regression formulae, with special reference to stature regression formulae of the Chinese. *Biometrika* 21: 303–321.

Trotter M, Gleser GC (1951) The effect of ageing on stature. *American Journal of Physical Anthropology, New Series* 9: 311–324.

Trotter M, Gleser GC (1952) Estimation of stature from the long bones of American Whites and Negroes. *American Journal of Physical Anthropology, New Series* 10: 463–514.

Trotter M, Gleser GC (1958) A re-evaluation of stature based on measurements taken during life and long bones after death. *American Journal of Physical Anthropology, New Series* 16: 79–124.

Bone Pathology and Antemortem Trauma

S M Black, University of Dundee, Dundee, UK

Introduction

The analysis and description of human remains for the purposes of assisting medicolegal investigations in assigning a personal identity to the deceased center around the premise that throughout an individual's life span, a variety of alterations to the body will occur that will be sufficiently unique to serve much as a fingerprint does for identification. The greater the number, variety, and severity of insults that a body endures throughout its lifetime, the more individual and distinctive is that person with regard to antemortem and postmortem comparison. Whilst many of the insults the body sustains may remain untreated or warrant no consultation with a clinician, the more significant the injury or trauma, the more likely it will be to leave an imprint on the skeleton and the more likely that it will warrant medical attention whether through the family doctor, the accident and emergency room, or the clinical specialist. Recourse to one or any combination of these three medical pathways will result in a formal recording of the incident and the initiation of a paper trail which will be vital to a successful investigative process and ultimately identification of the deceased. There are a variety of insults that manifest on the human skeleton and they generally fall under the headings of pathological conditions or the remnants of scars of previous traumatic injuries.

This article provides a brief overview of some of the bone pathologies and antemortem traumas that might be encountered by the forensic anthropologist and illustrates how these can be utilized to assist in the identification of the deceased. This article is not intended to be comprehensive, as only a selected few conditions can be introduced due to the restrictions of space. It is also important to realize that the types of traumatic injuries and the manifestation of pathological conditions are geographically distinctive and individual to a country, a continent, or a particular conflict. Therefore whilst some of the conditions discussed here may be typical of the northern hemisphere, they may prove rare elsewhere.

Bone Pathology

The interpretation of pathologies relies on the accurate differential diagnosis of the disease or condition presented. A pathological condition is not a static event and the presentation detected on the deceased is merely a "snapshot" of the condition at that particular moment. The condition may be in its early stages of presentation, it may be at its most active, it may be in a process of remission, or the investigator may simply be witnessing the scars of a healed and cured condition. Therefore it is important to realize that the same pathology can present in a number of forms dependent upon its phase of activity and the manner in which each individual will respond to that insult.

A pathological skeletal condition is first recognized as an appreciable alteration to the anticipated "normal" appearance of the bones and fundamentally results from an alteration to the normal equilibrium between bone formation and bone resorption. Bone is produced by osteoblasts and removed by osteoclasts and any interference with the status quo will result in an imbalance of their normal rate of activity or indeed an overabundance of one particular cell type. The appearance of excessive new bone formation can be as much a result of increased activity in osteoblasts as it is a decreased activity in osteoclasts and of course the opposite is equally true, where an appreciable alteration in bone loss can arise through an excessive stimulation of osteoclast activity or a reduction in normal formation rates. Whilst the addition and removal of bone can occur as a simple alteration in volume resulting in a bone simply becoming larger/smaller or more dense/rarefied, the reality is that abnormal stimulation of osteoblasts and osteoclasts tends not to result in a "normal" bone appearance and therefore there is not only a quantitative alteration that alerts the anthropologist to the presence of a condition but it is more likely that the qualitative appearance of the bone will be the first element to attract attention and highlight an abnormality.

Both systemic and local factors can influence cell activity and cell population density and will include aspects of endocrine control, invasion of pathogenic organisms, viruses, and fungi. As fundamentally every manifestation arises from the actions of only two cell populations (osteoblasts and osteoclasts), it is not surprising that different diseases can produce remarkably similar characteristics and a differential diagnosis will require that a number of factors be assessed.

The visual manifestation of skeletal disease can present as:

- abnormal bone formation (e.g., periostitis)
- abnormal bone destruction (e.g., osteoporosis)
- abnormal bone density or bone type (e.g., osteogenesis imperfecta)
- abnormal bone size and/or shape (e.g., achondroplasia).

The form and distribution of a condition may be classified as:

- solitary abnormality with a single focus
- bilateral multifocal abnormality
- randomly distributed multifocal abnormality
- diffuse widely distributed condition.

Any alteration to the quality or quantity of the bone will either be directly visible to the naked eye or may only manifest when the remains are subjected to additional forms of analysis, including imaging (radiology, computed tomography scans, etc.), microscopic examination, and chemical analysis.

The classification of bone pathologies is extremely variable but a simple classification is shown in **Table 1**. It is clear that many conditions will span more than one category and there is no satisfactory classification system that is specific to each condition. For example, leprosy is an infectious disease that can manifest as an arthropathy.

Table 1 General classification of bone pathologies

Infectious diseases, e.g., tuberculosis, leprosy, osteomyelitis
Circulatory disturbances, e.g., aneurismal erosion, osteonecrosis
Reticulo-endothelial and hematopoietic disorders, e.g., anemias, leukemia, myeloma
Metabolic disorders e.g., rickets, fluorosis, scurvy
Endocrine disturbances, e.g., pituitary dwarfism, hyperthyroidism, acromegaly
Congenital and neuromechanical abnormalities, e.g., hydrocephalus, kyphosis, spina bifida
Dysplasias, e.g., achondroplasia, osteogenesis imperfecta, osteopetrosis
Tumors and like lesions, e.g., benign tumors, fibroblastic tumors, malignant tumors
Arthropathies, e.g., osteoarthritis, rheumatoid arthritis, gout

Abnormal Bone Formation

Proliferative reactions that characterize bone hypertrophy encompass a vast array of clinical conditions, including hemorrhagic conditions, inflammatory reactions, tumorous growths, circulatory disturbances, metabolic disorders, endocrine disorders, and other less specific conditions.

1. An example of a solitary abnormality with a single focus would be button osteomata (**Figure 1**). These are benign neoplastic lesions of dense lamellar bone that almost exclusively occur on the outer diploic table of the skull, either in the frontal or parietal regions. This condition presents as small discrete raised areas of smooth bone of approximately 1 cm in diameter that are sharply demarcated and rounded in profile. They are more common in males and of greatest frequency in the fourth and fifth decades. These "buttons" also become more noticeable with advancing age as they are more clearly defined on a bald head than on a head covered with hair. As a result, these can be useful corroborators of identity if photographs of the deceased or missing person are available for comparison. They are not uncommon, being present in 1% of autopsy material, and are even well documented in archeological material.

2. An example of a bilateral, multifocal abnormality would be osteoarthritic change (**Figure 2**). There are three dynamic components involved in the skeletal manifestation of osteoarthritis and they involve both bone loss and bone addition. There is: (1) a breakdown of articular bone which can ultimately result in damage to the subchondral bone; (2) eburnation of the articular surface; and (3) new growth of cartilage and bone at the joint margins (osteophytes). Osteoarthritis is a progressive condition that is characterized by the number of joints that become involved as the condition develops, with the joints of the vertebral column usually the first to display perceivable symptoms, followed by the knee, first metatarsophalangeal joint, hip, shoulder, elbow, acromioclavicular and sternoclavicular joints. Although there is likely to be a hereditary factor involved in the manifestation of this condition, it is closely correlated with advancing age.

3. An example of randomly distributed multifocal abnormality is typical of an infectious condition such as syphilis where the periostitis in the long bones can become complicated by ulceration of the overlying skin which will result in additional bone morphological alterations. Diffuse non-gummatous periostitis leaves the bone thick and dense, affecting not only the periosteal surface but often the entire compact structure of the tubular diaphysis.

4. An example of a diffuse widely distributed condition would be periostitis, which can be a widespread inflammation of the periosteum that covers every bone in the human skeleton. The condition can be isolated and mild, e.g., local inflammation, or can be widespread and more distinctive, as would be found in hyperostosis with pachydermia.

Abnormal Bone Loss

As with the section above, specific examples of pathological conditions could be listed that would fit within each of the criteria concerning location, distribution, and type of manifestation, but it is clear that many conditions cross the boundaries resulting in a somewhat unsatisfactory and perhaps therefore relatively meaningless categorization of conditions. Therefore classification may have its practical uses

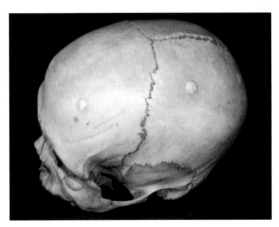

Figure 1   Button osteomata on the frontal and parietal bones.

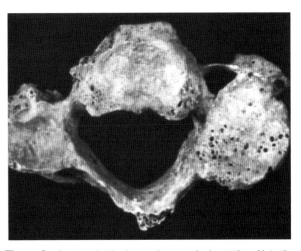

Figure 2   Osteoarthritic change in a cervical vertebra. Note the addition of bone around the superior articular facet and the margins of the body.

for differential diagnosis but within the limited scope of this contribution it would become little more than a meaningless list.

Osteopenia, osteoporosis, and osteolysis are the terms usually applied to an abnormal loss of bone. Osteopenia is a rather nebulous term that depicts a general loss of bone volume without direct specificity as to the cause. Conversely, osteoporosis depicts a normal quality of bone but an abnormal quantity. The classical understanding of osteoporosis is related to the postmenopausal condition in women where the amount of bone resorption surpasses bone formation and bone loss continues unchecked, resulting in an ultimate failure in the biomechanical properties of the structure. Osteoporosis is a widespread phenomenon that principally affects the cancellous structure and hence has implications for age-related fracture in the vertebral column, hip, and wrist. However, its involvement in the alteration of the biomechanical properties of compact bone should not be overlooked (**Figure 3**). Osteoporosis is naturally age-related but other predisposing conditions, surgical intervention (e.g., hysterectomy), and the side-effects of a variety of drugs can all lead to a rarefaction of bone volume.

Osteolysis can be a singular lesion or multiple discrete areas of bone loss and is easily visualized through infections such as leprosy or tuberculosis (**Figure 4**). Tuberculosis is a chronic infectious disease caused by either *Mycobacterium bovis*, which can be transmitted to humans from byproducts of cattle – normally milk or, more commonly, by direct transmission between humans through *M. tuberculosis* via respiratory contamination, with the primary focus being in the lungs. The bacilli circulate in the blood stream and locate within the skeleton, usually with preference for areas of hemopoietic activity, e.g., vertebral column, tarsals, ribs, and sternum. More than 40% of skeletal tuberculous lesions involve the vertebral column, perhaps because it represents the largest location of cancellous bone, but it is also known that the bacilli thrive under conditions of high oxygen tension and the vertebrae have a particularly well-developed arterial supply. In the column, the earliest detectable focus of blood-disseminated tuberculosis occurs in the region of the cartilaginous endplate at the anterior aspect.

Almost all pathological conditions can therefore be summarized according to:

- the amount of bone formed
- the type of bone formed
- the location of that new bone
- the amount of bone lost
- the location of the lost bone
- the overall shape and size of the resultant bone.

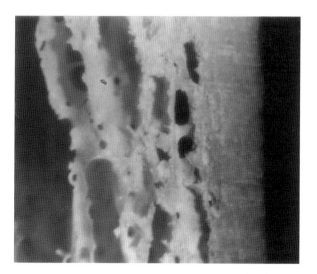

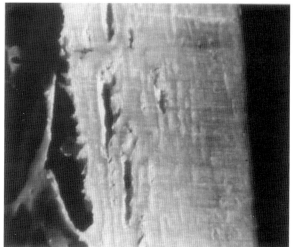

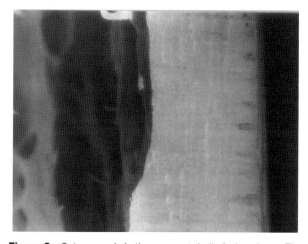

Figure 3 Osteoporosis in the compact shell of a long bone. The young individual at the bottom of the figure shows a dense cortex whilst with age it becomes more rarefied and lamellated.

The manifestation may be localized or widespread, single or multifocal, and occur within the range of minimal manifestation to gross representation. The pattern of manifestation will vary from individual

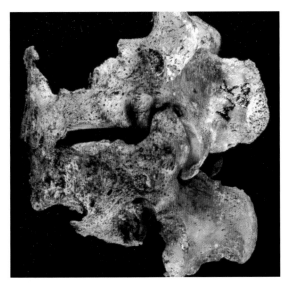

Figure 4 Tuberculosis in the vertebral column. The extensive lytic lesions in the bodies of the vertebrae result from abscess formation.

to individual, depending on the stage of progression of the condition when viewed and the degree of manifestation displayed by that individual. Therefore classification of pathological conditions is highly dependent on a number of specific factors that will govern the reliability of the differential diagnosis.

Antemortem Trauma

The extent to which trauma is displayed in the human skeleton is largely dependent upon a number of factors, including:

- the nature and severity of the trauma
- the time lapsed since the trauma was inflicted
- the degree and success of repair to that injury
- the presence/absence of infection subsequent to the injury.

Trauma generally arises through contact between the skeleton and external influences, although pathologies such as some of those considered above can lead to biomechanical insufficiencies, resulting in traumatic material failure. Rather than the trauma itself being the indicator of presence, often it is the remnants of a callus formation or the subsequent posttraumatic deformity that gives clues as to the condition that may have occurred. Forensic anthropologists are particularly practiced in the identification of recent and healed traumas that affect the skeleton.

Again, there are no clear boundaries between the classifications of antemortem trauma, but a broad grouping could include:

1. accidental trauma (e.g., fractures, dislocations)
2. traumas resulting from intentional and deliberate violence (e.g., gunshot injuries)
3. cultural/cosmetic-induced trauma (e.g., Chinese foot-binding)
4. therapeutic trauma (e.g., surgical intervention).

Fracture

It is clear that fractures can occur across all four categories above and can arise through both blunt, sharp, and crushing trauma scenarios as well as intentional breaks caused for therapeutic and even cosmetic purposes. Fracture is defined as a discontinuity or crack in skeletal tissue with or without injury to overlying soft tissues. Fractures arise when external forces exceed the normal sustainable plasticity of the structure when applied either directly or indirectly to the bone. There are a number of classifications for fractures but they tend to fall largely within five possibilities:

1. Tension fracture: these are generally associated with tendon attachments to bone and are frequently associated with athletic injuries and referred to as avulsion fractures. Complications following this form of fracture can include an impairment of the normal operation of the joint through the inability of the tendon to reattach to the appropriate location, dislocation of the joint, or necrosis of the attachment site of the muscle.
2. Compression fracture: these are the result of sudden and excessive impaction and have a variety of manifestations. This type of fracture is commonly seen in the vertebral column of osteoporotic individuals or following impact from an implement where radiating fractures can be seen emanating from the original compression area (**Figure 5**). If the bone is depressed, then this can result in a circular pattern of fracture around the initial impact site and this is most clearly seen in injuries to the skull.
3. Twisting or torsional fracture: in this situation the force is directed in a spiral orientation when one end of a limb is fixed and the other is free to rotate. Sports injuries are frequently of this nature and because the force is in a spiral direction, so is the pattern of the fracture.
4. Bending, angulating fractures: these are probably the most common form of fracture and occur as a result of the pressures of a fall or the response to an external force coming in contact with the bone. The maximum stress tends to occur at one specific area but a compensating tensile fracture can also occur on the opposing surface of the bone (**Figure 6**). In a young person where the bone is

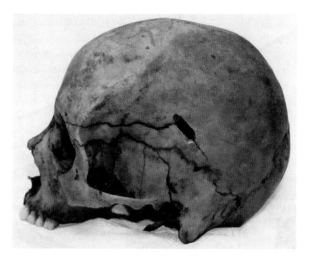

Figure 5 Tumbling bullet entry wound in the parietal bone. Note the radiating fracture lines that pass forwards into the frontal bone, backwards and inferiorly into the temporal bone.

highly mobile and elastic this can result in a "greenstick" fracture, where there is an incomplete transverse break in the bone and in this case the bone will subsequently heal with little residual evidence.

5. Shearing fracture: these occur when opposite forces are applied to bone in slightly different planes. For example, a Colles fracture of the wrist occurs when force is transferred up through the heel of the palm and the radius is sheared due to its firm attachment via the interosseous membrane.

Fractures are also classified with regard to the nature and severity of the distortion:

- A simple fracture involves a single clean break with only one separation of the bone (**Figure 6**).
- A comminuted fracture occurs when many fragments of bone are displaced. Comminuted fractures are more likely to result in poor alignment and bone shortening which allow easier detection of the fracture even after a considerable time has elapsed since the event. Of course, surgical intervention for fracture reduction and to address re-alignment issues can leave orthopedic hardware in the body and this is an obvious indicator of previous trauma (**Figure 7**).
- A compound or open fracture results when the overlying skin is broken, thereby giving potential access to factors leading to infection. Acute fracture complications can include shock, hemorrhage, fat embolism, thromboembolism, gas gangrene, and secondary infection with septicemia. Osteomyelitis is an inflammation of bone and bone marrow caused by pus-producing bacteria. Compound fractures are a common cause for osteomyelitis, usually

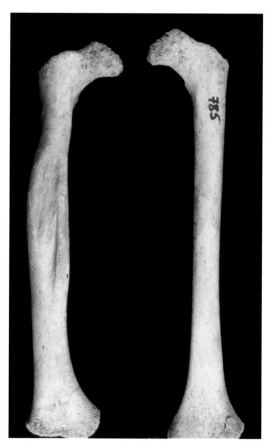

Figure 6 Fracture of the right femur of a juvenile. Note the extensive callus formation and overall thickening of the shaft. Misalignment has led to a foreshortening of the affected bone.

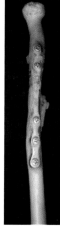

Figure 7 Fracture of the proximal one third of the shaft of the radius with orthopedic plating.

through introduction of either staphylococcal or streptococcal bacteria. The manifestation of acute osteomyelitis is usually most obvious in tubular long bones where there is abscess formation and necrosis. Sequestrae form when an area of necrotic bone becomes surrounded by living bone and at the same time detached areas of periosteum become stimulated to form new bone – an involucrum – which can become perforated by cloacae, which are channels through which the abscess can drain from the bone into the soft tissues and eventually perforate the skin to form a fistula.

- A simple or closed fracture does not involve an opening of the skin and therefore potential exposure to infection is significantly reduced.

Gunshot Trauma

The degree to which a bullet or trajectory will damage a bone is dependent on a number of factors, including the type of bullet, its velocity, distance from the target, angle of trajectory, and any deflections. When a bullet passes through bone a characteristic set of wounds is produced and these will be different if the bullet is passing through compact, cancellous, or diploic bone. For example, in the skull, when the bullet strikes the outer diploic table it indents the bone and punches through, resulting in a rounded defect with little, if any, beveling of the bone at the entry margin. As the bullet exits through the inner table, small fragments of bone are displaced, resulting in an internal beveling. Conversely, as the bullet passes out of the skull it will pass cleanly through the inner table and leave beveling on the outer table (**Figure 8**). As the bullet passes through the bone small fragments of metal may be stripped from it and these can often be detected on a radiograph, as can other forms of ballistic residue (**Figure 9**). If the bullet strikes the bone at an oblique shallow angle, a characteristic defect, often referred to as a "keyhole" defect, occurs.

Radiating fracture lines are caused by the impact and they will follow weaknesses in the bone

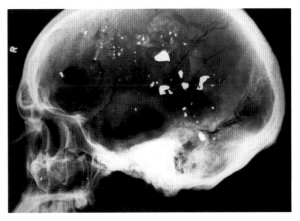

Figure 9 Metal fragments within the skull as a result of gun shot residue. Courtesy of M Warren, University of Florida.

microstructure. Fracture lines will stop when the energy dissipates or when they meet a foramen, a suture, or a preexisting fracture (**Figures 5** and **8**). If the ballistic energy is high, then fracture lines may meet a suture, follow it for a while, and then continue through the adjacent cranial bone. Concentric fractures are caused by an increase in intracranial pressure created as the soft tissue is compressed by the bullet. Extensive concentric fracturing occurs when gases expelled from the gun enter along with the bullet.

Sharp-Force Trauma

This includes all kinds of injury caused by a weapon or an implement with a sharp edge or point and generally results from stabbing-type injuries. The most common type of weapon is a knife, although other sharp implements such as axes or machetes combine a sharp edge with a heavy element, producing injuries that have both sharp and blunt impact features (**Figure 10**). It is not unknown for the tip of a knife to be snapped and remain embedded within the bone. When removed, the resulting wound is generally conical in shape with smooth edges. Axes, machetes, and other flat-bladed implements tend to produce elongated V-shaped grooves and valuable information can be gained about the weapon involved using scanning electron microscopy of the incised bone surface.

Amputations

Amputations can arise under a number of circumstances:

- natural accident
- surgical intervention
- war injuries
- social punishment/torture
- ritual.

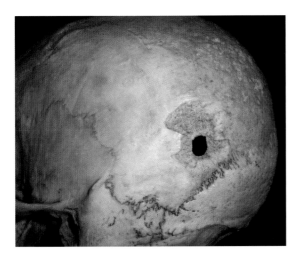

Figure 8 Gunshot exit wound in the occipital bone. Note the bevelling on the outer table but there is only one radiating fracture line halted by the lambdoid suture.

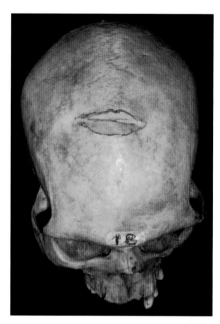

Figure 10 Machete injury to the top of the skull. The sharp impact of the blade can be seen in the center but the concentric depressed fracture that surrounds it is a clear indication of a heavy impact injury.

It is important to be able to separate a true amputation from a malunion following fracture and subsequent resorption of one section. Postamputation survival of less than 1 week will produce no detectable signs of healing. However, around 14 days postamputation, the severed bone end commences callus formation and therefore provides skeletal evidence of survival of the incident and the commencement of a healing process. The rounded end of the bone begins to smooth over and the medullary cavity becomes obliterated at the stump end (**Figure 11**).

Other mutilations such as intentional deformity (head-binding, foot-binding, etc.), scalping, defleshing, trephination, and crucifixion all leave their marker on the skeleton, as can traumas such as strangulation and decapitation. The list is virtually endless.

Summary

It is not possible to summarize adequately the range of pathologies and antemortem traumas that can be evidenced from the human skeleton in an article such as this and the list of suggested reading below will allow the subject to be considered in much greater detail and depth. Therefore just a few features have been selected for illustration to offer a flavor of the abundance of information that is available to forensic anthropologists to permit them to confirm the identity of the deceased through the route map of the insults and injuries of a lifetime. Pathologies and

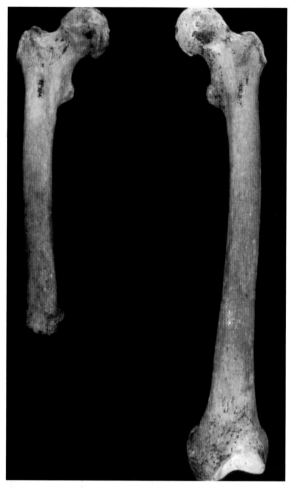

Figure 11 Amputation of the right thigh in the lower third of the shaft. Note the rounded stump indicating a considerable survival time after the event (in this specimen that was actually 55 years).

traumas are highly specific in terms of geography, often being indicative of a country or a continent, and patterns of antemortem trauma can be equally specific.

See Also

Anthropology: Overview; **Body Recovery**; **Deaths:** Trauma, Musculo-skeletal System

Further Reading

Aufderheide AC, Rodriguez-Martin C (1998) *The Cambridge Encyclopedia of Human Palaeopathology.* Cambridge, UK: Cambridge University Press.

Browner BO, Jupiter JB, Levine AM, Trafton PG (2002) *Skeletal Trauma.* New York: Saunders.

Di Maio VJM (1999) *Gunshot Wounds: Practical Aspects of Firearms, Ballistics and Forensic Techniques,* 2nd edn. Boca Raton, FL: CRC Press.

Nance EP (2001) *Skeletal Trauma: A Radiologic Atlas.* New York: Saunders.

Ortner DJ (2003) *Identification of Pathological Conditions in Human Skeletal Remains*, 2nd edn. New York: Academic Press.

Payne-James J, Busuttil A, Smock W (2003) *Forensic Medicine: Clinical and Pathological Aspects*. London: Greenwich Medical Media.

Rogers LF (2001) *Radiology of Skeletal Trauma*. London: Churchill Livingstone.

Scheuer JL, Black SM (2000) *Developmental Juvenile Osteology*. London: Academic Press.

Schwamm HA, Millward CL (1995) *Histologic Differential Diagnosis of Skeletal Lesions*. Maryland: Lippincott, Williams and Wilkins.

White TD (1999) *Human Osteology*. New York: Academic Press.

Cremated Bones

P Holck, University of Oslo, Oslo, Norway

Introduction

In most western countries, fire ranks as the fourth largest accidental killer, after motor vehicle accidents, falls, and poisoning. Victims of fire are commonly either the very young or elderly people. This may be because very young and elderly individuals are physically unable to escape from a fire and they may also have less tolerance for toxic gases. Most deaths are primarily due to smoke inhalation, lack of oxygen, and poisoning by carbon monoxide or other toxic gases. With the exception of mass deaths in fire accidents, heat is the direct and immediate cause of death in only a few cases.

The purpose of the investigation of cremations is not only to identify the victim but also to determine the circumstances leading to an accidental or intentional death, which makes it one of the most difficult forensic–anthropological tasks. Bone is commonly well preserved, but the level of preservation is closely related to temperature changes, and the characteristics of bone may be an indication of its thermal history. Because fire often reduces a skeleton to minute fragments of bones and teeth, termed cremains, the police investigation should be carried out in close collaboration with forensic anthropologists. An untrained person who is unfamiliar with cremated bones may not be aware of the information such pieces could produce. A famous letter from the renowned Swedish anatomist and anthropologist Carl Magnus Fürst to the chief inspector of antiquities in Stockholm, written in 1930, claimed that "cremated remains of human bones in burial urns are almost without any anthropological interest, especially in cases of such in a mass cemetery. From an anthropological point of view, therefore, these bones are of no scientific value." Unfortunately, this was a common attitude to forensic cases until a few decades ago.

Degrees of Burning

Since the intensity of temperature and oxygen supply are essential factors in the evaluation of body remains and in their possible identification, these factors are discussed first. When we study cremated bones, we soon discover that most of the material has been burnt to different degrees. Some of it is sooty, some is pale in color, almost chalky, and some does not seem to have been cremated at all. Relying on colors alone to indicate temperature may lead to error because the heat may have a local effect that is difficult to evaluate. The nature of the ground in which the bones are found should also be taken into consideration.

Even in large fires, the effect of the heat may be restricted to small areas as a result of draught, oxygen supply, and the size of the room. When studying forensic material, sometimes one part of the body of a corpse is completely charred and destroyed while another part is almost unburned (**Figure 1**).

From a technical point of view, the following factors are necessary for cremation: (1) a combustible material; (2) adequate ignition temperature; (3) sufficient supply of oxygen; and (3) technically suitable conditions. The human body contains both combustible substances, such as fat and proteins, and noncombustible substances, such as water and inorganic matter. When substances burn completely, they produce heat. When they do not, they need more heat. The thermal energy released when a substance burns is the positive heat of combustion, whereas the energy needed to burn a substance completely is the negative heat of combustion.

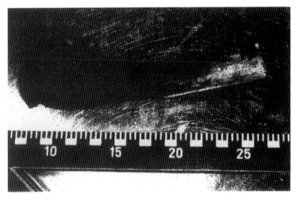

Figure 1 Local effect of fire on a thigh bone. Photo courtesy of P Holck.

Table 1 Distribution of combustible and noncombustible substances of a "normal" adult human body (70 kg), compared with that of a newborn baby (3 kg), with corresponding heat of combustion given in kcal kg^{-1}

	Substance	Weight (kg)	Heat of combustion (kcal kg^{-1})	Total (kcal)
Adult				
Combustible	Fat	11	8500	93 500
	Protein	13	5000	65 000
Noncombustible	Water	42	539	22 638
	Ash	4	200	800
Total		70		≈135 000
Newborn baby				
Combustible	Fat	0.3	8500	2500
	Protein	0.4	5000	2000
Noncombustible	Water	2.2	539	1200
	Ash	0.1	200	100
Total		3.0		≈3200

Reproduced with permission from Holck P (1997) *Cremated Bones. A Medical–Anthropological Study of an Archaeological Material on Cremation Burials*, 3rd edn. Oslo, Norway: University of Oslo, Anatomical Institute.

The total heat of combustion of a human body is the difference between its combustible and noncombustible substances (**Table 1**). Accordingly, cremation of a normal body creates surplus heat. However, a lean person will give out less surplus heat and in certain circumstances may be impossible to cremate completely (e.g., people who have suffered from weight-reducing diseases, such as cancer and tuberculosis). Infants and small children have a much lower body fat content than adults, and their released combustion heat produces only approximately 2% of what an adult body can produce. As a result, a child may be difficult to cremate (**Table 1**).

If the temperature is low and the supply of oxygen is reduced during cremation, combustible and toxic carbon monoxide will be formed instead of noncombustible carbon dioxide. In the first case, the flue gas will be dark, due to precipitation of carbon. To avoid this, modern cremations normally take place when the temperature of the incinerator has exceeded 650 °C – this is the ignition temperature of carbon monoxide.

Cremation and destruction of a human body require less heat than is commonly expected. The grade of burning depends on: (1) the temperature induced; (2) the duration of the heat; and (3) the oxygen supply. Finding melted substances, such as glass or metal, provides an idea of the temperature reached and may sometimes offer information that can assist in identification (e.g., surgical devices). It is known from modern domestic house fires that even cast iron can melt, and this indicates a temperature of more than 1550 °C. The remains of people who perish in such circumstances show great similarity to the most strongly cremated bones in archeological finds.

Classifying bones according to their different grades of cremation may therefore sometimes provide information about the temperatures and circumstances associated with the process that led to a person's death. Normally, five grades are used:

1. In grade 0 the bones are minimally affected by heat and show no external signs of having been burnt. However, this does not mean that the body has not been exposed to fire, but rather the soft tissues have all formed an insulating layer against the surrounding heat, which may have reached 150–200 °C for several hours. This may still be sufficient to destroy the collagen: this may be tested by placing bone pieces into an acidic solution such as 5% phosphoric acid. Grade 0 bones are more often found to be of interest in archeological finds than in forensic cases. However, destruction of cell material means that cremated bones are normally unsuitable for DNA analysis.

2. Grade 1 displays a bony surface of dull, grayish-black color, which may be a sign of incomplete burning due to a lack of oxygen. The changes in color can be followed deep into the bone. It is difficult to determine any upper temperature limit at this grade because carbon deposit depends more on oxygen supply than on temperature. It is, however, reasonable to assume that the temperature was not greater than 400 °C, since changes in the bone structure normally occur at this temperature.

3. Grade 2 indicates that the oxygen supply has been adequate but the heat-induced alterations to the structural nature of the bones are still moderate, probably due to shorter exposure rather than insufficient temperature. There are no longer signs of carbon deposit on the bone surface, but the interior of the bone may sometimes have a sooty appearance. The difference between grades 1 and 2 relates to the thickness of the compact layer. When heated between 400 °C and 700 °C, the color of the bone lightens from black to light gray and then to white. The hardness of the bone remains unchanged.

4. Grade 3 is most commonly found in archeological material. The bones have a cracked appearance and, when the surface is scratched with a sharp tool, a white stripe is left, unlike grade 2 bones. The stripe is an indication that the bones have reached temperatures in excess of 700 °C and that the organic matter (and water) has been completely removed. At this stage, the hardness of the bone increases considerably. There is

Table 2 Bone changes at different temperatures

	Temperature in °C	Changes in bone
Grade 0 ↓	100	Insignificant changes in bone and teeth. Collagen still intact
Grade 1 ↓	200	Only superficial color changes in bone and teeth. Considerable reduction of collagen. Nuclei (DNA) destroyed
	300	Weight reduction, loss of water. Modestly reduced volume. Collagen completely destroyed. Color: brownish/dark gray
Grade 2 ↓	400	Lowest solidity of the bone structure. Formation of microscopic fissures in the bone surface. Small cracks in the enamel of the teeth. Color: black/dark gray
	500	Deformation of the bone. Larger, net-shaped microscopic cracks in the bone surface. Color: grayish
	600	Further macro- and microscopic cracks in the bone surface. Formation of pyrophosphate (salts of heated phosphoric acid). Color: light gray
	700	Further reduction of the volume due to fusion of mineral crystals.
Grade 3 ↓		Liberation of water of crystallization. Previously formed pyrophosphate compounded with hydroxyapatite to whitlockite. Shrinkage and changes in lamellar construction of the Haversian systems
	800	Further shrinkage and deformation. Further fusion of the mineral crystals in the bone. Melting and crystallization of the dentine, but still without destruction of the dentine tubuli. Color: white/gray
	900	Marked macroscopic cracking of the bone surface. Destruction of the osteon structure. Further fusion of the mineral crystals. Cracking, melting, and destruction of the enamel of the teeth
	1000	Microscopic oval holes of various size in the bone surface. The dentine appears as ball-shaped formations with the tubuli still intact. Color: white, chalk-like structure
Grade 4 ↓	1100	Melting of the dentine tubuli
	1200	Total decomposition of the microstructure in bone and teeth

Reproduced with permission from Holck P (1997) *Cremated Bones. A Medical–Anthropological Study of an Archaeological Material on Cremation Burials*, 3rd edn. Oslo, Norway: University of Oslo, Anatomical Institute.

marked shrinkage due to fusion of mineral crystals in the bone, and the contents of α-tricalcium phosphate are transformed into β-tricalcium phosphate or whitlockite, which marks the transition from grade 2 to grade 3. When heating exceeds 800 °C, the lamellar pattern of the bone is lost, which reduces the efficiency of microscopic methods used in the examination. Also, bone shrinkage is more significant in this grade of cremation – up to 25% length reduction has been observed in human bones – which makes estimation of individual height unreliable.

5. Grade 4 is easy to recognize by the chalk-like appearance of the bones. At this extreme grade, the bones have been exposed to temperatures higher than 1100 °C. The nature of bone seems to have changed completely. The color is white, the weight is reduced, the bone has a porous, chalk-like consistency, and bones are mostly found as small, fragile fragments, often impossible to identify anatomically (**Table 2**).

Bones Commonly Found after Burning

When findings of cremated bones are examined, certain parts of the skeleton appear to be preserved more often than other structures. Bones from the neurocranium are commonly found as pieces of up to 10 cm in size, but bones from the facial skeleton are only occasionally found as such large fragments. This means that facial reconstructions of thermally decomposed bodies are unlikely to be possible. When an adult is exposed to temperatures of approximately 700 °C, the face becomes a skeleton within 15 min.

If the forehead is more or less intact, the frontal sinus should be examined and compared with X-rays of the presumed individual because the shape appears unique and thus this may be an important part of the identification work. Despite its thin and unprotected structure, the neurocranium is frequently found because of the insulating quality of the brain and cerebrospinal fluid. However, teeth, which are otherwise used to identify deceased persons, crack when they are exposed to heat. Enamel crowns are commonly lost while the roots remain intact; teeth of younger individuals usually resist heat better than those of elderly people. Thus, it is often not possible to use teeth of people exposed to fire for identification purposes (**Figure 2**).

The vertebral column is commonly well preserved: this may be related to the position of the body during burning. However, the sternum, ribs, clavicles, and scapulae are seldom seen in cremated material, probably because of their delicate shape and unprotected site in the body.

Pieces of long bones can be found as fragments which are several centimeters long. Phalanges are seldom found in burnt forensic material, as opposed

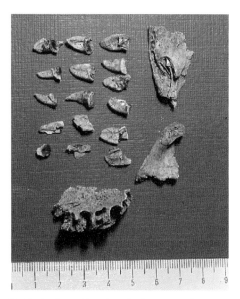

Figure 2 Typical remains of teeth after cremation: only the root dentine is preserved. Photo courtesy of NG Gejvall.

Table 3 Cross-section diameters of Haversian canals in humans and some domestic animals

Species	Average diameter (μm)
Humans	52.9–71.6
Cattle	47.9
Pig	32.8
Dog	21.2
Goat	21.2
Sheep	18.2
Goose	15.7
Hen	14.0
Rabbit	12.6

After Hunger H, Leopold D (1978) *Identifikation*. Berlin: Springer-Verlag.

to in archeological finds, where these bones are seen relatively often: this may be explained by the local influence of cool open air as opposed to indoor fires. Also, the pelvis is seldom found, despite its protected site in the body, with the exception of pieces from the most solid parts.

Human or Animal?

In both forensic and archeological cases, there may be doubt as to the provenance of the bones: are the pieces human or not?

Animals have much thicker, more compact bone than humans. Their trabecular units are a different size and shape, and this gives a heavier and more solid appearance than comparatively more porous and lighter human bones. The line between the spongy and the compact part of animal bone is also less distinctive than in human bones. Their outer/inner surface is often smoother and gives the examiner a feeling of unbreakable solidity.

Some experts recommend microscopic examination to distinguish human from animal bones of uncertain origin, because the human Haversian canals are much wider than those of animal bones (Table 3). In cremations, the examiner should pay more attention to macroscopic and morphologic–anatomic differences, even when limited, than to microscopic ones, because the bone shrinks and deforms, and can be very difficult to assess.

Determination of Sex

This is, of course, very important in all examinations. It should be based on common anatomical features,

even if macro- and microscopic techniques have also been applied. It should be kept in mind that sexing cremated bones is very difficult and uncertain and requires more material than any other examination. It is common for more than 50% of cremated bone material to remain undetermined. This may be surprising to the police and others unfamiliar with such examinations, but it is always better to present a smaller number of certain determinations than a more impressive series based on suggestions.

It is well known that the degree of sexual dimorphism varies between individuals and between different human races; nevertheless, the cremation process will sometimes emphasize sexually dimorphic criteria. Since larger and heavier parts of the skeleton, usually associated with men, are normally better preserved than smaller parts, some experts have suggested that sex criteria appear in cremated material as distinctly as in intact bones.

Measurements and sexing based on mathematical or statistical methods should be used with the greatest care. As previously mentioned, the original shape of the bones shrinks and deforms in an unpredictable way. In fact, distinguishing features that are supposedly certain, such as the narrow male sciatic notch, may change into a wide, female-appearing structure after cremation in an incinerator.

Estimation Of Age

Since there can be considerable miscalculations of certain age groups, especially in cremated material, the term "age determination" should be avoided. It is well known that the accuracy of age estimations in human skeletons decreases in proportion to age. This means that children's age may be determined with relatively high accuracy, whereas age estimations of older persons are connected with miscalculations of 10–15 years or more, if the age can be estimated at all.

Epiphyseal closure and tooth development are normally used to estimate skeletal age in children and young individuals. Adult age is frequently estimated on suture closure and root transparency of the teeth are frequently used, even though these criteria are associated with inaccuracy and individual variations. In cremations, however, tooth development is commonly unsuitable as a criterion of aging because heat easily cracks enamel and turns roots opaque.

Even the shape of the pubic symphysis can seldom be used as a criterion for age estimation because this part of the skeleton is rarely found preserved after exposure to fire. Neither is the morphology of the sternal end of the ribs helpful, because this part of the body normally appears skeletonized after only 20 min at a temperature of 700 °C.

Since so many methods for estimating age are unreliable, the skull sutures should be used to study age development when examining cremated bones, because skull pieces with sutures are often found. It is important to remember that the sutural pattern is controlled by biological factors alone, and unaffected by external, individual changes: the bones of the neurocranium undergo a slow process of fusion from early childhood to old age.

Cremated bones have one advantage: the cracking of the sutures allows for the study of their fractured edges as well as the skull surface. Their pattern changes with age, even before any sign of ossification can be seen on the external surface of the skull, and their total appearance may thus indicate the person's physical age to a relatively high degree of accuracy (**Figure 3**). By studying the suture of a young person, it can be seen that the only fusion of the skull bones is a thin zone near the internal lamina. This zone forms the first visible ossification of the suture at 10–12 years; it increases in thickness and reaches the external surface of the skull as the suture closes completely at old age.

Although anatomical determination of the examined skull fragments is often difficult or impossible, one is still able to give an indication of individual age because all the fractured edges undergo approximately the same age-related changes, even though the suture closure does not occur simultaneously. This is therefore a more reliable measure of age development than the sutural pattern seen on unburnt skulls. It is also important to consider the increasing thickness of the skull vault with age when aging cremated bones (**Figure 4**).

Theoretically, a rough estimation of age on postcranial parts of the skeleton can be assisted by studying the changes in the microstructures, because the width of the Haversian systems normally increases with age. However, the shrinkage of the bone

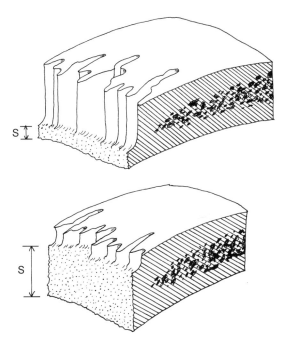

Figure 3 Age development of skull sutures. Top: a piece of the neurocranium from a young individual is shown with a short fractured ossification surface (S); bottom: the same surface is shown from an older person with a high fracture surface. Reproduced with permission from Holck P (1997) *Cremated Bones. A Medical–Anthropological Study of an Archaeological Material on Cremation Burials*, 3rd edn. Oslo, Norway: University of Oslo, Anatomical Institute.

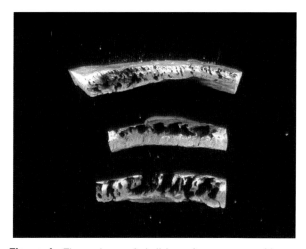

Figure 4 Three pieces of skull bone from persons of known age, with edges displaying an increase in the ossification line. Top: bone from an 85-year-old: complete closure of the suture (i.e., the ossification has reached the external surface of the skull); middle: bone from a 58-year-old: half of the skull bone is ossified; bottom: bone from a 37-year-old (bottom): only the internal lamina is ossified. Photo courtesy of P Holck.

substance, especially above 700–800 °C, may result in miscalculations.

The approximate age of children can sometimes be estimated by measuring the transversal diameter of the long bones, if these are preserved, in addition to examining the epiphyseal closure.

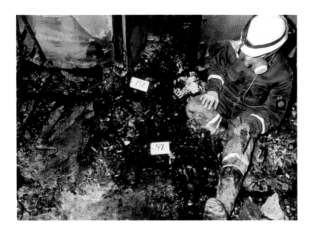

Figure 5 Situation from a mass disaster. Separation of cremated remains should, if possible, be executed by forensic anthropologists. Photo courtesy of the National Bureau of Crime Investigation, Oslo, Norway.

Height

In cremated material, it is not possible to estimate height with the same accuracy as in unburnt bone material. In cremations, long bones are rarely found to be complete and measurable; if they are, shrinkage must be considered. Also, correlations between the breadth, which is less often destroyed, and the corresponding length of the bone could theoretically be used and directly transferred to common anthropological tables (**Figure 5**).

Commercial Cremations

The first incinerator was constructed by the Italian professor Lodovico Brunetti and presented at the World Exhibition in Vienna in 1873. It attracted enormous attention, and after improvements made by the German engineer Friedrich Siemens, the first commercial cremation occurred in Germany in 1874. Two years later, the first crematorium was built in Milan, Italy, and soon most of the larger cities in Europe and the USA followed suit.

The frequency of cremations differs throughout the western world but may exceed 85% of all burials in some larger cities. Cremation is more prevalent in Protestant countries than in Catholic ones.

The incinerators are mainly of two kinds: electric or oil-heated. Because the normal body creates a certain surplus of heat during cremation, the temperature inside the incinerator will increase. It therefore starts at 650–700 °C, which is the lowest temperature for the prevention of formation of toxic and explosive gases. From the moment the corpse is placed inside, a sharp increase in temperature occurs (exothermal reaction), caused by the ignition of the most combustible parts of the body and surrounding materials

(e.g., the shroud and coffin, usually after 3–5 s), despite a constant supply of heat energy from the incinerator. After 40–50 min, the temperature will decrease during cremation of the less combustible parts of the body. However, the final temperature will be approximately 50 °C higher than the initial temperature after each cremation.

Because of the incinerator's increasing radiant heat, in addition to the higher temperature of combustion gases, some of the surplus heat will gradually disappear so that the final temperature increase will be 200–300 °C or more after a "normal" series of cremations during a work day. Each cremation normally lasts 1–2 h.

When the cremation ends, the bone remains are placed in a metal box to cool. There may still be large pieces of bone that are cracked and twisted but sometimes complete. The remains are then placed into a crushing machine to be transformed into the small bits appropriate for urns. The contents of urns are commonly called "ashes" but are actually bone fragments of several millimeters.

Unfortunately, some countries allow the ashes to be spread in nature as a sort of ceremony instead of a cemetery burial. Finds of such human bones can create many problems for police and forensic experts. Even pet animals are sometimes cremated, put into urns, and dispersed in the countryside.

Conclusion

The effect of fire on soft tissues and bones in a human body can be compared to a mechanical injury, where the depth of burning depends on temperature, the length of exposure, and the supply of oxygen to the part of the body in contact with the heat. The significance of the body's fat content has been mentioned previously. Also, the type of clothing influences the rate of burning.

Examinations of cremated bones are difficult, and the investigator must be very reserved, careful, and exact. It is difficult to make assured determinations of sex, age, and height, which are all important factors in the identification work of a forensic anthropologist.

However, some pathological changes and injuries can sometimes be found in cremated bones and these may lead to identification, although only 10% of modern western diseases cause changes in the skeleton. Cut marks can occasionally be seen and identified by their smooth and flattened edges, in contrast to the curved heat-induced cracking of bone; microscopic fractures can commonly be seen in the surface line of the impact area.

See Also

Anthropology: Overview; Bone Pathology and Antemortem Trauma; Autopsy, Findings: Fire

Further Reading

Holck P (1995) Why are small children so seldom found in cremations? In: Smits E, Iregren E, Drusini A (eds.) *Cremation Studies in Archaeology*, pp. 33–38. Amsterdam: Logos Edizioni, Saonara.

Holck P (1997) *Cremated Bones. A Medical–Anthropological Study of an Archaeological Material on Cremation Burials*, 3rd edn. Oslo, Norway: University of Oslo, Anatomical Institute.

Holden JL (1994) *Heat-Induced Physical, Chemical and Structural Alterations to Human Bone*. Victoria, Australia: Monash University.

Hunger H, Leopold D (1978) *Identifikation*. Berlin: Springer-Verlag.

Murray KA, Rose JC (1993) The analysis of cremains: a case study involving the inappropriate disposal of mortuary remains. *Journal of Forensic Science* 38: 98–103.

Richards NF (1977) Fire investigation – destruction of corpses. *Medical Science Law* 17: 79–82.

Ubelaker DH, Jacobs CH (1995) Identification of orthopedic device manufacturer. *Journal of Forensic Science* 40: 168–170.

Morphological Age Estimation

E K Simpson, Forensic Science Centre, Adelaide, SA, Australia

Introduction

Estimation of age from the skeleton is based on the knowledge that during a person's life his/her bones are constantly undergoing changes, and that these changes follow a chronological pattern. In the early stages the skeleton is characterized by the development and growth of bones and dentition, in the form of ossification centers and tooth buds. In childhood and adolescence, bones take shape and grow, and epiphyses develop and fuse with diaphyses. In the dentition, teeth grow and erupt, and deciduous teeth are lost and replaced by permanent teeth. When adulthood is reached, the basic skeleton is complete, but age changes are visible in the obliteration of sutures, changes in trabecular and microstructure of bone, and other degenerative changes.

When an attempt is made to estimate the age of skeletal remains, it is important to distinguish between age at death and time since death. Age at death is the estimation of the age of the person when he/she died, whereas time since death refers to the amount of time that has passed since the person died. Age at death can be estimated with reasonable accuracy, depending on the amount of skeletal material present, the parts of the skeleton that are represented, and the condition of the remains. Time since death is much harder to estimate due to the great variation produced by environmental factors such as burial depth, type of soil, and climatic and seasonal fluctuations. In this article, only the estimation of age at death will be discussed.

Estimation of age at death also needs to take into account the difference between chronological age and biological, or skeletal, age. Chronological age refers to the age of the individual measured in units of time (usually in months/years since conception or birth). Biological age refers to the age of a person based on the development and health of his/her bones in comparison to normal standards. A person who has suffered ill health throughout life and has not had access to regular medical treatment may appear at death to be considerably older in biological rather than actual chronological age. A person who suffered from a serious illness or from malnutrition during childhood may exhibit signs of a delay in maturation, and his/her bones will appear to be younger than the actual chronological age. When a skeleton is examined for the purpose of estimating age, it is only the biological age that can be interpreted. The relationship between chronological and biological (or skeletal) age is not constant, nor is it linear, which adds to the difficulty of estimating age. As a result, factors such as delays or advances in development and/or variability in the rate of degeneration on the skeleton need to be considered when estimating chronological age. For age estimation, sex and population of origin also need to be determined before attempting to age the skeleton. This is because population factors influence the aging process in individuals, as do differences due to sex.

Methods used in forensic anthropology to estimate age at death are usually based on population standards, generated from the major population groups around the world. However, individual variation between people from within the same population is often overlooked or underestimated. It can be difficult to estimate the age of an individual with accuracy when he/she is viewed in isolation from other specimens, as is usually the case in forensic situations. Variability in the skeleton arises through genetic and biological influences, and ultimately is the basis for our individuality, i.e., there is no such thing as an "average" individual. Over the years, scientific study has generated data that describe the central tendency of biological traits, for example, the most common age that epiphyseal union occurs in a particular bone. This average age has been established through the study of normal people – those who vary from the average to an acceptable level (nonpathological development). Therefore, when estimating the age of an individual, the scientist will always include an estimate of the possible variation due to age for that feature. This can be interpreted as an estimate of how closely the age of that person resembles the central tendency of the population. For example, estimating the age of a person using the rate of closure of cranial sutures is very variable, and age estimates are generally based on decades of development, with a standard error of about 5–10 years. It is for this reason that many researchers believe it is best to obtain an age estimate from as many sites as possible, and arrive at an overall age estimate based on a summary of all the findings.

Generally, seven age groups are used when assessing human remains. These are: (1) fetal (before birth); (2) infant (0–3 years); (3) child (3–12 years); (4) adolescent (12–20 years); (5) young adult (20–35 years); (6) middle adult (35–50 years); and (7) old adult (50+ years). Due to the amount of growth present in fetal, childhood, and adolescent years, estimation of age can usually be determined to quite a narrow range. Estimation of age of adults is complicated by individual variation in senescence, which is influenced by interactions between genes, culture and environment, and the individual. Often, it is only possible to assign a skeleton to a particular decade or period of life.

Estimating Subadult Age

There are a number of criteria that can be used to estimate the age of a subadult individual. These include eruption of the dentition, epiphyseal fusion, and measurement of the diaphyseal length of long bones. Estimation of fetal age is not always straightforward, due to variation in developmental factors. Consequently, relying on the size of bones as a means of estimating age has some associated problems. Modern research has established the existence of a close relationship between the development of the cervical vertebrae and age, which seems to be more reliable than some of the more traditional methods. Advances in medical imaging have also allowed better investigation of tooth germ formation and dental eruption.

The pattern of eruption of the dentition has been established through the study of development of teeth of people of known ages, generally through observations taken on longitudinal X-ray data. These studies have published findings on the times of formation, eruption, and loss of the deciduous dentition, and the formation and eruption of the permanent dentition. When estimating subadult age from the dentition, careful examination of the skull and comparison with the reference diagrams in the literature should enable an age estimation to be made.

Subadult age can also be estimated from the growth of long bones, in the fusion and union of the epiphyses, the ends of the bones, and in the overall length of the diaphysis, or shaft (**Figure 1**). A long bone usually has three centers of ossification – the diaphysis, which is the primary ossification center; and two epiphyses, the secondary ossification centers. Some long bones only have one epiphysis, but others, such as the long bones of both upper and lower limbs, have two epiphyses. Each epiphysis has a layer of cartilage called the epiphyseal plate, which lies between the epiphysis and the diaphysis. This is where growth of the long bone takes place. Cessation of growth occurs with the union of the epiphyses and the diaphysis. The stages of fusion between epiphysis and diaphysis have been carefully documented through research. A summation of the degree of epiphyseal fusion in different long bones in the body can be used to estimate age. The age at which epiphyseal fusion occurs varies according to population, sex, and individual differences. Females undergo epiphyseal fusion about 2–3 years earlier than males. Consequently the average female has a shorter period of growth and smaller body size than the average male. The last epiphysis to fuse is at the medial end of the clavicle. The average age at which this fuses is around 21 years of age. There is also a considerable variability, with reported findings of complete fusion at 18 years of age in some individuals, while other individuals aged over 30 years still had incomplete fusion.

Estimating Adult Age

Timing of cranial suture closure was one of the first techniques used to estimate the age of adult

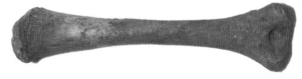

Figure 1 Neonatal right humerus. Note the unformed ends where the epiphyses are yet to fuse.

individuals. It is well known that the sutures between cranial bones ossify at different times during life. The sphenooccipital suture on the skull base is particularly useful for aging young adults, as fusion is completed in 95% of individuals between 20 and 25 years. The other cranial sutures show more variation in timing of closure. Sutures ossify on the endocranial surface before they ossify on the ectocranial surface, and this must also be taken into account when using this method. Overall, most researchers conclude that cranial sutures can be used to estimate age, but that their inherent variability makes them considerably less useful than other morphological characteristics.

Adult age can be estimated from the dentition based on patterns of wear and attrition; however this is fairly unreliable unless the individual is from a population whose pattern of wear is known to be fairly homogeneous. Other factors, such as variability caused by diet, pathology, or the use of teeth as tools must also be taken into account when estimating age from the dentition (**Figure 2**).

Estimation of age of adult skeletal remains can also be performed on the pelvis. The surface of the pubic symphysis shows degenerative changes during life. An understanding of the systematic osteological changes that the normal symphysis undergoes enables an estimation of age at death to be made. In young adults, the symphyseal surface is rugged in appearance and is characterized by horizontal ridges. By age 35, the sharp features of the surface are less defined, and a rim forms around the edge. The following years are characterized by progressive degenerative changes, including formation of a rough symphyseal surface,

and irregular borders. Until recently, the most commonly used method for estimating age using the architecture of the pubic symphysis was that of Todd, who described 10 stages of pubic symphysis change during aging. More recently, researchers Suchey and Brooks described six phases of degenerative change in the pubic symphysis. These phases are well described but still suffer the limitation of relatively arbitrary classification of a continuum of change in a biological structure.

Degenerative changes in the epiphyseal surfaces of the vertebrae, in the form of osteophytes, develop in individuals from about the mid-20s onwards. These signs of vertebral osteoarthritis can be used to estimate age by judging the severity of the lipping around the superior and inferior borders of the vertebrae. Using this method, an individual can be categorized as being from a particular decade of life at the time of death (**Figure 3**).

Recent Developments in Age Estimation

Since the 1980s, traditional morphological methods of age estimation have been supplemented by newer methods. These include histological and microradiographical examination of bone structure and the analysis of mitochondrial DNA of skeletal muscles. Age can be assessed histologically by counting the number of osteons and other structural factors of lamellar bone which have been found to be correlated with age. This technique has also revealed high variability in bone structure at the microscopic level, from factors such as nutritional status, sex, hormones, and mechanical loading. However, this method is also destructive, and as a result should only be performed when all other examinations have been conducted on the bone in question. Examination of microradiographs of bone has also been useful for estimating age. This technique is based on the correlation between increasing age and loss of bone through natural remodeling processes. While this method does not destroy bone tissue, interpretation is also subject to the same factors of variability seen macroscopically in bone. Other studies have been instrumental in verifying the validity and reliability of the traditional methods used to estimate age, for example, recent studies confirming the inherent variability in ectocranial suture closure and pubic symphyseal surfaces. Studies on the sternal end of the fourth rib suggest that this feature is a much more accurate and reliable method of estimating age. Other researchers have used larger sample sizes and more complex data-processing and statistical methodology to test and validate hypotheses originating from earlier research.

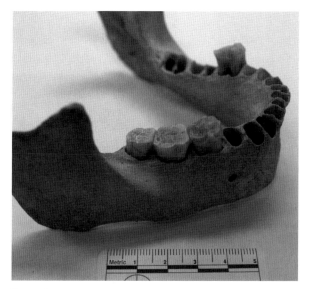

Figure 2 Mandible with worn molars as a result of an abrasive diet in addition to normal aging.

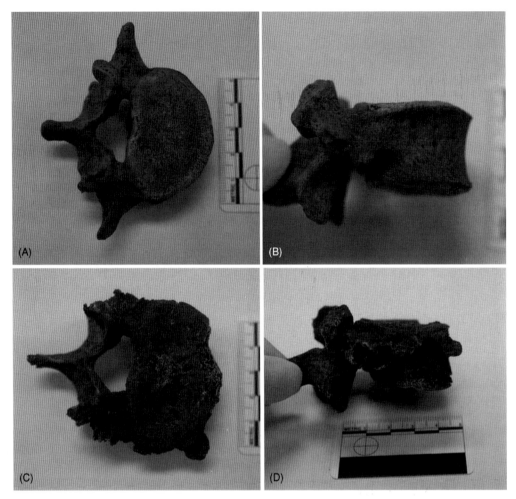

Figure 3 Contrast between a normal vertebra ((A) superior view, (B) lateral view, right side) and one showing age-related pathology ((C) superior view, (D) lateral view, right side). Note the superior and inferior lipping of the vertebral body margins, as well as the large osteophyte on the anterolateral region. Other degenerative changes can be seen on the superior surface, including pitting and Schmorl's nodes.

The above review has highlighted a number of methods for the morphological estimation of age. The choice and application of these methods will depend on the condition and completeness of the specimen being examined, and on the presumptive age estimation (adult versus subadult). Partial or incomplete skeletons may be restrictive in the amount of information available for assessing age. Complete skeletons are much more informative and age estimations based on this material are generally quite accurate and reliable. Most authors suggest using a multifactorial approach to age estimation for maximum reliability, but others propose selecting a single factor, such as the auricular surface of the ilium, with other anatomical regions given a lesser role. It is difficult to conclude which is to be preferred, but for the most part, the possibility of error due to method, technique, or inexperience is most likely to be reduced by applying as many different methods of age estimation as possible.

See Also

Anthropology: Overview; Archeology, Excavation and Retrieval of Remains; Taphonomy; Stature Estimation from the Skeleton; Bone Pathology and Antemortem Trauma; Cremated Bones; Pediatric and Juvenile; Sex Determination; Determination of Racial Affinity; Handedness; Role of DNA

Further Reading

Baccino E, Ubelaker DH, Hayek LA, Zerilli A (1999) Evaluation of seven methods of estimating age at death from mature human skeletal remains. *Journal of Forensic Sciences* 44: 931–936.

Bass WM (1995) *Human Osteology: A Laboratory and Field Manual,* 4th edn. Columbia, MO: Missouri Archaeological Society.

Dudar JC, Pfeiffer S, Saunders SR (1993) Evaluation of morphological and histological adult skeletal age-at-death estimation techniques using ribs. *Journal of Forensic Sciences* 38: 677–685.

Herschkovitz I, Latimer B, Dutour O, et al. (1997) Why do we fail in aging the skull from the sagittal suture? *American Journal of Physical Anthropology* 103: 393–399.

Iscan MY (2001) Global forensic anthropology in the 21st century. *Forensic Science International* 117: 1–6.

Iscan MY, Loth SR, Wright RK (1984) Metamorphosis at the sternal rib end: a new method to estimate age at death in white males. *American Journal of Physical Anthropology* 65: 147–156.

Iscan MY, Loth SR, Wright RK (1987) Racial variation in the sternal extremity of the rib and its effect on age determination. *Journal of Forensic Sciences* 32: 452–466.

Krogman WM (1978) *The Human Skeleton in Forensic Medicine*. Springfield, IL: CC Thomas.

Meindl RS, Lovejoy CO (1985) Ectocranial suture closure: a revised method for the determination of skeletal age at death based on the lateral-anterior sutures. *American Journal of Physical Anthropology* 68: 57–66.

Meissner C, von Wurmb N, Schimansky B, Oehmichen M (1999) Estimation of age at death based on quantitation of the 4977-bp deletion of human mitochondrial DNA in skeletal muscle. *Forensic Science International* 105: 115–124.

Murray KA, Murray T (1991) A test of the auricular surface aging technique. *Journal of Forensic Sciences* 36: 1162–1169.

Scheuer L, Black S (2000) *Developmental Juvenile Osteology*. London: Academic Press.

Schmitt A, Murail P, Cunha E, Rouge D (2002) Variability of the pattern of aging on the human skeleton: evidence from bone indicators and implications on age at death estimation. *Journal of Forensic Sciences* 47: 1203–1209.

White TD (2000) *Forensic Osteology*. San Diego, CA: Academic Press.

Yoshino M, Imaizumi K, Miyasaka S, Seta S (1994) Histological estimation of age at death using microradiographs of humeral compact bone. *Forensic Science International* 64: 191–198.

Pediatric and Juvenile

L Scheuer, Royal Free and University College Medical School, London, UK

Introduction

Forensic anthropology may be defined as the identification and analysis of human remains for medicolegal purposes. This procedure normally begins with the establishment of the four basic parameters of biological identity – sex, age, stature, and ethnicity – and, if successful, proceeds to the confirmation of personal identity. In the case of immature remains, both the demonstration of these factors and the techniques required are of an order different from those needed for adults. The forensic anthropologist can be called upon to confirm a suspected identity or assist in the identification of unknown skeletal remains from homicides, suicides, and unexplained or natural deaths. The forensic anthropologist's expertise has been used in identifying the remains of children who died as a result of mass disasters and war crimes and also those found in war graves.

There are also situations in which either the actual or the chronological age of a living child is unknown or the stated age is suspected as being incorrect. Most legal systems require an established age so that appropriate procedures may be observed, for example, when the statutory age for criminal responsibility has to be certified. In some countries, refugees arriving by sea or air who lack personal documents may be obliged to prove adult or dependent status in order to obtain a residence permit. It may be necessary for an official to assign an age and the forensic anthropologist may aid in this process.

This article is devoted primarily to the identification of juvenile skeletal remains, but aging in the living child and legal procedures are also discussed.

Remains of Dead Children

When skeletal or badly decomposed remains are discovered, investigating officers usually need to know immediately whether the remains are human, how long they have lain there, and how many individuals are represented. A competent forensic anthropologist should be able to establish if the remains are human, or indeed bone, although this depends on which parts of a body have survived. Parts of a polymer resin cast of a skeleton can at first sight be misleading and ribs of some mammals look remarkably like human ribs. However, only an osteologist experienced in juvenile anatomy can distinguish neonatal human bones from those of chickens and small rodents (**Figure 1**). The time since death cannot usually be determined by an osteologist or anthropologist; often, the specialized services of forensic archeology, palynology, entomology, or a specialized chemical laboratory are required. An estimation of the number of individuals represented should always start with the minimum number and only increase based on available evidence. A mixture of adult and juvenile bones, juvenile bones of very different sizes, and duplication of any one bone are some of the factors to be considered when assigning appropriate elements to different individuals.

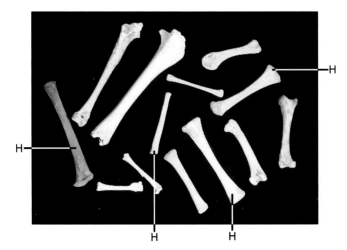

Figure 1 A mixture of perinatal human bones and chicken, duck, and rabbit bones. The human bones are labeled "H."

The next aim is to establish the biological identity of each individual through the assessment of sex, age, stature, and ethnic background. The purpose is to limit the search of the missing persons list, leading to the establishment of personal identity.

Of the four principal biological parameters, only the age can be estimated with any degree of reliability in juveniles. Although there are small skeletal morphological differences between the sexes from an early age, they are not significant for reliable determination of sex until after pubertal modifications have occurred. Therefore, sex determination is tentative at best. The age of most juveniles is so closely linked to stature that it is generally used to predict height, which is particularly variable during the pubertal growth spurt. It is difficult to establish ethnic identity from skeletal remains in the adult, and in the child it is even more difficult because sufficient data do not exist on which to base conclusions.

Age

The terminology applied to different periods of life varies both in different countries and as used by clinicians, skeletal biologists, and anthropologists. There are some commonly accepted definitions (**Table 1**), but other terms have a variety of meanings in different contexts (**Table 2**). Certain key ages in the life span of an individual are important legally, and the forensic anthropologist may be involved in determining whether these are relevant in a specific case. For example, is a dead baby a full-term infant, or is a runaway young person of an age to marry without parental consent? For the purposes of this article, juvenile is used to describe any stage of development before complete growth of the skeleton ceases at approximately 28 years of age.

Table 1 Definitions accepted by embryologists, clinicians, and pediatricians

Embryo	First 8 weeks after fertilization
Fetus	From 8 weeks of intrauterine life to birth
Preterm infant	Live birth <37 weeks (258 days) LMP
Full-term infant	Live birth from 37 to 42 weeks (259–293 days) LMP
Post-term infant	Live birth >42 weeks (294 days) LMP
Stillbirth	Infant born dead after 28 weeks LMP (UK definition)
Neonate	First 4 weeks of life
Infant	Birth to the end of the first year of life

LMP, last menstrual period of mother, a clinical timing. Fertilization dates are 2 weeks later.

Table 2 Some commonly used age terms with variable meanings

Perinate	Around the time of birth
Early childhood	First 5 years – often preschool age
Late childhood	From about 6 years to puberty
Puberty	Time of secondary sexual change – about 10–14 years in girls and 12–16 years in boys
Adolescence	Used by some authors synonymously with puberty and others as referring to behavioral and psychological changes at puberty
Young adult	Period from cessation of growth in height until final fusion of all other bones (see text)

Estimation of age of the juvenile uses the many incremental changes that occur during the period of growth and development. Growth consists of two main components: increase in size and increase in maturity. Although these elements are usually closely integrated, their relationship is not always linear. For example, an 8-year-old girl may be several centimeters taller than her friend of the same age. Similarly, two boys of the same height can be at different stages of skeletal maturity.

Biological Identity

When age is unknown, the concept of biological age is adopted as an indicator of how far along the developmental continuum an individual has progressed in terms of growth and development. Biological age may be expressed as dental age or skeletal age, depending on which elements of the skeleton are available to be employed in the estimation. Dental age may be estimated either from the times of eruption of teeth into the mouth or from the degree of their mineralization (Table 3). Skeletal age is estimated from the size and stage of development of the bones of the skeleton. Both methods require the unknown individual to be compared to a known standard, and this may introduce areas of incompatibility.

Dental Age

Estimation of age from the teeth has several advantages over skeletal aging. First, teeth normally survive inhumation better than any other part of the skeleton. There have been cases in which teeth were the only recognizable remains of an individual, either because of decay due to burial conditions or because there was an attempt to destroy a body by dismemberment or burning. Second, the development of the deciduous and permanent sets of teeth can be studied over the whole range of the juvenile life span, beginning in the embryonic period and lasting into early adult life. Finally, it is generally accepted that the relationship between chronological age and dental age is stronger than that between chronological age and skeletal age. Dental development is less affected than bone development by adverse environmental conditions, such as nutrition and disturbances of endocrine function. Additionally, the formation of all the deciduous dentition and part of the permanent dentition takes place before birth in a protected environment, whereas skeletal growth is exposed for increasing amounts of time to external influences. This is reflected in the increasing divergence between chronological and skeletal age, as environmental factors have more time to affect the growth of the skeleton.

Two aspects of tooth development have been used in the estimation of dental age: the emergence of teeth into the mouth and the stage of mineralization of their crowns and roots during development. Eruption is the continuous process by which a tooth moves from its crypt in the bone of the jaws to its position of occlusion in the mouth. Most studies are confined to actual emergence, which is wrongly referred to as eruption. In a skull or mandible, emergence is defined as the superior part of the crown of the tooth appearing level with the surface of the alveolar bone.

Estimation of dental age using mineralization stages of crowns and roots of developing teeth entails visualization from a radiographic image in order to view both erupted and unerupted teeth (Figure 2). Each available tooth is assigned a score based on the fractions of the crown and root that have developed, and then weighted scores are added to produce a total maturity score, which is plotted against age. It is a more accurate method of estimating age than emergence because emergence is an event whose exact time of occurrence is not accurately known, whereas the observance of mineralization indicates a defined point in the life span of all the developing teeth. However, mineralization has several disadvantages. First, it

Table 3 Some key stages in dental development

Age	Dental state
Birth	Deciduous incisor crowns 60–80% complete
	Deciduous canine crowns 30% complete
	Deciduous first molar crowns complete occlusal cap
	Deciduous second molar crowns separate cusps mineralized
	Crowns of first permanent molars just beginning to mineralize
2.5–3 years	All deciduous teeth emerged into the mouth
6–7 years	First permanent molars emerge into the mouth
8–12 years	Deciduous teeth replaced by permanent successors
12 years	Second permanent molars emerge into the mouth
18+ years	Third permanent molars (wisdom teeth) emerge into the mouth

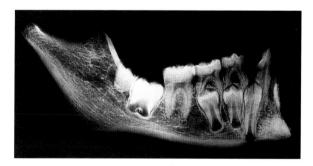

Figure 2 Radiograph of a damaged archeological hemi-mandible from a Romano-British skeleton from Peterborough, UK. The deciduous canine, first and second molars, and the first permanent molar are in occlusion. Visible unerupted teeth are the permanent canine, both premolars, the partially complete second permanent molar, and the incomplete crown of the third permanent molar. Reproduced from Scheuer L, Black S. "The Head, Neck and Dentition". In: *Developmental Juvenile Osteology*. p. 150. © 2000 with permission from Elsevier.

requires training and experience in reading the radiographs. Second, problems have arisen with the production of the standards of early infant and childhood stages because of the difficulties of radiographing very young children. Finally, there are many methodological problems that may cause discrepancies in results due to both sampling and the use of different statistical methods. In a forensic situation, when a presumptive age is urgently required, emergence may be the only practical way to obtain an estimate.

The study of dental microstructure, which involves counting perikymata (incremental lines on the surface of tooth enamel), can provide an even more accurate method of age determination. This method is independent of growth standards of a specific population, so it may prove relevant in individual forensic cases. Disadvantages are that it requires the services of a hard-tissue laboratory, experience in the technique, and it is very time-consuming and therefore expensive. One particularly pronounced incremental line, the neonatal line, can be of medicolegal significance in determining whether an infant was live-born or stillborn. It is formed very soon after birth and can be visualized by light microscopy if the child survived for about 3 weeks or by electron microscopy within 1 or 2 days of birth.

Skeletal Age

Aging a juvenile from skeletal remains requires both an understanding of the mechanism of bone growth and a detailed knowledge of the anatomy of the juvenile skeleton. Nearly all the elements of the skeleton begin development in prenatal life, and bone forms either directly in embryonic mesenchymal tissue or in an intermediate cartilaginous template of a future bone. Within each bone, osteogenesis starts in one location, the primary ossification center, and gradually expands until the precursor is totally replaced by bone. Most primary centers develop *in utero* and include the bones of the skull, the vertebral column, the ribs, sternum, the primary centers of the long bones of the limbs and their girdles, and the phalanges of the hands and feet. Many are recognizable by mid fetal life and most by birth (**Figure 3**).

Most postcranial bones also develop secondary ossification centers known as epiphyses, which are situated at the ends of long bones and at traction sites associated with irregular bones. Not all bones possess secondary centers; the major ones are those of the skull and the small bones of the wrist and ankle. The bones of the skull vault are formed from primary centers by a process of intramembranous ossification. The carpals and tarsals develop from a primary center that forms within a cartilaginous

precursor where the ossification front expands until it fills out the original template.

Nearly all secondary centers commence ossification after birth, although a few develop in the last few weeks of intrauterine life. In some situations, the state of maturity of a fetus can have medicolegal consequences. Visualization of the secondary ossification centers of the distal femur and the proximal tibia and commencement of ossification in the calcaneus and talus is usually accepted as signifying a full-term fetus.

Secondary ossification centers are separated from the primary center by a growth plate or physis, which is an area of cartilage that organizes further growth of the bone. They appear at a reasonably predictable rate in a well-documented pattern over a time period from the perinatal period until young adult life. When a skeletal element reaches its final size, the growth plate is totally replaced by bone as the epiphysis fuses to its primary center. As a general rule, the secondary centers of the limb bones that appear first are the last to fuse, whereas the late-forming epiphyses reach union with their primary centers in a shorter time period. In the major limb bones, early-forming epiphyses are found in the upper limb at the proximal humerus and distal radius and ulna and in the lower limb at the distal femur and proximal tibia.

The timing of fusion varies greatly in response to the function of the soft tissues with which the element

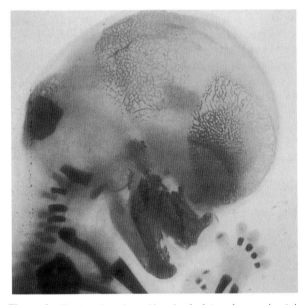

Figure 3 The head, neck, and hands of a fetus of approximately 14 weeks *in utero* showing the developing bones. The darker-colored bones are those developing from a cartilaginous template. The bones showing a network of trabecular bone are those developing intramembranously directly in mesenchyme. Adapted from Berkowitz BKB, Holland GR, Moxham BJ. *A Colour Atlas and Textbook of Oral Anatomy*, p. 247, © 1978, with permission from Elsevier.

is associated. For example, the skull and vertebral column that enclose the precociously developing nervous system reach union either before birth or in the early childhood years, whereas the epiphyses of the limbs fuse during the adolescent period when growth in height ceases. The timing of fusion is also significantly affected by the variability in onset of the adolescent growth spurt. The inability to sex juvenile remains until sexual dimorphism is well under way complicates the use of fusion times in this group until secondary sexual characteristics begin to show in the skeleton. This means that any estimated age bands have to be wider than if sex was known from other evidence, such as soft tissues.

There are a few sites in the skeleton that do not reach maturity until young adult life in the third decade. These include the jugular growth plate of the skull, the sacral vertebral bodies, the iliac and ischial epiphyses of the hip bone, the annular rings of the vertebral column, the peripheral epiphyses of the scapula, the costal notches of the sternum, and the epiphysis at the medial end of the clavicle.

From this brief description, it can be seen that by observing the stage of development of different parts of the skeleton, it should be possible to estimate the age of a juvenile from the perinatal to the young adult period (**Table 4**). Obviously, in the case of skeletal remains, accuracy depends strongly on which bones are available for study and on the stage of development of each particular bone. Greater accuracy will be obtained from those bones that show distinct changes in a relatively short period of time. For example, the fusion time of the pubic and ischial bones at their rami is quite variable, and fusion may take place at any time between the ages of 3 and 10 years; thus, this site is not very useful. The proximal

epiphysis of the tibia is preferred because it shows well-defined stages at certain ages (**Figure 4**).

Personal Identity

After a biological profile is established and a potential list of individuals is developed, the search for personal identity can begin. If successful, the individual can be positively identified by next of kin and can be given a name.

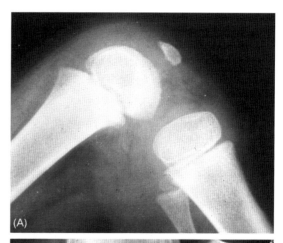
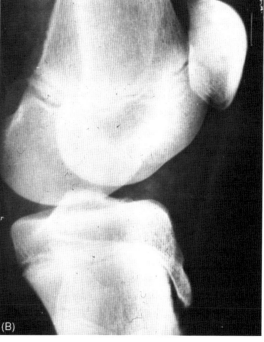

Figure 4 Lateral radiographs of juvenile knees. (A) A child between the ages of 5 and 9 years. The lower femoral and upper tibial epiphyses are small and separated from their diaphyses by wide growth plates. The patella is very small. (B) An adolescent. The epiphyses of the femur and tibia are much larger and overlap the ends of the diaphyses. The upper tibial epiphysis has developed its anterior tuberosity and the patella is of adult size. Reproduced from Scheuer L (2002) Application of osteology to forensic medicine. *Clinical Anatomy* 15: 297–312. © 2002 with permission from Wiley.

Table 4 Some key stages in skeletal development[a]

Birth	Lower femoral and upper tibial epiphyses present
	Calcaneus and talus start to mineralize
End of year 1	Skull bones develop diploe
	Anterior fontanelle fuses
	Two halves of mandible fuse at symphysis
	Vertebral half arches fuse posteriorly
By year 6	Four parts of occipital bone fuse around foramen magnum
	Vertebral centra and arches fuse in thoracic and lumbar column
Early childhood	Most early-forming epiphyses present
Late childhood	Most later-forming epiphyses present
Early adolescence	Late-forming epiphyses fuse
	Innominate fuses in the acetabulum
Late adolescence	Rest of long bone epiphyses fuse
Young adult	Late epiphyseal fusion of various elements

[a]This is a very abbreviated table and details can be found in the further reading section.

This step will rely on some feature that will separate individuals with similar biological profiles and that must match secure information from premortem sources. For instance, this may be a previous medical condition such as a fracture, a dental record, or a school record. Unfortunately, in the case of a young child, there may not have been enough time to accumulate any distinguishing features. Facial superimposition using a photograph of the missing person may prove useful, especially if there is a smile showing the anterior teeth.

The most important factor in the confirmation of identity from skeletal remains is DNA extracted from bones or teeth. This is only possible when an individual has been tentatively identified and samples can be matched with those from living relatives. It is also a technique involving the statistics of probability that is not easily understood by nonscientists or the general public. There may be problems with amplification and contamination, and methods are time-consuming and expensive. However, genetic investigation is a rapidly developing field that has the potential to produce many new techniques. It is currently possible to use breakdown products of the amelogenins, organic components of the enamel of teeth, for sex typing because these proteins are produced by a gene with copies on the X and Y chromosomes.

Unless the choice of personal identity rests on very secure evidence, it is important for the forensic anthropologist to resist any attempts to be pressurized into making an identification by the investigating authorities. The outcome can have profound legal and personal consequences. If a crime is suspected, it could mean the arraignment and trial of a suspect. In the case of any missing person, it can mean the end of painful uncertainty and possible eventual closure for grieving relatives and friends.

The Living Child

Occasionally, a forensic anthropologist may be called upon to aid a police surgeon, immigration official, or similar legal officer in examining a child whose stated age is under suspicion. Obviously, this situation will entail the most likely estimate of age because the actual chronological age cannot be proved if withheld.

In a perinatal infant, the weight and length of a normal-term baby are population-dependent. In the UK these are taken to be 2550–3360 g, 28–32 cm crown–rump length, and 48–52 cm crown–heel length. However, gestational age is also frequently estimated in the live newborn infant by an evaluation of the infant's neurological maturity.

In children, age may be estimated, as from skeletal remains, from both the teeth and the developmental state of the skeleton, although ethical considerations inhibit the use of some of the methods that can be freely applied to dead remains. Chief among these is the use of radiographs such as orthopantograms showing the total number of emerged and unerupted teeth or X-rays of the innominate bone, which would expose a young person to a considerable dose of radiation.

In older children, inspection of the mouth may be carried out by a dentist, odontologist, or anthropologist to observe the total number of emerged teeth. This can give a reasonably accurate estimate of age, especially between the ages of 6 and 12 years. Clinical emergence is judged from the time when the first part of the tooth is seen to pierce the gum or, on an X-ray, when resorption of the overlying alveolar bone is evident.

Skeletal development may only be viewed by means of some method of scanning. Cessation of growth in height at the end of adolescence may be gauged by an X-ray of the wrist because the lower radial and ulnar epiphyses are some of the last, easily accessible long-bone epiphyses to fuse. The state of the development of the dentition will give a more accurate estimate of age than the state of epiphyseal fusion because it is less subject to population variability or the vagaries caused by the timing of the adolescent growth spurt.

Legal Procedures

In the examination of either skeletal remains or a living child, the forensic anthropologist should be aware of various legal and political procedures. These often involve cooperation with other professionals, such as the investigative police team, the forensic pathologist, archeologists, or odontologist, with whom there should be agreement as to methodology. Each member of the investigation team needs to appreciate the others' skills and requirements and act accordingly. For instance, the anthropologist and the facial reconstruction expert need to have access to a skull that is as undamaged as possible, so the forensic odontologist must not resect parts of the jaw before others have had a chance to examine it.

The forensic anthropologist also needs to be aware of important issues such as confidentiality, continuity of evidence, and consent to treatment. In international situations, such as mass disasters and war crimes, there are additional matters concerning legal requirements in different countries and presentation of evidence that need to be taken into account.

Often, a written report by the investigating officer, the coroner, or procurator fiscal will be accepted, but sometimes a personal appearance at an inquest or other court is required. These proceedings may take months, or even years, after the initial investigation, when recall of a case may be difficult under the sometimes harassing conditions of a courtroom. Care must also be taken when giving evidence not to be drawn outside the areas of expertise by a lawyer trying to prove incompetence. It is advisable to ensure familiarity with the original report, which must be as detailed, accurate, and free from jargon as possible so that it may be understood by nonscientific personnel.

See Also

Anthropology: Stature Estimation from the Skeleton; Sex Determination

Further Reading

Demirjian A, Goldstein H (1976) New systems for dental maturity based on seven and four teeth. *Annals of Human Biology* 3: 411–421.

Dubowitz LM, Dubowitz V, Mercuri E (1999) *The Neurological Assessment of the Preterm and Full-Term Infant*. London: MacKeith Press.

Fazekas IGy, Kósa F (1978) *Forensic Fetal Osteology*. Budapest: Akadémiai Kiadó.

Hillson S (1996) *Dental Anthropology*. Cambridge, UK: Cambridge University Press.

Kraus BS, Jordan RE (1965) *The Human Dentition before Birth*. London: Kimpton.

Moorrees CFA, Fanning EA, Hunt EE (1963) Age variation of formation stages for ten permanent teeth. *Journal of Dental Research* 42: 1490–1502.

Scheuer L, Black S (2000) *Developmental Juvenile Osteology*. London: Academic Press.

Scheuer L, Black S (2004) *The Juvenile Skeleton*. London: Elsevier.

Sex Determination

C A Briggs, University of Melbourne, Melbourne, VIC, Australia

Introduction

Anthropology is employed in a forensic setting to help create a biological profile of unknown skeletal or decomposed remains in order to arrive at conclusions or inferences regarding provenance. Sex determination is one of the key questions addressed when formulating this profile – its knowledge immediately eliminates 50% of the population from the process of identification.

Sex-distinguishing characteristics of the skeleton are dependent on the existence of sexual dimorphism, due to the influence of sex hormones, the adaptations of the female to the function of childbearing, as well as cultural differences between the sexes. Although present to a degree at all ages, sexual dimorphism becomes most apparent after puberty when secondary sexual characteristics have fully developed. For this reason, sex can be most accurately ascertained in skeletons from mature individuals, although senility and pathology may influence these characteristics and therefore alter reliability in the aged. It is worth noting that sex determination is rarely based on any one skeletal feature alone. An expert forensic anthropologist is aware of the range of variation of sexual traits within the skeleton and the degree of overlap that normally exists between males and females. As with assessment of other parameters that lead toward a successful identification of the deceased, as many criteria as are available are assessed before coming to a definitive conclusion.

It is apparent that subtle race-related differences may exist in the degree of development of sexual characteristics within the skeleton, and there may also be geographic variation. Where possible, the racial affiliations of skeletal material should be ascertained at the same time as criteria used to determine sex are applied. As with sex-distinguishing characteristics, however, many racial traits do not appear fully until puberty, and even in adolescence they may not be completely formed. These racial and geographic differences may be partially overcome by carefully observing individual sex-distinguishing traits in a subsample of a specific population. For example, accurate measurement and recording of the articular surface of a long bone in a set number of separate skeletal remains may allow for the successful determination of sex, provided these measurements have been taken carefully, the population is sufficiently sexually dimorphic in size, and both sexes are represented. In this way trait-specific information for a given population group may be collected. This is particularly useful when only partial remains are available for examination due to taphonomic factors, such as predators or fire.

Principles of Sex Determination

The determination of sex is normally undertaken by examining appropriate elements of the skeleton and scoring a list of traits as male, female, or indeterminate. Each trait is scored separately and the overall results are weighted for a final assessment. Observations are generally made of the cranium or the bones of the postcranial skeleton, in particular the pelvis and os coxae. The modifications that occur in the pelvis at puberty generally provide a more reliable estimate of sex than do cranial measurements. Important sex differences begin to develop in the skeleton before birth and, while there are recent reports detailing sex-distinguishing characteristics in fetal, neonatal, and infant skeletal remains, it is not usually until the individual approaches the age of 14–16 years that decisions on sex differences can be made with any degree of confidence.

Morphological (visual) examination remains the quickest and easiest method of determining sex in the great majority of unknown skeletal remains and in experienced hands will result in 95–100% accuracy when the whole skeleton is available for assessment. The accuracy of such assessment is, however, only as good as the expertise of the examiner. Because of their less subjective nature, metrical analysis (particularly of the skull) as well as discriminant function analysis should also be applied because of their objectivity and reproducibility. Metrical methods use statistically determined discriminant functions with sectioning points, above or below which one or other of the two sexes will fall. The reliability and accuracy of metrical indices vary depending on the bones assessed and relate, in part, to the original data on which sectioning points were calculated. While various skeletal collections around the world have been used to provide data sets, the majority of indices are based on the Terry and Hamann-Todd collections in the USA, that were put together in the early part of the twentieth century. These two collections comprise skeletons of known race, sex, age, and stature, but are heavily biased toward whites and blacks from lower socioeconomic groups who lived in the central west of the USA at the end of the nineteenth century. In recent years, it has become apparent that, for a variety of reasons, the use of these formulae may be becoming less applicable when applied to modern populations and population groups different from those upon which the formulae are based. Such functions as are available should, therefore, be restricted in their application to those population groups from which the functions were originally derived. Nevertheless, the development of discriminant functions based on skeletal measurements has helped greatly in removing the subjective bias from sex determination. Their use tends to back up the morphological assessments made by the expert anthropologist and makes reliable sex assessment available to the less experienced.

The skeletal elements that are of most use in sex determination are listed below, in descending order of reliability:

- the pelvis: os coxae and sacrum
- the cranium
- the long bones: especially the femur, humerus, and tibia
- other bones, e.g., the sternum, clavicle, and calcaneus.

The accuracy of sex determination in adults is approximately as follows:

- entire skeleton: 100%
- pelvis alone: 95%
- skull alone: 90%
- skull and pelvis: 98%
- long bones: 80–90%
- long bones and skull: 90–95%
- long bones and pelvis: >95%.

In immature (prepubertal) skeletons the chance of a correct sex allocation is only 50% unless the pelvis is present, which improves the chances of correct sex allocation to about 75–80%.

Sex Determination from the Adult Pelvis

Morphological Determination

The pelvis in general and the pubis in particular have long been regarded as the best sources of information for determining the sex of an unknown individual. While sex differences begin to develop in the skeleton before birth it is not usually until about the mid-teenage years (particularly in western societies) that decisions on sex differences can be made with any degree of certainty. Both morphological and metrical characteristics may be used in this assessment. The morphological sex features of the pelvis and os coxae are listed in **Table 1** and illustrated in **Figures 1–3**. Reference casts of the pubic symphysis and auricular surface of both males and females have been developed and these may help with correct sex assignment. However, these are not useful unless the examiner has seen large numbers of symphyseal and auricular surfaces to be able to distinguish between age-related and pathological changes.

Metrical features of the hip bone also assist with sex assessment, especially the ischiopubic index. This is the length (in mm) of the pubis divided by the length of the ischium (in mm) multiplied by 100. In males the index ranges from 73 to 94 and in females from 91 to 115. However, as there may be some difficulty in locating the exact reference points, for example

Table 1 Sex-distinguishing features of the female pelvis

General morphology
Gracile and smooth (rugged with marked muscle attachments in male)
Overall shape
Female pelvis wide and shallow, with larger pelvic outlet (pelvis high and narrow in male)
Pubic bone
Wide and rectangular body of pubis (narrow and triangular in male)
Wide subpubic angle (narrow in male)
Ventral pubic arc (absent in male)
Curved ventral pubic concavity or lateral recurve (straight or convex in male)
Greater sciatic notch
L-shape in female (J-shape in male)
Auricular region
Preauricular sulcus frequently present (absent or slight in male)
Elevation of the auricular surface above the adjacent postauricular area (coplanar in male)

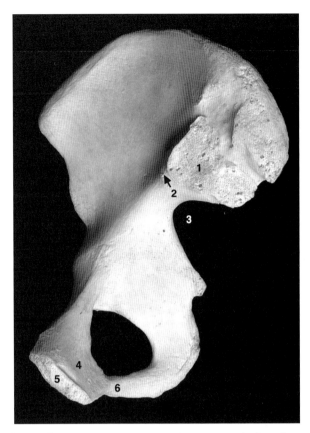

Figure 3 Hip bone. 1, auricular surface; 2, preauricular sulcus; 3, greater sciatic notch; 4, body of pubis; 5, symphyseal surface; 6, lateral recurve.

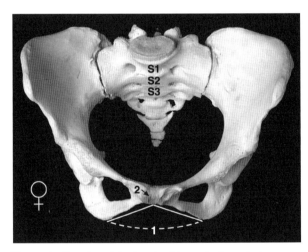

Figure 1 Female pelvis. 1, subpubic angle; 2, ventral arc.

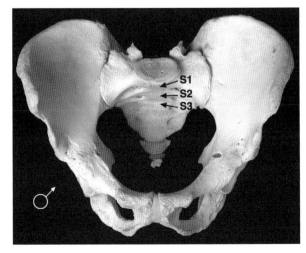

Figure 2 Male pelvis.

those within the acetabulum, this measurement is usually best performed by someone with knowledge of the anatomical landmarks.

Morphological characteristics of the sacrum (**Figures 1** and **2**) that are often quoted as assisting with sex determination are:

1. the relative width of the ala of the sacrum compared with the width of the first sacral body (1:1 in the female; 1:2 in the male)
2. the shape of the ventral (pelvic) concavity (flattened anterior contour from the first to the third sacral vertebra in the female; regular curve anteriorly from the first to the fifth sacral vertebrae in the male)
3. the extent of the auricular surface relative to the lateral masses of the second and third sacral vertebrae (limited to the lateral mass of the second sacral vertebra in the female; it extends on to the lateral mass of the third sacral vertebra in the male).

The sacrum is not always the most reliable of bones for sex assessment as it often shows variability in the number of segments present. For example, in prefixation of the vertebral column there is part-fusion of the first sacral vertebra with the last lumbar vertebra (sacralization of the fifth lumbar vertebra). The reverse of this, partial or complete separation of the first sacral vertebra (lumbarization of S1), is not uncommon.

Sex Determination from the Cranium

Morphological Examination

The factors that contribute to sexual dimorphism in the cranium are many, but the most important may be seen from the front and from the sides (**Figures 4** and **5**). A detailed tabulation of traits diagnostic of sex features in the cranium is summarized in **Table 2**, however some are noted here. The bones comprising the frontal view are generally smaller in the female, with smoother and less pronounced landmarks (**Figure 5**). The contour of the forehead, due to a more prominent frontal tuber, is higher and more vertical in the female than in the male; the superciliary arches are much less strongly developed than in the male; the orbits are higher,

more rounded, and relatively larger compared to the upper facial skeleton; and the orbital margins are sharper and less rounded than in the male. In the male the nasal aperture is higher and the nasal bones are larger.

One of the distinguishing sex characteristics seen from the lateral view (**Figures 6** and **7**) is the size and degree of projection of the mastoid process. Mastoid processes are larger and more prominent in males than females, and this may be determined by measuring the index of mastoid length to mastoid height (greater in males than females). In addition, the posterior end of the zygomatic arch extends its (supramastoid) crest further in males than females, often beyond the external auditory meatus.

Examination of the occipital region of the cranium is often worthwhile as it provides evidence of the robustness of the skeleton and hence a further clue as to sex. For example, the external occipital protuberance is much larger in the male, as are the occipital condyles, and the transverse (nuchal) occipital lines are more evident. The distance from the opisthocranion, from just above the external occipital protuberance (where the skull attains its greatest posterior

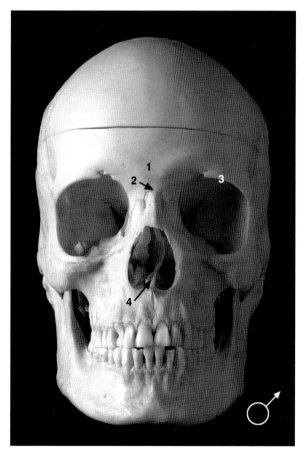

Figure 4   Male skull (view from front). 1, glabella; 2, nasion; 3, superior orbital margin; 4, nasal spine.

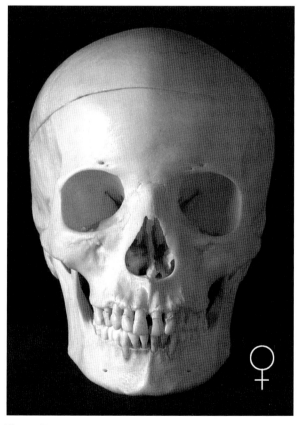

Figure 5   Female skull (view from front).

Table 2 Sex differences in the appearance of the skull

Trait	Male	Female
General size	Large	Small
Architecture	Rugged	Smooth
Supraorbital ridges	Medium to large	Small to medium
Mastoid processes	Medium to large	Small to medium
Occipital region	Marked muscle lines and protruberances	No marked muscle lines and protruberances
Frontal eminences	Small	Large
Parietal eminences	Small	Large
Orbits	Square with round margins	Round with sharp margins
Forehead	Sloping, less rounded	Vertical
Cheekbones	Heavier, project laterally	Light, more compressed
Palate	Large, broad, U-shape	Small, parabolic
Occipital condyles	Large	Small
Mandible	Large, high symphysis and broad ramus	Small, lower symphysis and smaller ramus
Chin shape	U-shaped	V-shaped
Gonial angle	Angled	Vertical
Gonial flare	Pronounced	Slight

From Clement and Ranson, 'Craniofacial identification in forensic medicine.' Hodder Arnold 1988.

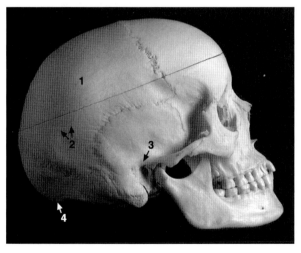

Figure 6 Male skull (view from side). 1, parietal tuber; 2, temporal lines; 3, supramastoid crest; 4, external occipital protruberance.

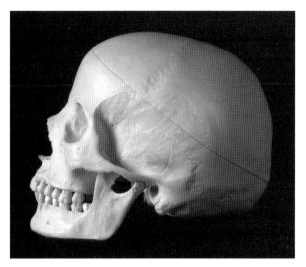

Figure 7 Female skull (view from side). 1, frontal tuber.

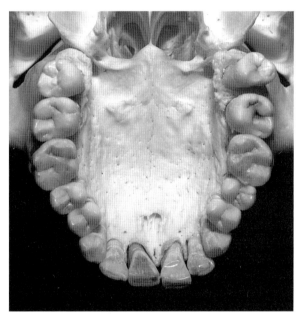

Figure 8 Palate.

extent) to the glabella, provides an index of maximal cranial length. Maximal cranial length is usually greater in males than in females.

Examination of the cranium from above reveals the ellipsoid shape of the cranial contour with the point of greatest maximal breadth of the vault at the parietal eminence (parietal tuber), a primary center of ossification and more prominent in females. While possessing few distinctive sex-related bony features, examination of this view of the skull is important as it may help confirm the racial affiliation of the deceased and allow application of the appropriate metric standards of measurement.

The inferior view of the cranium contains the hard palate of the maxilla and palatine bones (**Figure 8**). The width of the hard palate, as measured between the outside of the second molars, is quite variable,

Table 3   Discriminant function weights from cranial measurements in American white skulls of known sex

Measurement[a]	1	2	3	4	5	6
1	3.107	3.400	1.800		1.236	9.875
2	4.603	−3.833	−1.783		−1.000	
3	5.786	5.433	2.767			
4		−0.167	−0.100	10.714		7.062
5	14.821	12.200	6.300	16.381	3.291	19.062
6	1.000	−0.100		−1.000		−1.000
7	2.714	2.200		4.333		4.375
8	−5.179			−6.571		
9	6.071	5.367	2.833	14.810	1.528	
Sectioning point	2676.39	2592.32	1296.20	3348.27	536.93	5066.69
% correct	86.6	86.4	86.4	84.5	85.5	84.9

Adapted from Giles and Elliot (1963) Sex determination by discriminant function analysis of the crania. *American Journal of Physical Anthropology* 21: 53–68.

[a]The following measurements are multiplied by the above weights, the totals are summed, and the value compared with the known sectioning points:
1. maximum length (from glabella in the midline to opisthocranion).
2. maximum breadth (perpendicular to median sagittal plane, avoiding supramastoid crest).
3. basion–bregma height (midpoint on anterior border of foramen magnum to bregma).
4. basion–nasion maximum diameter.
5. maximum bizygomatic diameter.
6. basion–prosthion (basion to most anterior point on maxilla in median sagittal plane).
7. prosthion–nasion.
8. external palate breadth.
9. mastoid length.

although it tends to be broader and shallower in males than females.

Metrical Analysis

Some of the features of the skull useful in determining sex lend themselves to measurement in numerical units, whereas others may only be differentiated in terms of presence or absence, or degree of development. Measurements and discriminant function weights suitable for differentiating sex in adult American white and black crania are summarized in **Table 3**. Reported accuracy is between 82% and 89%.

Sex Determination from the Mandible

The lower jaw or mandible is a separate bone which articulates via its condylar processes with the squamous temporal bone of the cranium. It consists of two rectangular plates on each side, a horizontal plate called the body, and a vertical plate called the ramus (**Figure 9**). The body contains the teeth, within sockets in its alveolar process, while the ramus is for articulation and attachment of the muscles of mastication. On the body in the midline is the mental protuberance, with a median ridge above and an elevated triangular area below, representing the site of fusion of the two halves.

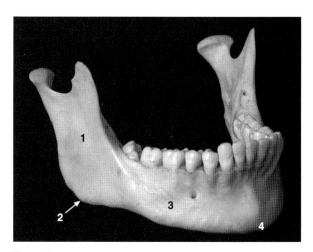

Figure 9   Mandible. 1, ramus; 2, gonion; 3, body; 4, gnathion.

Posterolaterally, the angle of the mandible is referred to as the gonion. It represents a point of intersection of lines drawn along the inferior and posterior borders of the bone. The gonion is often flared (gonial flare) or everted, particularly in males, by the attachment of a powerful muscle of mastication (masseter) and in these situations the bigonial breadth is widened. The ramus diverges above into condylar (behind) and coronoid (in front) processes, with an intervening mandibular notch. The coronoid process

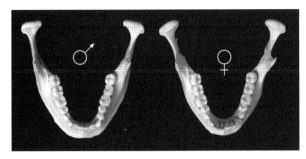

Figure 10 Male and female mandibles.

receives the tendon of temporalis, a very large muscle of mastication which, along with other masticatory muscles, may leave prominent impressions on the bone, especially in the male.

The mandible is often used to determine the sex of skeletal remains (**Figures 9** and **10**). In the male it is more robust, larger, and thicker, with greater body height and a broader ascending ramus. The gonial angle is less obtuse (less than 125°), the condyles are larger, and the chin is square, in contrast to a V-shaped chin in females. The bicondylar breadth, the direct transverse distance between the most lateral points on the two condyles, is usually greater in males.

Sex Determination from Other Bones of the Skeleton

In general the limb bones of females are more gracile and less well marked by muscle attachments than those of males. The articular ends of the bones are smaller and the shafts less robust. The above observations are reflected in the metrical features of the bones and to date almost all bones of the skeleton have been used in determining sex of an individual through statistical analysis. This is particularly the case with reference to the diameter of the articular ends of the humerus, radius, and femur, and to a lesser extent the circumferences of the long bone shafts. However, size differences between different population groups mean that sex determination from the limb bones is population-specific.

Special attention has been given to long bones such as the femur as this is the largest bone in the skeleton, it is surrounded by the largest limb muscle mass, and parts of it are likely to remain preserved even after prolonged incineration. The same comments may be made for the calcaneus, which is often protected due to the presence of footwear. In most populations the dimensions of femoral breadth and circumference, in particular the maximal diameter of the femoral head, tend to be more dimorphic than length. Similarly,

Table 4 Measures of selected postcranial bones and bony features

Bone	Females (mm)	Indeterminate (mm)	Males (mm)
Shoulder			
Scapula length	<129	140–159	>160
Glenoid cavity length	<34	34–36	>37
Clavicle			
Mean length	140		158
Humerus			
Vertical diameter head	<43	44–46	>47
Mean length	305		340
Mean epicondylar breadth	57		64
Radius			
Diameter of head	<21		>22
Femur			
Vertical diameter of head	<41.5	43.5–44.5	>45.5
Femoral length	439		477
Bicondylar width	<72	74–76	>78

measures of the maximal vertical diameter of the glenoid fossa of the scapula are greater in males than females. Sex differences are reported for other postcranial bones, including metacarpals, metatarsals, the ribs, vertebral bodies, and the clavicle; however, in most cases these have not been extensively studied, nor their reliability in assessing sex adequately tested. Nevertheless, because a skull may be damaged or removed from a forensic scene and a complete pelvis is not always present, knowledge of sex-related features of other skeletal elements is important.

Some measurements used to estimate sex in postcranial remains are indicated in **Table 4**. More details, including range and standard deviation, are presented in manuals of human osteology.

Sex Determination in Fetal and Juvenile Bones

Lack of availability (and hence of studies) of large samples of fetal and juvenile skeletal material of known age, sex, and race has made confident determination of sex of the isolated fetal or juvenile skeleton difficult. However, recent reports suggest that there may be detectable skeletal differences in sex between birth and 5 years, including a more prominent chin in boys, as well as an anteriorly wider dental arcade and deeper and narrower sciatic notch in boys than girls. These observations are, however, based on very small sample sizes and should therefore be viewed with caution.

Sex Determination from DNA Analysis

Where suitable samples of bone or teeth are available, DNA analysis provides a more objective assessment of sex identification. Perhaps the most famous recent identification case involving DNA analysis relates to bones found in a grave in Yekaterinburg in the Ural mountains in Russia. Comparison of both nuclear and mitochondrial DNA extracted from femora and tibiae, with blood samples taken from the ancestors of the Romanov family involving the maternal line to the Duke of Edinburgh, indicated that five of the nine skeletons located at this site were those of Tzar Nicholas, his wife, and three female children.

Conclusions

There are important indicators that appear throughout the life of an individual that allow for the determination of sex with a reasonable degree of accuracy. However, it is worth recognizing that there are always limitations on the information that a forensic anthropologist can provide toward a successful identification of an unknown deceased. It is appropriate to restate that sex of a set of skeletal remains should be determined not only from a single parameter, but from a battery of observations, and should never be made without justification. Each individual trait should be scored separately and the overall results weighted for a final determination. In this way, data can be viewed by independent reviewers, and more importantly, trait-specific information for the sample under analysis can be collected. This will come in useful when examining remains from a population group for which there are few or no baseline data or where the influence of factors such as minimal dietary intake has an effect on skeletal maturity and therefore on sex-related differences in the skeleton. In this way, population-specific traits can be assessed and determination of sex made with some confidence.

See Also

Anthropology: Stature Estimation from the Skeleton; Cremated Bones; Morphological Age Estimation

Further Reading

Bass WM (1995) *Human Osteology – A Laboratory and Field Manual.* Missouri Archaeological Society, special publication no. 2. Columbia: Missouri Archaeological Society.

Brothwell DR (1981) *Digging up Bones.* British Museum. Oxford, UK: Oxford University Press.

Fazekas IG, Kosa F (1978) *Forensic Foetal Osteology.* Budapest: Akademiai Kiado.

Iscan MY, Kennedy KAR (1989) *Reconstruction of Life from the Skeleton.* Alan R Liss.

Kolesnikov LL, Pashinyan GA, Abromov SS (2001) Anatomical appraisal of the skulls and teeth associated with the family of Tsar Nicolay Romanov. *Anatomical Record* 265: 15–32.

Krogman WM, Iscan MY (1986) *The Human Skeleton in Forensic Medicine.* Springfield, IL: Charles C Thomas.

Rathbun TA, Buikstra JE (eds.) (1984) *Human Identification: Case Studies in Forensic Anthropology.* Springfield, IL: Charles C Thomas.

Reichs KJ (ed.) (1986) *Forensic Osteology.* Springfield, IL: Charles C Thomas.

Schutowski H (1993) Sex determination of infant and juvenile skeletons: I Morphognostic features. *American Journal of Physical Anthropology* 90: 199–205.

Stewart TD (1979) *Essentials of Forensic Anthropology.* Springfield, IL: Charles C Thomas.

Suchey JM, Brooks ST, Katz D (1988) *Instructional Materials Accompanying Female Pubic Symphyseal Models of the Suchey-Brooks System.* Fort Collins, CO: France Casting.

Ubelaker DH (1989) *Human Skeletal Remains.* Taraxacum.

Wood WB, Briggs CA, Donlon D (2002) Forensic osteology. In: Freckleton I, Selby H (eds.) *Expert Evidence,* pp. 3601–3802. Thomson Lawbook.

Workshop of European Anthropologists (1980) Recommendations for age and sex diagnoses of skeletons. *Journal of Human Evolution* 9: 517–549.

Determination of Racial Affinity

M K Marks and J A Synstelien, University of Tennessee, Knoxville, TN, USA

Introduction

Racial assessment at autopsy may be straightforward in fresh remains. The task is more challenging with mutilated or fragmented remains where the focus shifts to hair form, melanocytes, DNA, or skeletal biology. In a decomposing or a skeletal stage the duty is nearly impossible without the collaboration of an experienced forensic anthropologist. This task is daunting due to intra- and interpopulation skeletal variation and the incongruence between the biology and sociology of race. Soft-tissue autolysis and putrefaction following death cause skin discoloration, distortion of facial features from gas accumulation and fluid loss, hair loss, and eventual skeletonization. As many homicide victims are concealed, deposited rurally, or curated to thwart discovery and identification, decomposition processes force assessment of race from diagnostic skeletal morphology.

Forensic anthropology provides a biological profile for the medicolegal community by estimating age, sex, race, stature, and ante-, peri-, and postmortem trauma. The medicolegal community has developed a reliance on this demographic evidence from forensic anthropology. Age and sex evaluations are achieved using established qualitative visual criteria and quantitative metric methods from skeletal and dental anatomy. Stature estimation involves measurements and formulated regression equations. Bone trauma is more difficult to interpret as it requires knowledge of perimortem biomechanical events. Assessment of racial affinity, the most challenging aspect of completing the biological profile, has become an integral and evolving part of the expertise of forensic anthropology.

Definition of Race

Biological and forensic anthropologists use the term "race" to reference a population that shares a common geographic and genetic history. What constitutes group membership varies between populations based on a mosaic of social, religious, economic, and physical attributes. How individuals classify themselves according to the chosen attributes constructed and accepted by their group is not universal. From a shared history, a unique combination of skeletal traits characterizes groups that may be absent or less frequent in other groups due to geographic distance and/or isolation. These differences provide the basis for identification and interpopulation comparison. Unfortunately, science has not deciphered the complex polygenic mechanism of inheritance of skeletal traits and how they correlate to soft-tissue similarities or differences.

Use of the term race has fallen out of favor amongst many biological anthropologists due to the historic and contemporary social misuse and abuse of racial categorization. Not immune from the stigma of the race concept elsewhere in the social sciences, the race notion specifically deepens the schisms (a) between forensic and biological anthropology and (b) within the discipline of anthropology. During the 1990s, a desultory attempt has been made to distance forensic anthropology from this sensitive issue by renaming the exercise as estimation of ethnicity, ethnic affiliation, racial ancestry, ancestry, population, etc. Ethnicity is a term of social and/or cultural identity that may or may not have a biological basis. The social and biological meanings of race are separate public and academic areas and should not be defined, compared, or contrasted in terms of each other. Whatever

criteria, motives, or incentives are used to define, delineate, divide, or unite contemporary populations – ethnic, social, religious, historic, economic, political – they are in no way scientific, irrespective of the means used in forensic anthropology.

Why is Race Important?

Concurrent with providing social self-identity, race is a significant variable in skeletal biological research. Regional populations differ in the degree of expressed skeletal sexual characteristics. This is particularly evident in the skull, where both sex and race traits are present. There is variation between populations in the age and rate of skeletal and dental maturation in children and adolescents. This is evident in the chronology of tooth emergence and appearance and fusion of long-bone epiphyses. Also, adult proportions vary between populations in torso length and between pectoral and pelvic limbs. Cognizance of this variation is critical when applying stature estimation formulae. Finally, some methods of adult aging are population specific, e.g., pubic symphysis, cranial sutures, and sternal rib ends. Comprehensive skeletal collections of known individuals are limited, and research standards on aging are generally based upon collections of individuals from the USA and Europe. Although multiracial, these collections are biased toward European and African descendants.

Besides routine, case-based human identification work, the increased involvement of forensic anthropology in human rights issues has raised critiques in the applicability of these standards to other populations. This is particularly important when the objective is war crimes prosecution. Additional legal implication for race assessment in US casework involves prosecution related to illegal excavation, curation, and sale of remains of American Indians in violation of the 1990 Native American Grave Protection and Repatriation Act (NAGPRA).

Historical and Modern Studies on Race

Colonial exploration and imperialism revealed an unsuspecting degree of human biological and cultural diversity. Prior to the 1960s, with limited understanding of genetic inheritance, these historical pernicious perceptions led to the conclusion that individuals more similar in appearance were more closely related than those dissimilar. Hence, systematic studies of human diversity placed local populations within classification schemes of relatedness. Early criteria included skin and hair color gradations, variation in hair form, and differences in proportions of facial features. These characteristics were viewed as non-evolutionary invariants and defined races as fixed types. Multiple classificatory schemes of races have been proposed with the traditional anthropological studies, recognizing Caucasoid, Negroid (African), Mongoloid (East Asian and the Native Americans), and Australoid (Australasians). These racial divisions were based on loosely distributed world population variation prior to the mid-fifteenth century when these regions were relatively isolated.

Today, research has shifted from type categorization to adapting/evolving populations. The human phenotype is highly responsive to the environment, and characteristics such as facial features, skin color, and body size and shape are biological adjustments through adaptation and chance genetic mutations that our ancestors have made to their particular geography. Anthropological research includes anthropometry of the body and head of living people, including measurement of height, weight, fat distribution, a variety of limb lengths, and body breadths and circumferences. Craniofacial anthropometry and craniometrics are particularly sensitive indicators of population history. Quantification of other complex traits includes skin color, dimensions of teeth, and fingerprint patterns. The level of genetic diversity in a population provides clues to past events affected by evolutionary forces, i.e., mutation, gene flow, and genetic drift. Molecular research on population relatedness evaluates genetic variation through world distribution patterns of classical genetic marker variants, for example, blood type, and allele frequency mapping of DNA marker variants, that is, nuclear and mitochondrial DNA sequence and/or Y-chromosome allelic variation, to calculate linear convergence estimations or group distances. In general, these studies support early visual appraisals of regional clustering while adding a temporal dimension by providing estimates of when regional lineages may have diverged.

Population Movement and Admixture

Clearly, races are not static entities – they continue to evolve. Today, it is the norm for people to travel and migrate. Over generations, many once-distinct social and biological borders became obscure. The physical characteristics attributed to race, be they soft, osseous, or dental, therefore, have gradually modified over time across the landscape. The popular concept of race includes the cultural dimension of self-identification. The US Census Bureau reflects self-identification through sociopolitical categories and not by anthropological or scientific design. In 1790, the first US census was collected in which free individuals were selected "White" or "Other" based on physical appearance. Slaves were counted separately. Growing diversity in the US has resulted in an increased number of social race categories in addition to national-origin groups. Also, for the first time the 2000 census allowed individuals to select multiple groups/races in consideration of the growing number of children and minorities who identify themselves as multiracial. Of the total population, 97.6% selected one racial category while 2.4% responded to the two or more categories (see Table 1). Of respondents selecting two or more races, 72% identified as White and another race.

The Hispanic population is the fastest growing group in the USA. Latin America has a complex heritage and many Hispanics and Latinos, ethnolinguistic categories indicative of Spanish speakers and people of Latin American descent speaking either Spanish, French, or Portuguese, e.g., Brazilians, do not identify with a particular racial group (see Table 1). Approximately 12.5% of the US population self-identified as Hispanic or Latino in the 2000 US census. The largest constituent of Hispanic speakers in the US are Mexican (66%) who identify themselves as either ethnic Mexican–American or Chicano. In terms of distribution, Hispanics and Latinos on the west coast of the USA are mostly of Mexican origin while those on the east coast are predominantly of Cuban and Puerto Rican origin.

In anthropological genetic studies of contemporary Americans, Mexican Hispanics display American Indian (36–58%) and White traits, and those of Cuban and Puerto Rican origin display combinations of White, American Indian (with contribution less than 21%), and African traits. The African contribution to the Hispanic population was similar in

Table 1 US population by racial category[a]

Race	Total population[b] (%)	Hispanic population[c] (%)
White	75.1	47.9
Black or African American	12.3	2.0
American Indian and Alaska Native	0.9	1.2
Asian	3.6	0.3
Native Hawaiian and other Pacific Islander	0.1	0.1
Some other race	5.5	42.2
Two or more races	2.4	6.3

[a]Race as defined by the US Census Bureau does not reflect biological race and is self-identified.
[b]Total US population is 281 421 906 individuals.
[c]Equals 100% total. The total number of self-identified Hispanics was 35 305 818, or 12.5% of total respondents.
Source: US Census Bureau, Census 2000.

Table 2 US citizens reporting two or more races[a]

Race	Total individuals selecting one race or in combination[b]	Individuals selecting one race	Individuals selecting in combination[b]
White	216 930 975	211 460 626	5 470 349
Black or African American	36 419 434	34 658 190	1 761 244
American Indian and Alaska Native	4 119 301	2 475 956	1 643 345
Asian	11 898 828	10 242 998	1 655 830
Native Hawaiian and other Pacific Islander	874 414	398 835	475 579
Some other race	18 521 486	15 359 073	3 162 413

[a]Race as defined by the US Census Bureau does not reflect biological race and is self-identified.
[b]In combination with one or more of the other listed races.
Source: US Census Bureau, Census 2000.

both regions at less than 17% with increasing tendency amongst Puerto Rican and Cuban descendants. The mixed expression of traits may be indicative of Latin American origins. Admixture in the African American gene pool with European Americans averages 20–25%. There is trace introduction of American Indian genes into the African American gene pool at less than 2.6%. Introduction of African genes into American Indian gene pool is slightly larger at 5%. American Indian admixture with non-Indian genes is estimated around 15%. Population estimates of admixture are region dependent within the USA providing wide ranges and estimates.

In the USA, when mixed traits of White and a minority group are present, the individual most likely identifies with the minority population as phenotypic characteristics, particularly Black, are generally dominant to White. In addition, increasing ethnic identity among Black Americans is confirmed by US census data where Blacks, like Whites, are less likely to report more than one race (see **Table 2**).

Craniofacial Morphology

Craniofacial detail has long been recognized as differentiating populations. Here, many traits are by-products of the entire developing craniofacial complex resulting from both genetic and environmental components. No region is independent during growth. All expand, remodel, and function interdependently as a result of soft-tissue development to provide unique cranial form, facial profile, and dental occlusal type. The expanding fetal, neonatal, and infant brain establishes head form and cranial base design. The base, in turn, provides a template for facial projection and proportion. The maxillary palate is an extension of the anterior cranial fossa and the palate perimeter, in turn, establishes the shape of the apical base of the maxillary dental arch.

Predispositions for retrusive and protrusive mandibular variation as well as the tendency for dental malocclusion types are a consequence of head form and facial morphology.

The experience of the skeletal biologist and familiarity with reference populations is key to establishing successful assessment. Only after years of study on numerous samples can the expert develop an appreciation for the inherent variation within and between populations to confidently diagnose race from craniofacial morphology. Skeletal features represent the same degree of continuum seen in any soft tissue and no single specimen will demonstrate every feature in the classic sense. Consultation by an experienced forensic anthropologist versed in regional variation is a must for accurate race diagnosis.

Table 3 is a generalized subset of the target visual variables utilized by anthropologists for racial estimation. As with soft-tissue gradations, this variation is subtle and subjective. As mentioned, target bony traits include facial structure and relative proportions, dental traits, and neurocranial morphology (**Figures 1** to **4**). Also, the traits in **Table 3** represent classic morphological expressions characteristic of each group. It is important to bear in mind that these traits are derived from combined sex designations and certain traits are more sex-sensitive than others. Finally, all traits are adult manifestations, i.e., postpubertal, beginning between the ages of 17 and 21 years, and not discernible on subadult crania.

Metric Craniofacial Indicators

When visual morphology is nondiagnostic, numeric analysis from crania and/or postcrania can provide assistance through a statistical comparative population approach. The success of metric methods is highly dependent on the investigator's familiarity

Table 3 Craniofacial indicators

Morphology	American Black	American Indian	American White
Face			
Profile	Projecting	Intermediate	Flat
Shape	Intermediate	Wide	Narrow
Orbits	Rectangular	Round	Angled
Nasal root	Low, rounded	Low, ridged	High, narrow
Nasal bridge	Low	Low	High
Nasal width	Wide	Medium	Narrow
Nasal spine	Small	Medium	Pronounced
Lower nasal margin	Round	Flat, sharp	Sharp, still
Teeth			
Palatal shape	Hyperbolic	Elliptical	Parabolic
Maxillary incisors	Spatulate	Shovel-shaped	Spatulate
Posterior occlusal surfaces	Crenulated	Simple	Simple
Vault			
Brow ridges	Nondescript	Nondescript	Pronounced
Muscle attachment	Nondescript	Nondescript	Pronounced
Sutures	Simple	Complex	Simple
Postbregma	Depressed	Straight	Straight
Texture	Smooth, sheen	Intermediate	Coarse, matte

Source: Adapted from (1) Gill and Rhine (1990) *Skeletal Attribution of Race*. Albuquerque: Maxwell Museum of Anthropology. (2) Byers SN (2002) *Introduction to Forensic Anthropology: A Textbook*. Boston: Allyn and Bacon.

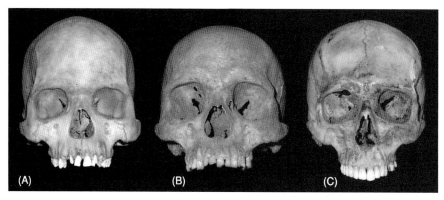

Figure 1 Frontal view of classic representatives of (A) American Black, (B) American Indian, and (C) American White female skulls. Note the subtle craniofacial variation listed in **Table 3**.

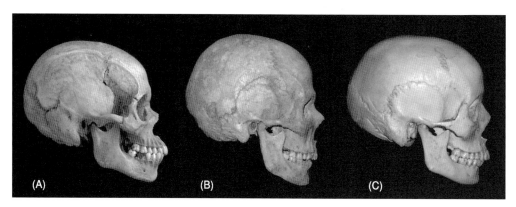

Figure 2 Right lateral view of classic representatives of (A) American Black, (B) American Indian, and (C) American White female skulls. Note the subtle craniofacial variation listed in **Table 3**.

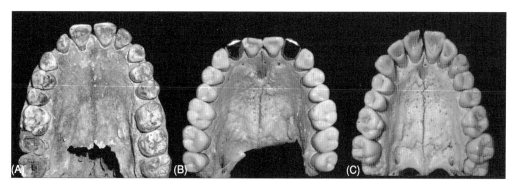

Figure 3 Palatal views of classic representatives of (A) American Black, (B) American Indian, and (C) American White male skulls. Note the respective parabolic, hyperbolic, and convergent tooth rows.

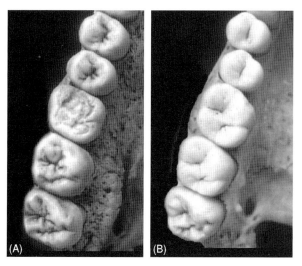

Figure 4 Occlusal view of classic representatives of (a) American Black and (B) American White male premolars and molars demonstrating complex and simple pit and fissure morphology.

with the population sample from which the comparative analysis is taken. Anthropometric studies have demonstrated skull size and shape, relative body proportions, and skeletal robustness differs between populations as well as between sexes within a population.

The Forensic Data Bank

In 1984, the National Institute of Justice sponsored the formation of the Forensic Data Bank within the Anthropology Department at the University of Tennessee. Essentially, the purpose of the Forensic Data Bank is the collection of metric skeletal data from contemporary populations. From this, a discriminant function-based, user-friendly computer program was created which generates a population classification based on cranial and/or postcranial metric measurements from complete or fragmentary

remains. Furthermore, the program provides sex and stature estimation. The current expanded edition, Fordisc 2.0, contains a known age, sex, and race database of approximately 1550 individuals from seven specific geographical regions. With the exception of many American Indians, all were born in the twentieth century. The African American or Black sample is drawn from across the USA as also are the American Indian and White samples, although a few Whites were European-born. Chinese, Japanese, and Vietnamese males were drawn from Hong Kong, Japan, and Vietnam, respectively. Additionally, historical craniological data from approximately 2500 individuals representing worldwide local populations established prior to European expansion are included. Six main geographical regions are included representing Europeans, Africans (sub-Saharan), Far Easterners (Japanese, Chinese), and Australo-Melanesians, Polynesians, and the Americans.

Fordisc results do not diagnose skulls by populations. Statistical classification within groups in the database is achieved by typical probabilities that allow the analyst to draw conclusions. The program is qualified through selection of reasonable populations for comparative analysis. Ongoing data collection in several regions of the world strengthen the prospect of program revisions to incorporate the expanding body of metric skeletal data.

Conclusions

The anthropologist's holistic consciousness provides a seamless integration of biological and social perspectives. Race is a complex construct that can be studied and debated and used and misused by those with sociological, anthropological, political, religious, educational, economic, or other agendas. Biological anthropologists studying population genetics, anthropometrics, and osteometrics have aptly demonstrated that the biology is no less complex. Forensic anthropologists assess race to deliver any and all evidence that may allude to victim identification. It is no less important than any other demographic variable we study. For success, the investigator must be familiar with the wide range of human skeletal variation. More than any other exercise in forensic anthropology, racial evaluation is an estimation based on subjective experience and objective measurement. No single trait can correctly evaluate race on a majority of occasions. Racial assessment reflects the recognition of a suite of skeletal traits most consistent and diagnostic with a specific population. Regardless of population, there is for now significant and subtle bone morphology that differentiates them. As human variation evolves, admixture will continue to morph new designs that will make group differentiation increasing by difficult and the most daunting task in forensic anthropology.

See Also

Anthropology: Archeology, Excavation and Retrieval of Remains; Stature Estimation from the Skeleton; Sex Determination; **War Crimes:** Site Investigation; Pathological Investigation

Further Reading

Dixon AD, Hoyte DAN, Ronning O (1997) *Fundamentals of Craniofacial Growth*. Boca Raton, FL: CRC Press.

Enlow DH, Hans MG (1996) *Essentials of Facial Growth*. Philadelphia, PA: WB Saunders.

Howells WW (1973) *Cranial Variation in Man: A Study by Multivariate Analysis of Patterns of Difference Among Recent Human Populations*. Cambridge, MA: Peabody Museum of Archaeology and Ethnology.

Krogman WM, Iscan MY (1986) *The Human Skeleton in Forensic Medicine*. Springfield, IL: Charles C. Thomas.

Molnar S (2002) *Human Variation: Races, Types, and Ethnic Groups*, 5th edn. Upper Saddle River, NJ: Prentice-Hall.

Ousley SD, Jantz RL (1996) *Fordisc 2.0*. Knoxville, TN: Forensic Anthropology Center, University of Tennessee.

Reichs KJ (1998) *Forensic Osteology: Advances in the Identification of Human Remains*. Springfield, IL: Charles C. Thomas.

Scott GR, Turner CG (1997) *The Anthropology of Modern Human Teeth: Dental Morphology and its Variation in Recent Human Populations*. New York: Cambridge University Press.

Stinson S, Bogin B, Huss-Ashmore R, O'Rourke D (2000) *Human Biology: An Evolutionary and Biocultural Perspective*. New York: John Wiley.

Handedness

M H Czuzak, University of Arizona, Tucson, AZ, USA

Introduction

The assessment of handedness from skeletal remains is based upon observable morphological asymmetry in the bones and joints of the pectoral girdle and upper extremity. The asymmetry results from hypertrophy of bony elements exposed to excessive forces or chronic loading, in accordance with Wolff's laws of bone remodeling. In theory, a right-handed person should exhibit stouter bones or modified joint surfaces, indicating overuse, on the favored right side. However, research suggests that such asymmetry is not always observable and, in some cases, the opposite side may be larger. Thus, in practice, the assessment of handedness is potentially troublesome.

Defining Handedness

"Handedness" describes the consistent, unequal use of one limb over the other in a certain set of prescribed tasks. The antiquity of handedness and its inextricable link to humanity continues to be a focus for anthropological reconstructions of past populations and characterizations of individual ways of life. The supposition of links between the behavior of handedness and its anatomical presentation, cerebral asymmetry, language, and manual manipulation is the basis of much of this research. Many assume that handedness is a readily observable phenomenon, that modern humans are mostly right-handed, that handedness is universally defined and measurable, that evidence of handedness in a few fossils represents that of the whole population, and that handedness is conclusively linked to brain laterality and thus brain complexity.

Humans are considered unique among animals because right-hand dominance is defined as a cross-cultural, population trait. According to traditional estimates, right-handers have comprised 90% of the human population throughout history. Many accept this as a standard ratio and use it to confirm observed asymmetries. However, current studies reveal that handedness is expressed in degrees and hand usage is rarely strictly unilateral. Additionally, differing definitions and problems in its measurement highlight some of the problems inherent in handedness assessment. For example, most use the task of writing as the main criterion for handedness assignation, even though it many not coincide with the limb choice for other activities. Many overlook, neglect, or forget the fact that the nondominant limb has the potential to undergo heavy loading during tasks not classically used to define "handedness." Such loading conditions could stimulate bone remodeling, thereby reducing anatomic asymmetry or even forcing the asymmetry in the opposite direction to that expected. In addition, preferential limb usage may vary according to the specific task and across the many joints or segments comprising the upper extremity, making assessment of "handedness" from skeletal remains far from certain.

In defining handedness, questions also arise as to which quality – power or precision – and which activity – active or passive – should be included in the task list. Traditionally, it seems that activities requiring more coordination and cerebellar involvement are deemed more important in the assignation of handedness, even though crude, assistive, passive activities may generate greater forces that affect the bones to a greater extent. Ultimately, the tasks used by the victim or victim's family to define handedness and those used by the anthropologist may not correspond, resulting in inconsistencies in the relationship between asymmetry and handedness.

Previous Research

Numerous studies unquestionably document morphological asymmetry in the skeleton. However, subsequent interpretations attributing such asymmetry to handedness are potentially flawed if the ante-mortem handedness pattern for the sample is not known and the researcher is relying on the assumed 90% frequency of "right-handedness." If handedness of the sample is "known," one must be critical of the task set used to define handedness. Overall, results have been mixed in the establishment of a link between asymmetry and handedness.

One of the earliest studies was performed by Schultz in 1937 in which he compared asymmetries in long bone lengths (upper and lower limbs) in humans and nonhuman primates. He found that the human arm bones exhibited a greater degree of asymmetry than those from the nonhuman primates. In addition, he noted a magnification of asymmetry in the upper limb relative to the lower limb that was suggestive of handedness but dismissed the link since it was contrary to his earlier fetal research.

Approximately 30 years later, T. Dale Stewart observed a difference in morphology of the right and left glenoid fossae while analyzing Korean War dead and in subsequent analysis of skeletons in the Terry collection. He reported that the right side of

the scapular glenoid exhibited increased beveling, dorsal inclination, and arthritic change. Handedness for both of Stewart's samples was not known. However, in 1980, Schulter-Ellis replicated Stewart's study using 10 cadavers of known handedness and corroborated his findings.

One of the strongest correlations between asymmetry and excess limb use was established by Jones and his colleagues in 1977. Upon analyzing humeral radiographs of 84 professional tennis players, they found a 28.4–34.9% increase in cortical thickness of the humerus on the "playing side." This study indicates the degree of loading and constancy of limb use necessary to result in asymmetry marked enough to allow one to postulate handedness confidently.

More recent studies attempting to document asymmetry in order to predict handedness have met with varying degrees of success. In 1986, Glassman and Bass attempted to test the relationship of the jugular foramen to limb asymmetry, a correlation used in the past to indicate handedness. Assuming that handedness is linked to cerebral asymmetry, the cerebral hemisphere controlling the dominant limb would require a greater blood supply and, by default, a larger drainage system. The venous drainage of the brain is primarily via the internal jugular veins, which pass through the jugular foramina of the skull. Though working with a skeletal sample of unknown handedness (the Terry collection), the authors demonstrated that the hypothesis is unfounded due to the lack of correlation between limb and jugular foramen asymmetry.

Roy and colleagues measured the anterior and posterior cortical bone thickness of the second metacarpal on plain radiographs of a large living sample for whom handedness was self-reported. They found a statistically significant correlation between handedness and several variables calculated from the cortical thicknesses. However, an earlier study performed by Garn and his colleagues on the cortical thickness of the second metacarpal in patients with chronic renal disease resulted in a paradoxical occurrence of asymmetry. Among the 227 individuals in the study, all exhibited a greater right-side cortical area, including the 19 self-reported left-handed individuals. The authors conclude that the paradoxical asymmetry may be specific to their particular sample or it suggests that left-handed individuals use the right hand more than suspected.

In a comprehensive study in 1998, Czuzak analyzed gross osteometric measurements, proximal and distal joint surface areas, midshaft cortical thicknesses, and osteoarthritic scores in the humeri, radii, ulnae, and first metacarpals of 39 cadavers. Right–left asymmetry was compared to handedness, which was assigned by next of kin. Interestingly, there was

Table 1 Summary of previous studies

Author	Year	Study	Findings
Schultz	1937	Compared human upper-extremity bone lengths with those of nonhuman primates in an attempt to compare degree of asymmetry between human and nonhuman primates	Human ($n = 753$) arm bones exhibited a greater degree of asymmetry than those from nonhuman primates ($n = 530$)
Garn *et al.*	1976	Examined the degree of cortical asymmetry of the second metacarpals in radiographs of 227 patients with chronic renal disease; handedness was self-reported by patients	Reported a paradoxical occurrence of asymmetry in the cortical thickness of the second metacarpal; all exhibited a greater right-side cortical area, even the 19 left-handed individuals
Stewart	1976	Compared the morphology of the glenoid cavity between the right and left sides and compared these to differences in humeral length using the Terry collection; handedness is unknown for this sample	Right glenoid exhibited increased beveling of the dorsal border and the entire face tended to be more dorsally inclined; these occurred often with greater right humeral length and right-sided arthritic changes
Jones *et al.*	1977	Compared radiographs of humeri of 84 professional tennis players	Humerus on the "playing side" exhibited marked hypertrophy in cortical thickness (34.9% males; 28.4% females)
Schulter-Ellis	1980	Tested Stewart's study using 10 cadavers of known handedness	Corroborated Stewart's findings
Glassman and Bass	1986	Studied the relationship of the jugular foramen to limb asymmetry (a correlation used in the past to indicate handedness) in the Terry collection; handedness is unknown for this sample	Demonstrated that the hypothesis is unfounded due to a lack of correlation between the sides of the larger structures
Roy *et al.*	1994	Measured the anterior and posterior cortical bone thickness of the second metacarpal on plain radiographs of a large living sample for which handedness was assessed by "personal impression"	Found statistically significant correlation of handedness to their variables calculated from the cortical thickness measures (cortical bone area, periosteal area, medullary area, and second moment of area)
Czuzak	1998	Compared asymmetry of the humeri, radii, ulnae, and first metacarpals using osteometric data, joint surface areas, midshaft cortical thickness, and osteoarthitic score on a sample of 39 cadavers for whom the handedness was assigned by next of kin	Frequency analysis revealed an overall trend of misclassification of handedness, with greater misclassification for the nonright-handed individuals, females, and when using joint surface area and cortical thickness data

an overall trend of misclassification of handedness based on skeletal asymmetries and the misclassification was exaggerated in nonright-handed individuals, females, and for measures of cortical thickness and joint surface area. As found by Garn, it is probable that these 39 individuals were also using their non-dominant limbs more than expected or defined by any handedness questionnaire (**Table 1**).

Handedness in Forensic Practice

The assignation of handedness is often not a typical feature of the forensic biological profile unless the skeletal asymmetry is so grossly obvious that it warrants remark. Such obvious asymmetry may be apparent in individuals experiencing excessive unilateral loading of a limb, as may occur in tennis players or baseball pitchers. Alternatively, unilateral disuse due to paralysis may also result in noticeable asymmetry. In these cases, postulation of handedness based on the observed asymmetry may be helpful in corroborating identification. However, since most individuals are

not exposed to excessive unilateral loads, asymmetry may not be as obvious. Assignation of handedness based upon minimal asymmetry and/or the assumption that 90% of individuals are right-handed may compromise identification of skeletal remains. Care must be taken not to overinterpret the remains.

Summary

From this brief overview, one may conclude that the concept of handedness is not as conspicuous as personal experience might suggest. There is no doubt that one limb is preferred/specialized to perform certain tasks but the opposite limb is never inactive. Humans are truly bimanual; unless incapacitated, the opposite limb assists the one performing the primary activity. The "nondominant" limb can even take over the activity during times of fatigue. Activities used to define handedness vary greatly, with no universally accepted set of tasks to guide researchers. Based on the ambiguity of handedness itself and the paucity of studies supporting its interpretation from skeletal remains, caution should be exercised in the assignation of handedness.

See Also

Anthropology: Stature Estimation from the Skeleton; **Autopsy:** Procedures and Standards

Further Reading

Czuzak M (1998) *Skeletal Asymmetry, Degenerative Joint Disease and Handedness in Humans.* Unpublished PhD dissertation. Tucson, Arizona: University of Arizona.

Garn SM, Mayor GH, Shaw H (1976) Paradoxical bilateral asymmetry in bone size and bone mass in the hand. *American Journal of Physical Anthropology* 45: 209–210.

Glassman D, Bass W (1986) Bilateral asymmetry of long arm bones and jugular foramen: implications for handedness. *Journal of Forensic Sciences* 31(2): 589–595.

Hellige JB (1993) *Hemispheric Asymmetry: What's Right and What's Left.* Massachusetts: Harvard University Press.

Jones HE, Priest JD, Hayes WC, Tichenor CC, Nagel DA (1977) Humeral hypertrophy in response to exercise. *Journal of Bone and Joint Surgery* 59A: 204–208.

McManus C (2002) *Right Hand, Left Hand: The Origins of Asymmetry in Brains, Bodies, Atoms and Cultures.* Massachusetts: Harvard University Press.

Roy TA, Ruff CB, Plato CC (1994) Hand dominance and bilateral asymmetry in the structure of the second metacarpal. *American Journal of Physical Anthropology* 94: 203–211.

Schulter-Ellis FP (1980) Evidence of handedness on documented skeletons. *Journal of Forensic Sciences* 25(3): 624–630.

Schultz AH (1937) Proportions, variability and asymmetry of the long bones of the limbs and the clavicles in man and apes. *Human Biology* 9(3): 281–328.

Stewart TD (1976) Evidence of handedness in the bony shoulder joint. *American Academy of Forensic Sciences Abstracts* (annual meeting Washington, DC) 124: 68.

Stewart TD (1979) *Essentials of Forensic Anthropology.* Springfield, IL: Charles C. Thomas.

Role of DNA

B Ludes and C Keyser-Tracqui, Institut de Médecine Légale, Strasbourg, France

Introduction

Deoxyribonucleic acid (DNA) is used by forensic scientists as a means of identification, for example of criminals and corpses and now it has also been found to be relevant in anthropology, in fields such as human evolution, population movements, and paleodiseases. In the 1990s, it became possible to extract DNA from very old tissues such as skeletal remains. Such DNA permitted discovery of aspects of past social organizations that were previously unknown or difficult to ascertain using conventional techniques. Some recent studies have shown that these analyses may become routine with well-preserved human remains but, in the majority of cases, many problems still remain, namely, in methodology, sampling procedures, and interpretation guidelines.

The DNA Molecules

Nuclear DNA

Every human cell, excluding red blood cells, has a nucleus that contains DNA, which carries the genetic information. DNA is made up of two complementary strands that are coiled together in a helix. These strands are composed of different subunits (bases): adenine (A), guanine (G), thymine (T), and cytosine (C), which pair together to form a very long chain. The DNA content of the nucleus in humans is divided into 23 pairs of chromosomes that are passed on to children by both parents, with each parent giving 23 chromosomes. Among these 23 pairs of chromosomes are 22 pairs of autosomes and one pair of sex chromosomes, XX for female, and XY for male.

Currently, it seems that only 10% of the human genome carries genetically relevant information which is essential for each individual. Since it appears that the remaining regions of the human genome are not subject to evolutionary pressure and selection mechanisms, they vary greatly from one person to another. This is the reason for the accumulation of mutations (single nucleotide changes) and rearrangements (deletions, insertions, and duplications) leading to the generation of a genetic diversity within noncoding regions. DNA polymorphisms consist of sequences repeated in tandem (e.g., short tandem repeats; STRs), present at specific sites (loci) on the genome. The number of these repeats varies from one person to the other, causing variations in size, known as alleles. Since each specific locus is present on both the chromosomes in a given pair (except for the XY pair of sex chromosomes), each person has one allele inherited from the maternal chromosome and one from the paternal chromosome. As a result, it is possible, through the analysis of the autosomal STRs, not only to identify (to a high degree of probability) an individual from a sample of DNA but also to test close familial relationships.

More recently, Y-chromosomal markers (STRs and biallelic markers) have also been used for human identification in forensic casework and paternity testing as well as for the study of human evolution. These markers are of special interest because they are haploid and paternally inherited; the fact that they do not undergo recombination offers the possibility of directly tracing male lineages back in time.

Mitochondrial DNA

Every human cell has a "second" genome, found in the cell's energy-generating organelle, the mitochondrion. Each mitochondrion has several copies of its own genome, and there are several hundred to several thousand mitochondria per cell. The entire DNA sequence of the human mitochondrial genome (16 569 nucleotides) was determined in 1981. The mitochondrial DNA (mtDNA) contains 37 genes, all of which are involved in the production of energy and its storage in adenosine triphosphate (ATP).

Apart from its maternal inheritance (fathers make no contribution to the mitochondria of their children) and lack of recombination (due to the lack of paternal mtDNA with which to recombine), two aspects of mtDNA make it particularly useful for the analysis of forensic and archeological material: (1) its high copy number, which increases the chance of survival of a few molecules in the face of molecular damage that may affect forensic or ancient biological samples; and (2) the fact that it accumulates mutations faster than nuclear DNA, resulting in the ability to discriminate between individuals or populations. Among the possible analyses of mtDNA, those concerning two hypervariable (HV) regions of the control region (specifically the noncoding regions HVI and HVII) are the most frequent, since they contain the highest degree of polymorphism.

Techniques

Analysis of restriction fragment length polymorphisms (RFLPs) and cloning of DNA fragments from ancient samples were the two techniques initially used in molecular anthropology. While highly efficient and reliable, these techniques often reach an impasse when the quantity of DNA available for analysis is very limited, or when the DNA is too severely damaged.

In 1985, a process was reported by which specific portions of the sample DNA can be amplified almost indefinitely. This has revolutionized forensic and ancient DNA analyses because the process, the polymerase chain reaction (PCR), has allowed the amplification of extremely low concentrations of DNA. Nowadays PCR is the most widely used technique in the field of molecular anthropology because even degraded DNA can be amplified and subsequently analyzed.

PCR amplification is achieved by denaturing the DNA sample into separate individual strands. Two synthetic oligonucleotide primers are then used to hybridize to the DNA sequence of interest and a heat-stable DNA polymerase extends these primers to create a complete and complementary strand of DNA. In this fashion, two new copies of the sequences of interest are generated. This process is typically repeated sequentially 25–40 times thereby creating millions of copies of the target DNA sequence. The amplified sequence can then be detected by gel electrophoresis.

Ancient DNA

The DNA molecule extracted from ancient preserved biological material, called ancient DNA (aDNA), is fragmented into small pieces ranging from only a few base pairs (bp) to a few hundred at most. Some of the bases may have undergone chemical changes and the DNA content available for analysis is extremely small, sometimes fewer than ten molecules per gram of bone.

Little is known about the optimum preservation conditions; temperature, pH, and moisture levels are probably the most important factors, followed by the degree of protection from the external environment. Burial in wet soil may be unsuitable for DNA survival, leading to extreme fragmentation of the DNA, and microbial activity and microenvironmental variation around bones also play important roles. There is no method available for the rapid screening of bones for indications of DNA survival, and there is no direct correlation between DNA content and the age of a bone. Nevertheless, the age limit for successful retrieval seems to be around 100 000 years.

Bone and teeth are the major sources of DNA in archeological studies. These tissues are more likely than soft tissues to persist, due to their physical durability, and conditions within the bone are relatively more favorable for the preservation of DNA. Compared to other organs, bones have low water and catabolic enzyme content which may allow a rapid mummification of the individual osteocytes or cementoblasts. The cell material is also abundant in compact bone with 20 000 osteocytes per cubic millimeter. The important characteristic of bone and tooth tissues is that their matrix is composed of crystalline calcium phosphate (hydroxyapatite), which is known to bind to double-stranded DNA. The binding of the DNA molecule to the bone matrix may play a role in the long-term protection of DNA from chemical breakdown. The hardness and the high hydroxyapatite concentration of tooth dentine may preserve DNA to an even greater extent than occurs in bone.

Applications of DNA Analysis in Anthropology

The main applications of these analyses are identification of sex of human remains, kinship analyses, the study of paleodiseases, and tracing the migrations of populations and their gene distributions. DNA data are also used to test the hypotheses of the origins of anatomically modern humans; in this context, comparisons have been performed with the Neanderthal DNA sequences.

Sex Identification

Identification of sex by morphological criteria is dependent on the survival of either skull or pelvis and assumes that their morphology has not been affected by any pathology. However, skeletal remains are frequently incomplete or ambiguous in juveniles and infants. DNA analysis provides an accurate and reliable method for the sex determination of human skeletal remains. These molecular investigations are based on the PCR amplification of repetitive DNA sequences from both X and Y chromosomes. For this purpose, the amelogenin gene (present in both sex chromosomes) is chosen since the sequences on the X and the Y chromosome are nonidentical. The number of repeats in the two chromosomes is different so that the PCR products show sex-specific size differences: the amplified products have 112 bp for the Y chromosome and 106 bp for the X product. Partial amplification failure of either the X or the Y template DNA can occur, but this failure occurs more frequently when larger sequences are amplified. For example, the amplification of three different PCR systems based on the amelogenin gene can be achieved in a single reaction using three primers. Primers 1 and 2 anneal to the X chromosome, while primers 1 and 3 anneal to the Y chromosome, which has a 64 bp deletion. The PCR product from the X chromosome has 195 bp and is larger than that from the Y chromosome, which has only 132 bp. These sequences are large and, in ancient samples, partial amplification may be responsible for the visualization of only one band in male samples (of 132 bp), the

other sequence located on the X chromosome being too large and possibly degraded for correct amplification. Another method is based on the hybridization of the PCR products with probes specific for the X and Y sequences but partial amplification failure has also been reported.

Kinship Analysis

The "genetic fingerprinting" techniques which have been widely employed in the identification of murder victims and sexual assault criminals and in settling paternity disputes have also been used widely for determining kinship within a group of burials. The DNA sequences used in kinship determination are called microsatellites, which are located in the intergenic regions and have no known functions. These STRs consist of a 2, 3, 4, or 5 bp sequence repeated 5–30 times. More than 10 000 STRs have been described in the human genome but only about 60 are used for identification purposes. The chosen STRs must be hightly polymorphic in the human population, and each marker has to be found in several versions. These alleles have different numbers of repeats and, therefore, their own diagnostic length. PCR primers are designed for each STR to yield amplification products of 100–450 bp; for analysis of ancient tissues, the smaller the products the better the identification. Except for monozygotic twins, no two living persons have exactly the same combination of STR alleles, so the examination of 16 polymorphic STRs allows the identification of a given person by their unique genetic fingerprint. The frequency of STR alleles is determined in various populations in order to calculate the probability of occurrence of a genetic profile more than once. For past populations not enough individuals are available for calculating the allele frequencies, but by increasing the number of studied STRs we can achieve the identification of human remains, within the burial group, to determine kinships. As an example, the present authors and coworkers have successfully extracted DNA from the skeletal remains of 62 individuals excavated from a burial site of the Xiongnu people, in northern Mongolia. Three types of genetic markers were used to determine the genetic relationships between the people buried in this necropolis. Results from autosomal and Y-chromosome STRs as well as from mtDNA analyses showed close relationships between several individuals and provided additional background information on the social organization within the necropolis as well as the funeral practices of the Xiongnu people.

Paleopathology

Recently, molecular biology has become a powerful tool for identifying bacterial, protozoan, and viral infections in ancient human remains. This approach has been extensively used for the detection of the *Mycobacterium tuberculosis* complex, *Mycobacterium leprae, Yersinia pestis, Plasmodium falciparum, Trypanosoma cruzi*, and the influenza virus. The study of residual bacterial DNA in skeletal or mummified tissue samples has allowed not only a confirmation of the diagnosis made, notably on bone lesions, but has also added to the progress in the knowledge of the history of some infectious diseases and of their prevalence in past civilizations. For instance, it has been proved, through DNA analysis of ancient tissue, that tuberculosis was present before European contact in the New World, and that infection with this mycobacterium was relatively frequent in ancient Egypt. Molecular detection of ancient microorganisms has also provided nucleic acid sequences that could be compared with those of modern isolates. Such comparisons of ancient pathogens with their modern counterparts at the DNA level may reveal the evolution of a pathogen over time and help to identify variations in its virulence. As an example, gene sequences of the 1918 "Spanish" influenza virus have been used to frame hypotheses about the origin of this pandemic virus, and to look for clues as to its virulence. It is likely that knowledge gained by studying these human pathogens will in the future be applied to prevent, or at least predict, the emergence of new infections with pandemic potential.

Evolution

Molecular biology also permits us to tackle ambitious goals, such as studying the genetic structure of extinct species and their relationship to contemporary species. A prime example, within the genus *Homo*, concerns the role of Neanderthals in the evolution of modern humans.

Neanderthals are a group of extinct hominids that inhabited Europe and the Middle East between about 230 000 and 30 000 years ago. Their proximity in time to anatomically modern humans has raised questions about the coexistence of these two hominid forms. It is controversial as to whether Neanderthals (1) should be regarded as direct ancestors of modern Europeans; (2) contributed, by hybridization, to the gene pool of modern humans before becoming extinct; or (3) evolved totally independently of *Homo sapiens*. The classical view emerging from anatomical and archeological studies has placed Neanderthals in a different species from *H. sapiens*. Furthermore,

analyses of molecular genetic variation in the mitochondrial and nuclear genomes of contemporary human populations have generally supported the view that Neanderthals were not related to modern humans. Nevertheless, the relationship between Neanderthals and modern humans remains enigmatic, so the retrieval of Neander DNA is still one of the major goals of researchers in the field of ancient DNA.

The first successful extraction of a mtDNA sequence from a Neanderthal was performed on the 40 000-year-old Neanderthal type specimen found in a limestone quarry in the Neander Valley, Germany. A few years later, a second mtDNA sequence from a Neanderthal child (dating to about 30 000 years ago) found in Mezmaiskaya Cave in the northern Caucasus was determined and found to be similar to the type specimen. Phylogenetic analysis placed these two Neanderthals from Germany and the Caucasus together in a clade that is distinct from modern humans, suggesting that their mtDNA types have not contributed to the modern human mtDNA pool. Two new mtDNA sequences, subsequently obtained from a Neanderthal individual (about 42 000 years old) from Vindija, Croatia and from a second Neanderthal individual from the Neander Valley (about 40 000 years old), made it possible to estimate the mtDNA diversity among Neanderthal specimens. This genetic diversity was comparable to that of contemporary humans and lower than that of the great apes. The newly obtained mtDNA sequences also confirmed the hypothesis that Neanderthals were a separate hominid species (*H. neanderthalensis*) rather than a subspecies (*H. sapiens neanderthalensis*) that contributed some genes to modern human ancestry. This hypothesis was further supported by a work based on Southern blot hybridization technique. Nonetheless, for some authors a comparison of Neanderthal and living human mtDNA with mtDNA from ancient fossils of anatomically modern humans was a crucial step for solving this question. This has recently been achieved by the typing of mtDNA HV region of two anatomically modern *Homo sapiens sapiens* individuals of the Cro-Magnon type found in a southern Italian cave and dated at about 25 000–23 000 years ago. The Cro-Magnon sequences fall within a genetic category shared by people today but not by Neanderthals, bolstering the theory that modern *Homo sapiens* replaced Neanderthals in Europe rather than interbred with them.

Human Migrations

Up until the 1990s, the study of human migration patterns was primarily accomplished using macroscopic examination of ancient and fossil bone specimens and analysis of genetic polymorphism in living populations. Now analysis of DNA polymorphisms can reveal the relationships between populations and thus allow past migrations to be identified. Since it is maternally inherited and evolves quickly, mtDNA has been used extensively for unraveling the ancient human migrations. However, since gene flow through the maternal lineage is expressed, current attempts to understand prehistoric human migrations also include the use of Y chromosomal nuclear markers. Moreover, because direct analysis of ancient samples is the unique tool for checking the conclusions based on genetic analysis of modern populations, analysis of ancient DNA research has also been used when possible to establish the time and route of major migrations in human history. Ancient samples from Native American archeological sites have been used, for example, to shed light on the peopling of the New World. This example represents, indeed, one of the more debated topics in the study of human migrations. It is generally accepted that the ancestors of Native Americans came from Asia across the Bering Strait; however, the timing, place(s) of origin, and number of waves of migration are surrounded by controversy. Analyses of mtDNA diversity among Native Americans (both contemporary and ancient) have revealed that nearly all of them belong to one of five mtDNA haplogroups: A, B, C, D, or X. Initially, the presence of haplogroups A, B, C, and D in Siberian and Mongolian populations led scientists to propose these areas as potential geographic sources of ancestral Native American populations. Recently, this notion has been strengthened by the discovery of haplogroup X in Altaian populations from southern Siberia. Furthermore, several studies on Y chromosome DNA polymorphism were performed to investigate male migrations to the American continent. It has been proposed that populations occupying the area including Lake Baïkal, the Yenissey River Basin, and the Altai Mountains were the source for dispersals of New World Y-chromosome founders. Nevertheless, questions concerning the number and timing of migrations into the New World remain, to date, unresolved.

Other issues, such as the expansion of Neolithic farmers into Europe or the role of male and female migrations in human history, have also been investigated through DNA analyses. By using autosomal, mitochondrial, and Y chromosome polymorphisms, it has been shown, for example, that Y chromosome variants tend to be more localized geographically than those of mtDNA and the autosomes. In other words, it seems that females have had a much higher migration rate than males. Patrilocality could be a good explanation: women moved much more frequently between groups than did men, leading to greater between-population differences for the Y chromosome.

Contamination, Interpretation Difficulties and Validation of Results

The importance of fossils in the field of anthropology has been somewhat reduced as it has became possible to study human history through the distribution and frequency of DNA sequences from present-day populations worldwide. A reconciliation of both approaches (paleontological and genetic) has come with the extraction and amplification of DNA from ancient specimens. However, technical pitfalls make ancient DNA studies liable to yield dubious results, particularly when human remains are studied.

Ancient DNA molecules tend to be damaged and consequently are refractory to most of the current procedures for nucleic acid analysis. Water and oxygen, which cause hydrolysis and oxidation of DNA, respectively, reduce the number and the size of the fragments that can be amplified. Under these circumstances, it is possible that DNA polymerase errors, as well as miscoding lesions in the template DNA sequences occur.

The difficulty in amplifying DNA in archeological samples may also result from the presence of inhibitors that interfere with the PCR reaction. Indeed, archeological specimens may contain low-molecular-weight compounds, most likely to be derived from the burial environment, which copurify with DNA and potently inhibit the activity of Taq polymerase employed in PCR.

Nevertheless, the main problem encountered in the analysis of ancient DNA is contamination of samples by modern DNA molecules. Because of the efficiency of PCR, even low levels of contamination with contemporary DNA will lead to erroneous results. Human remains are particularly difficult to work with, owing to the difficulty of identifying contaminating human sequences. Such contaminations may stem from a variety of sources, such as handling during excavation or removal of samples or contamination of reagents and glassware used during the extraction and analysis procedures.

All these problems can be overcome by the implementation of specific precautions in the preparation and handling of samples and solutions as well as experimental controls at the DNA extraction and amplification stages. To avoid contamination, all DNA extractions and PCR preparations involving ancient DNA samples should be performed in a laboratory room exclusively dedicated to ancient DNA analysis and physically separated from the main genetics laboratory. In each extraction and amplification step, a control sample (a sample with no tissue, bone, or extracted DNA sample) should be included and processed similarly. A strong inverse correlation between amplification efficiency and length of the ancient DNA to be amplified should be noted. Multiple extracts must be performed, preferably from different tissues of the same individual, and the results should be identical. The amount of damage likely to have been suffered by the ancient DNA should be determined. An estimation of the number of ancient template DNA molecules from which the PCR starts should be made to ensure the quality of ancient DNA sequences. The cloning of the PCR product and sequencing of several clones should be used to detect problems and to obtain a consensus sequence for the target. DNA extraction and amplification should be independently repeated in a different laboratory, and the results should be consistent across laboratories.

In addition to contamination, ancient DNA studies face other problems. Since the archeological and paleontological specimens used are valuable and available in limited quantity, the small amounts of DNA that could be extracted allowed typing of only a limited number of markers for each sample and the data obtained are not always highly informative. Moreover, only the remains that are discovered can be analyzed; this means many questions may never be addressed by ancient DNA methods. Finally, another drawback to using archeological materials is that it is often difficult to obtain anything resembling a population of individuals who lived together at the same time.

Conclusion

Molecular anthropology intertwines with a variety of disciplines, such as forensic genetics, anthropology, archeology, evolutionary studies, and paleopathology. From human remains, the molecular biologist attempts to understand issues such as the nature of societies that existed in the past, their cultural and ritual customs, their evolutionary histories, their migrations and interactions with other societies through trade, warfare, and acculturation, their impacts on the environment, their means of subsistence, and their diseases. However, technical pitfalls make the field liable

to give dubious results unless many precautions and experimental controls are implemented. Future developments such as the possibility of removing or repairing chemical damage in the ancient DNA would be welcome additions to this field.

See Also

Anthropology: Sex Determination; Determination of Racial Affinity; **DNA:** Basic Principles; Risk of Contamination; Mitochondrial

Further Reading

Brown K (2002) Ancient DNA applications in human osteoarchaeology: achievements, problems and potential. In: Cox M, Mays S (eds.) *Human Osteology in Archaeology and Forensic Science*, pp. 455–473. London: GMM.

Erlich HA (ed.) (1989) *PCR Technology: Principles and Applications for DNA Amplification.* New York: Stockton Press.

Greenblatt CL (ed.) (1998) *Digging for Pathogens: Ancient Emerging Diseases, their Evolutionary, Anthropological and Archaeological Context.* Balaban Publishers.

Hummel S (ed.) (2003) *Ancient DNA Typing: Methods, Strategies and Applications.* Berlin: Springer-Verlag.

Innis MA, Gelfand DH, Sninsky JJ (eds.) (1995) *PCR Strategies.* San Diego, CA: Academic Press.

Keyser-Tracqui C, Crubézy E, and Ludes B (in press). Nuclear and mitochondrial DNA analysis of Xiongnu population (III BC–II AD) from the Egyin Gol valley (Mongolia, peri-Baïkal area). *American Journal of Human Genetics* (in press).

Kimpton CP, Oldroyd NJ, Watson SK, *et al.* (1996) Validation of highly discriminating multiplex short tandem repeat amplification systems for individual identification. *Electrophoresis* 17: 1283–1293.

Martin RB, Burr DB (1989) *Structure, Function and Adaptation of Compact Bone.* New York: Raven Press.

Moretti TR, Baumstark AL, Defenbaugh DA, *et al.* (2001) Validation of short tandem repeats (STRs) for forensic usage: performance testing of fluorescent multiplex STR systems and analysis of authentic and simulated forensic samples. *Journal of Forensic Science* 46: 647–660.

Mullis KB, Ferré F, Gibbs RA (eds.) (1994) *PCR: Polymerase Chain Reaction.* Boston, MA: Birkhäuser.

Parsons TJ, Weedn VW (1997) Preservation and recovery of DNA in postmortem specimens and trace samples. In: Haglund WD, Sorg MH (eds.) *Forensic Taphonomy, The Postmortem Fate of Human Remains*, pp. 109–138. New York: CRC Press.

ASPHYXIA

A Walker and C M Milroy, University of Sheffield, Sheffield, UK

J Payne-James, Forensic Healthcare Services Ltd, London, UK

Introduction

The etymological meaning of asphyxia as derived from the Greek means "absence of pulsation." It has come to be used in modern forensic medical practice to refer to death or other clinical sequelae due to lack of oxygen. There are many different ways of classifying asphyxial death, and perhaps the simplest is to consider the possible practical effects by which asphyxia may occur. Asphyxial death can be applied to a number of mechanisms of death where respiration/ventilation is affected, including:

1. suffocation, where death is associated with deprivation of oxygen, either from a lack of oxygen in the surrounding environment or obstruction of the upper airway
2. smothering, more specifically where there is external obstruction of the upper airway
3. strangulation, which may occur by ligature or by manual pressure using one or both hands, when the term throttling may be used
4. choking, e.g., inhaling food
5. garrotting (commonly used to describe application of a ligature)
6. chest compression (due to fixation of the external chest wall as a result of crushing)
7. hanging (by another, deliberate self-harm, or autoerotic asphyxia).

It can be seen that several of these terms, and the mechanisms associated with them, may interrelate. Not all may be due to asphyxia alone; other factors, such as vasovagal stimulation, may contribute. Other terms such as neck compression may be used to cover external pressure on the neck, such as by an arm lock during restraint.

Overly rigorous use of terminology can however be misleading and the emphasis should be on having a clear description of the cause of deprivation of oxygen or prevention of respiration/ventilation and the findings associated with each episode. This article focuses on two areas of asphyxia – that of death in closed and confined spaces and the clinical findings in those who have survived assaults that could have caused asphyxial death.

Asphyxial Death

The investigation of such deaths has traditionally been founded on the so-called "classic signs of asphyxia." These signs have included congestion, cyanosis, edema, petechiae, and fluidity of blood. None of these signs is reliable or indeed diagnostic as an indicator of asphyxia as a mode of death. Petechiae are pinhead-sized hemorrhages seen in the skin, the sclera, and conjunctivae, and on mucosal surfaces in the mouth as well as the organs of the chest. Most characteristically they are seen on the outer and inner surfaces of the eyelids. In cases of manual strangulation petechiae may be florid. They are often absent in hanging and may occur in many nonasphyxia deaths. The proposed mechanisms of causation have included raised venous pressure and increased vascular fragility due to hypoxia. The latter explanation is not supported by their absence in many hypoxic deaths. They can appear rapidly in coughing bouts or retching and the most logical view is that they occur due to raised venous pressure. However, because they are common, when appropriately looked for, and occur in many different mechanisms of death, their presence must be interpreted with caution and in the context of the death with the surrounding circumstances.

The other "classic" signs are congestion, cyanosis, and edema, which are such common findings in many different modes of death as to have no specific diagnostic value. Fluidity of blood has more to do with the rapidity of death than the mode of death and has diagnostic value in determining the cause of death. It has been appropriately stated by Knight that abnormal fluidity of blood is part of forensic mythology and has no relevance in the diagnosis of asphyxia. In all cases of possible asphyxial death physical external and internal evidence of asphyxia may be present and must be taken into account with the known history and background prior to death.

Additional nonspecific features that may rarely be present include frank hemorrhage from orifices such as the nose and ear, and spontaneous evacuation of feces and urine.

Asphyxia with Confined and Enclosed Spaces

Deaths associated with confined and enclosed spaces present problems to the investigating pathologist, as there may be few or no diagnostic features at autopsy. Although the deaths are typically classified as asphyxial, there may be no features to make such a diagnosis. As with all deaths, but in particular with these deaths, the findings and surrounding circumstances need to be taken into account in determining the cause and ultimately the manner of the death.

Mechanism of Death

Suffocation is the most common term used for deaths associated with reduced availability of oxygen. It is also used in cases where other nontoxic irrespirable gases are encountered. In a person confined within an enclosed environment a number of factors may contribute to the collapse and death of the victim, including the lack of oxygen and the build-up of carbon dioxide. The presence of other irrespirable gases should be considered, especially in an industrial setting, such as mining. One well-recognized situation in which a hypoxic death occurs is where a young child, often playing a game trying to hide from others, enters a self-locking fridge or box and then has no mechanism of escape. No specific signs are seen and petechiae and other asphyxial signs are absent. Homicide victims may be placed in confined spaces. In one such case seen by one of the authors, the victim had been placed in a box trunk and left tied up but without any obstruction of the airway. The victim had abrasions where he tried to move in the box in his desperate struggle to try and get out. He had no asphyxial signs at autopsy.

Carbon dioxide may play an important part in deaths in enclosed spaces. In environments such as submarines a mechanism to remove carbon dioxide is present. Otherwise an increase in carbon dioxide will result in central nervous system depression and respiratory collapse. The normal concentration of carbon dioxide in air is 0.1%. If the concentration of carbon dioxide is raised but oxygen remains at 20%, death will still occur from breathing such a mixture of gases. This is illustrated when rapid entrance into an environment high in carbon dioxide results in almost immediate collapse. Carbon dioxide poisoning has also been postulated as a cause of death in infants placed in appropriate sleeping positions, when they are at risk of rebreathing carbon dioxide. Carbon dioxide is not *per se* directly toxic, unlike carbon monoxide, cyanide, and hydrogen sulfide. However, even nontoxic gases can be asphyxiating if too high a concentration is present in an enclosed space and rapid collapse may occur on entering such an environment. When multiple deaths are encountered it may be because colleagues go to the aid of a victim and are then overcome by the same gases.

One well-recognized situation where carbon dioxide poisoning occurs is in grain silos. The grain in the silo gives off carbon dioxide and, if a worker enters the silo before the carbon dioxide has been vented the worker may collapse on breathing the carbon dioxide.

Similar episodes of collapse and sudden death may be encountered where workers enter ships' holds or when cleaning or inspecting fuel tanks of ships. Some industrial tanks contain high concentrations of nitrogen. The mechanism of death in these cases appears to be a rapid cardiorespiratory arrest mediated through central brainstem receptors rather than slower hypoxic death. This mechanism of death has been compared to people dying of plastic-bag asphyxia. In these deaths no asphyxial signs are seen and death in these cases appears very rapid. In some planned suicides the placing of the plastic bag over the head has been accompanied by the use of helium, another irrespirable gas.

Methane in an enclosed atmosphere may be hazardous and can be encountered in a number of situations including mining, where methane production has long been recognized as a problem because of its explosive qualities (firedamp). It may also kill by oxygen deprivation. Methane, along with other gases, including hydrogen sulfide, may be produced in sewers.

Use of solvents in enclosed spaces may result in exposure, collapse, and death. Many different solvents are used in industry, many being halogenated hydrocarbons, which are also used as degreasers, cleaners, propellants, and for chemical synthesis. They have properties similar to general anesthetics.

Exposure to methylene chloride (dichloromethane) may result in the production of carboxyhemoglobin in the absence of combustion. In car-exhaust suicides, the typical finding is of very high carboxyhemoglobin concentrations. Lower concentrations may be seen in people with preexisting natural diseases where death takes place before higher levels are reached. However, with emission control technology being introduced on modern motor vehicles, carbon monoxide concentrations in exhaust fumes are significantly reduced. This has resulted in unsuccessful attempts at suicide, and in successful cases the absence of raised carboxyhemoglobin concentrations. In these cases death has been attributed to carbon dioxide poisoning. It has been proposed that the cause of death be given as "inhalation of automobile exhaust gases." Leakage of gasoline (petrol) into the vehicle cabin following automobile accidents has been reported as a contributory factor in deaths, where the victims were trapped, but had not sustained major injury.

Postmortem Investigation

For most of these types of asphyxial deaths there are typically no specific findings. Asphyxial signs are characteristically absent. The autopsy should be directed at excluding other nonnatural causes and the presence of natural disease, that may have contributed to death. Toxicological examination should be undertaken to exclude other causes and gases that can be measured. In confined spaces where machinery is being used products of combustion may contribute to death and carboxyhemoglobin should be measured. Solvents should be sought where appropriate, in consultation with a toxicologist where unusual gases may be suspected to obtain appropriate samples for analysis. No specific microscopic features are seen. Biochemical markers of hypoxia have not proven their value in casework.

The investigation of deaths in confined spaces often presents the pathologist with the task of proving the impossible as carbon dioxide, nitrogen, and similar gases cannot be measured at autopsy. The ultimate identification of the cause of death will involve other agencies such as the Health and Safety Executive (in the UK) carrying out investigations at the scene of the death to identify excess gases in the environment. Other cases, such as a young child found in a closed box, may be self-evident, though investigations should be directed at excluding other causes and criminal and civil proceedings may still be brought, necessitating a thorough inquiry.

Survivors of Asphyxia

The term might appear to be an oxymoron but there are a substantial number of cases in the clinical forensic setting where near-death has occurred as a result of some impairment of respiration and ventilation. In general the survivors are those who have been subject to a physical assault where breathing may have been impaired by pressure on the thorax (e.g., some restraint deaths) or on the neck, or by occlusion of the upper airways such as the mouth and nose. As with asphyxial deaths, additional mechanisms may come into play (e.g., physical damage to local structures such as the hyoid bone or thyroid cartilage) which may account for some of the physical signs seen. Additionally, unlike the decedent, the survivor's injuries will evolve over a period of time.

If the survivor was aware of the attack at the time (i.e., was conscious or not intoxicated through drugs and alcohol) there is the likelihood that signs of a struggle have taken place with the possibility of bruising, scratching, and other signs of struggle on both victim and assailant.

In many cases when an asphyxial mechanism is applied for only a short time the findings may be absent or minor. **Figure 1** illustrates the neck of a 40-year-old female subjected to two-handed manual pressure to the neck sufficient to render her unconscious. No petechiae, cyanosis, or swelling was observed. The only findings confirming the account (which had been witnessed) were two small curvilinear superficial abrasions with associated "skin lifts" caused by the assailant's fingernails.

Figure 2 shows the neck of a 38-year-old male around whose neck a ligature had been placed. The linear scratch overlaid with dried blood was caused

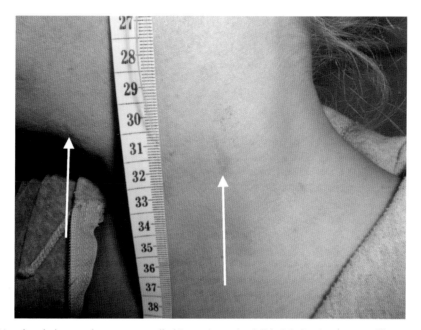

Figure 1 Victim of two-handed manual pressure applied to neck – only visible injuries are two curvilinear superficial abrasions – caused by fingernails. Photo courtesy of Dr Jason Payne-James.

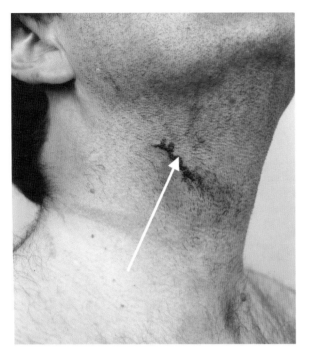

Figure 2 Residual red ligature mark – scratch caused by victim's own fingernails when trying to remove the ligature. Photo courtesy of Dr Jason Payne-James.

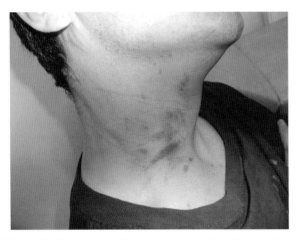

Figure 3 Red grouped, lined marks, caused by fingers of one hand gripping neck. Photo courtesy of Dr Jason Payne-James.

by a scratch from the victim's own fingernail as he tried (and succeeded) in pulling the ligature off. The ligature mark is clearly seen.

Figure 3 shows the neck of a man who had been throttled by an assailant single-handed. At the time of the assault the victim was intoxicated and was unable to defend himself. Others intervened, with witnesses indicating that the victim appeared cyanosed.

Figure 4A shows the plethoric complexion of a male who had been garroted to the point of near-unconsciousness on perhaps three occasions over an hour or so. The photograph was taken about 3 h after the events. He stated he had been unable to breathe on

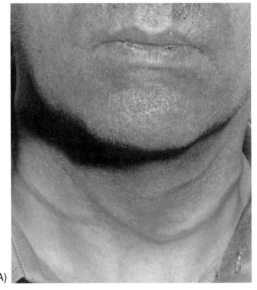

(A)

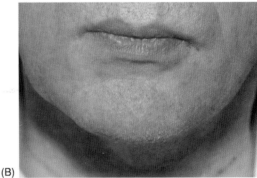

(B)

Figure 4 (A) Florid plethoric complexion caused by ligature application about three hours after event. (B) Same male approximately five days later with resolution of color. Photo courtesy of Dr Jason Payne-James.

each occasion. Initially it was considered that the color change between his face and neck related to an outside lifestyle. He advised that his skin was normally of normal color. No petechiae were distinguishable.

However, over the course of the next 5 days his face reverted to the color and appearance seen in **Figure 4B**.

His eyes on presentation (**Figure 5A**) exhibited marked conjunctival hemorrhages (just visible on this image) with no obvious edema.

By day 5 (**Figure 5B**), the conjunctival hemorrhages were more extensive with the start of breakdown of pigment. However, marked resolving edema could be seen in the infraorbital region, associated with evolution of periorbital bruising (there had been no blunt impact of any kind).

This series of photographs is consistent (although in extreme form) with the leakage of blood from blood vessels following constriction, and that all physical signs appear above the level of the constricting or obstructing force.

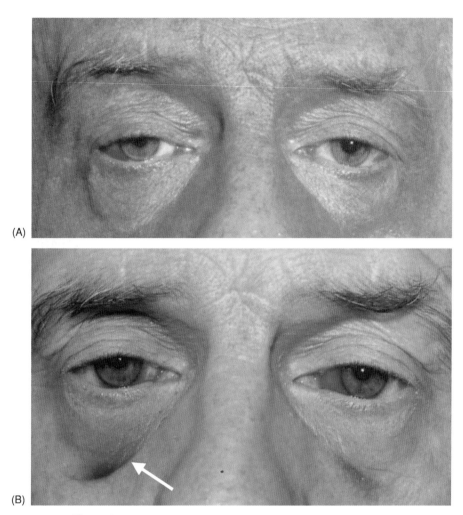

(A)

(B)

Figure 5 (A) Same person as **Figure 4**, note conjunctival hemorrhages at three hours. (B) At day five conjunctival hemorrhages still present but also has marked infraorbital edema. Photos courtesy of Dr Jason Payne-James.

Finally, **Figure 6** shows the change in appearance of the ligature mark over the same time period.

The effects of arm locks during restraint causing asphyxia can also create florid signs. A young Asian male was stopped by police and he attempted to swallow some drugs. An officer attempted to prevent this happening by placing him in an arm lock. The male subsequently said that he was unable to breathe and thought he was going to die. Examination (about 1 h after the incident) revealed marked petechiae, particularly in the periorbital region (**Figure 7A**). Further examination of the eyes, which initially appeared unremarkable (**Figure 7B**), revealed extensive and expanding conjunctival and subconjunctival hemorrhage (**Figure 7C**).

In addition to the external signs of asphyxia the clinician needs to be aware that some signs of asphyxiation may also be present intraorally. A male who had been held in an arm lock by club security for a number of minutes with only brief respite to gasp for air presented a few hours later with hoarseness and dysphagia. Intraoral examination showed petechial hemorrhage on the uvula associated with marked uvular edema. This took about 24 h to resolve.

Additional soft-tissue and bony injury is well recognized following blunt-force trauma to the upper airways (including hyoid bone and cartilaginous fracture). Although the damage itself may not be truly asphyxial, the subsequent soft-tissue swelling may precipitate upper-airway obstruction and potential asphyxiation. In any individual with persistent or marked anterior neck, throat, or mouth pain after potential asphyxial injury consideration should be given to further management (e.g., hospital admission for observation, administration of steroids) or investigation (imaging of the neck) to exclude or confirm more serious underlying pathology (**Figure 8**).

In particular it is appropriate to reexamine the living victims some days after the initial insult to

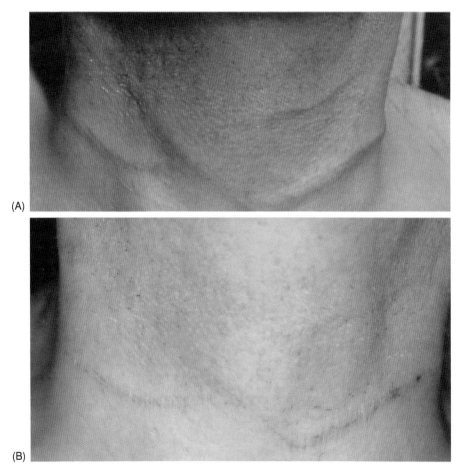

Figure 6 Ligature marks from male in **Figures 4** and **5** showing (A) initial and (B) subsequent appearance. Photos courtesy of Dr Jason Payne-James.

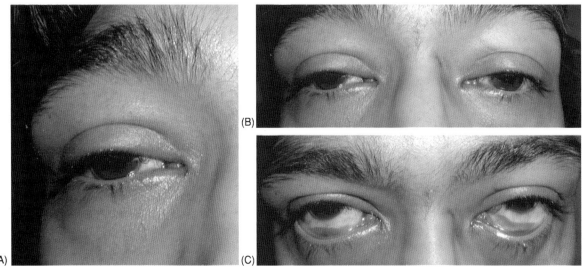

Figure 7 (A), Eye signs, following asphyxia secondary to restraint in neck lock. (B and C) illustrate conjunctival hemorrhage that remains occult until lower eyelash retracted. Photos courtesy of Dr Jason Payne-James.

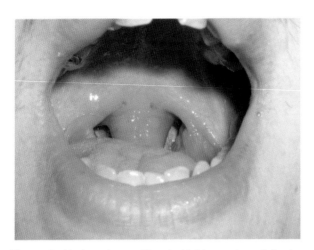

Figure 8 Uvular edema with petechial hemorrhage following neck compression. Photo courtesy of Dr Jason Payne-James.

record and determine the evolution of any relevant physical findings.

Summary

The diagnosis of asphyxial death or injury requires an understanding of the range of situations that it may encompass. The signs of asphyxial death may be nonspecific and may not conform to classically described patterns. The results of asphyxial injury in the living may overlap with other types of injury, such as blunt force applied to the neck, or the consequences of such injury and assault, such as vasovagal inhibition. In all cases a full and detailed assessment of the circumstances surrounding the death or injury is required

and then physical or autopsy findings must be interpreted in the light of those issues.

See Also

Carbon Monoxide Poisoning: Clinical Findings, Sequelae In Survivors; **Postmortem Changes:** Overview

Further Reading

Byard RW (2004) Accidents (with Cohle SD). In: *Sudden Death in Infancy and Childhood and Adolescence*, 2nd edn. Cambridge, UK: Cambridge University Press.
Byard RW, Wilson GWP (1992) Death scene gas analysis in suspected methane asphyxia. *American Journal of Forensic Medicine and Pathology* 23: 42–44.
Byard RW, Gilbert JD, Klitte A, Felgate P (2002) Gasoline exposure in motor vehicle accident fatalities. *American Journal of Forensic Medicine and Pathology* 23: 42–44.
Ely SF, Hirsch CS (2000) Asphyxial deaths and petechiae: a review. *Journal of Forensic Sciences* 45: 1274–1277.
Gill JR, Ely SF, Hua Z (2002) Environmental gas displacement. Three accidental deaths in the work place. *American Journal of Forensic Medicine and Pathology* 23: 26–30.
Gilson T, Parks BO, Porterfield CM (2003) Suicide with inert gases. *American Journal of Forensic Medicine and Pathology* 24: 306–308.
Saukko P, Knight B (2004) Suffocation and "asphyxia." In: *Knights Forensic Pathology*, 3rd edn. London: Arnold.
Schmunk GA, Kaplan JA (2002) Asphyxial deaths caused by automobile exhaust inhalation not attributable to carbon monoxide toxicity: study of 2 cases. *American Journal of Forensic Medicine and Pathology* 23: 123–126.

AUTOEROTIC DEATH

R W Byard, Forensic Science Centre, Adelaide, SA, Australia

Introduction

Autoerotic death is a term used when an individual has died during some form of solitary sexual activity from an accident caused by associated materials or equipment. A variety of terms have been crafted to describe this type of death including sexual asphyxia, sex hanging, asphyxiophilia, Kotzwarrism, auto-asphyxiophilia, hypoxyphilia, and erotized repetitive hanging. Many of these terms emphasize the role that

induced hypoxia from hanging often plays; however, death may also result from a variety of other traumatic events, including drowning, electrocution, crush asphyxia, and exsanguination, or more rarely from air embolism or volatile substance toxicity.

Although deaths from autoerotic activity have been reported for many years from a wide variety of cultures, there remains considerable confusion in recognizing cases and also in accurately determining the manner of death. Frequently articles in newspapers, often describing cases of adolescent boys in boarding schools, refer to bizarre "fainting games" with no acknowledgment of the likely sexual basis of the activity. Cases have also been presented at professional meetings where the use of bondage equipment in which the deceased become entangled was attributed to "Harry Houdini" escapology activity. Such deaths have also been incorrectly attributed to suicides and homicides. Certainly there are cases in which the manner of death is unclear; however, the majority of cases have readily identifiable features that enable an accurate diagnosis to be made.

One of the characteristic features, particularly in male practitioners, is evidence of concomitant paraphilias such as fetishism, bondage, or masochism. While these may provide useful clues as to the events leading up to death, they also demonstrate that the psychopathology underlying this behavior is complex, idiosyncratic, and often ill-understood.

Definition

Autoerotic death has been defined as accidental death occurring during solitary sexual activity in which some type of apparatus, material, or substance that was used to enhance the sexual stimulation of the deceased caused unintended death. Autoerotic asphyxial death then refers to the subset of cases where hypoxia is used to enhance orgasm. This definition precludes the use of the term for cases of natural death due to organic disease, where the intention has been to end life, where life has been terminated by another, or where more than one person is involved in the sexual activity, that is, in typical cases death is accidental, unexpected, and solitary.

Historical Background

Stimulation of sexual arousal by inducing cerebral hypoxia has been recorded in many societies for centuries. The Romans reported this type of activity among the Celts, and tribal groups as geographically separate as the Yaghans of Tierra del Fuego and the Inuit of northern Canada have engaged in similar behavior. It has been suggested that the Maya of Central America may also have known of this activity given that one of their goddesses, Ixtab, was a goddess of the hanged.

In the Middle Ages, the association between hanging and penile erection and ejaculation was well appreciated, as this was often seen at public executions. A folk superstition of the time held that mandrake plants grew under gibbets where the semen from hanged men had fallen and an etching attributed to Dürer shows a hanged man ejaculating. Reznick quotes an old English poem that graphically illustrates this event:

> In our town the other day
> They hanged a man to make him pay
> For having raped a little girl.
> As life departed from the churl

> The townsfolk saw, with great dismay
> His organ rise in boldest way
> A sign to all who stood around
> That pleasure e'en in death is found.

De Boisment, who described the first case in the medical literature in 1856 – that of a 12-year-old boy – also conducted a study of hanging executions in France. He found that 30% of the male prisoners either had erections or had ejaculated in their terminal moments. This may, however, merely represent a terminal neurophysiological reflex rather than an indication of sexual arousal as has been suggested.

Prior to this, considerable attention had been focused on the phenomenon by De Sade in his 1791 novel *Justine* and by the death of Frantisek Kotzwarra under unsavory circumstances. Kotzwarra was regarded as one of Europe's finest bass players and composed *The Battle of Prague*. He was found dead in a brothel having been left suspended by a prostitute for too long a time. A popular publication at the time entitled *Modern Propensities: or an Essay on the Art of Strangling* described such activities. Suspension has been a common practice in brothels since then, and hypoxia has been used as a treatment for impotence. The "Hanged Mans Club" in Victorian England dealt specifically with assisted sexual asphyxia. Peter Motteux, who translated Cervante's *Don Quixote* and Rabelais' *Gargantua and Pantagruel* around the turn of the eighteenth century, was also thought to have expired at the hands of a prostitute during an episode of assisted erotic asphyxia.

In the mid-twentieth century asphyxia during sex with a partner was allegedly popularized in parts of Europe by soldiers of the French Foreign Legion returning from war in Indochina. The general population was also introduced to the features and dangers of solitary sexual asphyxia in popular magazine articles with titles such as "The Orgasm of Death." Although there are numerous underground magazines, clubs, and brothels that deal with this activity the dangers are well recognized, with names such as "terminal sex" being used. It has been suggested that publicizing these deaths may result in clusters of cases due to adolescent copycat activity.

Autoerotic misadventure has also featured in popular literature in the writings of Beckett, Joyce, and Burroughs and has appeared in films such as *The Ruling Class*. Descriptions may be found on many Internet sites.

Psychological and Physiological Background

Autoerotic asphyxiation is classified as one of the paraphilias, disorders in which an unusual act or imagery is necessary to achieve sexual gratification. Other examples of paraphilias include masochism, sadism, pictophilia (using pornographic or obscene films or images), transvestophilia (cross-dressing), rapism (violent assault), kleptophilia (theft), telephone scatophilia (obscene phone calls), and klismaphilia (enemas). There is however, considerable overlap between autoerotic asphyxiation and certain of the other paraphilias. This reflects the complexity of the underlying psychopathology and demonstrates that human behavior represents a continuum and not a series of discretely packaged diagnostic entities. While voyeurism, pedophilia, coprophilia (preoccupation with feces), and mysophilia (preoccupation with filth) have been reported in practitioners of autoerotic asphyxia this appears to be coincidental, with no higher rates than in the general population.

Cross-dressing in cases of autoerotic practice varies considerably from a fetishistic obsession with a single item of female clothing such as underwear or shoes to complete transvestism with the wearing of panties, padded brassieres or clothing, female outer clothes, shoes, mascara, wigs and jewellery. Practitioners may have large collections of clothing that may also involve cisvestism, or the dressing in clothes that are archetypal to one's own sex. Examples of this include males wearing clothing typical of pilots, cowboys, or soldiers and females wearing harem or French maid outfits.

Although bondage often involves the participation of a second person quite elaborate rope bindings and knots that have been put in place by the victims on their own are often present. Terms such as cordophilia and ligotism have been suggested for cases where physical restraints are needed for sexual stimulation. Restraints have been found in as many as 51% of cases.

A factor in some cases of autoerotic asphyxia is the element of risk taking, with the potential for death being recognized as an added stimulus. Assessment of motives becomes even more difficult in cases where practitioners have been depressed, as suicide then becomes a distinct possibility.

One of the difficulties in determining why this behavior occurs is that most practitioners have no interest, need, or desire to elaborate on their reasons for pursuing what appears to be risky and bizarre activity. Victims have often been socially functional and successful in their careers with no hint of psychiatric illness. Most have been heterosexual with no history of unusual sexual activities; in fact their autoerotic activities have often been so successfully hidden from spouses and children that there may be reluctance to accept that this has occurred. Psychological reviews of fatal cases, while essential in their assessment, often obtain only second-hand or conjectural data, and interviews with practitioners have suffered from small populations and selection bias.

It has been suggested that hypoxia may produce a pleasurable effect and enhance the sensation of orgasm in certain individuals. Slang terms for sexual asphyxia such as "head rushing," "ecstasy," and "flying to the moon" suggest a not unpleasant sensation and Roland's comments in de Sade's *Justine* following a hanging episode support this:

> Oh Thérèse! one has no idea of such sensations, what a feeling! it surpasses anything I know! Now they can hang me if they want!

Incidence

It has been difficult to determine the precise incidence of this type of behavior as pathologists and law enforcement officers are usually only aware of cases where there has been an unexpected outcome. In the USA the death rate has been estimated at between two and four cases and in Scandinavia estimates of one to two cases per million of the population per year have been proposed. There appears to be further regional variability in incidence, however, as the rate in Australia does not appear to approach this. For example in South Australia with a population of 1.5 million there is one case every 1–2 years (a rate of 0.3–0.7 per million per year). This is unlikely to represent underreporting.

It is uncertain how practitioners learn about the various described techniques although fortuitous discovery while experimenting with bondage must account for a certain number of cases. Popular magazines and films have also raised awareness and a number of contact groups advertise through underground bondage magazines and the Internet.

Diagnostic Criteria

Certain characteristic features in typical cases of autoerotic death provide criteria for diagnosis. These are summarized in **Table 1**. Although all of these features are not always present there should be evidence of solitary sexual activity with death from the unintended effects of a device, apparatus, material, or substance that was integral to the activity. Assessment of the death scene may be compromised if family members or friends have taken steps to conceal the nature of the fatal episode. This usually occurs because of embarrassment about the circumstances of death, or concerns for the potentially damaging

Table 1 Features of fatal autoerotic deaths

Evidence of solo sexual activity
Private or secure location
Evidence of previous similar activity in the past
No apparent suicidal intent
Unusual props including ligatures, clothing, and pornography
Failure of a device or set-up integral to the activity
    causing death

effects that such a death may have on the reputation of the deceased.

Death Scene Features

While a classic case would be a male aged between 15 and 25 years who is found hanging in a secluded or secure place such as a bedroom, toilet, attic, basement, garden shed, or isolated area of woodland, many variations are now recognized. Males aged between 9 and 80 years, and females from 19 to 68 years have been involved, although female victims are exceedingly rare compared to males, with fewer than 30 cases reported.

Practitioners of either sex certainly have a reasonable expectation of privacy with doors often locked from the inside. There is no evidence of scene disturbance and no signs of inflicted injury from assault. The feet may be resting on the floor or ground.

Unfortunately the secure and secluded nature of the scene often results in delayed discovery of the body with subsequent decomposition. Purging of bloody fluids from the mouth or nose, swelling of subcutaneous tissues, and discoloration of skin have occasionally been incorrectly interpreted as evidence of assault prior to death.

Ligatures around the neck may have been padded with towels or soft material to prevent bruising or abrasions that may draw attention to the activity. Props and equipment used by males may be extremely elaborate and unusual and have included mock gibbets, scuba diving helmets, motor vehicles, tractors, and lifts. A case has been reported of an individual who suspended himself from a backhoe which he had named "Stone" and to which he wrote poetry. In another report, a male victim would chain himself naked to the back of his Volkswagen car and run along behind it. Crush asphyxia ensued when the chain became wrapped around the rear wheel dragging him in to the side of the vehicle. Other unusual devices have included a garbage tin into which a victim used to climb to compress himself.

More usual props include pornographic pictures or literature that have been carefully positioned so that they can be viewed by the victim during sexual

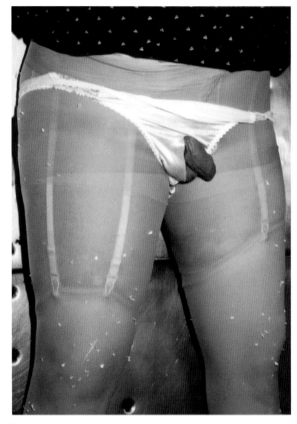

Figure 1 A victim wearing a dress with stockings, suspenders, pantyhose, and female underwear. The underwear and pantyhose had been cut to expose the genitals.

activity. Mirrors may be placed so that the victim can also see himself. There is a significant incidence of fetishism amongst male practitioners and victims are often found wearing female underclothes, dresses, or quite elaborate costumes (**Figures 1** and **2**). One victim had a photograph of a female face glued to his body. Other fetish items have included sanitary napkins, shoes, raincoats, and rubber and leather items. Rubber clothing may consist of rubber sheets or wetsuits, and cases have been described of victims making trousers out of car tire inner tubes or water bed liners. Another effect of wearing such heavy clothing is restriction of movement that may be augmented by other bondage equipment, elastic underwear, or bandages. One practitioner covered himself with mud because of the compressive effects that occurred as it dried. Vibrators and lubricating creams may also be present and a variety of devices including vegetables, shoehorns, wine bottles, traffic cones, and table legs have been used as rectal foreign bodies. Occasionally the victim will have photographs of himself wearing various items such as female clothing, wigs, or bondage gear placed within view of

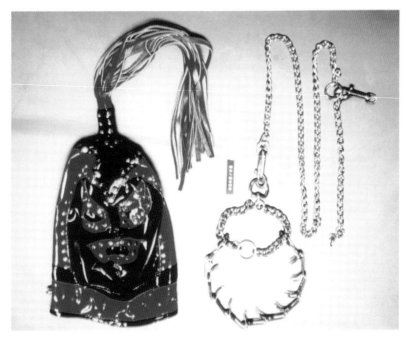

Figure 2 An elaborate mask with a dog collar found on a victim who had accidentally hanged.

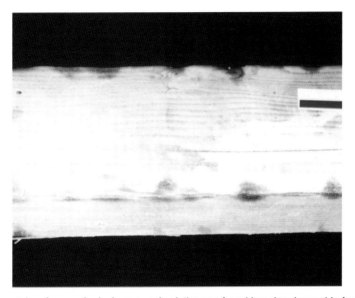

Figure 3 An overhead beam taken from a shed where a male victim was found hanging dressed in female underwear. At least six grooves were present from previous episodes.

the suspension point. Cases have also occurred where victims have taken videos of themselves during episodes. This may be particularly useful in assessing the fatal episode if it has been captured on film.

Pornography, unusual clothing, and devices used to cause real or simulated pain are all rare in female victims and bizarre props and fetishism have not been described. The paucity of death scene features in female cases may result in confusion with both suicide and homicide.

Given that the victim has usually engaged in this form of activity before, often for many years, there may be physical evidence of previous episodes at the scene. This may take the form of grooved overhead beams where ropes used for suspension have worn marks (**Figure 3**), or removed paint. Hooks or pulleys may be found in the walls or ceiling (**Figure 4**). One of the most unusual examples where there was clear evidence of similar episodes in the past involved a victim who would dress in female clothing and jump into a canal tied to a stone. He was found drowned tied to a stone; a number of nearby stones with remnants of clothesline attached to them were testaments to prior episodes. His self-rescue mechanism of

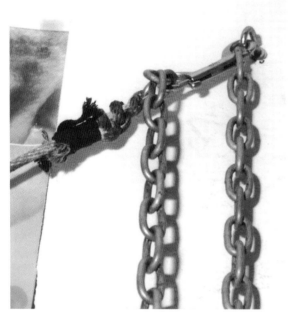

Figure 4 An elaborate series of chains and ropes attached to a wall hook enabled a victim to suspend himself while surrounded by pornographic pictures attached to the walls of the room. Literature pertaining to autoerotic activity was present in the room along with numerous other bondage items.

cutting the clothesline and gaining release had failed when he dropped his scissors.

Masochism has been found in 12% of cases with features including body piercing, particularly of the nipples, tongue, and genitals, or pinching of the genitals, nipples, or skin by clothes pegs, hairclips, or a rabbit trap (**Figure 5**). Given the recent popularity of body piercing among young people certain of these features are now less significant as markers of sadomasochism. Ligatures and metal washers may have been placed around the genitals and the buttocks and nipples may have been cut. There may also have been other forms of self-mutilation in the form of superficial stabbing, infibulation of the scrotum, or burning with cigarettes. Antemortem photographs of the deceased may show sadomasochistic features with simulated wounds.

Restraint is a common feature and may be achieved by a complex arrangement of ropes, chains, plastic tapes, or handcuffs which suggest ritualistic behavior (**Figures 4** and **6**). Cases have occurred where a victim has wrapped his face in plastic tape or rolled himself in plastic sheeting and then been unable to extricate himself from the asphyxiating situation. Devices to deliver electrical stimulation/shocks have been used.

Evidence of antemortem sexual activity may take a variety of forms with exposure of the genitals (**Figure 1**) and, less commonly, complete or partial nudity. A condom (**Figure 7**), cloth, handkerchief, or plastic wrap may be covering the penis in an attempt to prevent soiling, and the hands may be touching the genitals. While semen may be present this is not a particularly useful sign, as terminal ejaculation is not uncommonly seen in a variety of natural

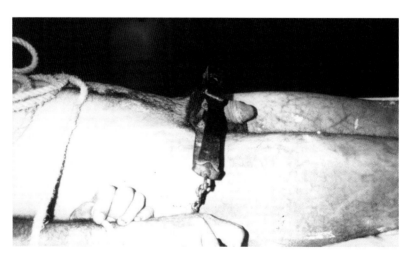

Figure 5 A rabbit trap had been applied to the suprapubic skin by a victim who was subsequently found hanging. There were no injuries to the genitalia.

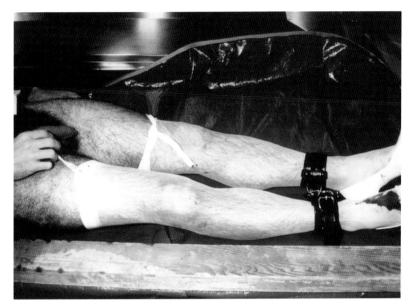

Figure 6 Binding of the legs with a leather belt in addition to the wearing of female underwear in another victim.

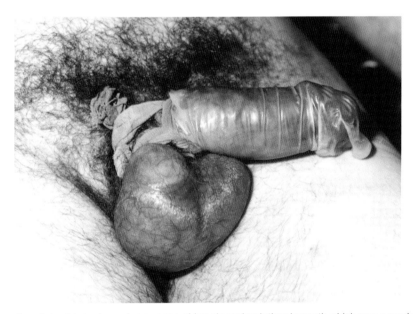

Figure 7 A victim was found dead in bed wearing a range of female underclothes beneath which was a condom tied with elaborate knots to the penis by lengths of pantyhose.

and non-natural deaths. Its presence certainly does not confirm that masturbation has occurred.

Fail-Safe Device

An important feature of many scenes may be the presence of a fail-safe mechanism to enable the victim to extricate him- or herself from a potentially dangerous

situation. This is not necessarily always present, however, as the potential for a lethal event may not have been perceived. Fail-safe mechanisms may be relatively simple and consist of the ability to stand up, thus relieving pressure around the neck from a ligature placed over the top of a door, or bending the legs, thus taking pressure off a ligature placed around the neck and tied to the ankles. Unfortunately if unconsciousness supervenes the victim's full body or leg weight may pull continuously on the ligatures maintaining pressure on the neck resulting in death.

Other self-rescue devices have consisted of keys to open locks holding restraining chains, knives to cut constrictive or suffocating plastic sheeting, or scissors or knives to cut restraining or suspensory ropes. Cases have occurred where all of these have failed when releasing equipment has been dropped, possibly as the victim has succumbed to the effects of worsening cerebral hypoxia. Rope nooses have also caught on hair and remained tight, and chairs or objects used to stand on have fallen over or been knocked out of reach.

Lethal Outcomes

Death most often results from cerebral hypoxia due to hanging when neck compression occludes major neck veins and arteries, or blocks the airway, or stimulates the carotid sinus reflex. Asphyxiation may be caused by suspension from abdominal ligatures or result from occlusion of the mouth and nose by rubber masks, tape, or plastic sheeting. Plastic bags have been placed over the head and objects such as plastic balls or sanitary napkins have been held in the mouth by female underwear or dog collars. Positional asphyxia with chest compression may result from wedging of a body into a tight space, and mechanical asphyxia has been achieved by tightly wrapping the body in blankets or sheets of plastic. Cases where death is due to causes other than compression of the neck, chest, or abdomen have been called atypical.

Inhalation of volatile substances such as chloroform, aerosol sprays, and dental anesthetic gas may be used to augment sexual activity and may also cause death from hypoxia due to central respiratory depression or aspiration of gastric contents, or from arrhythmias due to cardiotoxicity. While the container of volatile material may not be obvious at the scene, victims may still be wearing respirators or gas masks. In these cases headspace analyses should be performed on post-mortem blood and tissue specimens to check for volatile substances.

Less commonly, death may occur from exsanguination due to rectal trauma associated with foreign body insertion, or from peritonitis following perforation of the bladder after insertion of foreign bodies into the penis. Lethal trauma has followed the intrarectal discharge of a grease gun and fatal air embolism may occur after intravaginal foreign body insertion.

Electrocution has occurred in cases where a variety of devices have been used to electrically stimulate the victim. Characteristic electrical contact lesions with central areas of blistering surrounded by blanched areas and rims of hyperemic tissue may be useful in establishing the cause of death.

Death due to hyperthermia has occurred in a victim who was wearing a dress, female underwear, and seven pairs of stockings/pantyhose (**Figure 8**) on a day when the ambient temperature was at least 39 °C (102 °F). Medication which caused anhidrosis and hyperthermia in hot weather also contributed to the terminal episode.

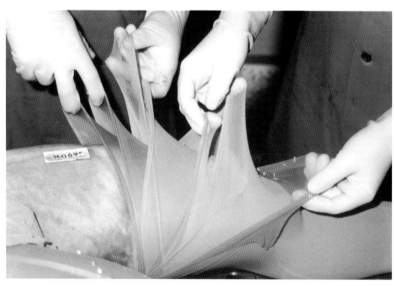

Figure 8 Multiple pairs of stockings and pantyhose worn by a victim who succumbed to hyperthermia.

Diagnostic Problems

One of the earliest problems with autoerotic asphyxial fatalities was confusion with suicide. As this may have considerable ramifications in terms of insurance payments clarification is essential. Usually review of the psychological status of the victim and the circumstances of death reveals no evidence of depressive illness or suicide; however, cases have occurred where practitioners have chosen to commit suicide using typical paraphernalia. Typical death scene features may be of limited assistance as mirrors and neck padding may be found in suicide.

Other difficulties have arisen when cases have been mistaken for homicides. This usually occurs when typical death scene features are not present, as with female victims, or where the death scene has been altered to disguise the true nature of the event. Cases have also occurred where an individual engaged in autoerotic practice was killed by another and where attempts have been made to disguise a homicide as an autoerotic accident.

Another problem that has arisen periodically has been the failure to distinguish deaths due to natural diseases while an individual has been masturbating from genuine cases of accidental death. Sudden death is a well-recognized complication of strenuous activity and cases are not infrequently seen in standard forensic practice where an individual engaged in some form of sexual activity has died. The usual scenario is a middle-aged or elderly male who dies while engaged in consensual sex and is found at autopsy to have extensive coronary artery atherosclerosis producing lethal ischemic heart disease. So well known are these type of cases that they have been termed "coital coronaries" or "la mort d'amour." Cases of natural death during solitary sexual activity must not be termed autoerotic death, no matter how unusual the devices or props may have been, as clear separation of accidental from natural deaths and suicides must be maintained if the term autoerotic death and its association with misadventure is to remain at all useful.

Further Reading

Blanchard R, Hucker SJ (1991) Age, transvestism, bondage, and concurrent paraphilic activities in 117 fatal cases of autoerotic asphyxia. *British Journal of Psychiatry* 159: 371–377.

Byard RW (1994) Autoerotic death: characteristic features and diagnostic difficulties. *Journal of Clinical Forensic Medicine* 1: 71–75.

Byard RW, Bramwell NH (1991) Autoerotic death: a definition. *American Journal of Forensic Medicine and Pathology* 12: 74–76.

Byard RW, Hucker SJ, Hazelwood RR (1993) Fatal and near fatal autoerotic asphyxial episodes in women: characteristic features based on a review of nine cases. *American Journal of Forensic Medicine and Pathology* 14: 70–73.

Franzini LR, Grossberg JM (1995) *Eccentric and Bizarre Behaviours.* New York: John Wiley.

Geberth VJ (1996) *Practical Homicide Investigation: Tactics, Procedures and Forensic Techniques,* 3rd edn. Boca Raton, FL: CRC Press.

Hazelwood RR, Dietz PE, Burgess AW (1993) *Autoerotic Fatalities.* Lexington, KY: DC Heath.

Hucker SJ (1990) Sexual asphyxia. In: Bluglass R, Bowden P (eds.) *Principles and Practice of Forensic Psychiatry,* pp. 717–721. Edinburgh, UK: Churchill Livingstone.

Knight B (1996) Fatal pressure on the neck, Chap. 15. In: Knight B (ed.) *Forensic Pathology,* 2nd edn., pp. 361–389. London: Edward Arnold.

O'Halloran RL, Dietz PE (1993) Autoerotic fatalities with power hydraulics. *Journal of Forensic Sciences* 38: 359–364.

Resnick HLP (1972) Erotized repetitive hangings: a form of self-destructive behavior. *American Journal of Psychotherapy* 26: 4–21.

Rupp J (1973) The long bug. *Journal of Forensic Sciences* 18: 259–262.

Sivaloganathan S (1984) Aqua-eroticum – a case of auto-erotic drowning. *Medicine Science and the Law* 24: 300–302.

Vanezis P, Busuttil A (1996) *Suspicious Death Scene Investigation,* pp. 147–151. London: Edward Arnold.

AUTOPSY

Contents

Procedures and Standards

P Saukko, University of Turku, Turku, Finland
S Pollak, University of Freiburg, Freiburg, Germany

This article is adapted from 'Postmortem Examination: Procedures and Standards' in *Encyclopedia of Forensic Sciences*, pp. 1272–1275, © 2000, Elsevier Ltd.

Introduction

The need to establish the cause and manner of death has always existed. It is vitally important to know whether a death is due to natural causes (i.e., where there are no signs of violence), an accident, by the hostile action of a community member or enemy troops, or, perhaps an act of God (i.e. unavoidable).

The historical development of postmortem procedures shows two distinct paths to our present-day systems. The earliest system, the external examination of a dead body, began in ancient China more than 2000 years ago. Even today, it is the prevailing method of postmortem examination in many parts of Asia. It is worth noting that at that time medical doctors did not participate in postmortem examinations, which were conducted by government officials.

The history of "necropsy," the investigative dissection of a dead body, or the more extensively used term "autopsy," literally, seeing for oneself, is much shorter. According to our present knowledge, the earliest anatomical dissections took place in the first known school of anatomy in Alexandria, Egypt, around 320 BC; the earliest medicolegal dissections were at the University of Bologna, Italy, between 1266 and 1275, and hospital autopsies came considerably later, in the fifteenth century.

External Postmortem Examination

According to Tao and coworkers, the early development of ancient forensic medicine originated in the period of warring states (475–221 BC) in China. The earliest known written instructions, dealing with investigations of the scene of death in cases of death by hanging, were engraved on bamboo slips and found in Yun-meng subprefecture in Hubei province in 1975 from a tomb dating from the Qin dynasty (221–207 BC). These documents also revealed that failure to report suicide to the authorities or any interference with the corpse before it had been examined were punishable offences. McKnight assumes that the interest in state-ordered and officially conducted forensic assessments dates from the time when the state first began to prosecute homicides. The system was developed further during the Song dynasty (AD 960–1279). The key decree establishing the inquest system was issued in AD 995, specifying that, in all unnatural cases of death or serious injury where there was any indication of foul play, the competent authority had to dispatch a government official who was to proceed immediately (within 4 h) to the scene to conduct an inquest (i.e., an investigation of a dead body or a wounded individual). Failure to do so was punishable. Particular attention was called to deaths in prison, as judicial torture to the point of death and subsequent cover-up were not uncommon. A reinquest, performed by officials of a neighboring subprefecture, was mandatory in all nonnatural deaths resulting from illegal acts. The use of official documents and prescribed forms to record the injuries in a body were introduced during the Song dynasty. They included a written request for a postmortem examination reporting the case to the higher authorities, external examination, and conclusions of the examination, including both a front and a back sketch of the body with drawings of the injuries. These were public documents, which had to be signed by the parties involved and certified by the official assigned to the case.

Many of the earlier publications on forensic medicine in ancient China have been lost but extensive information about investigative techniques acquired in the course of several centuries has been compiled in the oldest surviving systematic handbook of forensic medicine, the *His Yuan Chi Lu* (Collected Writings on the Washing-Away of Wrongs), written by Sung Tz'u (1186–249) and published in 1247. In 1440 the book was first published outside China in Korean and, thereafter, numerous translations of various versions of the book were published in Japan, Europe, and the USA.

The statutory basis for the English coronial system was established in September 1194 by article 20 of the Articles of Eyre, which stated: "In every county of the King's realm shall be elected three knights and one clerk, to keep the pleas of the crown." The resemblance between the English practices and the Chinese pattern has suggested a possible cultural influence, which, according to McKnight, may have existed through close contact with the Norman empire of Sicily and the cosmopolitan group of courtiers at the Sicilian court, especially under Roger II.

In continental Europe, the Justinian Code (AD 529–564) stated the principle that the function of medical experts is to assist the judiciary by impartial interpretation and opinion. The use of medical expertise (barber-surgeons) in the examination of violent deaths was also mentioned in the Canon law of 1209 by Innocent III and in the municipal laws, e.g., in Freiburg since 1220. The examination of violent deaths was carried out by barber-surgeons and was reported orally to the judges. Subsequently, the surgeons had to give expertise also on injuries of living persons.

Anatomical Dissection

The prerequisite for the idea of an autopsy was the knowledge of human anatomy. King and Meehan have quoted Sigerist, stating: "In all archaic civilisations the chief sources of anatomical knowledge were the kitchen and the cult." For example, the practice of haruspicy or hepatoscopy, the process of foretelling of the future by examining the entrails of sacrificial animals, was widespread in ancient times and practiced in Babylon in 3500 BC.

The history of autopsy shows three partly overlapping paths of development. The first lasted almost 2000 years from the first known school of anatomy in Alexandria around 320 BC, where human dissections were carried out, till the publication of the great textbook of anatomy *De Humani Corporis Fabrica* in 1543 by Andreas Vesalius (1514–1564), the "father of anatomy," marking the overthrow of traditional Galenic anatomy. The possibility of dissecting human bodies varied greatly at times. In Vienna the first anatomical dissection took place in 1404. In 1410, Pope Alexander died suddenly and was autopsied by Pietro D'Argelata. Pope Sixtus IV (1471–1484) issued a bill permitting studies on human bodies by students at Bologna and Padua. Felix Platter I, the famous anatomist in Basle, Switzerland, was said to have performed more than 300 autopsies since 1559.

Medicolegal Autopsy

Analogous to the external postmortem examination, the medicolegal autopsy was introduced as a result of the requirements of the judicial system. According to Singer, the earliest medicolegal dissections took place at the University of Bologna, Italy, from 1266 to 1275, though McKnight claims that there is evidence that autopsies had been performed in China several centuries earlier, but the Chinese did not continue this line of exploration. In France, Ambroise Paré performed the first medicolegal autopsy in 1562.

Our knowledge of the old autopsy procedures is rather scanty. With few exceptions, detailed written autopsy records mainly exist for relatively recent times. Exceptions are the reports of the autopsy of Emperor Maximilian II from 1576 and of Markgrave Jakob III of Baden, who died in 1590 and was autopsied by two professors of the Freiburg University in the presence of the personal physician of the deceased.

The principles of the modern medicolegal investigation were developed based on the codes of sixteenth-century Europe: the Bamberg Code (Constitutio Bambergensis) in 1507, the Caroline Code (Constitutio Criminalis Carolina) in 1532, and later the Theresian Code (Constitutio Criminalis Theresiana) in 1769.

The Austrian decree of 1855 contains detailed instructions in 134 paragraphs on the performance of medicolegal autopsy, and it is worth mentioning that even today this is valid legislation in Austria. The Prussian edict of 1875 is similar, although not as detailed. Both of these instructions can be considered as the culminating point of legislation, dealing with the performance of medicolegal autopsy.

Clinical Autopsy

Before the mid nineteenth century, autopsies were greatly affected by the prevailing medical concepts and the pathologist could not see what he did not know. The clinical autopsy, as we understand it today, took much longer to develop and first became meaningful after the introduction of modern concepts of pathogenesis of diseases by Carl von Rokitansky (1804–1878) and cellular pathology by Rudolf Virchow (1821–1902).

The concept of a "complete" autopsy changed over the centuries: at the beginning of the nineteenth century increased attention was paid to the actual autopsy technique. Prost, a French physician, insisted in 1802 that all organs of the body should be examined and declared that 3 h was the minimum length of time for a postmortem examination. In 1846 Rudolf Virchow, then a prosector in Berlin, insisted on regularity and method and definitive technique. The classical techniques that are still in use today are more or less modifications of those introduced by Rokitansky, Virchow, Ghon, and Letulle, among others.

In 1872 Francis Delafield's *A Handbook of Postmortem Examination and Morbid Anatomy* was published in New York, and German and English editions of Rudolf Virchow's book on autopsy technique were published in 1876.

The Present Use of the Autopsy

Objectives of Autopsy

An autopsy is a detailed systematic external and internal examination of a corpse carried out by a pathologist or one or more medicolegal experts to ascertain the underlying and possible contributing causes of death and, depending on the jurisdiction, also the manner of death. Before the pathologist can begin the examination, authorization to perform the autopsy on that particular body is necessary. An assessment of possible risks that may be involved with the autopsy must also be considered and necessary health and safety precautions taken. The autopsy and all related measures must be carried out in a manner consistent with medical ethics and respecting the dignity of the deceased.

An autopsy is performed to achieve one or more of the following objectives:

- to identify the body or record characteristics that may assist in identifying the deceased
- to determine the cause of death or, in the newborn, whether live birth occurred
- to determine the mode of death and time of death, where necessary and possible
- to demonstrate all external and internal abnormalities, malformations, and diseases
- to detect, describe, and record any external and internal injuries
- to obtain samples for any ancillary investigations
- to obtain photographs or retain samples for evidential or teaching use
- to provide a full written report and expert interpretation of the findings
- to restore the body to the best possible cosmetic condition before release.

In addition to the anatomical dissection there are two main types of autopsy:

1. The medicolegal or forensic autopsy, which is ordered by the competent legal authority (coroner, medical examiner, procurator-fiscal, magistrate, judge, or the police) to investigate sudden unexpected, suspicious, unnatural, or criminal deaths. Also unidentified bodies or deaths occurring in special circumstances, such as deaths in police custody or during imprisonment, are often subjected to a medicolegal autopsy. In most jurisdictions, permission of the relatives is not required and the medicolegal autopsy takes priority over the clinical.

2. The clinical (hospital) autopsy is to investigate the extent of a known disease and the effectiveness of treatment and it is sometimes also performed for medical audit or research purposes. Almost invariably, the consent of relatives is needed unless the deceased has given consent antemortem.

Medicolegal Autopsy

Further developments in medicolegal autopsy have been characterized and greatly influenced by the judicial system adopted in any given country, the main emphasis being on the detection and investigation of criminal and other unnatural or unexpected deaths. Due to different legislations, there exists great variation in the medicolegal autopsy rates and practices between countries. In addition to national measures to create guidelines and harmonize medicolegal autopsy, there has been an increasing international interest in achieving uniform and internationally recognized rules concerning the methods of carrying out autopsies. This has become imperative, especially with respect to human rights issues. The mass killings in Cambodia, Rwanda, Bosnia, and Kosovo should have made it quite clear, even to the general public, what implications a medicolegal investigation, or the lack of it, may have on human rights.

In May 1989, the United Nations Economic and Social Council adopted in its resolution 1989/65 the Principles on the Effective Prevention and Investigation of Extra-Legal, Arbitrary and Summary Executions, which had been created by cooperation with intergovernmental and nongovernmental organizations, in particular the Minnesota Lawyers International Human Rights Committee. Later, in 1991, the General Assembly of the United Nations endorsed the Model Autopsy Protocol of the United Nations.

The European Council of Legal Medicine (ECLM) is an official body, with its seat in Cologne, Germany, that deals with scientific, educational, and professional matters in Europe. It has delegates nominated by the national medicolegal associations from all European Union and European Economic Space (EES) member countries. Since the early 1990s the ECLM has also been active in this field and its document *Harmonisation of the Performance of the*

Medicolegal Autopsy was adopted by the General Assembly in London in 1995.

The Council of Europe is an intergovernmental organization that aims, among other things, to protect human rights and a pluralist democracy. It should not be confused with the European Union. The two organizations are quite distinct; however, all the European Union states are also members of the Council of Europe, which currently has 45 member states. In its 43rd Ordinary Session, the parliamentary assembly of the Council of Europe adopted recommendation 1159 (1991) on the harmonization of autopsy rules. Following this recommendation, a working party of international experts in legal medicine and law, with representation from Interpol as well as the International Academy of Legal Medicine, was established in 1996 under the Committee of Bioethics to make a proposal for the autopsy rules. Among the guidelines used in the work was the autopsy rule produced earlier by the ECLM. The working party finished its work in November 1998 and this new Pan European recommendation R (99) 3 on the "harmonisation of medicolegal autopsy rules and its explanatory memorandum" was adopted by the committee of ministers on February 2, 1999 at the 658th meeting of the ministers' deputies. Although the document is a "recommendation" by nature and hence not strictly legally binding, it has, however, legal implications because all 45 Council of Europe member countries have agreed to implement these principles in their national legislation.

Clinical Autopsy

Despite increasingly sophisticated investigative and imaging techniques, the clinical autopsy has been shown to have maintained its value and has remained an essential factor in the quality assurance of medical care. Regardless of this, there has been a progressive decline in autopsy rates throughout the world. The mandatory 20% autopsy rate required for accreditation of postgraduate training in the USA was withdrawn in 1971, on the grounds that each institution should set its own rate but that ideally it should be close to 100%. According to the World Health Organization (WHO) statistics published in 1998, the total autopsy rates in Europe in 1996 varied between 6% (Malta) and 49% (Hungary). In other parts of the world reported to the WHO, the rates varied between 4% (Japan) and 21% (Australia) (**Table 1**).

The reasons for this decline are many and complex: overreliance on new diagnostic techniques, lack of appreciation of autopsy work, poorly performed autopsies by inexperienced trainees without proper supervision, long delay of autopsy reports, economic factors, fear of malpractice litigation, to name just a few.

The standardization and harmonization of clinical autopsy have taken place primarily on the national level and professional organizations, for example, the Royal College of Pathologists, has published guidelines on autopsy practice for postmortem reports and audit. The quality of healthcare and quality assurance and audit has become increasingly important and these procedures have been introduced even for autopsies.

Autopsy Techniques

Both clinical and medicolegal autopsies may involve different strategies and techniques, depending on the questions they are expected to answer. Autopsy techniques in adults are generally different from those employed for pediatric autopsies.

Table 1 Reported information on autopsy rates 1996

Country	Autopsy rate (%), all ages
WHO region of the Americas	
Canada	20
USA	12
WHO European region	
Albania	Not available
Austria	27
Belgium	Not available
Bulgaria	25
Czech Republic	31
Denmark	32
Finland	36
France	Not available
Germany	8
Greece	Not available
Hungary	49
Iceland	38
Ireland	7
Israel	Not available
Italy	Not available
Luxembourg	Not available
Malta	6
Netherlands	8
Norway	9
Poland	9
Portugal	Not available
Romania	7
Spain	Not available
Sweden	37
Switzerland	19
United Kingdom; England + Wales	24
United Kingdom; Northern Ireland	11
United Kingdom; Scotland	15
WHO Western Pacific region	
Australia	21
Japan	4
New Zealand	16
Republic of Korea	Not available
Singapore	16

The scope of medicolegal autopsy is often much broader than that of clinical autopsy and may also include the investigation of the scene of death. All background information on the circumstances of death is of paramount importance for the choice of the right approach. In a medicolegal autopsy, the examination of clothing is often an essential part of the external examination, whereas in a clinical autopsy it is generally not. Both types of autopsy should consist of full external and internal examination of the body, including the dissection and investigation of all three body cavities.

The external examination An external description of the body includes:

1. the age, sex, build, height, ethnic group, and weight, nutritional state, skin color, and other characteristics of the deceased, such as scars or tattoos
2. a description of postmortem changes, including all essential details relating to rigor mortis, hypostasis, and decomposition
3. careful investigation and description of all body surfaces and orifices, including color, length, density, and distribution of hair, color of irises and sclerae, presence or absence of petechiae, or any other abnormalities or injuries. The examination should be carried out systematically and include head, neck, trunk, upper and lower extremities, and the back.

The internal examination Examination of the body cavities includes description of the presence of gas (pneumothorax), fluids (effusions or exudates) or foreign bodies, and the measurement of their volume, appearance of the internal surfaces, and anatomical boundaries as well as the location and external appearance of organs.

The classical autopsy techniques vary mainly in the order in which the organs are removed:

1. the organs may be removed one by one (Virchow's technique)
2. cervical, thoracic, abdominal, and pelvic organs can each be removed as separate blocks (Ghon's technique)
3. they may be removed as one single block, which is then subsequently dissected into organ blocks (Letulle's technique)
4. all organs are dissected *in situ* (Rokitansky's technique).

All organs must be dissected, the outer appearance as well as the cut surfaces described, and the weight of the major organs recorded. The hollow organs must be opened and their contents described and measured. All relevant vessels, arteries, and veins as well as ducts should be dissected. All abnormalities must be described by location and size.

Sampling Histological examination of the main organs should be performed in all autopsies. The need for further ancillary investigations may depend on whether the cause of death has been established with the necessary degree of certainty, and, if not, additional samples should be taken for toxicological or other investigations. For toxicology, this may include peripheral blood, vitreous humor, cerebrospinal fluid, bile, hair samples, or other relevant tissues. When retaining tissues, one has to take into consideration the possible restrictions depending on national legislation.

Special procedures Sometimes special procedures and modifications of normal dissection techniques are necessary. If there is suspicion of air embolism, chest X-ray should be performed before autopsy. Where neck trauma is suspected, the brain and the organs of the chest cavity must be removed before dissection of the neck to drain the blood from the area, to avoid artifactual bleeding. Postoperative autopsies may present various problems with medicolegal implications, such as complications of anesthesia, surgical intervention, or postoperative care. New radiological imaging techniques, such as magnetic resonance imaging (MRI) and multislice computed tomography (MSCT), have recently been applied to particular medicolegal problems, such as the investigation of charred or decomposed bodies as well as the visualization and analysis of patterned injuries. However, a detailed description of these special dissection procedures and techniques is beyond the scope of this article.

Autopsy Report

The report is an essential part of the autopsy. It should be full, detailed, and comprehensive. A medicolegal autopsy report, in particular, should also be comprehensible for nonexperts. In addition to the factual, positive and negative gross, microscopic, and analytical findings, the pathologist should conclude with a discussion of the significance of the findings. Where the findings are of uncertain nature and there are several competing causes, the pathologist should attempt to give an opinion as to their probability.

See Also

Autopsy: Medico-legal Considerations; Pediatric; Adult

Further Reading

Health Services Advisory Committee (1991) *Safe Working and the Prevention of Infection in the Mortuary and Postmortem Room.* London: HMSO.

King LS, Meehan MC (1973) A history of the autopsy: a review. *American Journal of Pathology* 73: 514–544.

Knight B (1990) The medieval coroner. *Medical Legal Journal* 58: 65–80; discussion 81–82.

Ludwig J (ed.) (2002) *Handbook of Autopsy Practice*, 3rd edn. Totowa, NJ: Humana Press.

Royal College of Pathologists (1993) *Guidelines for Postmortem Reports.* London, UK: Royal Collage of Pathologists.

Saukko P, Pollak S (2000) Postmortem examination: procedures and standards. In: Siegel JA, Saukko PJ, Knupfer JA (eds.) *Encyclopedia of Forensic Sciences*, pp. 1272–1275. San Diego, CA: Academic Press.

Singer C (1957) *A Short History of Anatomy and Physiology from the Greeks to Harvey.* New York: Dover.

Sung T (1981) The washing away of wrongs: forensic medicine in thirteenth-century China. In: *Science, Medicine, and Technology in East-Asia,* vol. 1. Ann Arbor, MI: Center for Chinese Studies, The University of Michigan.

Tao JJ, Cameron JM, Xu W (1988) A brief history of forensic medicine in China. *The Criminologist* 12: 67.

Medico-legal Considerations

S Cordner and H McKelvie, Victorian Institute of Forensic Medicine, Southbank, VIC, Australia

Introduction

Autopsies are a part of the health and justice systems that have generally been poorly understood by the community, including the medical profession in more recent times. As far as the general community is concerned, this is not surprising, given that many people are uncomfortable talking or thinking about death, and autopsies directly confront the physical mechanisms of death in a very intimate way. To a certain extent, this could also be true of doctors whose focus is on promoting health and prolonging life, and for whom the details of pathology practice and the purposes and outcomes of autopsies have been of limited interest. A definite lack of awareness about autopsy processes – amongst the public, clinicians, and some pathologists – was exposed during the inquiries into organ retention procedures in the UK (at the Bristol Royal Infirmary and

the Alder Hey Hospital in Liverpool), and subsequently in Australia and elsewhere in the world. The practice of not providing details to next of kin about autopsy procedure, including the retention of organs, and the fact of the retention itself, was seen as ethically and, in some instances, legally blameworthy.

When autopsy problems surface in the public domain as they do from time to time, they touch very sensitive nerves. Consequently, the problems often acquire a political dimension – aggrieved, recently bereaved relatives are easily identified with. Also, even ethically performed autopsies can readily be described in terms amounting to disrespect. What makes such description a false characterization is essentially the justification for the examination and the motivation or ethical stance of the prosector. It is easy, however, for an autopsy institution to adopt a defensive posture in relation to how it might handle the risk of problems surfacing in public. We would like to suggest that clarity about the principles that drive the institution, and the development of policies and procedures which give effect to those principles, enable a positive approach from the outset that also serves as the institution's best defense, should it come under scrutiny. Such principles might include what the World Health Organization suggested in a 1999 publication, *Ethical Practice in Laboratory Medicine and Forensic Pathology*:

> It is generally agreed that an autopsy is a procedure of ethical significance, as it interferes with the body. This significance is such that the community has a right to expect that systems are developed, within legal and resource constraints, and with community input and understanding, to ensure that the substantial potential benefits of performing an autopsy are realized and that the autopsy is not meeting only narrowly defined needs.

Thus, it is possible to conclude that simply performing an autopsy in a presumed natural-cause death to "find the cause of death" in fulfillment of an obligation in a coroner's or other act, writing a brief report which is not discussed with anyone, of which the family does not receive a copy, and the results of which are only of bureaucratic significance, does not meet this principle.

So, while this article relates to the medicolegal aspects of autopsies, these aspects are defined from more fundamental considerations and it is with these that we will be most concerned. This article will therefore provide an overview of the context and purposes for autopsies, and other aspects of their performance, including the role of pathologists.

What is an Autopsy?

"Autopsy" means "to see for oneself," and is also known as "a postmortem examination." One needs to distinguish the whole process of an autopsy from its physical performance. The former includes:

- familiarization with the medical record and/or the supposed circumstances of the death
- possible attendance at the scene
- using the results of the autopsy to contribute to reconstruction of the circumstances surrounding death or the reconstruction of the clinicopathological course of the patient's illness.

The actual performance of an autopsy entails a thorough external and internal examination of a body, using techniques similar to those employed during major surgery – certainly a modern, well-designed and well-built mortuary bears some resemblance to an operating theater. During a full autopsy all internal organs, including the brain, are removed, weighed, examined, and small samples taken for processing so they can be looked at under a microscope. Other tests may also be performed, including checking for the presence of drugs, chemicals, or toxic substances. In some cases it may be necessary to retain a whole organ for further examination, in order to investigate more fully how the person died.

In some instances partial autopsies may be undertaken. For example, where myocardial infarction or coronary artery atherosclerosis is suspected as the cause of death, a family may authorize an autopsy that is limited to examination of the chest cavity. However, the value of such limited examination is controversial. On the one hand, there is the view that the suspected cause of death may be "confirmed." On the other hand, this confirmation will always be suspect if all other possibilities, only discoverable by a full autopsy, are excluded.

The Importance of Autopsies

Forensic pathology is increasingly relied upon by judicial systems, even in countries with strong religious and cultural opposition to the performance of autopsies. There are very few, if any, countries in the world where no autopsies for forensic purposes are performed. The numbers and types of deaths investigated by autopsy vary considerably from country to country. While the disinclination on cultural or religious grounds to perform more autopsies than are absolutely necessary must be respected, this must be accompanied by caution.

In many countries, major reliance is placed on the external examination of a body by a local medical officer when investigating the cause of death. While this is clearly a reasonable screening process, it is only that. Without autopsies, there will be many cases where it will not be possible to say why death occurred: it will not be possible to disentangle and distinguish, say, between natural and accidental deaths or suicides and homicides. Even with autopsies, some cases remain enigmatic. There must be acknowledgment that coming to correct conclusions about the cause and manner of death based simply on history and external examination is a process which is inherently and substantially flawed. Judicial decisions based on conclusions about the cause and manner of death reached without the benefit of an autopsy will have a high rate of error.

Context and Purpose of Autopsies

There are normally two different contexts in which an autopsy is performed: in a hospital, or as part of a medicolegal (forensic) investigation.

A hospital autopsy is usually performed to answer questions that the family and the deceased person's doctors may have about the course of the illness, cause of death, and/or any coexisting conditions. (These are important purposes, but institutions undertaking such autopsies should also seriously consider what capacity they have to bring about some of the additional benefits associated with autopsies, see below.) In most jurisdictions a hospital autopsy must be authorized by the deceased person, before death, or by the next of kin after death. This issue of consent to hospital autopsies constitutes the main medicolegal consideration in this context.

Depending on the death investigation system in operation, a medicolegal autopsy is authorized by a coroner, medical examiner, investigating magistrate, police, or other responsible official. These autopsies are to meet particular needs, which normally are to:

- identify the deceased
- determine the medical cause of death
- determine how the death occurred.

Again the same caveat applies as for hospital autopsies in relation to delivering other potential benefits.

The circumstances in which a medicolegal autopsy is carried out vary from jurisdiction to jurisdiction. However, they normally include some or all of the following:

- homicide or suspected homicide
- sudden, unexpected death, including sudden infant death
- violation of human rights such as suspicion of torture or any other form of ill treatment

- suicide, or suspected suicide
- suspected medical malpractice
- accidents, whether transportational, occupational, or domestic
- occupational disease and hazards
- technological or environmental disasters
- death in custody or death associated with police or military activities
- unidentified remains.

This list is taken from the Recommendation on the Harmonization of Medicolegal Autopsy Rules adopted by the Committee of Ministers of the Council of Europe (no. R (99)3).

During the course of meeting the (relatively narrow) needs of both the hospital and the medicolegal autopsy, the autopsy itself or tissue or information gained from the autopsy may be of further value. The examples are given as follows:

1. For hospitals and clinicians. Providing an accurate cause of death and characterizing the pathology are essential components of clinical audit (i.e., a process to ensure that illness is being correctly diagnosed and treated). Information from autopsies also contributes to the characterization of poorly understood diseases, and the evaluation of new medical therapies, new surgical techniques and procedures.
2. For families. Diseases with genetic components may be identified so that accurate reproductive and other healthcare advice can be provided, if requested, to close family members. Also, having a cause of death provides a factual basis for counseling relatives, particularly in relation to anxiety that any action or inaction on the relatives' part contributed to the death. (These issues commonly do not surface as problems until some time after death.)
3. For administering justice. Where the issues to be decided in the civil and criminal justice systems relate to matters of illness, injury, and death, it is invaluable to be able to compare objective medical evidence with the apparent circumstances of the death and confirm or establish identity.
4. For public health. The most obvious contribution autopsies make to public health is via medical and paramedical education and research. Another contribution is through provision of more accurate causes of death, allowing mortality statistics to be a more accurate source of information for formulating government health policy. Also, investigating deaths of vulnerable individuals behind closed doors, such as in hospitals or prisons, contributes to public confidence in, and accountability of, those institutions. Information from autopsies

may also be used as an early-warning system for issues of public health and safety, contributing to the prevention of disease and accidents.

Role of the Pathologist

To whom does the pathologist owe a duty? The answer to this question can sometimes be confused because the subject of the pathologist's examination is dead. The issues for most other doctors are clearer because there is a living patient. However, there is at least the argument to be made (and it is the instinctive feeling of many pathologists) that a duty is owed to the deceased, or at least to the memory or reputation of the deceased, that the true cause and circumstances of the death be revealed. If such a duty is doubted, a stronger case can be made that the forensic pathologist has a duty to the community at large, because of the trust that the community (including the deceased's relatives) has in the integrity of the medical profession generally. On that basis the forensic pathologist has a duty not to collude in wrongly hiding or obscuring the cause and circumstances of death.

The forensic pathologist's broad duty is to make sure that the cause and circumstances of the death are revealed. As with other health professionals, the more specific content of the forensic pathologist's duty is to exercise at least a reasonable degree of care and skill in his/her work, i.e., in the production of valid and useful observations and conclusions. In assessing what is a reasonable degree of care and skill, reference can be made to the practice of colleagues of similar training and expertise. However, such practice is substandard if it does not produce reliable and valid results. What this means in practical terms requires an understanding of the basic aims of the autopsy. These are:

- to discover, describe, and record all the pathological processes present in the deceased that could contribute to understanding the cause and circumstances of the death
- to relate these processes to the known medical history of the deceased to draw conclusions about the cause of symptoms and signs observed in life, and then to draw conclusions about the cause of death and other medical and nonmedical factors contributing to death
- to contribute to the reconstruction of the circumstances surrounding the death. Where these circumstances are important or likely to be in dispute, this will require consideration of the scene of the death as well as the relevant autopsy

observations, many of which may be of trivial medical consequence

- in accordance with good medical practice, to record all the relevant observations and negative findings, and to retain specimens, so that another pathologist at another time is in as good a position as possible to come to his or her own conclusions about the death
- on completion of all of the scientific and medical tests, to complete an autopsy report that contains the results of the autopsy findings together with the results of any specialist tests that may have been undertaken. In medicolegal cases, this report may be used, together with witness statements, to arrive at a legal finding with respect to the death. The pathologist may also be involved in giving evidence at any subsequent legal hearing into the death (an inquest) or other proceedings, such as a murder trial or civil proceedings relating to the death.

In terms of attendance in court, there are many pitfalls awaiting practitioners as they give evidence of their observations and conclusions. The pitfalls, or the mistakes that can be made, occur in the following areas:

- providing opinions that are at the edge of, or beyond, the expertise of the witness
- providing opinions that are based on false assumptions or incomplete facts
- providing opinions based on incomplete or inadequate scientific or medical analysis
- where failures of communication occur between expert witnesses, police, and lawyers
- providing opinions that are biased, consciously or unconsciously, in favor of one side or other in the proceedings.

The giving of evidence may be the culmination of the pathologist's work in a particular case and there is an obligation to bring to this task the same reasonable care and skill as to other aspects of the practitioner's craft. After all, it is on the basis of the evidence that important decisions will be made affecting the life and liberty of accused persons (in criminal matters) or affecting liability and compensation (in civil matters).

Managing the Mortuary

As has been alluded to, the autopsy is a unique procedure in medicine. Virtually all other procedures in almost every other aspect of medicine are performed for the benefit and with the consent of the individual. In a forensic pathology context, the deceased person's body has been taken out of the control of the relatives

and the autopsy is often performed without the express consent of the deceased person (whilst alive) or the next of kin. These two factors alone place a heavy responsibility on forensic pathology systems to ensure that the autopsy is carried out in a dignified way with appropriate respect for the deceased person and the interests of the next of kin. This obligation is often expressed in relevant legislation dealing with autopsies. In discharging this obligation the following should be considered carefully:

- facilities and equipment available for the receiving and proper storage of bodies and the subsequent performance of autopsies
- facilities for the viewing of bodies by relatives
- the performance of the autopsy competently within a reasonable time of receipt of the body
- the ability of next of kin, or other properly interested parties, to be represented by an appropriately qualified person at the autopsy
- the reconstruction of the body after the autopsy
- the availability of the body for funeral purposes within a reasonable time
- the provision of the formal report within a reasonable time and its availability to next of kin and properly interested parties.

In managing the mortuary, considerable responsibility is usually given to scientific and technical staff. Historically, problems have arisen when financial relationships have developed between funeral directors (or undertakers) and mortuary staff. Such relationships are intended to ensure that the mortuary delivers funeral business to a particular undertaker, which is normally to the detriment of the next of kin. Other problems include the handling of personal property arriving with the deceased at the mortuary. This includes clothing, jewelry, and, not infrequently, considerable quantities of money. Unless the mortuary has well-documented and reliable procedures to record such property, false accusations against the mortuary can easily be made and will be difficult to refute. Such allegations, if not properly refuted, will adversely affect the reputation and credibility of the mortuary, its staff, and its work.

Retention of Tissue Samples and Whole Organs for Diagnostic Purposes

To a large extent the pathologist performing an autopsy must be relied upon to use appropriate discretion to conclude what tissue is necessary to be retained for the purposes of the autopsy. This may include both small samples of tissue and whole organs. Diagnosis is the main reason why whole organs removed at autopsy may be retained. The necessity for this is well established. If it is suspected that there is pathology which is complex, not visible with the naked eye, otherwise difficult to find or particularly important to characterize in detail, then larger parts, the whole organ or numbers of organs, may need to be retained. For example, the examination of a fresh brain is much less satisfactory in terms of diagnostic yield than examination after formalin fixation. Efforts to speed fixation, for example with microwave techniques, have not been widely accepted or adapted. In medicolegal contexts, tissue or organs may need to be retained in case a pathologist later instructed by an interested party, or the defense, would be assisted by having access to it. It may only be in this way that the first pathologist is able to put the second pathologist in the best possible position to come to his or her own views about the death. Sometimes, retention for later more careful examination is necessary because of shortage of time at the autopsy or the need to involve treating or interested clinicians.

However, the pathologist's discretion to retain tissue must be tempered by family sensitivity to the issue of organ retention. The recent controversy has highlighted to pathology services the need to provide next of kin with information about the reasons for retaining tissue and/or organs (for hospital autopsies) to seek their consent, and involve them in decisions about their disposal once diagnostic testing is completed. (Indeed, the Human Tissue bill introduced into the UK parliament in early 2004 purports to make failure to obtain appropriate consent to retention of tissue a criminal offense.) In accordance with the wishes of the family, and where practicable, arrangements may be made to reunite organs with the body before burial or cremation. In other instances, organs may be returned for separate disposal, or with family approval, disposed of by the pathology service by its normal procedures (usually incineration as medical waste).

With respect to retention of smaller tissue samples, in most cases it seems that families are less sensitive about and are more accepting of histology blocks and slides being retained by pathology services on an ongoing basis (for accreditation purposes and in medicolegal cases, in the event of further testing or evaluation being required by a court). (In any event, in the UK, if the Human Tissue bill is passed, consent will also be required from next of kin for retention and storage of these samples.) In places where this issue is not regulated, it would be prudent for pathology services to develop and publish policies to deal with those families who are concerned about all forms of tissue retention. In this context, it is normal for the following tissue samples to be retained

(where the relevant equipment and expertise are available):

- Some small specimens are retained for various tests relevant to the particular case, the results of which are available as part of the pathologist's file in the case. (The testing may be toxicological, microbiological, biochemical, immunological, endocrinological, tissue culture, histological, radiological, forensic odontological, anthropological, neuropathological, or genetic (molecular biological). Either macroscopic or microscopic photography may be employed to advance the characterization of the pathology and the recording of any of the testing. Models or casts may also be created to advance these as well.)
- Small samples of all internal organs examined are also retained to be made into histology blocks and slides for later examination under the microscope to detect conditions not visible to the naked eye, or to characterize and/or record pathology visible with the naked eye. Increasingly, these samples are required to be kept for specified periods for laboratory accreditation purposes.
- If toxicological analysis is required, then samples of blood, urine, bile, liver, and stomach contents may be retained. In special toxicological or biochemical circumstances, other fluids or tissue may be retained, e.g., lung (inhalation of volatiles), vitreous humor (alcohol level, glucose, ketones, electrolytes), kidney, hair, bone, fat, skin, or other organs or tissues.
- To cover the possibility of later requests, a small sample of blood may be retained in all nontoxicology cases.

Conclusion

The very nature of an autopsy, as well as its substantial potential benefits, makes it a significant event. In this context, the community has a right to expect that systems are developed to ensure that the wider benefits are being realized and that autopsies are not meeting only narrowly defined needs. Plainly, community understanding and input are required to ensure that autopsy procedures and the systems developed to realize their wider value accord with the law and reflect current values. This was repeatedly made clear by public concern voiced when autopsy issues reach the public domain, as in the recent "organ retention scandal" in the UK, with parallel concerns in Australia and elsewhere. The court of public opinion may not exhibit much in the way of merciful qualities. In any event, the days of "pathologist knows best," if not gone, are rapidly disappearing.

Autopsy institutions would do well, whatever the strict legalities might allow, to act on principles and follow policies which are in advance of local public expectations.

See Also

Autopsy: Procedures and Standards; Pediatric; Adult; **Death Investigation Systems:** China; Japan; Nordic Countries; Certification of Death and the United Kingdom System; United States of America

Further Reading

College of American Pathologists website at www.cap.org
El Nageh MM, Lineham B, Cordner S, Wells D, McKelvie H (1999) *Ethical Practice in Laboratory Medicine and Forensic Pathology.* World Health Organization regional office for the Eastern Mediterranean, series 20. Alexandria, Egypt: World Health Organization.
Royal College of Pathologists of Australasia Position Statement on Autopsies. Available online at http://www.rcpa-manual.edu.au/uploadedmedia/rcpaautopsypolicy.pdf.
Royal College of Pathologists of Australasia website. www.rcpa.edu.au.

Pediatric

H F Krous, Children's Hospital and Health Center, San Diego, CA, USA
T S Corey, University of Louisville School of Medicine and Office of the Kentucky Medical Examiner, Louisville, KY, USA

Introduction

The autopsy examination may be thought of as the final history and physical conducted by a physician. It represents the last examination by a trained specialist – thus it further represents the last opportunity to document findings and procure necessary samples for laboratory testing. The autopsy examination should never be conducted as a "black box" exercise in which no information is provided. Just as in the living patient (in whom a "history" and physical are routinely conducted), a thorough postmortem examination includes a detailed account of both the recent or immediate events leading to death (the postmortem equivalent of the "history of present illness") and an account of prior pertinent events and findings (the postmortem equivalent of "review of systems, past medical history, and social history").

Because the autopsy represents the last time the patient/decedent will be examined, adequate documentation of all findings is important. It is recommended that findings be documented in multiple forms, to provide a clear representation to persons reviewing the case days, months, or years later. Most cases should be documented diagrammatically, photographically, and in written form. Many cases should be documented radiographically as well. Written documentation may take many forms, depending on the style and philosophy of the particular office and the individual pathologist. Either detailed checklists or dictated descriptive reports may suffice. Whatever the preferred style, it should be kept in mind that the goal of the written record is to allow independent interpretation by adequate description of all pertinent findings. Further documentation by photographs, radiographs, and diagrams provides other forms of illustrative documentation, and thus these serve as further records of the findings on which the pathologist relied to render medicolegal opinions. Adequate sampling of tissues for histological examination and proper procurement of tissues or fluids necessary for ancillary testing further allow adequate investigation and documentation. In general, a postmortem investigation will include three elements: (1) scene examination/investigation; (2) case history review (**Table 1**); and (3) autopsy examination. Each of these is assessed and given proper weight by the pathologist rendering an opinion regarding cause and manner of death. The individual components of a complete autopsy will vary depending on the individual case. Specific tests necessary in one particular scenario may not be germane to another case. In general, most cases will require the following components:

- gross examination and dissection
- microscopic examination of tissues
- toxicologic screening of blood and/or other body fluids.

Table 1 General definitions

Prematurity	Delivery at less than 37 weeks' gestation
Low birth weight	Birth weight less than the fifth percentile expected for gestational age
Gestational age	Age at birth measured from the first day of the last menstrual period
Postconceptional age	Total age measured from the estimated day of conception and including the postnatal age
Postmaturity	Delivery at or after 42 weeks' gestation
Neonatal period	First 28 days of life
Early neonatal period	First 7 days of life
First trimester	First 12 weeks of gestation
Second trimester	12th to 24th week of gestation
Third trimester	24th to 42nd week of gestation

Of course, there are always exceptions – for instance, microscopic examination is of no value in severely decomposed remains, and toxicologic evaluation may not be relevant in cases involving a long hospitalization interval between the precipitating event and death. In pediatric postmortem examinations, additional testing not usually undertaken in investigations involving autopsies on adults may be necessary. Such specialized tests may include postmortem metabolic screening, and radiographic skeletal surveys.

General Dissection

Gross Examination

Although the autopsy of an adult and child share certain similarities, there are important differences. The lethal diseases of infancy differ significantly from those of older children and adults, and not infrequently may require some specialized dissection techniques. The external appearance, developmental features, nutritional state, and measurements and weights of the organs and body are critically important in infants. Standard external measurements in infants and young children, in addition to the routine length and weight obtained in all postmortem examinations, may include head circumference, chest circumference, abdominal circumference, crown–rump length (CRL), and foot length. Also in addition to the weights of major organs routinely recorded in the postmortem examinations, the weights of the thymus and adrenals are recorded. Weights and proportions taken at autopsy examination are easily compared to standard tables and charts available in many reference texts.

External examination   Regarding the gross description of the external body surface, examination of the infant requires notation of some parameters not routinely mentioned in older children and adults. These unique descriptors include the following:

- condition of the cranial sutures and fontanelles
- distribution of the scalp hair (premature babies may display hair over the forehead and face)
- formation and location of the ears (low-set ears may be seen as a part of Potter's facies due to oligohydramnios)
- patency of nares (newborns are typically obligate nose-breathers)
- developmental quality of the facies (abnormal facies are seen in many congenital syndromes and diseases)
- configuration of hard and soft palates

- development of nails (abnormalities are seen in ectodermal dysplasias)
- configuration of palmar creases (simian creases are seen in a higher percentage of some chromosomal abnormalities, including some trisomies)
- development of solar creases (assessment of gestational maturity)
- patency of anus.

Developmental characteristics and growth parameters are important not only to the accurate identification of certain syndromes, but may also provide clues to underlying metabolic disorders. Because many congenital syndromes may be difficult to recognize in early infancy, frontal and lateral photographs are recommended in the event that consultation with a medical geneticist is necessary.

It is important to demonstrate the spectrum and ages of all injuries not related to medical therapy by observations, diagrams, photographs, gross dissection, and microscopic examination as indicated.

Adequate gross description of injuries includes description of location in relation to stable anatomic landmarks; documentation of size, shape, and color of the injury; and proper use of terminology to define blunt-versus-sharp-force injuries. The eyes should be carefully examined to rule out the presence of conjunctival and scleral petechiae. The nasal and oral cavities should be carefully examined with an otoscope (if available) to document any injury of the mucosal surfaces. Often, it is necessary to place additional incisions along the longitudinal axes of the extremities and dorsal trunk to document blunt-force trauma. Extensive subcutaneous dissections of the chest, abdomen, and back, and limbs, if required, can assist in the identification of occult trauma. The posterior soft-tissue dissection may be accomplished through a "double Y"-shaped incision, with the first Y over the scapular region and the additional Y inverted over the buttocks.

Body weight and length   The reference tables for the body weight and length are found in standard reference texts. The weight and external measurements are obtained after the body is undressed and all paraphernalia have been removed.

Body measurements   The crown–heel length (CHL) is the length measured from the top of the head to the bottom of the heels with the infant fully extended in a supine (face-up) position. The CRL is measured when the infant is supine and is the distance between the top of the head and the bottom of the buttocks when the hips are flexed vertically. The head circumference is more accurately described as the occipitofrontal circumference (OFC). The OFC is the maximum circumference of the head and is taken by positioning the measuring tape at the frontal and occipital prominence. The foot length should be obtained when estimation of gestational age is in question in a neonate. Microscopic examination of the skin, lungs, and kidneys assists in determining gestational age.

Internal examination   The internal examination of the thoracic and abdominal cavities is undertaken in the same manner as that conducted in older children and adults. The procedure begins with the standard Y-shaped incision over the thorax, extending down to the symphysis pubis. An oval incision is extended around the umbilicus, which is kept in continuity with the urachal remnant, umbilical arteries, and bladder.

Body cavities and serosal surfaces   The organs are examined first *in situ* – as they sit in the body cavities. The volumes and appearances of fluids in the body cavities are described. These fluids may provide information relative to the presence or severity of disorders, including cardiac failure, infections, hepatic dysfunction, renal disease, or thoracic duct injury. During the *in situ* inspection, the pathologist assesses the anatomic relations of the vessels and major organs. Specific areas of note in the examination of the infant include the distribution of the great vessels, the rotation of the gut, and the locations and relative sizes of the thymus, the liver, and the spleen.

The presence and distribution of petechial hemorrhages on the parietal and visceral serosal surfaces are noted. Petechiae limited to the thoracic cavity are a frequent and important positive, but not pathognomonic finding in sudden infant death syndrome (SIDS). Conversely, petechiae in the thoracic and abdominal cavities may signify a disturbance in coagulation, oxygenation, or acid–base imbalance.

Removal of the neck, thoracic, and abdominal organs   The complete tongue is removed in continuity with the hyoid and other neck organs, including larynx, proximal esophagus, and thyroid and parathyroid glands. After removal of the thymus gland and isolation of the carotid arteries, the tongue, neck organs, thoracic, abdominal, and pelvic viscera are removed *en bloc*. This technique maintains important anatomic relationships and aids in ensuring recognition of anomalies such as total anomalous pulmonary venous connection below the diaphragm, as well as high airway obstruction or foreign bodies.

Examination of the head   Examination of the head is a routine element of the autopsy in any case of sudden unexpected infant death, as an infant may be the victim of homicidal blunt head trauma without any external signs of trauma. After reflection of the scalp, any injuries visible on the inner aspect of the scalp should be documented. The cranial cap should be removed by, or under the direct observation of, the pathologist (rather than the autopsy assistant), so that parafalcine subdural hemorrhages are not missed, and so that artifactual subarachnoid blood is not overinterpreted.

Routine examination of the spinal cord is preferred, and is especially critical in cases of suspected shaking. The spinal cord and supporting musculoskeletal elements should be examined via a posterior approach in order to eliminate artifacts of dissection.

In cases of intracranial trauma, the globes and optic nerves should be examined to rule out hemorrhages of the retina, optic nerve sheath, and perineural sclera. The globes are easily removed via a superior approach through bone windows in the orbital plates. A superior approach ensures adequate optic nerve preservation.

Organ weights and measurements   Organ weights are best noted while the organs are in a fresh state. The measured organ weights should be compared to the tabulated expected weights of infants with the same CHL, rather than with infants with the same weight or postnatal age. Since infant body weight can change dramatically over a short time, it is not a reliable reference for comparing organ weights. Also, since prematurely born infants will have postnatal measurements that differ from those of infants born at term, the infant's age at death is unsatisfactory for comparison of organ weights.

Cardiac valve circumferences and ventricular myocardial thicknesses may be measured for comparison to standard reference charts.

Microscopic Examination

Except in cases of severe decomposition, microscopic examination of tissues is a standard part of a complete infant autopsy. It is worth remembering, however, that microscopic sections in cases with decomposition may still yield valuable information, hence, it must be kept in mind in special circumstances. Standard sections of all major organs are routinely submitted. In the infant, these sections will be more numerous than in the standard adult autopsy. To complement the usual heart, lungs, liver, and kidney, sections in infant autopsies include three sections of the heart (right ventricle, left ventricle, and septum), and sections of each pulmonary lobe, the thymus, spleen, skin, muscle, tracheal ring, adrenal, and costochondral junction. Additionally, the pathologist is encouraged to sample all grossly recognized pathologic processes.

Accurate pathologic diagnoses are made from optimal gross observations and high-quality microscopic sections. High-quality sections can be achieved when tissues are adequately and appropriately fixed, thinly cut, and optimally stained. All sections should be stained with hematoxylin and eosin (H&E) and other stains when indicated. Ideally, the number of sections per glass slide should be as few as economically feasible. Again, recommended blocks unique to the infant/young child include a cross-section of the larynx, the thymus, the costochondral junction of a rib, two to three sections from the heart, and sections from each lobe of the lungs. The tissues are to be fixed in 10% buffered formalin with a fixative volume to tissue ratio of 10:1.

If central nervous system pathology is suspected or the cause of death is uncertain, the brain should be fixed in 10% or 20% formalin prior to examination. Addition of a small amount of glacial acetic acid to the formalin will increase the firmness of the parenchyma, and thus facilitate sectioning.

It is important to demonstrate the spectrum and ages of all injuries not related to medical therapy by observations, diagrams, photographs, gross dissection, and microscopic examination as indicated. If timing of an injury may be important, the injury should be sampled for microscopic examination, as dating of a contusion by color is imprecise and often inaccurate.

Microscopic examination of the thymus, costochondral junction, and adrenals is recommended since they provide histopathological evidence of the alleged duration and/or severity of illness before death and allow comparison of the autopsy findings with the clinical history and death scene investigation findings. Each of these organs will show involutional changes secondary to stress from any cause over a relatively short period of time.

Discretionary microscopic sections include both hippocampi, midbrain at the inferior colliculi, pharyngeal soft tissue rostral to the hyoid, diaphragm, gastroesophageal junction, distal ileum with ileocecal valve, and colon.

Microscopic examination of the cervix, vagina, distal rectum, and anus is indicated when abnormalities or injuries are grossly identified. Postmortem dilation of the anus, with exposure of the pectinate line, should not be misinterpreted as trauma.

Toxicology and Postmortem Chemistry Studies

Postmortem toxicology studies may be invaluable in establishing a cause of death. Since the presence of many substances cannot be discerned at the time of gross autopsy examination, appropriate specimens must be obtained and retained for subsequent analysis if indicated. Obtaining blood and urine samples is mandatory, and collection of brain and liver samples is recommended. If retained, brain and liver should be frozen at $-20\,°C$. When the death appears unnatural or suspicious, then collection of cerebrospinal fluid, bile, vitreous humor, gastric contents, and kidney tissue should be considered.

If a closed head injury is suspected, vitreous humor should not be collected until the pathologist has examined the globes to rule out retinal hemorrhages. Therefore, it is preferable to delay collection of vitreous humor until the cranial contents and vault have been examined.

Essentially all toxicology specimens require refrigeration. Blood should be stored at $4\,°C$ and not frozen. The preservative, sodium fluoride, should be added to the blood sample. In general, other liquids and tissues may be retained in a frozen state.

Routine toxicologic screening analyses include (but are not necessarily limited to) alcohol, cocaine, narcotics, and amphetamines, and many commonly prescribed and over-the-counter drugs including acetaminophen (paracetamol), diphenhydramine, and many others. Other tests may be performed as required or indicated by the history and/or pathological findings. Results of toxicological analysis should be interpreted in light of specimen source, laboratory procedures, standard toxicological reference ranges, and clinical history and death scene investigation findings.

Vitreous humor is very useful in the postmortem evaluation of the hydration status of the decedent, as vitreous electrolytes are stable for a longer period of time than those in blood. Urea nitrogen and creatinine are quite stable in the early postmortem period. Previous studies have shown that infants dying of acute dehydration display statistically significant elevations of vitreous sodium and urea nitrogen values, thereby allowing its diagnosis.

If the globes are to be examined to rule out retinal hemorrhages, then consultation with an ophthalmologic pathologist, if available, prior to collection of vitreous fluid is recommended. We recognize that many institutions do not have access to an ophthalmologic pathologist; therefore, the prosecting pathologist must exercise careful judgment as to the best course of action to obtain and preserve important diagnostic data. The vitreous fluid may be collected using a 20-gauge needle attached to a 5-ml or 10-ml syringe. The needle is inserted at an angle of 45°, lateral to the iris, and directed medially. The aspirated fluid should be clear and colorless. Care must be taken to prevent the needle tip from abutting the retina on the medial side.

Microbiology

All cultures and other microbiologic tests initiated prior to the infant's death should be completed in the original laboratory. Results of these studies should be reported to the forensic pathologist performing the postmortem examination.

In selected jurisdictions, microbiologic studies can be initiated in a hospital setting prior to reporting the death to the medical examiner. This is encouraged where allowed, but it is important to remember that, in other jurisdictions, no studies can be initiated until the medical examiner assumes jurisdiction and authority over the body.

During the initial stages of the autopsy, a blood culture may be collected by sterile technique. Other microbiology specimens are collected as dictated by the history and physical findings noted during the autopsy. It is recommended that blood be collected from the left heart in order to reduce the chance of postmortem contamination from intestinal flora. Direct touch preparations obtained from involved organs may be retained for Gram stain determinations or for evaluating the presence of inflammatory infiltrates. Whenever indicated, serum is retained and frozen to permit the serological identification of suspected pathogens.

Microbiologic studies, when indicated, include analysis for aerobic and anaerobic bacteria and viruses. Serum for serological analyses and tissues collected for viral cultures may be kept frozen until subsequent analysis.

When investigating deaths occurring suddenly and unexpectedly in an outpatient setting, the pathologist must remember that the body has often been exposed to room temperature conditions for an unknown postmortem interval. Previous studies have shown that the proportion of positive blood cultures increases in a linear fashion with increasing postmortem interval. Cautious interpretation of positive culture results is advised if multiple organisms are recovered, or if a site of infection is not demonstrable histologically.

Spinal Fluid by Cisternal Tap

Blind puncture of the cisterna magna is not recommended if there is a possibility of central nervous system trauma. If, however, infection of the central nervous system is suspected and trauma has been excluded, then a cisternal tap may be performed. The skin of the lower posterior skull and upper neck is sterilized with Betadine followed by 70% isopropyl alcohol or other technique. Using a sterile needle (spinal, or at least 4 cm (1½ in) long), the midline at the level of the second cervical posterior spine is punctured, angling upward 10°, aiming for the foramen magnum. Usually, a slight "give" will be felt when the needle enters the subdural space. Deeper penetration should be avoided. Typically, 5–10 ml of sterile spinal fluid can be aspirated. If trauma of the central nervous system cannot be excluded prior to intracranial examination, then, if indicated by examination, a direct culture of the meninges may be obtained upon removal of the skullcap. The meninges are incised with a sterile blade, and a sterile swab is then inserted between the meninges and the cortical surface.

Examination of the Middle Ears

The middle ears may be a source of sepsis. To examine the middle ears, remove the petrous portions of the temporal bones. Incise the lateral aspect of the petrous ridge where it is continuous with the temporal bone with bone scissors or, if necessary, a mechanical saw. Incise the bone near the sella: extend the incision anteriorly and laterally to meet the lateral incision. After these incisions are completed, the petrous bone may be removed, exposing the middle-ear cavity. Take cultures of purulent exudates if they are present.

Storage and Transportation

If specific microbiologic transport containers are unavailable for use, place tissue samples for bacterial, mycobacterial, fungal, or viral cultures in sterile containers to which 1–2 ml of preservative-free sterile saline solution has been added. Refer the sample for analysis as quickly as possible after collection.

Microbiologic results should be interpreted in light of clinical history, death scene investigation results, premortem culture results if available, specimen source, collection technique, multiplicity of organisms isolated, and the pathogenicity of the isolated organisms, as well as appropriate current medical literature.

Metabolic Disorders

Metabolic disorders must be kept in mind, especially in those cases where a cause of death is not apparent upon completion of the gross postmortem examination. Defects in fatty acid oxidation are the most common of these disorders associated with sudden unexpected death in infancy and early childhood.

A defect of fatty acid oxidation causing an infant's death is suggested by any or all of the following features:

- acute life-threatening events (ALTEs)
- fasting hypoglycemia
- myopathy
- previous sibling affected with ALTEs, myopathy, or Reye's syndrome
- family history of "SIDS."

It is imperative, therefore, that the autopsy pathologist is aware of the medical history and carefully examines the tissues for evidence of lipid accumulation, and collects appropriate samples for definitive biochemical tests. Screening for multiple metabolic disorders can be performed if a blood standard card is collected. In cases of sudden unexpected infant death, it is recommended that two such cards be collected – one may be submitted for metabolic screening while the other may be retained as a standard in case issues of paternity or other questions arise subsequently.

The cut surfaces of the liver, heart, and muscles may be pale yellow, alerting the pathologist to fatty infiltration and the necessity to collect appropriate material for further analysis. However, in some cases postmortem tissues may not be grossly abnormal; therefore, it is recommended that routine metabolic screening be performed in all suspected SIDS cases.

Even microscopic examination of skeletal and cardiac muscle, liver, and kidney with routine H&E staining may reveal little, if any, cytoplasmic lipid. Therefore, if the history suggests a disorder of fatty acid oxidation, then staining of frozen sections of fresh tissues with oil red O may be performed. Because the laboratory results of histochemical staining of frozen tissues become available some time following the postmortem examination, it is recommended that tissues and fluids from patients suspected of having a fatty acid oxidation disorder be collected and stored in an appropriate fashion, as described below. If further investigations do not suggest a particular defect, those materials can eventually be discarded.

Due to advances in technology, it is now possible to screen for the major metabolic defects from a blood sample collected on a blood standard card. If an abnormality in β-oxidation of fatty acids is discovered on screening, suggesting medium-chain acyl-coenzyme A dehydrogenase (MCAD) deficiency, then confirmatory testing for the various

mutations can be performed on retained blood, or even on paraffin-embedded tissue.

Urine

Analysis of abnormal fatty acid metabolites in urine is a diagnostic tool that may be used to detect a disorder of mitochondrial fatty acid oxidation. Only 0.1 ml is required. Most of the defects present with dicarboxylic aciduria; the only exceptions are CT and CPT deficiencies. Some defects (e.g., MCAD deficiency) have, in addition, a characteristic excretion pattern of acylglycines and acylcarnitines. Unfortunately, urine is often not available at postmortem examination; in a recent study of SIDS, urine was found to be present in only 40% of subjects even when the bladder was opened at autopsy. Personal experience of both of the authors has shown urine to be absent in the overwhelming majority of SIDS cases. However, swabbing the bladder wall with a cotton ball often provides sufficient material for metabolite analysis. If collected, urine and swab samples should be stored at –20 °C.

Blood

Blood is conveniently and safely stored on blood standard cards, which are now widely commercially available. After the blood has dried, the card may be placed in a glassine envelope or other suitable container, and stored in a cool, dry place. If a wet specimen is desired, collect 20 ml of blood into a tube with anticoagulant, then centrifuge it and store separately the plasma and cells at –20 °C. Such samples (both wet and dry) are useful for making a postmortem diagnosis of MCAD deficiency, the most common disorder of fatty acid oxidation. In such cases acylglycine and acylcarnitine conjugates are present. Blood may also be used to assist in the diagnosis of other metabolic disorders, since abnormal metabolites are likely to accumulate in the plasma.

Vitreous Fluid

Vitreous fluid has been postulated as a useful alternative body fluid for the detection of abnormal metabolites in the diagnosis of diseases presenting with organic aciduria. Analysis of this fluid for metabolites has not been evaluated completely, but a number of metabolic disorders have been identified by this means, including MCAD deficiency and glutaric acidemia type II. As stated earlier, vitreous humor should be collected after the cranial contents have been examined. If there is evidence of traumatic injury, the case should be discussed with the pathologist who will perform the microscopic examination of the globes prior to collection of vitreous.

Skin Biopsy

For genetic studies and for the evaluation of some defects that cannot be performed in other tissues, a small skin biopsy specimen should be collected under sterile conditions into tissue culture medium containing 1% dimethyl sulfoxide and frozen at −70 °C. Skin stored in such a manner can often be successfully cultured.

With an appropriate protocol of collection, storage, and sample analysis, it should be possible to ensure correct diagnosis of disorders of fatty acid oxidation presenting to the pathologist. Appropriate counseling of affected families will lead to pre-symptomatic sibling diagnosis of these frequently treatable disorders, which, in turn, can prevent the catastrophic metabolic consequences of the disorders.

Additional Procedures

Photographs, radiographs, and collection of trace evidence are encouraged when warranted by the investigation of the scene where the infant was found lifeless, the findings of the deputy coroners or medical examiners, or the pathological abnormalities identified during the postmortem examination.

Photography

Photographs include the case number, and a measuring device (ruler). A color code may be included when appropriate, for example, with bruises. Photographs include distant "scanning" photographs, and closer, detailed "spot" photographs of the injury or finding of interest. In the closer views, the lesion should largely fill the frame of view of the camera. The camera is held perpendicular to the body surface, so that distortion of the injury or finding is minimized. If a pattern injury is being documented, it is important to have the scale in the same plane, and immediately adjacent to the pattern injury. Documenting the injury in this way will allow future computer-generated overlay comparisons with possible items. The field of view should be considered – although the pathologist or photographer may be accustomed to seeing various dissecting instruments, blood on the autopsy table or cutting board, and other such items, these will be distracting, if not frankly disturbing to others who view the photographs later. The field of view should be "coned down" as much as possible to eliminate such distracting findings. Additionally, the background or surroundings should be cleaned of blood and tools. Further, distracting findings such as genitalia, medical hardware, or autopsy incisions may be covered with surgical towels, so that the photograph concentrates only on the physical finding of interest. Photographs showing normal body cavities and organs are of diagnostic value in excluding disorders, and enhance effective consultation by pathologists not performing the postmortem examination. They are also useful adjuncts in testimony provided during depositions and trials.

Radiography

Use of radiographs as part of the pediatric autopsy examination has several purposes and benefits. First, radiographs serve as yet another form of documentation of findings seen by the pathologist at the time of examination. Radiographic examination allows the documentation of natural normal or abnormal osseous findings. In cases of possible physical abuse, radiographs may detect otherwise occult fractures of the extremities. In cases involving abandoned newborns, radiographs document the presence of air or gas within the lungs, gastrointestinal tract, and body cavities. These findings, along with others, are used by the pathologist in rendering an opinion regarding the central question of live birth versus stillbirth. In years past, whole-body radiographs or "baby grams" were seen as helpful adjuncts to the autopsy, but these are of limited value, as this type of study does not allow the visualization of small but important findings such as injuries to the metaphyseal regions, known as classic metaphyseal lesions. Rather than a single-view "babygram," a skeletal survey, consisting of multiple views of the head, torso, and each extremity, is recommended. The skeletal survey identifies and more finely characterizes abnormalities, and allows detection of subtle but important findings such as classic metaphyseal lesions. The radiographs are appropriately permanently marked with case identifiers. If any questions or concerns arise, these studies should be interpreted with the assistance of a radiologist with expertise in pediatric and forensic medicine.

Trace Evidence

Trace evidence is to be collected in compliance with national, state, and county investigative and police policies and procedures. Proper identification and chain of evidence need to be maintained at all times. These specimens are to be collected and retained by approved methods. Examples of trace evidence that may be routinely collected by law enforcement agencies include: identification prints (of the soles of the feet in the neonate), scalp hair standards, identification photographs, and a DNA standard card. Other trace evidence will be collected as dictated by the circumstances of the individual case.

See Also

Children: Sudden Natural Infant and Childhood Death; Non-inflicted Causes of Death; **Imaging:** Radiology, Pediatric, Scintigraphy and Child Abuse

Further Reading

Buchino JJ, Dimmick JE (2001) The role of the pediatric pathologist. In: Stocker JT, Dehner LP (eds.) *Pediatric Pathology*, 2nd edn., pp. 3–4. New York: Lippincott/ Williams and Wilkins.

Byard RW (2004) *Sudden Death in Infancy, Childhood, and Adolescence*, 2nd edn. Cambridge, UK: Cambridge University Press.

Byard RW, Krous HF (2001) *Sudden Infant Death Syndrome. Problems, Progress and Possibilities*. London: Arnold.

Collins KA (2003) Sudden infant death syndrome. In: Froede RC (ed.) *Handbook of Forensic Pathology*, 2nd edn., pp. 105–110. Northfield, IL: College of American Pathologists.

Corey TS (2003) Investigation of child abuse. In: Froede RC (ed.) *Handbook of Forensic Pathology*, 2nd edn., pp. 125–138. Northfield, IL: College of American Pathologists.

Fierro MF (2003) Infanticide, abandoned newborns, and feticide. In: Froede RC (ed.) *Handbook of Forensic Pathology*, 2nd edn., pp. 111–124. Northfield, IL: College of American Pathologists.

Graham M (1998) The role of the medical examiner in fatal child abuse. In: Monteleone JA (ed.) *Child Maltreatment: A Clinical Guide and Reference*, 2nd edn., pp. 531–558. London: GW Medical.

Kleinman PK (1998) Postmortem imaging. In: Kleinman PK (ed.) *Diagnostic Imaging of Child Abuse*, 2nd edn., pp. 242–247. London: Mosby.

Schulz DM, Giordano DA, Schulz DH (1962) Hearts of infants and children. Weights and measurements. *Archives of Pathology* 74: 464–471.

Stocker JT, McPherson TA (2001) The pediatric autopsy. In: Stocker JT, Dehner LP (eds.) *Pediatric Pathology*, 2nd edn., pp. 5–17. New York: Lippincott/Williams and Wilkins.

Adult

J A J Ferris, Auckland Hospital, Auckland, New Zealand

Introduction

The purpose of this article is to review the practical aspects of the adult forensic or medicolegal autopsy. It is important to recognize that in many cases a careful analysis of the interrelationship between the medical history and any prescribed treatments may provide important information required for the accurate reconstruction of the circumstances of death. In contrast to the hospital autopsy, which has as its primary object the evaluation of natural disease processes and correlations with clinical presentation, evolution of disease processes and effect of medical and surgical treatments, the adult medicolegal autopsy (forensic) has as its principal aims the determination of a series of distinct but often interrelated objectives:

1. to determine the identity of the deceased, including a description of the weight, length, physique, racial characteristics, and any physical abnormalities
2. to determine the time and place of death
3. to determine the mode of dying and the time interval between the episodes of assault and death
4. to determine the medical cause for death
5. to document in detail any and all injuries to the body and direct the photographing of such injuries
6. to determine the manner of death (murder, suicide, natural causes, etc.)
7. to collect and preserve evidence that might link an assailant with the victim
8. depending on the rules governing the consent for autopsy, to retain tissues and organs that may be required for evidential purposes
9. to collect samples that may be required for further specialist forensic examinations such as microbiological, toxicological, and DNA analysis
10. to provide a complete written report documenting all of the autopsy findings and an expert interpretation of these findings
11. to restore the body to a cosmetic condition that is in keeping with the religious and cultural traditions of the family.

In most jurisdictions the medicolegal autopsy is performed on the properly authorized instructions of a legal authority such as a coroner, medical examiner, procurator fiscal, or magistrate. The pathologist must ensure, prior to the postmortem examination, that all of the available details of the circumstances of the death are provided. The history of the circumstances of death may require modification of the autopsy procedures and will often focus attention on a particular aspect of the postmortem examination.

The actual postmortem examination has two distinct but equally important phases: the external and internal examinations.

Documentation of Findings

Comprehensive notes are essential and if dictation is used the tapes should be retained as required by the local judicial standards. Handwritten notes and diagrams must also be retained in a master file.

Pathologists are required to document all of their findings and the format of their record and autopsy protocol is often dictated by the jurisdiction in which the case is being investigated. This may be in the form of a standard preprinted format. Such printed formats, however, do not allow for the wide variations and extent of descriptions required in the forensic autopsy and should be strongly discouraged. As with the autopsy examination, the report format should allow for flexibility but should include all of the information derived from the autopsy examination, including the negative findings since in the forensic autopsy these may be as significant as positive findings. This degree of flexibility and variability of report format is readily accommodated with any of the modern forms of computer-based word-processing systems.

Most hospital autopsy reports catalog the findings based on organ systems such as respiratory system and cardiovascular system. This form of protocol is principally of value in correlating disease and treatment but may be very difficult for lawyers and lay juries to understand. A much easier format to present in court, and certainly easier for the nonmedical individual to understand, is to document the findings anatomically in much the same way that the dissection is performed. The report can be divided in to, "Head," "Neck and Chest," and "Abdomen." For example, documentation of a stab wound through the chest wall, right lung, and heart is much easier to visualize than to expect a lay juror to link apparently unrelated injuries to the skeletal system, the respiratory system, and the cardiovascular system. It is important to remember that the underlying purpose of a forensic autopsy is to communicate the findings to all of those whose role is the investigation of the death.

An autopsy protocol is provided in **Figure 1**; the key to any such report is complete and comprehensible documentation.

Autopsies should only be conducted in mortuaries that have adequate facilities and safety procedures. Since in many cases a full medical history may not be available, in order to protect all the staff and attendees from the possibility of infection, universal safety precautions should be applied. Photographic and X-ray facilities should be available and there should be adequate space for the examination, documentation, and if necessary, temporary storage of exhibits, and clothing.

Handling and Preservation of Evidence

It is appropriate to assume that almost all cases of trauma or unnatural death, be they murder, motor vehicle accident, or industrial accident, may be eventually the subject of either a criminal investigation or civil litigation. Because of the sophistication and extreme sensitivity of modern forensic science techniques, any material related to such cases that may be required for examination in a forensic science laboratory must be handled in such a way that it is free from contamination. The purpose of these forensic examinations may be to determine if a known and unknown sample had a common origin and it becomes the responsibility of any individual who has possession of these samples to ensure that they are properly identified, preserved, and packaged for transportation. Failure to do this may result in loss or deterioration of the exhibit and an inability to prove continuity of the sample may result in its inadmissibility in court. The normal packaging, labeling, and transportation of tissue and body fluid samples in a hospital environment will meet most of these requirements. However, problems tend to arise in connection with clothing and other nonbiological samples.

Any clothing on the body must be removed carefully, preferably without cutting, and placed in appropriate bags for drying and storage. Although it is usually not the role of the pathologist to carry out detailed examination of clothing, it is often valuable for the pathologist to identify damage such as cuts or bullet holes and relate these to injuries and marks on the body.

Each item must be separately identified in such a way that this marking does not interfere with or destroy the evidence to be examined. If it is not possible to mark the items directly, they must be placed in appropriate containers and each container sealed and marked for identification.

Every effort must be made to preserve the object (such as clothing) in the condition in which it was found. To prevent decomposition, items that are stained with blood and other body fluids need special handling. Wherever possible they should be air-dried before packaging, otherwise they should be packaged in paper containers and transferred as soon as possible to a special storage area. Blood, body fluids, and internal organ samples should be refrigerated or sent immediately to the laboratory for testing and storage.

Every item recovered must be properly packaged and labeled with the following information:

- what the item is (blood, urine, bullet)
- where it was taken from (bullet from left chest cavity)

- when it was taken (8:30 p.m., July 4, 2004)
- who took it.

The initials or signatures of all persons who have had custody of each item should be placed on the label. When samples are handed over to a police officer or investigator, a record of the name of the person to whom the exhibits are handed must be maintained by the autopsy facility, together with the date and time that the exhibits were handed over. Records of all the procedures involving the handling of autopsy exhibits in relation to any particular case should be retained as a permanent record and also incorporated in the autopsy report. Special sample kits are frequently available from forensic laboratories which take into account the particular sampling needs and technical requirements of that laboratory.

Identification

How was the body identified to the pathologist and what were the date and time of this identification?

External Examination

This phase of the autopsy may provide the only opportunity to collect contact trace evidence and

---

REPORT OF AUTOPSY

Department of Forensic Pathology
Institute of Pathology
165 St. Judes Road
Ardbeg
Tel: 08-3124-785

Date of Examination   _____

Commenced at   _____

Coroner   _____

Autopsy Number   _____

Coroner's Number   _____

Deceased's Name   _____

Age   _____   Sex   _____

Date of Death   _____

Estimated Time of Death   _____

PRINCIPAL PATHOLOGICAL FINDINGS:

1. Major disease or injury directly leading to death.

2, 3, 4, etc. Other major findings.

CAUSE OF DEATH:

Part 1 *a.* Terminal Event (i.e. Bronchopneumonia)
  due to or as a consequence of

  b. Underlying disease process or injury.
  due to or as a consequence of

  c. Underlying disease process or injury.

Part 2 *a.* Conditions contributing to death but not directly related to the disease process listed under Part 1.

Date: _____   Signed: _____

Figure 1 Standard autopsy protocol.

document and photograph injuries. It is at this stage of the postmortem examination that the nature, extent, and direction of the later internal examination may be decided. In some special cases the autopsy may be limited to external examination only without full internal examination. This should only occur in exceptional circumstances since most forensic pathologists have encountered many cases where subsequent full internal dissection has revealed injuries or disease that have significantly altered the course of the case investigation.

At the end of each postmortem examination the pathologist should be able to state that there was no evidence of any natural disease process which could have caused or accelerated death or caused collapse. If any such disease was found, then its role in the death should be considered and either included or excluded as a factor. Limited external examinations

---

Autopsy Report
Page 2

General Preamble:

This should include the names of all of the persons present such as police officers, witnesses, staff etc. and their roles. In routine non-criminal cases such a name list may not be required.

Identification:

How was the body identified to the pathologist including the date and time.

External Examination:

All external features should be listed as described above, including any possible identifying marks, scars or tattoos.

External injuries should be listed separately and in some cases the **internal injuries** should be described separately from the remaining of the internal examination.

SPECIAL EXAMINATIONS SUCH AS RADIOLOGICAL EXAMINATION, LASER SCANNING, OR SPECIAL FINGERPRINT STUDIES:

The results of any specialized examinations of the body should be included in the autopsy report and the phase of the autopsy examination at which any such examinations were made should be noted.

EXHIBITS:

At this point in the documentation, all external exhibits should be listed and the person to whom the exhibits were handed should be named, i.e.

The following samples were taken from the body and handed to

1.
2.
3.

INTERNAL EXAMINATION:

Head:

Scalp: Presence or absence of bruising on its under surface.

Skull: Thickness and density. Distribution and direction of fractures. Dura.

Brain: Weight, meninges. Location and extent of injuries, hemorrhages or natural disease. Cerebral vessels.

Spinal Cord: Was it examined?

Pituitary Gland:

Figure 1 Continued

should only occur with the full consent of the pathologist and authorizing legal authority and such decisions should only be made in the light of pathology staff health concerns, religious or cultural traditions of the next of kin, or resource constraints. Limiting the extent of postmortem examination should never be simply for the convenience of the parties involved.

The external examination should document and detail everything on the outside of the body, including the clothing, evidence of medical treatment, scars, tattoos, and all injuries. Patterns of blood stains on the skin and clothing should be recorded, as well as all other marks on the clothing that might correlate with patterns of injury. In all cases of suspicious death and in most cases of motor vehicle accidents the clothing should be examined prior to removal from the body for trace evidence. Routine stripping of all bodies admitted to a forensic mortuary facility by anyone other than a pathologist or qualified mortuary staff is inappropriate and may result in the loss of vital evidence.

Autopsy Report
Page 3

Neck and Chest:

    Neck Musculature: Presence or absence of bruising.

    Hyoid Bone and Laryngeal Cartilages: Presence or absence of fractures.

    Thyroid Gland: Size and colloid content.

    Pharynx and larynx: Presence of foreign material.

    Rib cage: Presence or absence of fractures.

    Pericardial Sac and Pleural Cavities: Presence and amount of blood or effusions.

    Trachea and Main Bronchi: Presence or absence of blood, froth, mucus, etc.

    Lungs: Separate weights. Presence or absence of emphysema, pneumonia, embolism, or infarction. Extent of inflation or collapse and the amount of edema fluid.

    Heart: Weight, general size. Extent of dilatation of each chamber. Condition of valves and valve orifices. Thickness of right and left ventricles in millimeters and an assessment of the degree of hypertrophy. Presence or absence or scarring or infarction. The condition and distribution of the coronary arteries and the location of areas of stenosis or thrombosis. Old or recent?

    Aorta and Great Vessels: (peripheral veins if required).

    Esophagus:

    Diaphragm:

Abdomen:

    Peritoneal Cavity:

    Stomach and Duodenum: Contents, presence or absence of ulcers.

    Intestines:

    Liver: Weight, presence or absence of cirrhosis or fatty change.

    Gallbladder and Bile Ducts:

    Spleen: Weight. Appearance of capsule and cut surface.

    Pancreas:

Figure 1 Continued

A complete general external examination of the body is required, including:

1. documentation of height and weight
2. distribution and grading of rigor mortis
3. distribution of postmortem lividity, with a comment on any areas of pressure pallor
4. secondary lividity
5. apparent degree of fixation
6. hair color, eye color
7. presence or absence of petechial hemorrhages on the conjunctiva, eyelids, and face
8. appearance of the ears and nose
9. presence of blood or vomitus in both the nose and mouth
10. nature of dentition
11. presence of any foreign material
12. appearance of the neck, trunk, limbs, and external genitalia, including a list of needle marks, scars, tattoos, and skin rashes.

Autopsy Report
Page 4

Mesenteric and abdominal lymph nodes:

Adrenal Glands: Cortical lipid content, presence or absence of hemorrhage.

Kidneys: Separate weights. Subcapsular surfaces. Evidence of cortical thinning and or scarring.

Bladder and Ureters: Presence and approximate amount of urine.

Uterus, Tubes and Ovaries or Prostate Gland and Testes:

Skeleton:

List any bone disease or evidence or old or recent fractures.

EXHIBITS:

TOXICOLOGY RESULTS:

OTHER LABORATORY TESTS:

MICROSCOPIC EXAMINATION:

COMMENTARY:

Date: _____   Signature:

Figure 1 Continued

Any evidence of medical treatment or resuscitation, including endotracheal and nasogastric tubes, airways or surgical marks, or incisions on the body should be fully documented. It is strongly advised that all such evidence of medical intervention should remain undisturbed until the body has been viewed by a pathologist and that all medical appliances should remain with the body until that time.

Injuries should be described separately.

External Injuries

Since documentation of injuries is a key part of the autopsy examination, it is usually advisable to shave the scalp hair so that all scalp wounds can be visualized. Palpation of scalp wounds through the hair is not sufficient and will not allow for the recognition and documentation of patterned scalp bruises. These should be listed systematically by anatomical location and numbered. The exact location should be related to a particular part of the body, i.e., head, right arm, front of trunk, left leg, and the specific site of injury should be measured from a fixed part of the body, i.e., sternoclavicular joint, elbow, ankle.

The description should include the size, shape, color, and nature, i.e., bruise, abrasion, laceration, stab wound.

For example, a horizontal linear abrasion 6.0 cm long on the left side of the neck extending from a point 5.0 cm below the chin to the left jaw angle; or a stab wound 1.8 cm long situated on the left side of the chest, 4.0 cm below and 3.0 cm to the right of the right sternoclavicular joint. (This wound was directed downwards to the left at approximately 45° to the horizontal, gaping by 5.0 mm with a narrow rim of abrasion 1.0 mm wide. Its medial end curved vertically downwards and was pointed. Its lateral end was rounded.)

Internal Injuries

In some circumstances, it is appropriate to describe the internal injuries separately from the general internal examination, e.g., when relating to the effects of stab wounds which may have passed through several organ systems. The same may apply to gunshot wounds. This decision should be based on the ease of a nonmedical person's ability to understand the extent of internal injury.

Internal Examination

The nature and extent of internal examination in a forensic autopsy are similar to that for the hospital autopsy, although the order in which the body cavities will be examined is determined by the nature of the case and the needs of the particular investigation. For example, it is important that the brain be removed before dissecting the neck structures in a case of suspected neck injury.

The chest and abdomen are usually opened by a Y-shaped incision from the tip of the shoulders to the sternomanubrial joint and then carried vertically downwards to the symphysis pubis. In hospital cases the Y-shaped incision is often made below the breasts. This is inappropriate for a forensic autopsy, since it does not allow for proper examination of the neck structures. The chest plate is removed as a triangle, including the costal cartilages and the sternum. Whether the internal organs are removed as a single block or in separate organ groups will depend on the practice and training of individual pathologists and the needs of the particular case.

In practice, it is often best to remove the neck and chest organs as a single block and then, after ligating the jejunum, the liver, spleen, pancreas, stomach, and duodenum can be removed as a separate block. The gastric contents should be described and appropriate samples of body fluids taken for toxicological analysis as required. The aorta and retroperitoneal tissues can then be removed and the pelvic organs may be left *in situ* for further dissection if required.

Access to the brain is achieved by a coronal incision across the top of the scalp from behind each ear. If this incision is well behind the vertex, reflection of the scalp is often made easier and the final cosmetic result much better. It is important to expose the posterior subscalp tissues so that all subscalp and galeal injuries can be recorded.

A pathologist must be prepared to defend any decision not to undertake a particular part of the postmortem examination, including histological examination and radiology.

Special Dissection Techniques

As far as possible, all special dissections should be performed in a bloodless field, i.e., the brain should be removed before neck dissection, and in pelvic dissections the pelvis should be elevated after the thoracic and abdominal organs have been removed by placing a block under the lumbar vertebrae. Representative sections from all areas of injury should be taken and labeled specifically for the site of origin. It is also important that photographs should be taken at all stages of these dissections and the autopsy report should reflect the nature and extent of the special dissections that have been performed.

Anterior neck dissection   This should be performed in all cases of suspected neck injury.

- The skin should be reflected to expose the sternomastoid muscles and the external jugular veins. This is best achieved with lateral neck incisions extending from the mastoid processes vertically downwards and then carried anteriorly and medially below the sternoclavicular joints to the midline below the manubrium. In many jurisdictions such incisions are unacceptable and it may be necessary to perform the traditional Y-shaped incision from the front of the shoulder to the sternum. Unfortunately, in cases of severe obesity this will not allow a good exposure of the higher anterior neck structures. The other traditional opening incision under the breasts should not be used for careful neck dissection.
- Layer-by-layer dissection of the neck musculature *in situ* should commence with reflection of the sternomastoid muscles and by incising their sternal and clavicular insertions. The omohyoid, sternohyoid, and sternothyroid muscles should then be removed to expose the thyroid gland.
- The thyroid gland should next be removed to expose the cricothyroid muscle and any bruising or injury to the hyoid bone or laryngeal cartilages should be noted and sampled.
- Next, identify the common carotid arteries and their bifurcations and note any associated adventitial bruising or hemorrhage.
- Incise the digastric muscles, free the tongue from the mandible, and remove the neck structures by retracting on the tongue. Do not hold or compress the laryngeal structures.
- Finally note any injury or bruising on the posterior pharyngeal or laryngeal structures or on the anterior surface of the cervical vertebrae.

Posterior neck dissection   This is a valuable technique to examine for posterior neck injury or to expose the vertebral arteries either for angiography or for evidence of traumatic subarachnoid hemorrhage.

- Expose the posterior neck musculature by a vertical midline posterior incision with bilateral extensions at the level of the occipital protuberance.
- Perform a layer-by-layer dissection from above downwards, cutting the splenius capitis, the semispinalis capitis, the posterior insertion of the sternocleidomastoid muscle, and the trapezius.
- The vertebral arteries are seen within a deep triangle formed by the superior oblique muscle laterally, the rectus capitis posterior major medially, and

the upper border of the posterior arch of the atlas with the inferior oblique muscle covering the lower border of this bony arch.
- The first cervical nerve may be seen immediately below the vertebral artery crossing the upper border of the posterior arch of the atlas.

This is a difficult dissection and, if the body has been lying on its back for some time after death, the tissues may be edematous and very congested due to lividity. If necessary, leave the body on its front for at least 30 min after dissecting the skin before continuing to expose the deeper neck structures.

Facial Dissection

In suspected cases of smothering, facial fractures, or other facial injury, this technique allows for a good demonstration of the extent of injury in the periorbital or maxillary areas. It also allows for the reconstruction of the facial tissues after dissection without significant disfigurement. Dissect only one side of the face at a time.

- Join the inferior ends of the coronal scalp incisions to the upper lateral extensions of the chest incisions.
- Dissect forwards, incising the external auditory canal and in a vertical plane dissect off the skin to expose the parotid gland and the zygomatic arch and then dissect anteriorly, superficial to the fatty tissue over the facial musculature.
- Carefully enucleate the eye from behind the skin flap, taking great care not to buttonhole the eyelids or to perforate the eyeball.
- Dissect along the margin of the mandible to the midline and dissect off the lips by cutting through the buccal mucosa behind the skin flap.
- Complete the dissection by exposing the lateral aspects of the nasal bones and nasal cartilage.
- It is most important that the lateral dissection should not be extended across the midline to allow for a vertical line of fixation of the facial structures essential for the reconstruction of the face without disfigurement.

Pelvic Dissection

This technique is essential in any case of alleged pelvic injury, rape, or sodomy. Using this technique it is possible to visualize and photograph not only mucosal injuries to the vagina and rectum but also perivaginal and perirectal injuries and injuries to the sphincters and the muscle floor of the pelvis. Speculum examination alone does not provide this degree of visualization.

- In order to ensure a bloodless field, all of the internal organs, except the pelvic organs, should be removed and the pelvis should be elevated by placing a block under the sacrum.
- Extend the abdominal incision vertically downwards to the root of the penis or clitoris and reflect laterally to expose the symphysis pubis and pubic rami.
- With a saw, cut through the superior pubic rami and then extend the saw cut downwards and medially through the inferior pubic rami. Removal of this central wedge of bone will expose the bladder and urethra intact.
- Open the urethra into the bladder and then dissect off the bladder and urethra to expose the anterior wall of the vagina.
- Open the vagina and expose the cervix. At this stage it will be possible to visualize the state of the hymen and any old or recent vaginal injuries. It is also possible to take additional vaginal swabs if necessary.
- Next, dissect the vagina from the anterior surface of the rectum and remove together with the uterus, tubes, and ovaries.
- The final stage is to open the anus and rectum and then remove them to display the posterior aspect of the floor of the pelvis.

Exhibits

At this point document all internal samples such as blood, urine, and gastric contents as in the external exhibit list and check against the list of exhibits prepared by the individual responsible for receiving all of the exhibits.

Toxicology Results

Since these results are not necessarily going to form a part of the evidence of the forensic pathologist in homicide cases, such results should not be automatically included in the autopsy report.

Other Laboratory Tests

Biochemistry results, microbiology and viral studies, and diatom studies should be included if they form a part of the opinion as to the cause or manner of death.

Reports by special consultants such as neuro-pathologists should either be appended to the autopsy report or incorporated into the report.

Microscopic Examination

In most cases microscopic examination of all of the major organs should be carried out. Histology will not only confirm the gross findings but will allow for the evaluation of natural disease processes and in the case of injuries allow for an assessment of the age of the injury and compare it with other injuries to the body. While the accurate timing of injuries may be difficult, this microscopic comparison may be very important in the overall evaluation of the significance of injuries.

Summary Opinion or Commentary

The purpose of the commentary is to combine a medicolegal opinion of the autopsy findings with an explanation of the disease or injury processes leading to death. This should be written in such terms that the findings and conclusions can be readily understood by a nonmedical person and yet should be scientifically accurate. Such a commentary should be able to be read out in court so that a jury will have a complete understanding of the medical aspects of the case, the significance of any injuries, and how these relate to the death and any assault.

This commentary should start with a statement as to whether or not the death was natural and, if unnatural, whether or not there was any natural disease that may have contributed to the death. It should be possible for the pathologist to state that there was no natural disease to cause or accelerate death or to cause collapse, and if the pathologist cannot make this statement, he/she should explain why.

The next part of the commentary should explain the disease process or injuries which directly led to the death and should represent a simple explanation of the sequence of events already listed in the "Principal Pathological Findings" shown on the front page of the report and also listed under Part 1 of the "Cause of Death" (**Figure 1**).

Any contributory conditions or injuries should be described next and how these may or may not have contributed to death or the assault.

Any other major disease processes should be explained and if they did not play a part in the death, this should be stated.

Did the toxicological analysis reveal any findings such as evidence of alcohol intoxication which could have contributed to death?

See Also

Autopsy: Medico-legal Considerations; Pediatric

Further Reading

Burton JL, Rutty GN (2001) *The Hospital Autopsy*, 2nd edn. Oxford, UK: Oxford University Press.

Code of Practice and Performance Standards for Forensic Pathologists (2004) The Home Office Policy Advisory Board for Forensic Pathology and The Royal College of Pathologists. www.rcpath.org.

Gordon I, Shapiro HA, Berson SD (1988) *Forensic Medicine – A Guide to Principles.* London: Churchill Livingstone.

Knight B (1983) *The Coroner's Autopsy.* London: Churchill.

Knight B (1996) *Forensic Pathology,* 2nd edn. London: Arnold.

Ludwig J (2002) *Handbook of Autopsy Practice,* 3rd edn. Totawa, NJ: Humana Press.

Pounder DJ (2000) Autopsy. In: Siegel JA, Saukko PJ, Knupfer GC (eds.) *Encyclopedia of Forensic Sciences,* vol. 3, pp. 1155–1161. London: Academic Press.

Royal College of Pathologists (2002) *Guidelines on Autopsy Practice.* Royal College of Pathologists. www.rcpath.org.

Rutty GN, Ryan JM (2002) *Essentials of Autopsy Practice.* London: Springer Verlag.

Saladino AJ, Dailey ML (1978) The problem-oriented postmortem examination. *American Journal of Clinical Pathology* 69: 253–257.

Wagner, Scott A (2004) *Color Atlas of The Autopsy.* Boca Raton, FL: CRC Press.

Infectious

K Kibayashi, Saga Medical School, Saga, Japan

Introduction

The infectious autopsy, or high-risk autopsy, is defined as the postmortem examination of a deceased person who has had, or is likely to have had, a serious infectious disease that can be transmitted to those present at autopsy, thereby causing them serious illness and/or premature death. Many infectious diseases present autopsy prosecutors and laboratory personnel with risks for postmortem acquisition of infections (**Table 1**). The prevalence of human immunodeficiency virus (HIV) infection, hepatitis B, and hepatitis C in forensic autopsy populations is much higher than in the general public because of an overrepresentation of intravenous drug abusers among decedents subjected to autopsy. In addition, these infectious diseases and tuberculosis are frequently asymptomatic or clinically undiagnosed and may be present without morphological evidence at autopsy. In fact, occupational infections of HIV, hepatitis B virus (HBV), hepatitis C virus (HCV), and *Mycobacterium tuberculosis* have been realized as a serious concern among forensic autopsy workers. In forensic investigations, however, autopsy

of the victims is deemed essential to determine the cause and manner of death even when the deceased person had highly contagious pathogens. Furthermore, forensic autopsy plays an important role in diagnosing such infectious diseases and thus provides vital information on the epidemiology and pathogenesis. This section reviews the current state of our knowledge of the frequently concerned occupational infections, HIV infection in particular, and provides preventive measures, including postexposure managements.

HIV Infection

Background

Since the first case reports of acquired immunodeficiency syndrome (AIDS) appeared in 1981, HIV infection and AIDS have become a global pandemic with an estimated 42 million people living with the virus worldwide in 2002. Although many countries have developed national strategies to prevent HIV infection, the number of infected people is still increasing, notably in sub-Saharan Africa, where

Table 1 Infectious diseases and agents that can be transmitted at autopsy

Viruses
Human immunodeficiency virus (HIV)
Viral hepatitis (hepatitis B virus, hepatitis C virus)
Human T-cell lymphotropic virus (HTLV)
Viral hemorrhagic fevers (Lassa, Marburg, Ebola, and Crimean-Congo hemorrhagic fevers)
Rabies
Smallpox
Bacteria
Tuberculosis
Meningococcal infections
Streptococcal infections
Anthrax
Plague
Tetanus
Legionnaires' disease
Typhoid fever
Paratyphoid
Tularemia
Diphtheria
Erysipeloid
Glanders
Scrub typhus
Fungi
Blastomycosis
Coccidioidomycosis
Protozoon
Toxoplasmosis
Prion
Creutzfeldt–Jakob disease

Table 2 Risk factors of human immunodeficiency virus (HIV) infection

Unprotected sexual contacts (homosexual and heterosexual)
Intravenous drug abuse
Transfusion of blood or blood products
Newborn baby of mother at risk of HIV infection
Occupational exposure to blood or body fluids (healthcare and autopsy workers)

29.4 million people are infected with the virus. Currently, two types of HIV are known: HIV-1 and HIV-2. HIV-1 infection constitutes the majority of patients in the world. HIV-2 infection is primarily seen in West Africa. Both types of HIV are transmitted through sexual contact and exposure to infected blood or blood components and perinatally from mother to neonate (**Table 2**).

HIV infection is diagnosed by detecting antibodies specific to the virus, or by detection of the virus itself, through the p24-antigen, by nucleic acid-based tests, or if necessary by culture and virus isolation. HIV-infected individuals develop an antibody response to HIV proteins, and detection of these antibodies is the basis of screening assays. The usual combination of diagnostic assays is an initial screen with enzyme-linked immunosorbent assay (ELISA) followed by confirmatory testing of reactive specimens with a Western immunoblot. ELISA is a reliable screening method with high sensitivity and specificity. A false-negative result can occur if the patient has not yet seroconverted, following acquisition of HIV infection, during the so-called window period. The other cause of a false-negative is very advanced HIV disease, when the patient may lose the ability to make HIV antibodies. Following the occasional detection of HIV-2 outside the geographical regions with the highest prevalence of HIV-2, HIV-2 detection has been incorporated into many commercial ELISA systems.

HIV primarily infects $CD4^+$ T-lymphocytes and cells of the monocyte/macrophage lineage. The loss of $CD4^+$ T lymphocytes plays a role in the pathogenesis of immune deficiency related to HIV infection. As the number of $CD4^+$ T-lymphocytes declines, immune dysfunction eventually becomes apparent in infected persons. Following transmission, there are three clinical stages of infection: (1) primary infection; (2) a clinically latent asymptomatic period; and (3) clinical progression leading to AIDS. AIDS is defined by a $CD4^+$ T-lymphocyte count of less than 200 cells per μl or the clinical or histopathological presence of opportunistic diseases indicative of profound immunodeficiency.

HIV and Forensic Autopsy

In forensic autopsy, the prevalence of HIV infection is considered to be higher than expected from health statistics, mainly because intravenous drug abusers are one of the risk groups of the infection, and their lifestyle brings them into the medicolegal jurisdiction. The detection of HIV infection, identification of route of infection, and diagnosis of AIDS have medicolegal significance to determine and document the cause and the manner of death. Autopsy could also reveal clinically undiagnosed infectious diseases and neoplasms other than the primary cause of death and help in epidemiological studies, quality assurance activities in assessing diagnostic, or treatment modalities. For example, the forensic autopsy is the only means of determining the range and prevalence of opportunistic diseases and has an immediate impact on patient management where the hospital autopsy is rarely performed. The forensic autopsy of asymptomatic persons who died of unsuspected causes of death other than AIDS has contributed to the understanding of the pathogenesis of HIV disease progression. Furthermore, the identification of HIV-infected subjects at autopsy affords the opportunity for surviving sexual or needle-sharing partners to undergo early testing and counseling and to commence an early therapeutic intervention, thus avoiding further dissemination of infection within the community.

At autopsy, collection of blood and tissue samples is of value for the diagnosis of HIV infection and AIDS. Because immunoglobulins are less likely to be affected by postmortem changes, HIV antibody testing is effective in serum samples taken from bodies even with putrefaction due to prolonged postmortem intervals. A study shows that ELISA is consistently repeatedly positive in cadaveric sera from AIDS patients, with postmortem intervals ranging from 5 h to 58 days; a false-positive result is not observed in specimens from noninfected persons despite prolonged postmortem intervals producing hemolysis. Histopathological diagnosis of AIDS is made according to the criteria in HIV-infected persons with specific opportunistic infections, neoplasms, or AIDS dementia complex (**Table 3**). Legal guidelines for HIV testing and reporting to public health authorities, where applicable, should be followed. Pathologists should maintain the confidentiality of HIV status on autopsy reports to the greatest extent possible.

The potential for occupational transmission of HIV is a serious concern among pathologists and mortuary staff as well as laboratory personnel who may deal with postautopsy samples. In clinical settings, most occupational HIV infections among healthcare providers are the result of needlestick or other sharps

Table 3 Opportunistic infections, neoplasms, and acquired immunodeficiency syndrome (AIDS) dementia complex in AIDS

Opportunistic infections
Viruses
Cytomegalovirus disease and retinitis
Progressive multifocal leukoencephalopathy (papovavirus infection)
Herpes simplex (chronic ulcer, bronchitis, pneumonitis, or esophagitis)
Bacteria
Recurrent pneumonia
Mycobacterium tuberculosis (pulmonary or extrapulmonary)
Mycobacterium avium complex or *M. kansasii* (disseminated or extrapulmonary)
Mycobacterium, other or unidentified species (disseminated or extrapulmonary)
Recurrent *Salmonella* septicemia
Fungi
Candidiasis of esophagus, bronchi, trachea, or lungs
Cryptococcosis (extrapulmonary)
Histoplasmosis (disseminated or extrapulmonary)
Coccidioidomycosis (disseminated or extrapulmonary)
Protozoa
Pneumocystis carinii pneumonia
Toxoplasmosis of brain
Cryptosporidiosis (chronic intestinal)
Isosporiasis (chronic intestinal)
Neoplasms
Kaposi's sarcoma
Lymphoma
Cervical cancer of uterus, invasive
AIDS dementia complex
HIV encephalitis
HIV leukoencephalopathy
Diffuse poliodystrophy
Vacuolar leukoencephalopathy
Cerebral vasculitis
Other
Wasting syndrome

HIV, human immunodeficiency virus.

injuries. A small number of HIV seroconversions following mucous membrane or nonintact skin occupational exposure have also been reported. A scalpel injury during hospital autopsy and seroconversion thereafter in a pathologist has also been reported. Although the estimated risk of HIV infection following occupational exposure to blood or body fluids is only 0.3%, the risk of transmission in a specific situation is likely to vary, depending on the circulating viral titer in the source case, volume of blood injected, depth of penetration, and immune status of the exposed person.

The corpses of infected persons remain potentially contagious with HIV even after a prolonged postmortem interval and have no safe time at which they cease to be an infective risk. Viable HIV is successfully isolated from the blood of nonrefrigerated cadavers at least 36 h after death and of refrigerated cadavers kept at 2 °C at least 17 days postmortem. Autopsy specimens such as blood, body fluids, and fresh tissues are also a potential source of infection. An experimental study shows that HIV suspended in serum remains infectious for several weeks at room temperature (20–28 °C); infectivity remains evident for several days even when dried on a glass coverslip. HIV is inactivated after being exposed to commonly used chemical germicides. A solution of sodium hypochlorite (household bleach) is also an effective germicide; concentrations ranging from 500 ppm (1:100 dilution of household bleach) to 5000 ppm (1:10 dilution of household bleach) are effective depending on the amount of organic material (e.g., blood, mucus) present on the surface to be cleaned and disinfected.

Forensic pathologists can safely examine patients with HIV infection by using well-established techniques for autopsy performance. However, creating a zero risk of blood exposure due to cut or needlestick injuries is not a realistic possibility in routine forensic practice. The prophylactic effect of antiretroviral drug is proved by a clinical trial in which treatment of HIV-infected pregnant women with zidovudine significantly reduced the rate of transmission of HIV to their babies. A three-drug regimen, including two nucleoside analog reverse transcriptase inhibitors and a protease inhibitor, effectively reduces the HIV replication in blood. Based on these rationales, postexposure prophylaxis with at least two antiretroviral drugs is recommended for individuals who have been exposed to blood infected with HIV. All antiretroviral drugs are associated with adverse events, especially gastrointestinal symptoms. Pathologists who have suffered a significant parenteral or mucous membrane exposure should carefully weigh the low rate of becoming infected with HIV and the adverse events of chemoprophylaxis.

In forensic autopsy, the identification of HIV-infected patients is difficult without knowing clinical information or the result of preautopsy serological testing. Chemoprophylaxis should be considered when the percutaneous blood exposure occurred during autopsy of individuals with gross clues of HIV infection such as generalized ill appearance, lymphadenopathy, or needle tracks. Chemoprophylaxis should be initiated promptly, preferably within 1–2 h postexposure, to maximize the chance of efficacy. This means that forensic pathologists cannot afford the time to consult individuals who have expertise in antiretroviral therapy once the exposure event has occurred. Although the frequency of occupational exposure of HIV-infected blood in forensic autopsy must be quite low and HIV is not highly infectious, forensic institutions should communicate in advance with the local hospital regarding the postexposure chemoprophylaxis. Postexposure counseling and follow-up intervention by experienced care providers familiar with the special medical and psychologic needs are also essential for exposed persons.

Hepatitis Viruses

Acute viral hepatitis is caused by one of the five viral agents: (1) hepatitis A virus; (2) HBV; (3) HCV; (4) hepatitis D virus; and (5) hepatitis E virus. In these, HBV and HCV can be transmitted by occupational percutaneous inoculation or transmucosal exposure to blood or body fluids of infected cadavers at autopsy. HBV and HCV are more infectious than HIV; the risk of infection following a percutaneous exposure to infected blood is 5% for HBV (HBeAg-negative source), 19–30% for HBV (HBeAg-positive source), and 1.8–10% for HCV, as compared to 0.36% for HIV. The most feared complication of viral hepatitis is fulminant hepatitis (massive hepatic necrosis): the mortality rate of fulminant hepatatis is greater than 80% in patients with deep coma. Fulminant hepatitis is a rare event and is primarily seen in HBV infection. Over 90% of individuals with acute hepatitis B have a favorable course and recover completely. However, acute hepatitis C has a poor prognosis, with at least 80% of infected individuals progressing to a carrier state leading to chronic liver disease with cirrhosis and even hepatocellular carcinoma.

Effective vaccines and specific immunoglobulins are widely employed to offer protection against HBV infection. For preexposure prophylaxis against hepatitis B, all personnel involved in autopsy work should have their HBs antibody status checked and should receive hepatitis B vaccine. Postexposure prophylaxis with hepatitis B immunoglobulin and/or hepatitis B vaccine should be considered for exposure to HBV after evaluation of the vaccination and the vaccine response status of the exposed person. No equivalent vaccine or immunoglobulin has been developed against HCV infection to date.

Tuberculosis

Tuberculosis caused by *Mycobacterium tuberculosis* usually affects the lungs, although in up to one-third of cases other organs are involved. Beginning in the mid-1980s in many industrialized countries, the number of tuberculosis case notifications, which had been falling steadily, stabilized or even began to increase. A major factor in this upsurge is an epidemic of tuberculosis among immunocompromised persons with HIV infection and the emergence of multidrug-resistant strains. Transmission of *M. tuberculosis* usually takes place through the airborne spread of droplet nuclei produced by patients with infectious pulmonary tuberculosis. It is estimated that staff of laboratories and autopsy rooms are between 100 and 200 times more likely than the general public to develop tuberculosis.

Because infectious aerosols are likely to be present in autopsy rooms, such areas should be at negative pressure with respect to adjacent areas, and the room air should be expelled directly to the outside of the building. Downdraft autopsy tables, ultraviolet irradiation to the air, and high-efficiency particulate air filtration are also recommended in autopsy rooms. The mask is particularly important to prevent tuberculosis. These masks should not be the standard surgical masks, but instead a high-efficiency particulate air-filtered respirator (N-95 respirator). Cutting into tissues, especially lungs, is particularly hazardous. Inflating both lungs with formalin and postponing dissection for 48 h can reduce the spread of infectious aerosols. All persons involved in autopsy work should have periodic purified protein derivative (PPD) skin testing. For individuals with latent tuberculosis infection identified by PPD skin test, intervention with isoniazid greatly reduces the risk of progressing to active disease.

Risk Reduction: Infection Control

Healthcare providers in hospitals can reduce their risk of exposure to blood and body fluids through the use of basic safety measures, barrier precautions, and technologically safer instruments. In 1985, a set of infection control guidelines known as "universal precautions" was issued to prevent or minimize the risk of occupational exposure to bloodborne pathogens. Universal precautions are based on the premise that all patients are potentially infectious, and include: (1) the use of gloves for procedures where contact with blood and body fluids might occur; (2) the use of masks and protective eyewear when splatter of body fluids is anticipated; and (3) the use of gowns or other protective garments when clothing is likely to be soiled. In 1989, another system of infection control procedure called "body substance isolation" was proposed, which implemented barrier precautions to all moist body substances, including tissue and feces, not just certain body fluids and blood-tinged body fluids. Both universal precautions and body substance isolation emphasize the prevention of sharp injuries and the use of barrier protection to avoid exposure to potentially infectious materials, and neither requires labeling of patients or specimens for implementation. In 1996, guidelines for isolation precautions in hospitals were developed, which synthesized the major features of universal precautions and body substance isolation into a single set of precautions called "standard precautions," and added transmission-based precautions designed to reduce the risk of airborne, droplet, and contact transmission in hospitals.

Forensic autopsy workers can minimize their risk of occupational infections by following the policy of standard precautions:

1. All cadavers should be treated as potentially infectious, regardless of their known infectious states, as should all surfaces and equipment used during autopsy.
2. All fluid and tissue specimens should be considered potentially infectious.
3. Postmortem procedures for all patients should include complete protective wear for anybody in the autopsy room who is at risk for fluid or tissue contamination.
4. Instruments and surfaces contaminated during postmortem procedures should be decontaminated with an appropriate chemical germicide.
5. All specimens should be put in a well-constructed container with a secure lid to prevent leaking during transport. Requisition forms attached to the cadaver or specimens need not contain any reference to the patient's infectious status, since standard precautions procedure should be used by all mortuary attendants and laboratory personnel.

Autopsy precautions should be directed at the prevention of sharps injuries, mucocutaneous contact with body fluids, and aerosol inhalation. Exposure may be prevented by using appropriate gloves, goggles, or face shield, cap, gown, apron, and shoe covers. The rate of occupational injury sustained during performance of autopsies is reported to be one in 11 autopsies performed by residents and one in 53 autopsies performed by staff pathologists. Injuries to the hands are most common, particularly on the palmar surfaces of the thumb, index finger, and middle finger of the nondominant hand, which typically retract tissue during autopsy. Metal and synthetic mesh gloves mitigate the risk of scalpel injuries, but may not protect against needle punctures. Additional measures, such as the use of round scalpel blades, blunt-tipped scissors, and placement of towels over sharp bony projections, are recommended. A vacuum-equipped oscillatory saw should be used to remove the calvarium to prevent aerosolization of bony dust and pathogens. In high classifications of airborne infections, a high-efficiency particulate air-filtered respirator or a powered air-purifying respirator should be worn. Training and education in the prevention of sharps injuries, respiratory protections, and adherence to standard precautions help to prevent occupational infections at autopsy.

Postexposure Management

For postexposure management, wounds and skin sites that have been in contact with blood or body fluids should be washed with soap and water; mucous membranes should be flushed with water. No evidence exists that using antiseptics for wound care or expressing fluid by squeezing the wound further reduces the risk of bloodborne pathogen transmission. Serology testing of the source and the exposed person for HIV, HBV, and HCV should be examined. Baseline serology for the exposed person will show the individual to be previously uninfected by any of the viruses and the existence of protective immunity for HBV. Occupational exposure should be considered an urgent medical concern to ensure timely postexposure management and administration of hepatitis B immunoglobulin, hepatitis B vaccine, and/or HIV chemoprophylaxis (**Table 4**).

Table 4 Transmission, risk of infection, and pre- and postexposure prophylaxis of postmortem-associated acquisition of infections

	HIV infection	Hepatitis B	Hepatitis C	Tuberculosis
Transmission	Bloodborne	Bloodborne	Bloodborne	Airborne
Risk of infection	0.3%	5% (HBeAg-negative source) 19–30% (HBeAg-positive source)	1.8–10%	High
Preexposure prophylaxis or precaution[a]	None	Hepatitis B vaccine	None	Negative-pressure N-95 respirator PPD skin testing Isoniazid
Postexposure prophylaxis or intervention	Antiretroviral drugs	Hepatitis B immunoglobulin Hepatitis B vaccine	None	

HIV, human immunodeficiency virus; HBeAg, hepatitis Be antigen; PPD, purified protein derivative.
[a]All bodies should be placed into standard precautions.

Prevention of Other Infections

Creutzfeldt–Jakob disease (CJD) is a neurodegenerative disease that is caused by infectious proteins called prions. CJD typically presents with progressive dementia and myoclonus, and usually results in death within a year of onset. Sporadic, genetic, and infectious forms of CJD have been recognized. Accidental transmission of CJD appears to have occurred with corneal transplantation, contaminated electroencephalogram electrode implantation, and surgical procedures. Epidemiological studies show no increased risk for healthcare workers. Because prions present at highest levels in the neural tissue, the main concern for infection in the context of autopsy is accidental parenteral inoculation with neural tissues at autopsy and neuropathological examinations. Precautions against possible infection should be taken to the autopsy of patients with rapidly progressing dementia; the brains of patients with CJD frequently have no recognizable abnormalities on gross examination. Prions are extremely resistant to common inactivation procedures. Inactivation of prions is not completed with formalin, but only with formic acid in formalin-fixed tissues. Autoclaving at 132 °C for 5 h or treatment with 2 N NaOH for several hours is recommended for sterilization of instruments.

Viral hemorrhagic fevers (Lassa, Ebola, and Marburg hemorrhagic fevers) are endemic in sub-Saharan Africa, but can be imported into other countries by infected international travelers. Prosecutors have died of autopsy-transmitted viral hemorrhagic fever. Moreover, the potential use of Ebola hemorrhagic fever, anthrax, and plague as biological weapons is of great concern. Strict standard precautions should be used at autopsy of bodies suspected with these infectious diseases. Negative-pressure rooms and high-efficiency particulate air-filtered respirators are also recommended in cases of viral hemorrhagic fever and plague.

See Also

Autopsy: Procedures and Standards; Medico-legal Considerations; **Occupational Health:** Autopsy

Further Reading

Centers for Disease Control and Prevention (1992) 1993 revised classification system for HIV infection and expanded surveillance case definition for AIDS among adolescents and adults. *MMWR. Morbidity and Mortality Weekly Report* 41(RR-17): 1–19.

Centers for Disease Control and Prevention (2001) Updated US Public Health Service guidelines for the management of occupational exposures to HBV, HCV, and HIV and recommendations for postexposure prophylaxis. *MMWR. Morbidity and Mortality Weekly Report* 50(RR-11): 1–52.

Claydon SM (1993) The high risk autopsy. Recognition and protection. *American Journal of Forensic Medicine and Pathology* 14: 253–256.

Council on Ethical and Judicial Affairs, American Medical Association (1992) Confidentiality of human immunodeficiency virus status on autopsy reports. *Archives of Pathology and Laboratory Medicine* 116: 1120–1123.

Crowe S, Hoy J, Mills J (eds.) (2002) *Management of the HIV-Infected Patient.* London: Martin Dunitz.

Garner JS (1996) Guideline for isolation precautions in hospitals. The hospital infection control practices advisory committee. *Infection Control and Hospital Epidemiology* 17: 53–80.

Inglesby TV, Dennis DT, Henderson DA, *et al.* (2000) Plague as a biological weapon. Medical and public health management. *Journal of the American Medical Association* 283: 2281–2290.

Johnson MD, Schaffner W, Atkinson J, *et al.* (1997) Autopsy risk and acquisition of human immunodeficiency virus infection. A case report and reappraisal. *Archives of Pathology and Laboratory Medicine* 121: 64–66.

Kibayashi K, Mastri AR, Hirsch CS (1996) Neuropathology of human immunodeficiency virus infection at different disease stages. *Human Pathology* 27: 637–642.

Kibayashi K, Ng'walali PM, Mbonde MP, *et al.* (1999) Neuropathology of human immunodeficiency virus type 1 infection: significance of studying in forensic autopsy cases at Dar es Salaam, Tanzania. *Archives of Pathology and Laboratory Medicine* 123: 519–523.

Klatt EC, Noguchi TT (1988) The medical examiner and AIDS. Death certification, safety procedures, and future medicolegal issues. *American Journal of Forensic Medicine and Pathology* 9: 141–148.

Knight B (1996) *Forensic Pathology,* 2nd edn. London: Arnold.

Libman H, Witzburg RA (eds.) (1996) *HIV Infection. A Primary Care Manual.* Boston, MA: Little, Brown.

Nolte KB, Taylor DG, Richmond JY (2002) Biosafety considerations for autopsy. *American Journal of Forensic Medicine and Pathology* 23: 107–122.

Scaravilli F (ed.) (1993) *The Neuropathology of HIV Infection.* London: Springer-Verlag.

AUTOPSY, FINDINGS

Contents

Drug Deaths

S B Karch, Berkeley, CA, USA

Introduction

Deaths from natural or traumatic causes display specific anatomic features. The anatomic findings associated with drug abuse are rarely specific, nor are the toxicological findings that accompany them. Drug-takers are at increased risk for a variety of lifestyle diseases, including hepatitis, tuberculosis, and human immunodeficiency virus (HIV). If drugs are present at the time of death in an HIV-infected person, and they frequently are, then it is often difficult or impossible to determine whether HIV-related infection or drug abuse was actually the cause of death.

Even if no lifestyle diseases are evident, postmortem blood measurements are difficult to interpret and may be misleading. This situation comes about mainly because of issues related to drug tolerance. Very high blood drug concentrations do not necessarily prove that drugs were the cause of death, and the demonstration of very low drug concentrations does not rule out drug involvement, because anatomic changes favoring sudden death may persist long after drug use is discontinued. Before drawing any conclusion based upon postmortem drug measurements, the effects of a very long list of confounding variables must be considered. Given the nonspecific nature of the death certification process, investigators must supplement information derived at autopsy with the results of toxicological testing and scene investigation.

Accurate death certification begins with a thorough account of what was observed at the scene and an inquiry into the decedent's past medical history. Knowledge obtained from such an inquiry may, in fact, prove more useful than findings from the postmortem examination. Reliance upon only the autopsy, or only the toxicology testing, to the exclusion of the other sources of information, is almost certain to result in an inaccurate or completely mistaken diagnosis.

Scene Investigation

Overview

The type of drug most likely to be responsible for death varies by location. Even in the same city, certain drugs are more popular within some population subgroups than within others, a circumstance that may be of some diagnostic value. In San Francisco, methamphetamine is most popular within the gay community, but that is not the case elsewhere. While the death of a 40-year-old male methamphetamine user in San Francisco would not be very surprising; the death of a 22-year-old woman from methamphetamine poisoning, in Baltimore would rightly be viewed as suspicious.

A thorough investigation may reveal which drugs were taken and how they were administered. Were needles or smoking implements at the decedent's side? Are pill bottles in evidence? There is a good chance they will be absent, because the scene is likely to have been disturbed. It is almost the rule, rather than an exception, that friends of the decedent will have either stolen any remaining drugs or attempted to sanitize the scene so that it appears drugs were not involved in the death. Inspection of nearby trash bins may provide useful information. Even when friends or relatives make an effort to conceal the decedent's drug use, the attempts are unlikely to be sophisticated, and traces of drugs such as cocaine can, without too much difficulty, be detected on table and counter tops.

It is also important to obtain documentation about how the deceased had been behaving just prior to death. Was the individual a known drug-user, recently released from jail? Was the individual a binge drug-user? Any one of those factors could have decreased the decedent's level of tolerance and converted a "recreational" dose of drug into a fatal one.

Drug-Specific Considerations

Needle-exchange programs are increasingly common, but most addicts are still forced to reuse syringes. It is likely that a syringe found at the side of a decedent will have been used many times previously. It follows that any drugs found in the syringe may, or may not indicate use by the decedent.

Much of the illicit drug supply is delivered by "body packers," transporting drugs concealed in their body cavities. Quantities in excess of one-half kilogram can be concealed in this fashion. Drugs are recovered when the courier arrives at his/her destination and takes a laxative. If one of the packets ruptures, death is the predictable result. Laxatives, passports, and foreign currency are likely to be found nearby, and readily suggest the cause of death. What at first sight might appear to be a case of ritual mutilation may, in fact, be a drug dealer's effort to reclaim drugs remaining in the body of a dead courier.

Psychotic drug-takers are an increasing problem. Some die alone, in their home or hotel room, their psychotic behavior evidenced by the destruction of their surroundings. Some may barricade their door against imaginary enemies. Taken in excess, stimulant-type drugs cause hyperthermia, both as a consequence of increased physical activity, and because of impaired heat dissipation. Accordingly decedents are often to be found in the shower, with cold water running, or surrounded by wet towels and ice cube trays.

If the drug user becomes psychotic in public, physical restraint will be needed, if not to protect the drug user, then to protect others. If death occurs during the struggle, the lethal outcome will be attributed to the process of restraint itself and to police misconduct. Unless the scene investigation is conducted appropriately, and the results made available to the pathologist prior to the autopsy, the actual cause of death may never be determined.

When death occurs during a police confrontation, a number of specific observations need to be recorded, but the most important function of the scene investigator is to notify the pathologist of the situation immediately. Most (though not all) psychotically agitated individuals who die suddenly are suffering from a syndrome known as excited delirium. This syndrome is associated with distinct, measurable neurochemical alterations that can be detected after death, but only if the brain is removed and frozen within 12 h. Standard protocols must be put in place to ensure that responsible authorities are notified as

soon as possible. Having notified the responsible authority, other measures to be taken include the following.

1. The ambient air temperature and the temperature of the body at the scene must be measured. Not all patients with stimulant toxicity are hyperthermic, but many are, and if the temperature is never taken, the proof is never obtained.
2. The means of restraint and the position of the deceased must be documented, not only with photographs, but also with the testimony of as many witnesses as possible. This documentation is especially vital if application of a chokehold is alleged. If a chokehold is applied effectively, it will lead to loss of consciousness in 15–20 s. If a witness insists that the struggle lasted much longer than 15 s, then application of a chokehold becomes an unlikely cause of death.
3. The records of the paramedics and emergency field workers should be obtained, including records generated in the emergency ward. An electrocardiogram, even if only a one-lead rhythm strip, may help make the diagnosis of long QT syndrome or other heritable channelopathy. Recording of pulse occimetry data is now routine in many jurisdictions. If the percentage oxygen saturation during resuscitation and transport has been recorded, it may be possible to rule in or out death from "positional asphyxia."
4. Chemical incapacitating agents have little effect on the psychotically agitated, and their use is to be discouraged. However, if these agents have been used, the canisters must be collected and weighed, so the amount of spray discharged can at least be estimated. This is possible because the weight of all containers leaving the factor is very similar, and because officers must record each use of the spray. There is no assay for the measurement of pepper spray (the most widely used such agent in the USA) from biological matrices, but capsicum and other chemical incapacitating agents can easily be recovered from clothing and from skin, using methanol swabs. If the chemical agent cannot be recovered from facial skin, then it is reasonable to assume that the spray never entered the lung, and if it did not enter the lung, it cannot be the cause of pulmonary toxicity.
5. If resuscitation was attempted, investigators must thoroughly document what happened at the scene, and what efforts were made in the emergency room. It is especially important to know what measures were taken to establish an airway. Multiple attempts at laryngeal intubation can result in laryngeal bruising. If the history of intubation is

not recorded, bruising might be falsely attributed to manual strangulation.

Postmortem Examination

Deaths related to stimulant and opiate abuse tend to follow a stereotyped pattern. This pattern has been recognized for more than a century and consists mainly of pulmonary and cerebral congestion. Nonetheless, there are some key differences between opiate-related and stimulant-related deaths. The differences are mostly explained by the observation that stimulants tend to exert direct cellular toxicity while opiates do not. As a consequence, most of the anatomic changes observed in opiate abusers are secondary either to the materials injected along with their drugs, or to the occurrence of "lifestyle" diseases, such as HIV and hepatitis.

External examination of opiate abusers is much more likely to disclose sclerotic veins, or "track marks," because the diluents and excipients found in heroin are less water-soluble than those found in cocaine and methamphetamine and, therefore, are more toxic to veins. However, the practice of simultaneously injecting cocaine and heroin is now so common that nearly all intravenous drug users will have evidence of chronic injection injuries. Most of the materials used to "cut" heroin display a pattern of birefringence that can easily be seen under low power magnification. Crystals found in the kidney and liver tend to be smaller than those found in the lung, since the lungs themselves will have acted to sieve out the particles. Each of the different cutting agents has a characteristic pattern of birefringence that is unique and identifiable.

If petechiae or bruises are present, they should be photographed, if only because petechiae can form after death. If the absence of petechiae is not documented initially, false charges of incompetence or "cover-up" may result. A careful neck dissection is the only way to determine whether a chokehold or neck compression has been applied, but the thoracic organs and the brain must be removed before commencing the dissection. Removing the other organs first will prevent postmortem bleeding into the soft tissues of the neck. If this precaution is not taken, it may be falsely concluded that neck injury had occurred.

Hemorrhage around the larynx, and the presence of facial petechiae, can be evidence for strangulation, but they may also simply be an artifact, the result of unsuccessful attempts at establishing an airway. Bruising within the larynx, in the absence of bruising of the long muscles of the neck, is virtual proof that bruising was the result of attempted medical intervention, not assault.

Other external markers include "crack thumb," a callus seen on the medial aspect of the thumb, secondary to repeated use of butane lighters to heat crack cocaine (**Figure 1**). Burns on the lower lip, a consequence of smoking hot glass "crack pipes," are also common (**Figure 2**). Excoriations of the anterior chest wall are usually a sign of chronic opiate abuse. Heroin and other opiates (though not fentanyl and other synthetic drugs) cause mast cells to release histamine, and can result in intense pruritus.

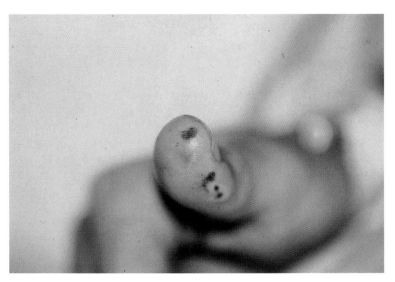

Figure 1 "Crack thumb." Disposable butane lighters are often used to heat crack pipes. If used repeatedly, the lateral aspect of the thumb becomes calloused.

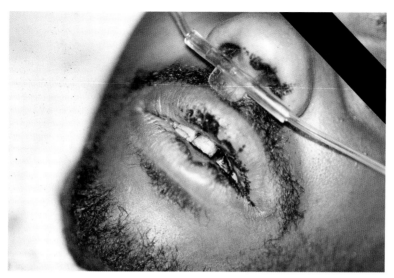

Figure 2   "Crack lip." Frequent smokers of crack cocaine often burn their lips on the improvised pipes they use for smoking.

Crack lung is an increasingly common finding, with little to distinguish it from other types of pulmonary anthracosis. Emphysematous changes may be marked as well. Pulmonary edema is almost inevitably present, but the mechanism remains unknown. Edema fluid in cases of opiate overdose is usually high in protein content and tends to froth and foam like egg white. If the agonal period was prolonged, capillaries will have ruptured, leaving the fluid blood-tinged. Terminal aspiration is exceedingly common, and if the drug concentration of the stomach contents was high, then drug may redistribute through the lungs into heart blood, resulting in falsely elevated postmortem drug concentrations.

The heart must be carefully weighed and left ventricular wall thickness measured at several different locations. Multiple sections, particularly of the left ventricle and septum, should be retained for histologic examination. Increased heart size may only become apparent after the heart has been weighed, and the result compared to the weight predicted by standard nomograms. When such comparisons are made, the hearts of long-term stimulant abusers will be found to be at least 10% above predicted norms. Heart size is an independent risk factor for sudden cardiac death and the measurement may prove to be a very significant factor in determining the cause of death.

A number of other changes are commonly seen in chronic abusers, though they are not invariably present. Opiates impair gut motility, and obstipation is almost diagnostic for opiate abuse, although the frequency of this finding appears to be decreasing, perhaps because the opiates are being used along with other illicit drugs, like cocaine, that stimulate the gut. Infiltration of the portal triads, with lymphocytes and plasma cells, can be seen in either opiate or stimulant injectors. It seems increasingly clear that the infiltrates represent underlying infection with hepatitis C. Enlargement of the periportal lymph nodes is an unexplained but common finding in heroin users, but not in users of cocaine or methamphetamine. The nodes (especially in the gastroepiploic area) themselves will often be found to contain high drug concentrations.

Postmortem Toxicology

Postmortem redistribution is defined as the movement of drug down a concentration gradient after death. The redistribution process begins immediately and continues indefinitely, but the greatest changes occur within the first 24 h. Redistribution is much more likely to occur if a drug has a large volume of distribution, and also more likely if the drug is sequestered in either the lung (fentanyl), or liver (propoxyphene).

The process of postmortem redistribution accounts for the fact that postmortem blood testing is an extremely unreliable process. Blood concentrations measured in otherwise unspecified "heart blood" (or worse still, blood pooled in the thorax or abdomen) should be considered simply as a qualitative measurement, proving only that drug is present. Blood should be taken from the femoral vessels, but if they are not ligated first, aspiration of more than 20 ml of blood may yield blood from the liver or inferior vena cava, where concentrations of many drugs would be much higher than samples obtained elsewhere in the body.

Perimortem aspiration of stomach contents is very common, and can lead to very high drug concentrations within the bronchial tree. Simple diffusion out of the bronchi then allows drugs to traverse thin-walled pulmonary vessels. If aspiration occurs into the left lung, simple diffusion can result in high drug concentrations in cardiac blood. As a consequence of drug redistribution, blood samples obtained from different parts of the body are likely to contain different concentrations of the same drug. Methamphetamine concentrations in left heart blood are 1.9–2.6 times higher than blood samples taken from the right ventricle at the same time. Drug concentrations in the pulmonary artery blood may be 6–10 times as high as the concentrations in heart blood. Cocaine levels in the subclavian vessels fall after death, but concentrations in heart and femoral blood rise. Measurements of drug concentrations in left heart blood are especially likely to be misleading.

Measurement made in the bile is problematic. Some drugs concentrate in the bile, and if drug concentration is high in the bile, then postmortem liver concentrations will increase. However, if drugs have been used several days before death, they are unlikely to be detected in blood or urine, but may well still be present in bile.

A widely held misconception is that the site of administration can be determined by measuring drug concentration at that site. Drugs circulate throughout the body and appear in all body secretions. Cocaine recovered from vaginal swabs does not prove that the cocaine was applied vaginally, any more than cocaine recovered from nasal swabs proves it was applied nasally. In theory, the presence of extravasated drug might be used to identify an injection site, but only if drug was also measured in multiple skin samples from other parts of the body, and a substantial difference was demonstrated.

No valid scientific evidence exists to support the notion that the cause of death can be determined by consulting a reference table, or by comparing postmortem testing results with results from clinical therapeutic drug monitoring. Tolerance to both stimulants and opiates emerges rapidly, and even the presence of massive amounts of drug does not prove that a particular drug caused death, or even that the massive amount of drug detected at autopsy was nearly so massive during life.

If a drug's effects decrease as the dose is held constant, or escalating doses of drug are required to produce the same effect, tolerance is said to exist. Except in certain special, albeit very important circumstances, the degree of drug tolerance cannot be assessed after death. Multiple studies have shown that postmortem concentrations of drugs like cocaine,

heroin, and methamphetamine are indistinguishable in those dying of drug toxicity, and those where the presence of drug is only an incidental finding (i.e., a heroin user who is murdered). Cross-tolerance to other opiates is limited, unpredictable, and cannot be assumed to exist. A chronic pain patient being treated with high doses of methadone, for example, might experience fatal respiratory depression after a much smaller dose of morphine.

Tolerance secondary to chronic stimulant abuse is associated with changes in dopamine receptor numbers and density, and the diagnosis of stimulant-associated excited delirium can be inferred from appropriate receptor measurements in appropriately preserved brain tissue. Lack of tolerance can be proven by the failure to demonstrate drugs in hair. The detection of drug in blood or other tissues, but not in the hair, proves that there has been no recent drug use. None of the exhumed Shipman murder victims in the UK had detectable morphine in their hair, though substantial amounts were detected in blood and liver tissue. The absence of morphine in the victims' hair proved that the decedents had no tolerance, and disproved suggestions in Shipman's medical records that some of the decedents were illicit drug takers.

The results of early studies suggested that postmortem morphine concentrations above $300\,ng\,ml^{-1}$ were proof of toxicity. But values well in excess of $300\,ng\,ml^{-1}$ may be seen as incidental findings in trauma victims who happen to be heroin abusers. One way to address this problem is by hair testing. Hair morphine levels can be used to identify which decedents were tolerant at the time of death and which were not. Morphine concentrations in the hair of active heroin users are much higher than those in abstinent users, and concentrations in overdose deaths are comparable to those seen in abstinent users. Although postmortem hair sampling is not yet a routine procedure, hair samples should be at least

Table 1   Some factors affecting postmortem drug measurement

- Age
- Bacterial metabolism
- Chiral variation
- Drug interactions
- Circulatory status
- Genetic polymorphism
- Glycolization
- Hepatic disease
- Hydration
- Kidney function
- Muscle wasting
- Protein binding
- Site dependence
- Tolerance
- Volume of distribution

collected and stored. Information derived from their analysis could be invaluable if questions about drug abuse should arise at some later date.

Conclusion

Pathologists responsible for determining the cause of death must integrate measurements and observations submitted by a small army of specialists. These specialists are likely to know far more about their individual fields than the certifying pathologist. However, none of these other specialists are physicians, and none are skilled in the process of differential diagnosis. While toxicologists and entomologists can reliably detect the presence of billionths of a gram of drug in blood samples or insect larvae, they are unlikely to know about the effects of hemorrhagic shock on plasma volume, or the proximity of the stomach to the liver. Attempts at directly relating postmortem blood drug concentrations to outcomes only seem reasonable to those unaware of just how many variables need to be considered (**Table 1**). It is the forensic physician's job to keep all these variables in mind.

See Also

Substance Misuse: Medical Effects; Cocaine and Other Stimulants; Herbal Medicine; Heroin; Substitution Drugs; Sedatives; Miscellaneous Drugs; Urine Analysis; Hair Analysis; Alternative Body Fluids Analysis; Patterns and Statistics; Crime

Further Reading

Ely SF, Hirsch CS (2000) Asphyxial deaths and petechiae: a review. *Journal of Forensic Science* 45: 1274–1277.

Hilberg T, Rogde S, Morland J (1999) Postmortem drug redistribution – human cases related to results in experimental animals. *Journal of Forensic Science* 44: 3–9.

Karch SB, Stephens BG (1999) Drug abusers who die during arrest or in custody. *Journal of the Royal Society of Medicine* 92: 110–113.

Karch SB, Stephens B, Ho CH (1998) Relating cocaine blood concentrations to toxicity – an autopsy study of 99 cases. *Journal of Forensic Science* 43: 41–45.

Karch SB, Stephens BG, Ho CH (1999) Methamphetamine-related deaths in San Francisco: demographic, pathologic, and toxicologic profiles. *Journal of Forensic Science* 44: 359–368.

Kitzman DW, Scholz DG, Hagen PT, et al. (1988) Age-related changes in normal human hearts during the first 10 decades of life. Part II (Maturity): a quantitative anatomic study of 765 specimens from subjects 20 to 99 years old. *Mayo Clinic Proceedings* 63: 137–146.

Messerli FH, Ketelhut R (1993) Left ventricular hypertrophy: a pressure-independent cardiovascular risk factor. *Journal of Cardiovasccular Pharmacology* 22(Suppl. 1): S7–S13.

Messerli FH, Soria F (1994) Ventricular dysrhythmias, left ventricular hypertrophy, and sudden death. *Cardiovascular Drugs Therapy* 8(Suppl. 3): 557–563.

Messerli FH, Nunez BD, Ventura HO, et al. (1987) Overweight and sudden death. Increased ventricular ectopy in cardiopathy of obesity. *Archives of Internal Medicine* 147: 1725–1728.

Moriya F, Hashimoto Y (1999) Redistribution of basic drugs into cardiac blood from surrounding tissues during early-stages postmortem. *Journal of Forensic Science* 44: 10–16.

Pounder DJ (1993) The nightmare of postmortem drug changes. *Legal Medicine* 163–191.

Pounder DJ, Adams E, Fuke C, et al. (1996) Site to site variability of postmortem drug concentrations in liver and lung. *Journal of Forensic Science* 41: 927–932.

Raven KP, Reay DT, Harruff RC (1999) Artifactual injuries of the larynx produced by resuscitative intubation. *American Journal of Forensic Medicine Pathology* 20: 31–36.

Spiehler V, Brown R (1987) Unconjugated morphine in blood by radioimmunoassay and gas chromatography/mass spectrometry. *Journal of Forensic Science* 32: 906–916.

Sterrett C, Brownfield J, Korn CS, et al. (2003) Patterns of presentation in heroin overdose resulting in pulmonary edema. *American Journal of Emergency Medicine* 21: 32–34.

Tagliaro F, De Battisti Z, Smith FP, et al. (1998) Death from heroin overdose: findings from hair analysis. *Lancet* 351: 1923–1925.

Tashkin DP (2001) Airway effects of marijuana, cocaine, and other inhaled illicit agents. *Current Opinion in Pulmonary Medicine* 7: 43–61.

Wetli CV, Mash D, Karch S (1996) Cocaine-associated agitated delirium and the neuroleptic malignant syndrome. *American Journal of Emergency Medicine* 14: 425–428.

Postmortem Drug Measurements, Interpretation of

B Levine and K A Moore, Office of the Chief Medical Examiner, Baltimore, MD, USA

Introduction

Toxicological examination plays an important role in death investigation. The primary mission of the postmortem toxicology laboratory is to assist the medical examiner or coroner in determining the cause and manner of death. The most obvious use for postmortem forensic toxicological analyses is in suspected drug intoxication and poisoning cases. Drug intoxications are not readily diagnosed at autopsy. In intravenous drug deaths, a recent injection site may be observable, and oral intoxications may be inferred from a large amount of unabsorbed tablet fragments in the stomach contents. However, other common anatomic findings such as pulmonary congestion and edema are nonspecific. Investigation of the scene where a death occurs may indicate the causative agent or agents. For instance, items such as medicine containers, syringes, or gas cylinders from the scene should be reported to the toxicology laboratory. Nevertheless, the function of the toxicology laboratory is to identify the substances present in the submitted postmortem specimens. Once these substances are identified and confirmed by an alternate analytical technique, they are quantified in appropriate specimens to determine whether these drug concentrations caused or contributed to death.

Toxicological investigations are important in deaths other than drug intoxications. For several reasons, many medical examiners' or coroners' offices routinely perform screening analysis for drugs on all homicides: many homicides are drug-related; the abuse of drugs may provide a motive for homicide; and an individual under the pharmacologic effects of drugs has a greater chance of committing or falling victim to homicides. Therefore, a drug-of-abuse screen provides answers to many of these questions.

In certain accidental deaths, impairment issues may have significant forensic relevance. Comprehensive testing for both therapeutic and abused drugs is routinely requested in driver motor vehicle fatalities to ascertain the potential role of drugs in the accident. Obviously, the well-documented role of alcohol in many motor vehicle accidents requires that alcohol testing be performed in these cases. However, drugs being taken therapeutically as prescribed may also be a factor in an accident.

Toxicological analyses may even be important in deaths due to natural causes. For instance, deaths from seizures occur with or without anatomic findings. The failure to identify anticonvulsant drugs in blood may indicate undermedication or noncompliance. Conversely, the presence of anticonvulsant drugs with no prior seizure history may require investigation. Patient compliance may also be an issue in deaths of individuals being treated for depression or mental illness.

This article will discuss the interpretive aspects of these analytical results. The techniques used to generate these analytical data will be discussed elsewhere. This article will include a number of subsections. There will be a discussion of specimens and the interpretive value of each. This will be followed by a discussion of how the analytical process impacts the interpretation of results. This is followed by a discussion of interpretive issues and complications associated with the finding of ethanol and/or postmortem cases.

Specimens Used for Analytical Toxicology

Blood

The single most important specimen to be collected is blood. Unlike clinical specimens where serum or plasma is tested for drugs, postmortem blood specimen analysis is performed on whole blood. As a result, the interpretation of postmortem blood concentrations using clinical serum or plasma data is fraught with difficulties. Blood should be obtained during all inspections and limited or complete autopsies. Ideally, two blood specimens should be collected, one from the heart and the other from a peripheral site, such as the femoral or subclavian veins. Quantification of drugs in blood is better correlated with toxicity or fatality. Blood quantifications must be interpreted in light of available history. A high concentration of a drug or a group of drugs in the blood of an individual with suicidal intent, a suicide note, and no anatomic cause of death at autopsy would be consistent with a suicidal drug or multiple drug intoxication. A large ratio of parent-to-metabolite concentrations may indicate an acute death. A therapeutic concentration in postmortem blood in an individual treated in the hospital for several days may indicate much higher concentrations at an earlier time. Often, hospital laboratories perform drug testing on urine specimens without associated blood quantifications. Therefore, the postmortem laboratory should obtain hospital blood specimens so that toxicity can be assessed. Of course, the clinical picture as documented by the hospital is extremely critical to this overall assessment.

In certain situations, heart blood can be contaminated either by trauma or from the release of drugs from tissue sites; in these cases, the alternate blood specimen can be used for interpretation of results. Blood from subdural or epidural clots should also be collected. These specimens could be useful when there is a period of time between an event and death.

Bile and Urine

Two useful postmortem specimens that should be collected in every case, if available, are bile and urine. The utility of urine in postmortem cases is similar to its uses in other types of drug testing.

Many drugs and metabolites are present in higher concentration in urine than in blood. Drugs also remain in the urine for days or longer after use. Moreover, bile can concentrate certain drugs such as opioids and benzodiazepines. However, the presence of drugs or metabolites in bile or urine will indicate exposure, but assessment of toxicity or impairment is usually impossible. The best that can usually be concluded is that the drug or drugs were used some time in the recent past, hours to days, depending on the drugs' pharmacokinetics profile.

Liver

In the absence of blood, liver is a useful alternative specimen for drug quantification. Drug metabolism occurs in the liver, so parent drugs and their metabolites may be present in higher concentrations in the liver than in the blood, thus making detection easier. Furthermore, many drugs, such as the tricyclic antidepressants, are sequestered in the liver.

Stomach Contents

In overdose drug ingestions, stomach contents can provide easy identification of the substance or substances taken if intact tablets are present. A large amount of drug would also be present in the stomach contents, thus facilitating analytical identification. Estimating the amount of drug in stomach contents may also give information about the intent of the decedent. For instance, if the amount of drug present in the stomach contents is inconsistent with the amount that should be present following proper therapeutic use, it may be suggestive of an intentional overmedication. There is one important caution in interpreting stomach contents quantifications: the presence of a large amount of drug or drugs in the stomach contents does not mean that drug intoxication has occurred. This must be combined with the quantification of the drug or drugs in the blood or liver, since stomach contents are unabsorbed material and substances must be absorbed before toxicity can occur.

Analytical Procedures

Although this article will not be discussing the analytical process, there are aspects of the analytical process that must be considered in the interpretation of ethanol and drug results. For instance, it is impossible for a toxicology laboratory to test for all available drugs when performing comprehensive drug testing. Instead, a laboratory's routine testing procedures are established to identify a large number of therapeutic and abused drugs or drug classes. Not every drug available can be detected in a routine testing protocol; even within a drug class, some drugs may be identified and others may not. A result of "no benzodiazepines detected" may indicate that an immunoassay was performed and the response was less than the cutoff calibrator. However, many benzodiazepines differ in their response in the immunoassay. Each laboratory must determine the type of testing offered based on available resources; however, it is crucial for the laboratory director to understand the capabilities of the routine testing procedures used by the laboratory. These facts reinforce the need for a drug history when a case is submitted. If the suspected agent is not identified routinely, then the medical examiner or coroner must decide as to the importance of this drug measurement in the ultimate certification of death. When the information is important, the toxicology laboratory may perform special testing in-house or send the specimen to a reference laboratory for testing.

It is also important that the laboratory be aware of the sensitivity or detection limits for the drugs included in the routine comprehensive testing procedures. Some drugs may only be detected in toxic or overdose amounts. This would be sufficient if the question concerns drug intoxication. However, if the issue involves drug compliance or impairment from therapeutic use of the drug, then the routine testing procedures may be inadequate. In those cases, additional testing would be required.

Ethanol

When ethanol is consumed before death, the interpretation of blood ethanol concentrations in postmortem specimens is similar to the interpretation of blood specimens in living individuals. According to multiple scientific studies, a blood ethanol concentration of $0.08 \, \text{g dl}^{-1}$ indicates that all individuals would show some impairment due to ethanol. This impairment would manifest itself in reductions in judgment, attention, and abilities in multitasking events. As the blood ethanol concentration increases, more overt symptoms of alcohol impairment would be observable. There are individual differences to these effects. In general, at a given blood ethanol concentration, less impairment will be demonstrated in a chronic drinker than would be displayed by the occasional or social drinker. A blood ethanol concentration at or above $0.40 \, \text{g dl}^{-1}$ can be consistent with causing death due to ethanol intoxication in the absence of other pathological findings. There are a number of published tables that correlate ranges of blood ethanol concentrations with effects.

In cases where there is a period of time between an injury and death, analysis of the more common postmortem blood specimens may not reflect the blood ethanol concentration at the time of injury, since ethanol metabolism will continue during the period of survival. In those cases, analysis of other specimens such as hospital admission blood or other samples collected closer to the time of injury would be more relevant in determining the role of ethanol in an injury. If no antemortem specimens were collected, blood from sequestered hematomas, such as subdural, epidural, or intracerebral blood, may better approximate the blood ethanol concentration at the time of injury. The theory behind this practice is that ethanol is not metabolized to the same extent as would occur in circulating blood. Nevertheless, the development of these hematomas is not instantaneous; as a result, the blood ethanol concentration will not be homogeneous. Moreover, the water content of the clot may differ from the water content of the circulating blood, further complicating the interpretation of the measured ethanol concentration.

The interpretation of postmortem ethanol concentrations is complicated by the potential artifactual increase in ethanol concentrations after death. For example, in trauma cases, blood from the heart, a common site of postmortem blood collection, may be contaminated by stomach contents. If there is any residual ethanol remaining in the stomach contents, this will cause an artificial increase in the heart blood ethanol concentration when the stomach contents come in contact with the heart. In these cases, blood from a peripheral site (e.g., femoral vein), away from the site of trauma, should be collected and analyzed for ethanol.

Although most embalming fluids contain methanol and do not contain ethanol, these fluids may also be a source of ethanol contamination if the specimens are not collected prior to embalming. If the issue of ethanol consumption arises after a body is embalmed, it is recommended that some of the embalming fluid be obtained and analyzed for the presence of ethanol to determine its contribution to the postmortem blood concentration.

Bacteria, yeast, and molds can, under proper conditions, produce ethanol. A number of substrates can be converted into ethanol by these microorganisms. Glucose is the primary substrate that may be converted into ethanol; therefore, any tissue with high concentrations of glucose or glycogen is susceptible to postmortem ethanol production. Blood, liver, and muscle are examples of specimens with high sugar concentrations in which significant concentrations of ethanol attributed to postmortem formation have been measured. Conversely, urine and vitreous humor are ordinarily free of the combination of glucose and

microorganisms necessary to produce ethanol. Other substrates for ethanol production include lactate, ribose, and amino acids. The mechanism of ethanol production from sugar is glycolysis, which is the first step in the normal breakdown of glucose.

There are a number of factors that can or should be considered when determining whether measured ethanol occurred due to antemortem consumption of alcohol or microorganism activity. For example, witnessed drinking by the decedent prior to death is obviously significant. While there is often an underestimation of the amount of ethanol consumed, the observation that the individual was drinking is usually reliable. Unfortunately, drinking history immediately prior to death is often unavailable, especially in the case of unattended deaths.

Although conditions for a body to putrefy or decompose may vary tremendously, there are a number of common characteristics of a decomposed body. The most striking trait is the foul odor associated with the body. Bloating, discoloration, skin slippage, and insect infestation are also common features associated with decomposition. Insect infestation, such as with maggots, is frequently present in decomposed bodies and is often helpful in ascertaining the length of time that an individual has been dead. When signs of putrefaction are present, postmortem production of ethanol must be considered as possible if not probable. Unfortunately, the amount of ethanol produced is highly variable between decedents; two bodies kept in the same conditions for the same length of time can produce widely different amounts of ethanol. This issue is further complicated if the individual had actually been drinking prior to death. In that scenario, the postmortem alcohol measured might be due to both antemortem consumption and postmortem formation.

When the body absorbs ethanol, it distributes according to the water content of each tissue or fluid. For example, since a given volume of vitreous humor and cerebrospinal fluid contains more water than an equal volume of whole blood, their ethanol concentrations will typically be higher than the blood ethanol concentration after equilibrium has been reached. Conversely, liver and brain will typically have lower ethanol concentrations than the blood ethanol concentration after equilibrium is achieved.

The distribution of ethanol between these specimens can provide a strong indication as to whether the measured ethanol resulted from drinking or decomposition. For example, one approach to multiple specimen analysis is to analyze blood, vitreous humor, and urine. In the postabsorptive phase of alcohol metabolism, the vitreous humor to blood ethanol concentration ratio is about 1.2 and the urine to blood ethanol concentration ratio is about 1.3, although there are wide variations in these ratios. The liver to blood ethanol concentration ratio is approximately 0.6; the average brain to blood ethanol concentration ratio is approximately 0.7–0.9. If the measured postmortem ethanol concentrations yield similar ratios to those established for these specimens, then it is reasonable to conclude that the measured ethanol resulted from drinking. Moreover, vitreous humor and urine are two specimens that are relatively resistant to the putrefactive process and thus are not sites generally associated with postmortem ethanol formation. If the blood ethanol concentration is positive and the vitreous humor and urine ethanol concentrations are negative, this is a strong indication that the ethanol concentration in the blood is the result of decomposition.

Microorganisms that produce ethanol may also be capable of producing other volatile substances. One of these volatile substances is acetaldehyde. However, since acetaldehyde is also a metabolite of ethanol, its identification in biological specimens cannot be used as a marker for decomposition ethanol production. Another volatile commonly seen as a putrefactive product is n-propanol. n-Propanol and n-butanol are not identified in individuals drinking alcoholic beverages and, therefore, are good markers for decomposition ethanol formation. In vitro studies have identified other volatile substances that may be produced during the decomposition process. Volatiles that have been identified include acetone, isopropanol, t-butanol, isoamylalcohol, and n-amylalcohol. In a manner similar to ethanol formation, the specific volatile or volatiles produced is dependent on putrefactive conditions.

In addition to identifying unique products of postmortem formation, one can also assay for products unique to ethanol consumption. Ethylglucuronide, a phase II metabolite of ethanol, would not be produced by microorganisms and would indicate ethanol production before death.

A number of studies have been performed that describe the production of ethanol in postmortem blood. These studies can be summarized by the following conclusions:

1. When ethanol is produced postmortem, the ethanol concentration is usually less than $0.07 \, \mathrm{g \, dl^{-1}}$.
2. Production of ethanol concentrations greater than $0.10 \, \mathrm{g \, dl^{-1}}$ has been reported.
3. The production of ethanol due to decomposition is variable and is dependent on the species of microorganism present, the available substrate, time lapse since death, and the temperature and other environmental conditions.

Although urine has been shown to be generally immune to the effects of postmortem production of ethanol, several studies have indicated that the combination of glucose in the urine, a condition that often occurs in diabetics, and a *Candida albicans* infection can result in the production of large amounts of ethanol. Both components are required for ethanol production to occur and it will not occur in the absence of either the glucose or the microorganism. This can be demonstrated in the laboratory by performing serial analyses of the urine for ethanol over several days and observing the increase in ethanol concentration over time.

Drugs

In many respects, the interpretation of postmortem ethanol concentrations is much simpler than the interpretation of postmortem drug concentrations. First, the pharmacokinetics of ethanol is less complicated than the pharmacokinetics of drugs. The route of ethanol administration is almost always oral. Ethanol distributes according to the water content of the fluid or tissue; as such, distribution ratios between fluids and tissues have been well established. These ratios can then be used to determine the individual's absorption status (absorptive or postabsorptive). At ethanol concentrations associated with drinking, elimination is zero-order, that is, the blood ethanol concentration decreases by a constant amount per hour; this allows an estimation to be made of an ethanol concentration at an earlier time. By contrast, drugs can be administered by a variety of routes, including oral, smoking, snorting, intravenous, or intramuscular. The pharmacokinetics of a particular drug may be different depending on the route of administration. For instance, delta-9-tetrahydrocannabinol (THC), the active component of marijuana, is metabolized differently depending on whether the marijuana is smoked or ingested orally. Oral ingestion of THC produces higher concentrations of the hydroxy metabolite in the plasma than does the smoking route.

Drugs distribute to different extents throughout the body. Due to extensive plasma protein binding, some drugs remain mostly in the vasculature; other drugs are sequestered in specific tissues or distribute throughout the body. Most drugs are eliminated by first-order kinetics, with elimination half-lives varying between hours and days among drugs. Even a particular drug may show significant variation between individuals, depending on the individual's age, gender, health status, or genetics. Some drugs are converted to active metabolites that must be incorporated into the overall interpretation.

Given these pharmacokinetic differences between drugs and between individuals, the prediction of a dose based on postmortem measurements is not reliable. Even the measurement of total body burden, that is, measuring the concentration of a drug in a tissue and multiplying by the tissue weight, has limited utility in predicting dose. One would need to measure the parent drug and all metabolites to reach a useful number. If a drug accumulates or is taken chronically, the measured amounts may reflect prior usage. Moreover, even within a tissue group, such as muscle, there are differences in concentration as a function of tissue site.

Correlating effects with postmortem measurements is also more complex with drugs. The effects of ethanol are generally correlated with the blood ethanol concentration. For a number of drugs, a therapeutic range has been determined. These ranges have been collected from therapeutic drug-monitoring data and represent plasma concentrations where optimum therapeutic benefit combined with minimal toxicity is achieved. It cannot be overemphasized that postmortem blood is highly variable in terms of homogeneity and hematocrit and that the use of clinical serum data alone to interpret postmortem blood concentrations should be done with caution. Antiepileptic drugs, some cardioactive drugs, and some antidepressant drugs would be examples of drugs where therapeutic ranges have been established in living individuals. Unfortunately, only a small number of therapeutic drugs have therapeutic ranges associated with them. Furthermore, none of the illicit drugs encountered by the postmortem forensic toxicologist have normal ranges established.

In an attempt to provide assistance in the interpretation of postmortem drug concentrations, a number of tables have been compiled. These tables may list therapeutic, toxic, and lethal concentration ranges for a large group of therapeutic or abused drugs. These compilations may be based on antemortem pharmacokinetics studies, literature references of poisonings that were successfully treated, or case reports of fatalities. It must be strongly emphasized that these tables are at best a guide or a starting point when interpreting postmortem drug concentrations. First and foremost, postmortem blood is often quite different than blood collected from living individuals. The pH of postmortem blood is generally acidic. The hematocrit of postmortem blood can vary widely, depending on body position and collection techniques. Postmortem blood is not homogeneous. When a drug is first absorbed, the blood closest to the site of absorption will have the highest drug concentration while blood remote to this site will have the lowest drug concentration. As the drug distributes, differences in concentration between blood sites is reduced. There are also postmortem factors that contribute to heterogeneity. Therefore, the use of these tables may lead to erroneous conclusions when used to interpret postmortem blood results.

Postmortem Redistribution

One of the early assumptions in the interpretation of postmortem drug analysis was that, at death, drug pharmacokinetics stopped. That is, drug absorption, distribution, and metabolism ceased once the individual died. Therefore, specimens could be collected some time after death and the analytical data generated reflected the situation at death. Unfortunately, over the past 25 years, it has become well established that this assumption is not valid in a large number of circumstances. In general, blood concentrations of many basic drugs such as tricyclic antidepressants and antimalarial drugs are site-dependent. The heart blood drug concentration will usually exceed the drug concentration in blood from peripheral sites such as the subclavian, iliac, or femoral veins. One explanation for this observation is that, after death, drugs bound to tissues during life will be released into the surrounding blood. For instance, digoxin, a cardiac glycoside used to treat congestive heart failure, accumulates in the heart. After death, the drug releases into the heart blood, causing an increased drug concentration in the postmortem heart blood. Subsequent analysis of this sample will result in an elevated digoxin concentration. If this concentration were interpreted in terms of clinical therapeutic drug-monitoring data, the concentration would suggest that toxicity due to digoxin was involved in the case. Studies indicate that vitreous humor digoxin analysis provides more meaningful interpretive information in these cases.

Drugs may be released from other tissues as well. Tricyclic antidepressants were among the first group of drugs where this postmortem redistribution phenomenon was documented. During life, tricyclic antidepressants are sequestered in the liver; after death, the drugs are released from the liver into the nearby blood. Studies have also indicated that these drugs release from the lung during the postmortem interval. Subsequent movement into the heart blood can lead to elevated drug concentrations when this specimen is measured. It is recommended that, in addition to quantifying the drug in a peripheral blood specimen, the liver should also be quantitated. Liver tricyclic antidepressant concentrations are 10–50 times higher than are blood concentrations. Since these concentrations are so high, loss of the drug during the postmortem interval would not be as significant in terms of reflecting the liver concentration at death. By comparing the liver and blood concentration ratios, one can better interpret the analytical findings.

Besides the distribution of absorbed drug, a number of studies have documented that, after death, unabsorbed drug from the stomach contents can distribute into fluids and tissues. This has been demonstrated with barbiturates and tricyclic antidepressants.

There are a number of other general observations with regard to the postmortem redistribution phenomenon. Drugs with high volumes of distribution and which are sequestered in tissues (e.g., tricyclic antidepressants or phenothiazines) exhibit the potential for postmortem redistribution. Redistribution follows the concentration gradient, that is, movement from an area of high concentration to an area of low concentration. Not all drugs display this phenomenon. Finally, the interpretation of postmortem blood concentrations must be made in the context of the specimen location.

Postmortem Decreases in Drug Concentrations

In addition to spuriously elevated drug concentrations in blood that result from postmortem redistribution, some drugs continue to be broken down after death. That means that the drug concentration measured at the time of sample collection may be significantly lower than the drug concentration that would have been measured immediately at death. Drugs that break down after death are associated with certain functional groups. Drugs that have a nitro group, such as clonazepam and flunitrazepam, will be reduced to their amino analogs after death. N-oxides such as chlordiazepoxide are also unstable postmortem. Sulfur-containing compounds may also display postmortem instability. Hydrolytic enzymes retain activity after death; therefore, ester compounds may be susceptible to their activity. The ester most commonly encountered in postmortem forensic toxicology that displays this characteristic is cocaine. Cocaine contains two ester moieties. After death cocaine is hydrolyzed almost exclusively at the phenyl ester by plasma pseudocholinesterase to yield ecgonine methylester. The rate of hydrolysis has been shown to be dependent on blood pH and temperature, with higher temperatures and pH increasing the rate of hydrolysis. The loss of cocaine in unpreserved blood can be dramatic. Acidifying blood to pH 5 inhibits chemical hydrolysis and 2.0% sodium fluoride inhibits enzymatic hydrolysis. These conditions resulted in no cocaine loss over 200 days at refrigerated (4 °C) and frozen (−15 °C) temperatures and for at least 60 days at room temperature.

Postmortem bacterial activity may also cause a decrease in drug concentration. For example, bacterial enzymes can hydrolyze the glucuronides of morphine, leading to decreased concentrations of the glucuronides and increased concentration of free morphine.

Even if the measured blood concentration of a drug or drugs reflects the concentrations at death, interpretation of concentrations by itself is problematic. Often, there is an overlap between therapeutic and toxic concentrations of drugs. One reason for this overlap is tolerance. Tolerance is defined as the effect that results from the chronic use of a drug where a larger dose becomes necessary to achieve the original desired effect. Tolerance is usually acquired and develops more rapidly to some drug effects than to other effects. Tolerance may result from a number of mechanisms. Pharmacokinetic tolerance refers to the change in drug disposition with continued drug use. This may refer to a reduction of drug reaching a target organ or an alteration in metabolism. Learned tolerance refers to a reduction in drug effects due to learned compensatory mechanisms. Cross-tolerance may also occur within a drug class and between drug classes with similar pharmacological effects. There is cross-tolerance between central nervous system (CNS) depressants such as barbiturates and benzodiazepines.

The prototypical example of tolerance affecting the interpretation of drug concentrations is with opioids such as morphine, methadone, oxycodone, and fentanyl. A blood concentration that would produce toxicity in an opioid-naive individual may not produce toxicity in an opioid-dependent individual. Blood opioid concentrations in patients receiving them for pain often overlap the concentrations found in addicts. There is also an overlap in blood opioid concentrations between dependent individuals who die of opioid intoxication and those who die from other causes. The proper interpretation of postmortem blood opioid concentrations requires knowledge of a number of factors:

1. Were there any other findings that could account for death?
2. Were opioids prescribed for medical reasons?
3. Was the decedent an opioid abuser?
4. Was the abuser being treated for this addiction?

It is only with this additional information that a meaningful interpretation of the analytical findings can be made.

Drug Interactions

A significant factor complicating the interpretation of postmortem ethanol and drug concentrations is the presence of multiple drugs in the same case. The effects of a particular drug may be affected by the concomitant use of ethanol or other drugs. These interactions can be additive, synergistic, potentiating, or antagonistic. An additive effect indicates that the total effect of a drug combination is the sum of the effects of the individual drugs. A synergistic effect means that the total effect of the drug combination is greater than the sum of the effects of the individual drugs. Potentiation is defined as an increase in the effect of a toxic substance acting simultaneously with a nontoxic substance. Antagonism refers to the canceling of effects of one drug by the simultaneous administration of another drug.

A number of interactions between ethanol and drugs have been characterized. For example, a synergistic effect in CNS depression is seen when ethanol and barbiturates are co-administered. Studies evaluating the behavioral effects of the combination of benzodiazepines and ethanol indicate an additive depressant effect on most measures of performance. In general, the behavioral effects of the benzodiazepines are very similar to those of ethanol and the two drugs in combination exacerbate the overt effects and apparent intoxication of each drug alone. When ethanol and opioids are co-administered the CNS depression and behavioral impairment are, at minimum, additive. This means that even if a group of these drugs is present in apparently therapeutic amounts, the combination of these drugs with or without ethanol may be sufficient to account for death.

The pharmacokinetics of a particular drug may also be affected by simultaneous use of ethanol and/or other drugs. The cytochrome P450 (CYP) system is a group of enzymes that are involved in the phase I metabolism of most drugs. Drugs that are metabolized by the same isozyme will compete for binding sites on the isozyme, leading to decreased metabolism for the drug with lower enzyme affinity. Although there are 12 CYP gene families, there are a smaller number of isozymes that are responsible for most drug metabolism. Therefore, it is quite possible that two co-administered drugs may be metabolized by the same isozyme. The drug that has a reduced metabolism will be detected in higher concentrations in the blood, possibly leading to toxicity. Therefore, an elevated postmortem concentration may be due to a decrease in metabolism as opposed to an overmedication. This has great significance in assigning a "manner of death."

Drugs that induce or inhibit drug metabolism may be another example of a pharmacokinetic drug interaction. The barbiturates have been known for a long time to be a CYP inducer. Enzyme induction leads to a decreased blood concentration of the drug affected by this induction. Conversely, enzyme inhibition leads to an increased concentration of the affected drug. Cimetidine and ketoconazole inhibit oxidative drug metabolism by forming a tight complex of the ferrous ion of CYP.

There are also genetic differences in drug metabolism. For example, individuals may be fast or slow metabolizers of a particular drug. Acetylation of procainamide to N-acetylprocainamide and demethylation of dextromethorphan show biphasic distribution of metabolic rates. Thus, the interpretation of parent to metabolite ratios must be interpreted in the context of these differences.

The combined use of ethanol and cocaine results in the formation of a unique metabolite, cocaethylene, by means of a transesterification process that occurs in the liver. The half-life of cocaethylene is slightly longer than cocaine, it is more toxic than cocaine, but it exhibits the same type and degree of CNS stimulation as cocaine. Therefore, the overall toxicity due to cocaine is increased when it is used in combination with ethanol.

Histologic Evidence of Drug Toxicity

As mentioned earlier, most deaths due to drugs are not associated with specific anatomic findings that enable the pathologist to assign the drugs as the cause of death. There are examples of drugs causing death as a result of specific damage to tissues that may be observed histologically. Methylenedioxymethamphetamine (MDMA, ecstasy) causes rhabdomyolysis and renal tubular breakdown. Another example of a drug causing tissue damage is acetaminophen (paracetamol). Acetaminophen intoxication demonstrates a multistage profile. The initial stage that occurs up to 1 h after ingestion produces nonspecific symptoms such as nausea, vomiting, and anorexia. This is followed by a period of apparent improvement; however, abnormal liver function tests do occur. Within 3–5 days of ingestion, hepatic necrosis occurs due to the formation of a toxic metabolite that binds to hepatic DNA. If untreated, death results from this liver necrosis. Postmortem blood analysis would most likely be negative for acetaminophen. Nonetheless, the death is due to liver necrosis caused by acetaminophen toxicity. This "drug death" would be identified by the pathologist during gross and microscopic examination of the body and not by the toxicologist performing a drug analysis.

Histologic evidence of toxicity can also be observed after the chronic abuse of drugs. Fatty liver, cirrhosis, cardiomyopathy, and pancreatitis are common findings in chronic abusers of ethanol. There are also cardiovascular changes such as scarring that may be observed in chronic cocaine abusers.

Conclusion

Postmortem ethanol and drug results, like clinical laboratory results, cannot be interpreted in isolation. Rather, they must be interpreted in the context of the particular case. If the analytical methods used do not identify a particular analyte of interest, then a final report of "no drugs detected" may be misleading. The interpretation of a blood ethanol concentration is dependent on the absence or presence of putrefaction. A particular blood morphine concentration will have different meanings based on the presence or absence of acute trauma and on the prior use history of the decedent. Certain drug concentrations may be artificially increased during the postmortem interval. Conversely, an unstable drug may be reduced in concentration during the postmortem interval. Finally, drugs may work together to produce toxicity that would not occur if the drugs were not taken in combination.

See Also

Autopsy, Findings: Postmortem Drug Sampling and Redistribution; **Drug-Induced Injury, Accidental and Iatrogenic**; **Pharmacology of Legal and Illicit Drugs**; **Substance Misuse:** Cocaine and Other Stimulants; Heroin; Sedatives; Miscellaneous Drugs; Alternative Body Fluids Analysis

Further Reading

Barnhart FE, Bonnell HJ, Rossum KM (2001) Postmortem drug redistribution. *Forensic Science Review* 13: 101–128.

Baselt RC, Cravey RH (1977) A compendium of therapeutic and toxic concentrations of toxicologically significant drugs in human biofluids. *Journal of Analytical Toxicology* 1: 81–98.

Baselt RC, Cravey RH (eds.) (1980) *Introduction to Forensic Toxicology.* Foster City, CA: Biomedical.

Corry JEL (1978) Postmortem ethanol production. *Journal of Applied Bacteriology* 44: 1–56.

Dalpe-Scott M, Degouffe M, Garbutt D, Drost M (1995) A comparison of drug concentrations in postmortem cardiac and peripheral blood in 320 cases. *Canadian Society of Forensic Sciences Journal* 28: 113–121.

Garriott JC (ed.) (2003) *Medicolegal Aspects of Alcohol.* Tuscon, AZ: Lawyers and Judges.

Havier RG (2001) The interaction of ethanol with drugs. *Forensic Science Review* 13: 101–128.

Levine B (ed.) (2003) *Principles of Forensic Toxicology.* Washington, DC: AACC Press.

Levine B, Smith ML (1990) Stability of drugs of abuse in biological specimens. *Forensic Science Review* 2: 147–157.

O'Neal CL, Poklis A (1996) Postmortem production of ethanol and factors that influence interpretation – a critical review. *American Journal of Forensic Medicine and Pathology* 17: 8–20.

Parker JM (1975) Postmortem drug level changes. In: Winek CL (ed.) *Toxicology Annual 1974,* pp. 151–165. New York: Marcel Dekkar.

Prouty RW, Anderson WH (1990) The forensic science implications of site and temporal influences on postmortem blood drug concentrations. *Journal of Forensic Sciences* 35: 243–270.

Stead AH, Moffat AC (1983) A collection of therapeutic, toxic and fatal blood concentrations in man. *Human Toxicology* 3: 437–464.

Stevens HM (1984) The stability of some drugs and poisons in putrefying liver tissues. *Journal of Forensic Science Society* 24: 577–589.

Winek CL, Wahba WW, Winek CL Jr, Balzer TW (2001) Drug and chemical blood-level data 2001. *Forensic Science International* 122: 107–123.

Postmortem Drug Sampling and Redistribution

D J Pounder, University of Dundee, Dundee, UK

Introduction

The sample most commonly used for postmortem toxicology is blood, and the analysis most commonly performed is for ethanol. Tissue samples other than blood may be used for alcohol analysis when blood is not available, because of the condition of the body, or to provide corroborative or additional data for interpretation. For the analysis of therapeutic drugs and drugs of abuse, blood is invariably the sample of choice, but for some poisons other tissues such as liver, kidney, or hair may be the optimum samples. In general the purpose of a postmortem analysis for drugs is to determine as accurately as possible the concentration of the drugs that existed in blood at the time of death, in order to assess the likelihood of drug toxicity, and in particular whether the death can be explained by the drug concentration found. Invariably, the blood sample obtained for analysis at autopsy is taken many hours or days after death. During this interval between death and blood sampling, drug concentrations in blood, and other biological fluids and tissues, may change significantly. This is true for most, if not all, drugs. The causes of these postmortem drug changes are complex. An increasing awareness of their importance over the past few decades has resulted in significant changes in the way in which blood samples are obtained at autopsy and how the drug concentrations in those blood samples are interpreted. An understanding of postmortem drug changes underpins both the rationale for the method of postmortem blood sampling for analysis as well as the rationale for the interpretation of the analytic results. Drug and metabolite concentrations in postmortem blood are interpreted by comparison with previously reported concentrations corresponding to therapeutic, toxic, and fatal conditions. Pharmacokinetic data obtained from drug studies in living volunteers cannot be applied directly to analytical results obtained from a postmortem blood sample.

Postmortem Drug Redistribution

Although clinical pharmacokinetics cannot be applied directly to postmortem toxicology, it provides a good starting point for an understanding of the most significant of the postmortem drug changes, namely postmortem drug redistribution. Volume of distribution (V_d) is an important clinical pharmacokinetic concept. The V_d is a theoretical volume that does not correspond to any physiological space. It is the hypothetical volume of body fluid that would be necessary if the total amount of drug in the body were distributed at the same concentration as in plasma. The V_d is expressed as liters per kilogram of body weight. For a drug that distributes to plasma only, the V_d approximates $40 \, ml \, kg^{-1}$. A V_d of $160 \, ml \, kg^{-1}$ implies a drug with extracellular distribution only. For a drug that has total body water distribution and can enter cells, for example, ethanol, the V_d approximates $640 \, ml \, kg^{-1}$. Some drugs have an apparent V_d greater than that of total body water and for these drugs, tissue depots sequester the high drug concentration. The V_d of several commonly encountered drugs are set out in **Table 1**. If a drug has a high V_d then this indicates that, in life, it concentrates in tissue depots, such as the liver and the lungs. Following somatic death, the death of the cells of these tissue depots of drug permits passive diffusion of the drug along concentration gradients within the body. Since at death the concentration of drugs with a high V_d is lower in blood than in solid organs such as lung and liver, drug diffuses from the solid organs into blood to raise the blood drug concentration significantly.

Postmortem drug redistribution is the postmortem elevation of drug concentrations in blood as a result of diffusion from drug depots in solid organs. To permit this postmortem diffusion process, factors must come into play that allow for the release of the drugs from their binding sites in the solid organs.

Table 1   Volume of distribution (V_d) of commonly encountered drugs

Drug	V_d $(l \, kg^{-1})$
Acetaminophen (paracetamol)	0.75–1
Amphetamine	3–5
Amitriptyline	18–22
Aspirin	0.15
Caffeine	1
Cocaine	1.2–1.9
Diazepam	0.95–2.0
Digoxin	5–7
Imipramine	11–16
Lysergic acid diethylamide (LSD)	0.27
Methadone	5
Morphine	3.2 (i.v.)
Phenylcyclidine (PCP)	5.6–6.8
Trazadone	0.89–1.5
Triazolam	0.8–1.3
Trimipramine	20–50

These are likely to be complex physicochemical changes occurring as part of the processes of autolysis and, later, putrefaction. Changes in pH, the tissue-binding characteristics of the drug, and cell membrane integrity are all probable elements. Cell death itself brings to an end any energy-dependent drug-concentrating systems. The loss of cell membrane integrity is paralleled by the release of intracellular enzymes from the solid organs into the blood. It is this phenomenon that results in the artifactual postmortem elevation of cardiac myocyte and hepatocellular enzymes. If such large molecules as these enzymes pass rapidly into the blood postmortem, then it is hardly surprising that much smaller drug molecules do so. Postmortem drug redistribution into blood is well established within hours of death and is typically marked by the time of autopsy which is commonly a day or even 2–3 days after death.

Drugs are weak acids or bases and in solution they become ionized when they lose or gain a hydrogen ion. The degree of ionization of a compound depends on both its specific pK_a and on the pH of the solution in which it is dissolved, a relationship described by the Henderson–Hasselbalch equation. Since the lipid-soluble form (nonionized) of a weak electrolyte is the species that crosses cell membranes, organic acids are more likely to diffuse across membranes when they are in an acid environment whereas a basic environment favors diffusion of bases across membranes. In this way drugs become trapped in the compartment in which they are more ionized because ionized (polar) compounds do not easily cross cell membranes. In life, intracellular fluid is more acidic than extracellular fluid, with the result that bases cross the cell membrane and are trapped in the intracellular compartment. One consequence of this relative partition is a higher V_d. After somatic death there is a sharp decrease in blood pH as a result of continuing cellular metabolism with carbon dioxide accumulation until available oxygen is exhausted and then there is anaerobic metabolism of glucose to lactic and pyruvic acids. In the minutes immediately following somatic death this very rapid fall in blood pH may cause redistribution of some drugs. There is some evidence that significant increases in blood morphine concentration occurring in the minutes after death are a result of the repartitioning of the drug consequent on pH changes.

The solid organs, which provide the most significant drug depots for postmortem drug redistribution, are those that combine a high drug concentration with a relatively large mass and an association with large blood vessels. The liver, the lungs, and the heart are the organs most responsible. Skeletal muscle, although amounting to about 30 kg of a 70-kg body, tends to have drug concentrations similar to or only a few fold greater than blood. Many drugs concentrate in liver at levels 50-fold or more than in blood. It was for this reason that liver was used historically for postmortem screening for drugs. Drug diffuses from the liver postmortem into the inferior vena cava and thence the right heart, superior vena cava, and contiguous neck and subclavian veins. In life, the lungs receive the entire blood flow from the right ventricle and therefore drug distribution into and accumulation in this tissue are very rapid. Compounds that specifically accumulate in the lungs are basic amines, for example, imipramine, amphetamines, methadone, and chlorpromazine. These exogenous basic amines are thought to be removed from the blood by the same carrier-mediated sodium-dependent transport systems that remove the endogenous amines 5-hydroxytryptamine and norepinephrine (noradrenaline) from the pulmonary circulation. For these drugs the ratio of lung tissue to blood concentration in life may be as high as 200 and this very large gradient provides the basis for postmortem drug redistribution into the pulmonary vessels and thence the cardiac chambers, as well as directly into the adjacent thoracic aorta. Cardioactive drugs, such as diltiazem, a calcium-channel blocker, and digoxin, are concentrated in the myocardium in life and after death show postmortem redistribution from the myocardium into cardiac blood. The endothelial cells of capillaries heavily concentrate some drugs such as phenobarbital. Postmortem release of drugs from endothelial cells into the blood is potentially very rapid. Certainly endothelial cells are shed into the blood during the first day postmortem.

Postmortem drug redistribution from solid organs into the blood occurs by passive diffusion, as described by Fick's first law of diffusion, which states that the rate of diffusion is proportional to the concentration gradient across the diffusion barrier. Although drugs diffuse most readily along the vascular tree within the blood itself, anatomical structures such as the diaphragm and the wall of the aorta do not in practice provide major diffusion barriers. Diffusion is temperature-dependent but refrigeration of the body is not a significant factor in the early postmortem period since it typically requires 18 h or more for the core body temperature to fall to that of the environment, and drug redistribution is well underway within hours of death. However, refrigeration will slow the rate of continuing drug redistribution if autopsy is delayed for days, although this is not of practical significance. Diffusion is time-dependent also, and empirical studies on cadavers with repeated blood sampling over many hours shows increasingly dramatic rises in blood drug concentrations.

Movement of drug within the blood is not only a result of diffusion since there is also natural postmortem movement of blood within the vessels providing some physical transport of drugs. These postmortem movements of blood are associated with pressure changes resulting from rigor mortis and putrefactive gas formation. The extent of this postmortem blood flux is also influenced by the degree of fluidity of the blood in the individual case. Following death there is loss of vascular tone in the arterial tree so that blood pools in the small peripheral vessels with a relative emptying of the larger arteries. During the first 24 h postmortem there is reflux of blood from the heart into the superior vena cava and the associated neck veins as a consequence of rigor mortis involving the heart muscle. With the increase in intraabdominal pressure accompanying early putrefaction, there is blood reflux from the abdominal aorta into the thoracic aorta, from the inferior vena cava into the right atrium and contiguous superior vena cava, and reflux from the left cardiac chambers into pulmonary veins. With the resolution of rigor mortis, which is the result of muscle putrefaction, the heart chambers are emptied of blood and there is flow into peripheral arteries with associated slight movements of venous blood. Gravitational phenomena related to body position and the tendency of blood movements to occur along the most linear natural anatomical trajectories are additional features that cause the pattern and extent of blood flux to be highly variable from case to case. In general, femoral venous blood can be expected to be influenced least by the postmortem movement and mixing of blood.

Empirical observations on drug-poisoning fatalities as well as experimental small-animal models have shown that there is a common general pattern of postmortem drug redistribution into blood. Lowest drug concentrations are found in blood from peripheral veins such as the subclavian and femoral veins. High drug concentrations are found in blood samples from the aorta, the superior vena cava, and the cardiac chambers, and the highest drug concentrations are found in the pulmonary vein and the suprarenal portion of the inferior vena cava. The latter two vessels drain blood from the lungs and the liver respectively. Thus, the lowest drug concentrations are found in blood samples from sites distant from the torso, which contains the organs in which drugs are most heavily concentrated, while blood samples from the heart or major vessels of the torso have much higher drug concentrations because of their proximity to these organs. This is not to say that the drug concentration in blood from peripheral sites – such as the femoral vein, simply because it is the lowest concentration – is unchanged from the time of death. Rather the drug concentration in peripheral blood is the closest available approximation to the drug concentration in blood at the time of death, but even so may be two- or threefold of that concentration. The difference in drug concentration between torso samples and peripheral venous blood samples is commonly several-fold and occasionally 10- or 20-fold. The preferred autopsy blood-sampling site for toxicological analysis is the femoral vein or the contiguous external iliac vein. Empirical cadaver studies suggest that the subclavian vein, although a peripheral venous site, is less reliable.

Postmortem drug redistribution accounts for the commonly observed fact that drug concentrations in blood vary significantly between blood samples taken at the same time from different anatomical sites in the one corpse. Overall drug concentrations in all blood samples postmortem increase with postmortem interval but the changes are most marked in torso blood samples. Consequently, the between-sample variability in drug concentration increases with postmortem interval. Although drug concentrations in peripheral venous blood, particularly femoral venous blood, increase least in the postmortem interval, they still do not represent precisely the drug concentration at the time of death but rather the best approximation available. Femoral venous blood is the best available postmortem blood sample, but is the best of a bad lot.

Some variability in drug concentrations between blood-sampling sites in cases of drug overdose is seen in life. During drug absorption, there is distribution of the drug from the blood to the tissues and this distribution phase lasts from 30 min to 2 h for most drugs. During this period there can be a sizeable difference between arterial and venous drug concentrations and this may be reflected in site differences in

postmortem blood drug concentrations where a person has died during the absorptive phase. In both animal models and human case studies of drug overdose, drug concentrations in arterial blood are sometimes as much as twice that of venous blood. This phenomenon may be a contributory factor in causing the postmortem drug concentration differences seen in acute drug overdose deaths, but it has a relatively minor impact when contrasted with the phenomenon of postmortem drug redistribution.

Postmortem drug analyses are performed on whole blood because postmortem blood clotting and red cell lysis makes it impossible to obtain a plasma sample, the usual matrix for drug analyses in the living. Within an hour or less of death, blood clotting is initiated throughout the vascular tree and, at the same time, clot lysis is initiated. The two processes occur simultaneously and the effectiveness of the clot lysis will determine whether the blood at autopsy is clotted, or completely fluid, or partly clotted and partly fluid. As a result the amount of blood clot present in a postmortem blood sample varies from body to body, and from site to site within the same body. When fibrin clot is present it always entraps large numbers of erythrocytes, so that the clot is relatively red-cell-rich. For drugs with an unequal distribution between erythrocytes and serum, the proportion of red cells and blood clot in a postmortem blood sample submitted for analysis may influence the drug concentration. For most drugs this is not an important factor in practice. For some drugs, such as chloroquine, which has an erythrocyte to serum drug concentration ratio of 32:1, the erythrocyte content of the postmortem blood sample might dramatically affect the drug concentration. The blood obtained from limb vessels is most likely to be fluid and largely devoid of clots, reflecting the approximately inverse relationship between the endothelial-derived fibrinolytic activity and the diameter of the vessel from which the blood was obtained. The uncoagulable fluid blood often, but not universally, present in limb veins provides as homogeneous a sample for analysis as can be hoped for. Thus far there is no proven correlation between the differences in hemoglobin concentration of postmortem blood samples and the differences in the concentrations of drugs detected.

Stomach Contents

Unabsorbed alcohol and drugs present in the stomach at the time of death passively diffuse into surrounding tissues, organs, and blood vessels in the postmortem period. Direct diffusion of alcohol, drugs, and poisons from the stomach contents through the stomach wall, diaphragm, and blood vessel walls to contaminate blood in the cardiac chambers and surrounding great vessels can be a significant problem, particularly with respect to alcohol analysis. It is a further reason to avoid sampling torso blood for the quantitative analysis of alcohol and drugs. Unabsorbed drug in the stomach also diffuses into the adjacent liver. The gastric contact area on the inferior surface of the liver is centered on the left lobe. There is both empirical and experimental evidence that drug levels in the left lobe of the liver may rise significantly postmortem as a consequence of drug diffusion from gastric contents. For this reason a liver sample for analysis should be taken from deep within the right lobe, the site most protected from this effect by distance and tissue mass.

A common autopsy finding is contamination of the airways by gastric contents as a result of agonal vomiting or passive postmortem reflux following relaxation of the esophageal sphincter at death. Any drugs or alcohol present in this material contaminating the airways diffuse readily into the blood within the cardiac chamber and the great vessels of the heart, including the pulmonary vessels, superior vena cava, and aorta. Spurious analytic results for alcohol and drugs resulting from this postmortem artifact are readily avoided by taking the blood sample from a peripheral vein.

Bacterial Activity

The bacteria, which break down the body tissues during decomposition, are also able to degrade some drugs. As a result the concentrations of susceptible drugs in blood may decrease during the postmortem interval. Drug lability to bacterial degradation is related to the presence of one of three chemical structures in the drug. Oxygen bonded to nitrogen but not to carbon or sulfur renders a drug labile. This occurs with nitro-groups bonded to either an aromatic nucleus or to a nonaromatic structure and also occurs with oximes and with N-oxide structures, e.g., chlordiazepoxide. A second vulnerable structure is sulfur in a chain bonded as a thiono-group (C=S, P=S), e.g., malathion. The third vulnerable group of compounds is the aminophenols, which have OH and NH_2 groups on the same aryl nucleus. Structures possessing a primary arylamine group, which are not phenolic or are phenolic but do not possess such an amine group, or have a substituted amine group, for example acetaminophen (paracetamol), are all stable. The stability of drugs generally reflects the stability of chemical structures in which carbon bonds with oxygen and nitrogen, nitrogen bonds with hydrogen, and sulfur bonds with oxygen. Sulfur forming part of a heterocyclic ring causes some instability to putrefaction, e.g., dothiepin and the phenothiazines. The observation that the degradation of these latter drugs is variable suggests that the bacteria capable of degrading them are less widely encountered than those capable of breaking down the other labile chemical structures. While the lability or stability of a drug to putrefactive bacterial degradation may be generally inferred from its chemical structure, anomalies have been observed, for example thiopental would be expected to be labile but is stable, and bendrofluazide would be expected to be stable but is unstable. Furthermore, a drug with a high V_d and a labile chemical structure can be expected to show postmortem redistribution effects, with increases in blood drug concentration, as well as later putrefactive degradation, with decreases in blood drug concentration, both of which are anatomical site- and time-variable.

Ethanol is formed postmortem by microbial action. A wide variety of bacteria normally present in the gut, and responsible for putrefaction, can generate ethyl alcohol in blood and other tissues. Also, yeasts, such as *Candida albicans*, may be responsible for postmortem alcohol production. Ethanol synthesis takes place by a pathway opposite to that of ethanol catabolism in the living body. The necessary alcohol dehydrogenase and acetaldehyde dehydrogenase enzymes are provided by the microorganisms while the carbohydrate substrates glucose and lactate are present in blood and tissues. The anatomically isolated position of the vitreous humor of the eye protects it from bacterial putrefaction. For this reason analysis of vitreous humor is useful to corroborate a postmortem blood alcohol and assist in distinguishing antemortem intoxication from postmortem alcohol production. Urine is similarly useful because it normally contains little or no substrate for bacterial conversion into ethanol, except as a consequence of some pathological abnormality, particularly diabetes mellitus.

Autopsy Sampling

In practice postmortem blood samples for quantitative toxicological analyses should be obtained from the femoral vein or the contiguous external iliac vein. Ideally, the sample should be obtained as soon as possible after death. Obtaining such a sample at the scene of death is good practice. If the sample is obtained at autopsy then it should be taken at the very start of the dissection. The femoral vein can be exposed through an incision in the groin, or the external iliac vein exposed through the normal autopsy abdominal incision. The blood sample should be obtained by a needle and syringe and not by severing the vessel and allowing the blood to flow into an open container, or to pool in the tissues or pelvis before collection. Prior to taking the sample the vessel must be ligated or clamped proximally, to avoid drawing blood from the immediately contiguous common iliac vein and the inferior vena cava. When a large volume of postmortem blood sample is needed for drug screening, that is to say qualitative rather than quantitative analysis, the sample may be obtained from anywhere. Best practice is to obtain a large volume of torso blood sample for qualitative analysis and a necessarily smaller volume of femoral venous blood for subsequent quantitative analysis. Sequestered hematomas, such as intracerebral hematomas and subdural hematomas, can be analyzed for alcohol and drugs, and give an indication of their presence in the body at the time the hemorrhage occurred – information that is useful if there has been a significant survival time. All blood samples should be labeled with their specific anatomical site of origin. Blood specimens should be preserved by adding 2% wt/vol sodium fluoride to the container. This inhibits microorganism production of ethanol, conversion of cocaine to ecgonine methyl ester by cholinesterases, and enzymatic loss of other esters such as 6-acetylmorphine. Preservatives are generally not required for other specimens.

For the purpose of corroborating a blood alcohol analysis on femoral venous blood, a sample of vitreous humor from the eye together with a urine sample, if the bladder contains urine, should always be taken. Urine is obtained directly from the unopened bladder by needle and syringe. Vitreous humor is obtained by direct aspiration from each eye using a small-volume syringe and a needle inserted adjacent to the outer canthus at an angle of 45° to the sagittal plane. Gentle suction avoids contamination with retinal fragments and typically produces 2–3 ml of slightly viscous fluid from each eye.

If stomach contents are retained for the purposes of assessing whether a death has occurred acutely following a drug overdose then the sample is best obtained last during the autopsy procedure, to avoid the possibility of contaminating other samples. The volume of the gastric contents should be measured at autopsy and a representative aliquot or the entire sample submitted for analysis. If the analytical laboratory has a preference for liver tissue analysis then the sample should be obtained from deep within the right lobe to minimize diffusional effects from stomach contents. Bile is easily collected by needle and syringe from the gallbladder at autopsy and, historically, has been most often used in the determination of opiates in general and morphine in particular. Many drugs are concentrated in bile.

In addition to liver, the tissues commonly collected for postmortem toxicological analysis are lung, brain, and kidneys. Lung tissue is a useful sample where there has been inhalation of volatile substances such as toluene. Brain, as a result of its high fat content, tends to accumulate lipophilic substances such as chlorinated hydrocarbons and other organic volatiles and should be sampled when these toxic compounds are suspected. Where heavy-metal poisoning is suspected, the kidney is a useful sample because heavy metals are concentrated there. Hair and fingernails are also the specimens of choice in assessing chronic heavy-metal poisoning such as from arsenic, mercury, and lead. Keratin is present in large amounts in hair and nails and is a rich source of cysteine. Heavy metals bind to sulfhydryl groups on the cysteine molecule to form a covalent complex. Numerous therapeutic drugs as well as drugs of abuse have been detected in head hair. Segmental analysis of occipital head hair, which grows at a rate of about 1 cm per month, can be used to assess chronic drug usage.

When the body is decomposed, has been embalmed, or is a case of exhumation, so that no blood sample is available, then the generally favored tissue sample for drug analysis is skeletal muscle. The sample is usually taken from the anterior thigh as a matter of convenience because this is the most readily accessible large muscle bulk in a supine cadaver. Any limb muscle would suffice but torso muscle, particularly the psoas, should be avoided because of the risk of postmortem drug diffusion from the stomach contents and viscera.

Where a body is maggot-infested the samples taken for toxicological analysis should include the maggots. Drugs present in a corpse are ingested by the maggots and sometimes concentrated within them. Furthermore, the maggots can be technically easier to analyze than the decomposing tissue of the corpse, which contains many putrefactive compounds that interfere with chromatographic analysis. Maggots can be killed with hot water, dried with paper toweling, and stored frozen. Drugs may also be detectable in the empty pupal cases left on the corpse after the flies have emerged.

All specimens, appropriately labeled, should be stored, sealed at 4 °C, and then transferred to –20 °C if long-term storage is necessary.

See Also

Autopsy, Findings: Postmortem Drug Measurements, Interpretation of; **Drug-Induced Injury, Accidental and Iatrogenic**; **Pharmacology of Legal and Illicit Drugs**; **Postmortem Changes:** Electrolyte Disturbances

Further Reading

Barnhart FE, Bonnell HJ, Rossum KM (2001) Post-mortem drug redistribution. *Forensic Science Review* 13: 101–128.

Pounder DJ (1994) The nightmare of postmortem drug changes. In: Wecht CH (ed.) *Legal Medicine 1993*, pp. 163–191. Salem, NH: Butterworth.

Pounder DJ, Jones AW (1998) Measuring alcohol postmortem. In: Karch SB (ed.) *Drug Abuse Handbook*, pp. 356–374. Boca Raton, FL: CRC Press.

Organic Toxins

O H Drummer, Victorian Institute of Forensic Medicine, Southbank, VIC, Australia

Introduction

Previous articles have reviewed various applications of toxicology used in forensic and legal medicine with a focus on synthetic and semisynthetic drugs. Naturally occurring toxic substances or organic toxins are more frequently encountered in forensic cases than might initially be considered and are often regionally specific depending on the availability of the plant, animal, or other sources of such substances. Ethanol and carbon monoxide (CO) are some of the most common substances, and are considered elsewhere in this encyclopedia. Other organic toxins include hydrogen cyanide, methanol, hydrocarbons, and other volatile substances, plant poisons, and animal poisons including venoms.

It would be impossible to list, let alone discuss, all organic toxins that come under this classification. Consequently, this article outlines some of the more significant organic-based poisons not covered elsewhere and illustrates their relevance to forensic and legal medicine.

Volatile Substances

Those toxins of a volatile nature of most importance are listed in **Table 1**.

Alcohol

Alcohol (as ethanol) is produced by the fermentation of cereals and fruits, and is a common substance produced in decomposing bodies. When present in specimens obtained from putrefying bodies, it is often difficult to establish whether any ethanol was present at the time of death since up to at least 0.2 g per 100 ml can be produced in the right circumstances. When available, vitreous humor can be used to determine the respective likelihood of the source of ethanol since it is much more protected from bacterial contamination postmortem.

Carbon Dioxide and Carbon Monoxide

These gases are important asphyxiants in forensic cases. When persons are exposed to CO, its presence can be determined spectrophotometrically as a complex bound to hemoglobin. The percentage bound to hemoglobin (% saturation) is a relatively stable adduct blocking the ability of hemoglobin to store and hence mobilize oxygen. Percent saturations over 20% are dangerous, while percent saturations over 50% are often fatal. In medicolegal cases, it is most often associated with death by suicide from exhaust gases from motor vehicles, or from inhalation of gases in fires. In fires, it is toxic at a lower saturation (<30%) due to the presence of other asphyxiant gases (carbon dioxide, hydrogen cyanide, and hydrogen chloride).

In some situations of apparent CO death from inhalation of motor vehicle gases, CO may not be present. Motor vehicles fitted with emission controls will often not produce significant CO once the engine is warm; rather the large amounts of carbon dioxide present are sufficient to cause death from simple asphyxiation (lack of oxygen) and/or metabolic acidosis, particularly if ventilation is poor. CO should always be considered in "strange" indoor deaths if fuel

Table 1 Important volatile organic toxins encountered in forensic medicine

Organic toxin	Source
Ethanol (alcohol)	Fermentation of specimens, decomposing bodies, numerous alcoholic beverages, methylated spirit
Carbon dioxide	Automobiles and other internal combustion engines, compressed gas
Carbon monoxide	Automobiles and other internal combustion engines, fires
Cyanide (hydrogen and inorganic salts)	Cyanotic bacteria, gases from fires and cyanide salts
Methanol	Alcoholic drinks, metabolism of pectins, industrial solvent
Other volatile substances	Methane (natural gas), propane (liquefied propane gas), butane (lighter fluids), automotive fuels, aviation fuels, solvents, and miscellaneous gases

heaters or open fireplaces are operating, particularly if ventilation is poor.

CO can be easily measured by differential spectrophotometry by virtue of the unique spectrum produced by the adduct with hemoglobin. A number of commercial instruments are available to measure CO. In postmortem specimens, putrefaction or otherwise altered blood can best be measured by gas chromatography either directly or by conversion to methane. While carbon dioxide can be measured by chromatographic means, given its presence in air there can be no value in measuring this gas in specimens, particularly in the postmortem situation.

Cyanide

This substance is highly toxic and should always be considered as a potential poison in unsolved cases, particularly in deaths of persons with occupations associated with laboratories (such as chemists and biochemists). Inorganic salts (potassium and sodium salts) have electroplating and metallurgical applications, while the gas has been used as a fumigant and insecticide as well as a warfare agent.

In forensic cases, the gas (hydrogen cyanide) appears most commonly in persons exposed to fires, particularly those that involve burning plastics. When this occurs, toxic blood concentrations may be as low as $0.5 \, mg \, l^{-1}$. Fatal exposure to inorganic salts generally leads to much higher blood concentrations of cyanide, often well over $2 \, mg \, l^{-1}$. Cyanide will be gradually "lost" in specimens stored for prolonged periods. This occurs through both volatilization and inactivation by tissues. Cyanide can be produced in blood and other specimens by the action of cyanogenic bacteria. Therefore, it is recommended to analyze specimens as soon as possible after collection or to store specimens frozen at $-60 \, °C$ until analysis.

Methanol

This poisonous alcohol is fortunately rare in forensic cases due to its relative scarcity in many parts of the world. However, if consumed, it is very toxic at doses over $10 \, ml$, largely due to its metabolism to formaldehyde and formic acid. Blood concentrations vary widely and will of course depend on the time from ingestion; however, fatal concentrations are often over $100 \, mg \, l^{-1}$ (0.01%). Trace amounts of methanol are produced following the metabolism of pectins contained in fruit and it is present in trace amounts in most alcoholic beverages. In this situation, blood concentrations are usually much less than $100 \, mg \, l^{-1}$. The metabolism of methanol is inhibited by co-consumption of ethanol. Consequently, methanol may accumulate to toxic levels in alcoholics whose blood alcohol concentration is continuously above 0.02%.

Methanol is measured by techniques similar to those of ethanol.

Other Volatile Substances

A number of other volatile substances are encountered in forensic cases. These usually occur through abuse of volatile substances and consist of hydrocarbons such as butane from lighter fluid refills, liquefied propane gas (LPG), automotive and aviation fuels, and a variety of domestic and industrial solvents. Abuse occurs by inhalation of the substance contained in a plastic bag or similar container, or through direct injection into the oral cavity through a pressurized can. Inhalation of these central nervous system depressants can lead to anoxia, heart rhythm abnormalities, or even a direct effect on the vagal reflex, leading to a cardiorespiratory arrest. Long-term use can lead to cognitive deficits and adverse behavioral changes. Occasionally volatile substances can be detected in accidental exposures through inhalation of fumes from fires, and explosions, including aviation incidents.

Toxicologically these substances are detected by use of headspace gas chromatographic techniques similar to that of ethanol. When exposure to volatile substances is suspected it is advised to provide a sample of lung fluid, or better, a whole tied-off lung. This provides a better opportunity for detection of substances that can readily dissipate on storage.

Plant-Based Toxins

Nicotine and Related Alkaloids

Nicotine is arguably the most common plant-based poison used in the community. While its main use is in tobacco-related products, it has also been used as an insecticide (as solutions of sulfate salt). A number of proprietary products now contain nicotine to wean people off tobacco, including chewing gum, nasal sprays, and transdermal patches. Nicotine is highly toxic, causing stimulation of the parasympathetic nervous system. Toxic doses cause pinpoint pupils, vomiting, excessive salivation and sweating, tachycardia, hypertension, and eventually convulsions and cardiorespiratory failure. It is easily absorbed orally, through inhalation of aerosols or smoke, or through dermal exposure. Consequently, significant exposure can be readily attained. Poisoning cases are still seen in tobacco workers who absorb the alkaloid through their skin, persons who inhale aerosols from spraying crops with nicotine solution, persons using multiple skin patches, and in children who eat nicotine-containing gum or patches.

A number of related substances are known that produce similar effects to nicotine by mimicking the effects of acetylcholine. These include muscarine from ingestion of *Amanita muscaria* mushrooms, atropine, and hyoscine (scopolamine) found in deadly nightshade (*Atropa belladonna*) and in many *Datura* spp. (or *Brugsmansia* spp.) (angel's trumpets, thorn apple), and lobeline found in lobelia plants.

The ancient poisonous weed hemlock (*Coniine maculatum*) is a relatively widespread biennial herb that contains a chemically related substance to nicotine, known as coniceine. This substance (and related substances in the plant) produces similar effects to nicotine at low doses (i.e., it stimulates the autonomic nervous system), but it causes paralysis at higher doses, resembling the effects of a narcotic.

Many deaths have been reported from these nicotine-like alkaloids. Most of the substances listed here are measurable by modern gas chromatographic techniques. Extraction from alkalinized blood and chromatography on a nonpolar to medium polar column will achieve adequate detection limits for nicotine, atropine, hyoscine, and coniceine.

Digitalis Glycosides

Digitalis glycoside digoxin and digitoxin are potent cardiotonics found in *Digitalis* spp. (foxglove). Digoxin is available in tablet form and is prescribed to persons with congestive heart failure and atrial fibrillation. The glycosides are very toxic if blood concentrations exceed about $5 \mu g\, l^{-1}$, so regular therapeutic drug monitoring is necessary. Other plants have substances that behave similarly to digoxin. Oleander is a free-flowering bush widely grown in eastern Australia, known botanically as *Nerium oleander*. Another plant, sometimes known as yellow oleander, is *Thevetia peruviana*. Both plants belong to the family Apocynaceae. Oleander contains a toxic substance that acts as a cardiac glycoside, of which oleandrin is the main active chemical. The content of oleandrin in dried leaves is about 0.13%, although this toxic substance is also found in the stems and flowers. The toxic activity in these plants varies from season to season. The toxic principles in oleander are not destroyed by heat, such as during boiling. Oleandrin has a similar activity on the human heart as digitalis glycosides. Digoxin and oleandrin act to increase heart actions (mainly force of contraction), and in higher doses affect the ability of the heart to function properly. Adverse effects include nausea, vomiting, visual disturbances (color hallucinations), headache, cardiovascular disturbances, salivation, abdominal pain, mydriasis (dilated pupils), and peripheral neuritis.

Death can occur with serious poisoning. Death is associated with abnormal heart rhythm leading to cardiovascular collapse.

Immunoassay screening assays used to monitor digoxin have substantial cross-reactivity with oleandrin.

Once exposure to oleander poisoning has been determined, the administration of antibodies to digitalis glycosides (Digibind) will reverse the effects of toxic substances in oleander.

Psilocybin

One of the more common poisonings in certain parts of the world is exposure to "magic mushrooms." Psilocybin is found in *Psilocybe* spp. and in some *Panelous* and *Concybe* genera. Psilocybin is converted metabolically to psilocin, the main active indole alkaloid. This substance interacts with serotonin ($5HT_{1A}$ and $5HT_{2C}$) and norepinephrine (noradrenaline) receptors in the brain. Psilocin causes anxiety, disorientation, depersonalization, psychosis, and hallucinations. Other adverse effects include severe nausea, vomiting, cardiovascular side-effects, hyperthermia, dilated pupils, and convulsions. These effects usually last for about 2 h and can be extremely intense and frightening.

Psilocin can be measured by high-performance liquid chromatography with electrochemical detection, gas chromatography–mass spectrometry, or liquid chromatography–mass spectrometry (LC-MS). If urine is used, conjugates should be hydrolyzed first to increase detectable alkaloid.

Ricin

One of the most toxic plant substances is the toxalbumins found in the castor-oil plant (*Ricinus communis*), *Jatropha multifida* (Jatropha fruit) and other Jatropha genera (active: ricin), and rosary pea (*Abrus precatorius*) (active: abrin). These lectins, consisting of two polypeptide chains, bind to intestinal cell walls and inhibit ribosomal protein synthesis. Ingestion of castor-oil seeds is a relatively common childhood poisoning episode, although seeds without broken seed coats are much less toxic. Symptoms include hypotension, severe gastrointestinal pain, acute pulmonary edema (if inhaled), and tissue necrosis. Kidney and liver failure is common. Adverse symptoms are often delayed for one to several days. A number of deaths are known from ingestion of these toxins. Antidotes are not known. A number of other lectins from other plant species are also toxic. Purified ricin from the castor-oil plant has been implicated in attempted poisonings and terrorist activities. Its analysis has been largely restricted to immunological procedures.

There is a multitude of other plant-based poisons, some of which are listed in **Table 2**. Of particular note are cocaine, tetrahydrocannabinol (*Cannabis sativa*), and morphine (opium poppy). These common plant poisons are covered elsewhere.

Animal-Based Toxins

The variety of animal toxins is enormous. Venomous or poisonous animals are ubiquitous and widely distributed throughout the animal kingdom and found in almost all continents and oceans. Animals can either secrete toxins (venomous) or be toxic if consumed (poisonous).

Table 3 provides a short list of such land and marine animals and the toxic substances associated with their toxic actions.

In the seas and oceans one of the most common forms of mortality is envenomation by one of the numerous forms of poisonous jellyfish. Many of the toxins used are unknown but are believed to be

mainly polypeptides that cause ion channel disturbances in smooth and skeletal muscle as well as serious immune responses. One of the more unusual forms is the Irukandji syndrome, in which many of the symptoms resemble catecholamine toxicity such as anxiety, sweating, piloerection, hypertension, and tachycardia. Pathologically, there are often few signs of envenomation.

Another relatively common source of mortality is ingestion of toxins contained in mollusks, crab flesh, and other related organisms. This is known as paralytic shellfish poisoning (PSP) or neurotoxic shellfish poisoning (NSP). These toxins include saxitoxin, palytoxin, and others such as tetrodotoxin. They all act to interfere with ion permeability in membranes.

A form of fish poisoning that is a significant public health issue is that of ciguatera poisoning. This is caused by ingestion of the ciguatoxins that accumulate in the food chain in warm-water fish. While rarely fatal, they have the potential to be so by their effect on sodium ion channels in nerves. These toxins are high-molecular-weight heat-stable polyethers with

Table 2 Important plant-derived organic toxins encountered in forensic medicine

Organic toxin	Source
Cocaine	*Erythroxylon coca*, and certain pharmaceutical preparations
Coniine and related alkaloids (coniceine)	*Conium maculatum* (hemlock)
Digitalis-like glycosides	Digoxin (and digitoxin), foxglove plant (*Digitalis* spp.), cane toad (*Bufo marinus*), oleander (*Nerium oleander*), yellow oleander (*Thevetia peruviana*)
Ibogaine	*Tabernanthe iboga*, licit and illicit sources as hallucinogen and for treatment of addictive behavior
Morphine and related alkaloids	Opium poppy, pharmaceutical preparations, heroin, codeine
Nicotine	Tobacco products, patches and other pharmaceutical preparations, insecticide products
Ricin and abrin	*Ricin communis*, castor-oil plant, industrially used in immunology, *Jatropha* spp., *Abrus* spp.
Psilocybin	*Psilocybe* spp., *Panelous* spp., *Concybe* spp. of mushrooms
Scopolamine	*Hyoscyamus niger* (henbane), *Datura stromonium* (jimsonweed), and other plants
Strychnine	*Strychnos nux vomica*, rodenticides

Table 3 Important animal-derived organic toxins encountered in forensic medicine

Type of poisoning or envenomation	Toxin and source
Jellyfish envenomations	Wide-ranging types of jellyfish can cause serious envenomation. Often caused by polypeptides, leading to abnormal sodium and calcium ion permeability, particularly in smooth muscle and heart; many toxins are not identified
Paralytic shellfish poisoning or neurotoxic shellfish poisoning	Saxitoxin, palytoxin, and other toxins found in bivalve mollusks, crab flesh and other marine species
Puffer fish poisoning, and related poisonings	Tetrodotoxins found in fugu (Japanese puffer fish). Tetrodotoxins are also used by the blue-ringed octopus, found in the skin of Central American frogs, the cutaneous glands of the Californian newt, in some marine fish with spiny fins, some shellfish, and many other marine species
Ciguatera poisoning	Ciguatoxins are found in larger tropical fish, leading to "fish poisoning"
Snake, spider and scorpion bite envenomation	Largely protein-based substances or polypeptides leading to hemolytic, neurologic, renal, and cardiovascular abnormalities

a potency that is unlikely to allow ready analytical detection in victims.

Tetrodotoxin and related toxins (maculotoxins) are the main poison in puffer fishes, a delicacy of the Japanese, as well as in the blue-ringed octopus, the skin of Central American frogs, in the cutaneous glands of the Californian newt, in some marine fish with spiny fins, some shellfish, marine gastropods, and many other marine species. Symptoms of poisoning include nausea, vomiting, blurred vision, muscular weakness, and paralysis of respiratory muscles. Mortality is high from this toxin.

Many other marine animals can inflict serious envenomations or cause poisonings.

A number of toxins mentioned above can be detected by the use of microtiter radioimmunoassay or enzyme-linked immunosorbent assay tests using antibodies raised against the toxin. More recently, LC-MS has been used to identify toxins in both the organism and specimens taken from the victim.

Bee and wasp stings are prevalent through many parts of the world and are arguably one of the leading causes of death from envenomation, for example, *Hymenoptera* wasp stings. The sting of the common European honey bee *Apis mellifera* can cause anaphylactic reactions in susceptible persons. Anaphylaxis is potentially serious and can often lead to death. The risk is increased with multiple stings. Symptoms may range from local swelling and pruritus to marked edema leading to bronchospasm, dyspnea, and cardiorespiratory collapse.

Venomous snakes are a major cause of serious to fatal envenomation throughout much of the world, particularly the USA, Australia, and Asia. The large number of dangerous species precludes any detailed review here; rather the reader should refer to relevant texts.

Snake venoms are complex in nature, comprising chiefly proteins. These proteins are often enzymatic in nature, including proteolytic enzymes, thrombin-like enzymes, collagenases, phosphoesterases, and phospholipases. These proteins are capable of causing local and systemic tissue damage. In some species, polypeptides act on the postsynapse to block the effects of endogenous neurotransmitters (e.g., acetylcholine nicotinic receptors) and in others affect movement of ions through the sodium channel.

Venomous spiders and scorpions are another large and dangerous group of animals that inflict many serious and often fatal envenomations every year. These venoms are again often proteins or polypeptides in nature, although some exceptions exist. The measurement of tissue specimens for snake, spider, and scorpion venoms is largely restricted to immunological tests. In some countries, kits are available to allow the detection of toxins resulting from snakebite, or at least to exclude snakebites as a cause of death when there is little or no pathology, or the circumstances do not allow unequivocal proof of an envenomation.

See Also

Alcohol: Breath Alcohol Analysis; Blood and Body Fluid Analysis; Acute and Chronic Use, Postmortem Findings; **Carbon Monoxide Poisoning:** Clinical Findings, Sequelae In Survivors; Incidence and Findings at Postmortem; **Toxicology:** Methods of Analysis, Antemortem; Methods of Analysis, Postmortem

Further Reading

Amdur MO, Doull J, and Klaassen CD (1995) *Casarett and Doull's Toxicology*, 5th edn. New York: Pergamon Press.

Baselt RH (2000) *Disposition of Toxic Drugs and Chemicals in Man*, 5th edn. Foster City, CA: Year Book Medical.

Ellenhorn MJ, Schonwald S, Ordog G, Wassrerberger J (eds.) (1997) *Ellenhorn's Medical Toxicology*, 2nd edn. Baltimore, MD: Williams and Wilkins.

Mebs D (2002) *Venomous and Poisonous Animals: A Handbook for Biologists, Toxicologists, Toxinologists, Physicians and Pharmacists*. Boca Raton, FL: CRC Press.

Meier J, White J (1995) *Handbook of Clinical Toxicology of Animal Venoms and Poisons*. Boca Raton, FL: CRC Press.

Ménez A (ed.) (2002) *Perspectives in Molecular Toxinology*. Chichester, UK: Wiley.

Moffatt AC (ed.) (2003) *Clarke's Isolation and Identification of Drugs*, 3rd edn. London: Pharmaceutical Press.

Sutherland SK, Tibballs J (eds.) (2001) *Australian Animal Toxins*, 2nd edn. Melbourne, Australia: Oxford University Press.

Williamson JA, Fenner PJ, Burnett JW, Rifkin JF (eds.) (1996) *Venomous and Poisonous Marine Animals: A Medical and Biological Handbook*. Sydney, Australia: University of New South Wales.

Fire

B Marc, Compiegne Hospital, Compiegne, France

Introduction

Recent studies have concluded that house fires, which are more frequent than any other fires, cause fire-related injuries in 3–5% of fires and fire-related deaths in 1–2% of fires. In all international studies, the rates of injury and death related to house fires are highest among minority and low-income populations. Children and the elderly represent a disproportionate percentage of fire victims. Victims under the age of 10 years or over the age of 70 years constitute most fire fatalities in all developed countries.

The rate of injuries is higher for fires that begin in bedrooms or living areas, that are started by smoking, defective electrical wiring, faulty or misused heaters, children or adults playing with fire, or that occur in very old houses. From various sources, cooking (1 in 3) and smoker's materials (1 in 5) seem to be the main sources of fire.

Most deaths in fire are attributed to a combination of smoke inhalation and burn injury. Moreover, half of the victims aged 18 years and older test positive for alcohol or other substances. These epidemiologic considerations lead to forensic guidelines for forensic doctors and crime-scene investigators faced with examinations of fire victims.

Etiology and Pathology of Fire Fatalities

A variety of factors may lead to fire fatalities. Most frequent are smoke inhalation and burn injury. In flame burns, there is actual contact between the body and the flame, with scorching of the skin progressing to charring. Flash burns are caused by initial ignition from flash fires that result from the sudden ignition or explosion of hydrocarbon fuels or fine-particulate material. Typically, the initial flash is of short duration, a few seconds at most. All exposed surfaces are burned uniformly. If the victim's clothing is ignited, a combination of flash and traditional flame burn occurs. Extremely high radiant-heat temperatures can cause burns in seconds. Air temperatures above $1500\,°C$ will cause second-degree burns on bare skin in less than 10 ms.

The extent of the burn is indicated as a percentage of total body surface area affected by thermal injury. This is determined by the classic "rule of nine": the head (9% of body surface), the upper extremities (each 9%), the front of the trunk (18%), the back (18%), each lower extremity (18%), and the perineum (1%).

Burns are also described according to their characteristics as from superficial to full-thickness burns. They are classified as first-, second-, third-, or fourth-degree burns. In first-degree (superficial) burns, the skin is erythematous without blisters. The skin is intact, with some injury of the epidermic cells and dilated congested vessels in the dermis. Second-degree (partial-thickness) burns can be either superficial or deep. The external appearance is a moist, red,

blistered lesion. There may be blistering. Destruction of the striatum granulosum and corneum, and edema at the dermal–epidermal layers are present. Deep second-degree burns show a complete disruption of the epidermis and destruction of the basal layer.

In third-degree (full-thickness) burns, there is coagulation necrosis of the epidermis and dermis with destruction of the dermal appendages. The extended lesions usually have a leather-like appearance. The lesions may be white, brown, or black. In fourth-degree burns, incinerating injuries extending deeper than the skin are present.

Both the size of the burn surface and the degree of burns, as well as the area in which the injury is inflicted, can play a direct role in the prognosis. Clothes worn by the burn victims can play a protective role but can also ignite and add more lesions if the clothes are highly flammable.

Toxic Gases and Death from Smoke Inhalation

Examination of victims who have died from smoke inhalation usually reveals soot in the nostrils and mouth as well as burns, and coating of the larynx, trachea, and bronchi at autopsy.

Thermal burns of the tracheobronchial tree are rare but hot air, whether dry or moist, can produce a rapidly fatal obstructive edema of the larynx. Moreover, the inhalation injuries of the lungs are frequently chemical injuries caused by combustion of toxic substances.

Absence of soot at external examination does not necessarily mean that the individual was dead before the fire started, since analysis of blood for carbon monoxide and hydrogen cyanide can reveal lethal levels.

Most victims of house fires die from carbon monoxide or at least are affected by it. In enclosed areas, in addition to carbon monoxide, hydrogen cyanide is responsible for death from smoke inhalation.

In 3857 fatalities of aviation accidents, occurring from 1991 to 1998, 41% were associated with fire, whereas 59% were not related to fire. There were fewer fire-related fatalities and associated accidents in the (carbon monoxide hemoglobin or COHb $\geq$ 10% and CN($-$) $\geq 0.25\,\mu g\,ml^{-1}$) category than that in the (COHb $<$ 10% and CN($-$) $< 0.25\,\mu g\,ml^{-1}$) category (**Figure 1**).

In house-fire victims, carbon monoxide and hydrogen cyanide, singly or combined, are probably not solely responsible for the deaths that occur in badly burned victims (a minority of fire victims). In fact, the significantly higher carboxyhemoglobin in unburned or scarcely burned victims (most fire victims)

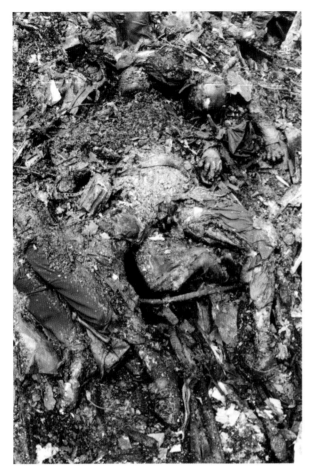

Figure 1 Accidental death by fire: bodies of victims of the Concorde air crash in August 2001 retrieved in their seats with their belts fastened (note the body with shoes and seatbelt almost intact).

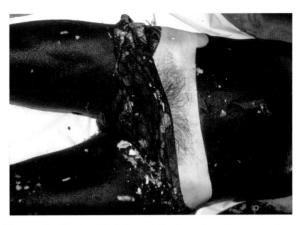

Figure 2 Smoke inhalation victim in a fire. The body does not show any major burns but its uncovered parts are darkened by soot. The skin appears white after partial removal of the underwear.

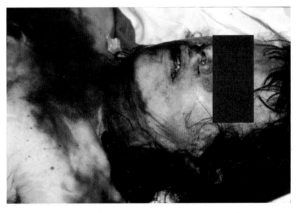

Figure 3 Smoke inhalation. The victim, poisoned by hot fumes, carbon monoxide, and hydrogen cyanide, had inhaled toxic fumes before her death. A percutaneous blood puncture allowed immediate blood analysis of her carbon monoxide and hydrogen cyanide concentrations.

indicates that carbon monoxide alone or combined with hydrogen cyanide plays a major role in the cause of death (**Figure 2**). Victims aged over 60 years often die either with carboxyhemoglobin concentrations below 60% or with a high concentration of hydrogen cyanide and a low concentration of carboxyhemoglobin. Carbon monoxide levels of 30% or 40% and even 20% may cause death if the victim suffers from an underlying disease such as severe coronary atherosclerosis.

The livor mortis, the muscles, and internal organs, as well as the blood, will have a cherry-red coloration but carboxyhemoglobin concentrations must be measured in blood sampled at autopsy.

If required, samples may be taken from the right ventricle at the scene of the fire and carbon monoxide levels rapidly obtained, following the guidelines of the US medical examiners. Results obtained for carbon monoxide concentration, using a detection method employed in emergency units, must be confirmed by reference methods. In a large series of data (from 1992 to 2002, in a population of 1.5 million inhabitants), in collaboration with a French national reference laboratory, first results have been confirmed by autopsy samples analyzed using a reference method (**Figure 3**). Their results give accurate answers to two questions: (1) Could death have occurred before the fire began? (2) Did the victims die from smoke inhalation?

A complete external examination of the body takes place near the scene of the fire. According to the results, criminal or fire investigations can immediately follow, keeping as many options open as possible for the police inquiry.

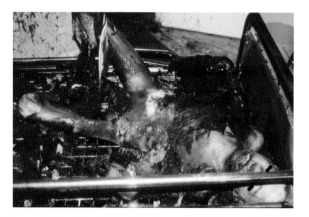

Figure 4   Accidental death by fire: a disabled man in bed was unable to escape from flames. Death was attributed to extensive burns in a living person at the time of fire. The victim's blood carbon monoxide concentration was high, but not lethal: his carboxyhemoglobin level was 32%.

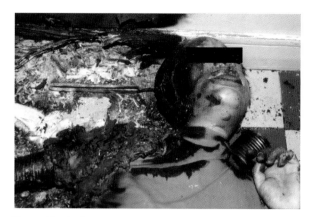

Figure 5   Accidental death by fire: aerosol burning with flash fire on the left side of the skull, face, neck, and shoulder.

Accidental Deaths by Fire

Accidental deaths by fire mostly involve children and elderly people playing with or using matches and lighters. Disabled adults are often involved in accidents with fire, as they may be unable to escape if a fire begins (**Figure 4**). Alcohol-related fires are also frequent in cases of alcoholic smokers (causing a fire in bed) or alcoholics using, for example, a fuel heater. Electric faults in old houses or renovated ones are also frequent. Electric faults may occur in industrial areas where high-voltage current is used. In car fires, often after a traffic accident, fire involves flammable hydrocarbon liquids. The flash point of hydrocarbons is the temperature at which sufficient fuel has evaporated to sustain a brief flash of fire, often started by an electrical device in the car. With hydrocarbon fuels, it is the vapors from evaporation that burn, not the fuel. When the vapor ignites, it raises the temperature of the hydrocarbon, causing increased and rapid evaporation of fuel and thus sustaining the fire. The flame in a flash fire moves out in all directions from the point of ignition. The temperature in flash fires from hydrocarbon fuels is 500–975 °C. Within a very short time of ignition, the oxygen level falls dramatically while carbon dioxide and carbon monoxide gases increase.

Fires in confined spaces such as a room can produce a phenomenon called a flashover, often involving a gas heater or device. Once a fire starts, it produces radiant heat, hot gases, and smoke. Initially, the fire and hot gases begin to heat the ceiling and adjacent upper walls and then objects in the lower portion of the room. In turn, the combustible materials in the room begin to give off flammable gases.

Adults may also be involved in accidents caused by the flammability of many aerosol cosmetics and household products; this can be attributed to the use of hydrocarbon propellants in combination with alcohol solvents. Products such as hairspray, deodorants, air fresheners, bug bombs, tire sealant, solvents, paints, and cleaners are propeled out of their aerosol gases, many of which contain propane, butane, isopropane, or isobutane. All these common products can generate dense, flammable vapors, creating a path for fire or explosion. When vapors spread throughout an enclosed space, they are subsequently ignited by an ignition source, and an explosion or flash fire may result. For example, a fatal case of burns by flash fire which caused the death of a 41-year-old woman when she used an air-freshener spray in a kitchen has been reported (**Figure 5**). The aerosol propellant gas consisted of a mixture of propane and butane and was ignited by the flame of a gas heater. Ignition resulted in a flash fire, extensively burning the woman.

Suicidal Deaths by Fire

Self-immolation is dramatic death by fire, and mainly occurs in adults between the ages of 20 and 40 years, who are suffering from significant mental disorders or have a history of alcohol or substance abuse. Immolation is rare. Suicide attempts usually pour a flammable liquid on themselves, generally gasoline, and set themselves on fire. The use of a flammable liquid is the most common method of immolation. The liquid container and matches or lighter are usually present at the scene. Victims should be examined for fingerprints. Generally, such suicide attempts present third-degree burns over most of their body, with the burns concentrated on the front part of the body. In a large proportion of cases, death by immolation is not immediate and parasuicides may be taken to intensive-care burn units. A particular pattern of suicide can be evidenced by miniepidemics of suicide, influenced by local or national events or by mimicking the method of suicide. Clusters of suicide have been well documented in particular communities.

The medical examiner at the fire scene or the forensic pathologist at autopsy should retain portions of clothing for the analysis of volatile substances. The clothing should be placed in a container with a screw-top cap since volatile material may escape through a plastic bag. Soil from under the immolation victim may also be sampled by scientific police for analysis of the presence of volatile substances. In deaths caused by self-immolation outdoors or in a large room, as in accidental flash fires, burns are the main cause of death and low carbon monoxide concentrations are found. When immolation occurs in motor vehicles, the victims often present with both anterior burns (the back is protected by the car seat) and elevated carbon monoxide levels.

Homicidal Deaths and Fire

Analysis of inflammable substances to determine whether death has occurred before or after burning is of paramount importance for judicial inquiries. Carboxyhemoglobin saturation and paraffin hydrocarbons can be detected in the left-heart blood, when burning has been the cause of death. In contrast, very low carboxyhemoglobin saturation and the absence of hydrocarbons in the left-heart blood determine that the victim was set on fire after death, in an attempt to dissimulate that death had occurred before. Interpretation of accelerants in the blood of cadavers found in wreckage after fire is important to decide whether accelerants containing petroleum components had been used and whether the cadavers had been exposed to fire before or after death. Accelerants in the blood of cadavers found after fire are analyzed by a combination of gas chromatography and mass spectrometry (GC–MS) in cases where accelerants are suspected of being used to start a fire. In homicidal deaths, where victims are burned to hide the method of death, accelerants cannot be detected in the blood, soot cannot be found in the airways, and carboxyhemoglobin concentrations are not higher than those found in smokers. When soot cannot be detected by the naked eye in the airways of a victim found in the debris of a fire, when the carboxyhemoglobin concentration in the

blood is no higher than in a smoker, the analysis of accelerants in the blood seems to be helpful in determining the cause of death and in confirming whether inflammables were used.

Identification of Fire Victims

Identification of deceased fire victims may be simple as, in many fire deaths, thermal injuries to the body are poor: death is caused by smoke inhalation. In such victims, identity can readily be established by personal identification (hair, teeth, tattoos, scars), photographs, and fingerprints. If a body is destroyed to such a degree that facial structures are mutilated and no fingerprints can be obtained, ante- and postmortem comparisons need to be made. It must be stressed that antemortem elements are fundamental for any reliable identification, using accurate comparison of various elements ante- and postmortem. Positive identification of victims is done by comparing ante- and postmortem criteria: scars and tattoos (**Figure 6**), jewelry, radiographs, dental radiographs, and DNA probes if necessary.

Dental identification is carried out by a forensic odontologist, using ante- and postmortem documents, dental charts, and X-rays of the jaws compared with the dental X-rays and charts of the individual who is believed to be the deceased. Radiography of jaws and teeth can provide one of the most reliable sources of information for comparison between ante- and postmortem conditions leading to definitive evidence in cases of identification since teeth and dental restorations are resistant to destruction by fire and are therefore very important in identification.

At autopsy, X-rays can be obtained to compare the postmortem X-rays with antemortem X-rays of the suspected individual, searching for a past fracture, an orthopedic material, and any bone pathology. Various radiographic examinations can provide a reliable source of comparison between ante- and postmortem conditions. Fractures, metal material, and peculiarities may be accurate criteria for postmortem identification.

Nowadays postmortem forensic identity uses polymerase chain reaction (PCR) to identify fire victims. To identify carbonized corpses and victims of large accidents, the analysis requires relatives of crash victims to give blood for analysis. DNA extracted from blood from the cardiac chamber or from any human remains of the decedent is analyzed using PCR and the results from all loci typing of the corpse are then compared with that of the alleged biological parents, which would confirm genetic compatibility.

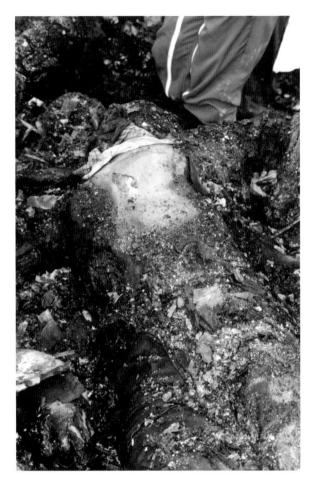

Figure 6 Large blue tattoo on the skin of the trunk of a crash fire victim: Concorde air crash in August 2001.

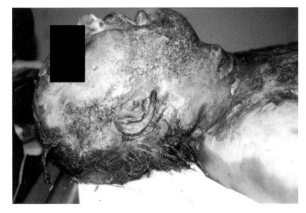

Figure 7 A homeless alcoholic, found dead in a fire, was extremely drunk (blood ethanol concentration: 2.10 g l^{-1}).

Autopsy Findings in Fire Victims

Mortality is predominantly determined by the total body surface area burned and by inhalation injury. Inhalation burns can be diagnosed clinically and confirmed by means of autopsy: upper-airway, major-airway, and parenchymal burns. Major-airway burns are always seen in conjunction with either upper-airway or parenchymal injury. Extensive surface burns, parenchymal injury – and secondary pneumonia if the victims survive a short delay – all contribute to the significant mortality.

Fatal residential fires account for 10% of all accidental deaths in developed countries, with one-fourth of the deaths involving elderly people. Significantly more fires killing elderly people were caused by faulty or misused electrical items in the house, particularly electric blankets and heating devices. The fire-related fatality rate is highest among older persons. Alcohol is not a factor in fatal fires involving older adults. This differs from fatal fires involving the young and middle-aged adults. Ethanol or substance use

may increase the risk of fire-related injury or death (**Figure 7**). From the records of all fatalities from fire reported to the US state medical examiner's office, blood assay results for ethanol were positive in 29.5% of fatalities of fire, and blood or urine assay results for substances of abuse were positive in 14.6% of fatalities. The most commonly detected illicit substances were cocaine, benzodiazepines, barbiturates, and cannabinoids. Forty percent of all the fatalities due to fire involved persons younger than 11 or older than 70. In contrast, 75% of drug-positive fatalities and 58% of ethanol-positive fatalities in fire involved persons between the ages of 21 and 50, suggesting that inebriation may impair the ability to escape from fire. Substance abusers in mid-life are at higher risk of injury or death in a fire.

A not uncommon external examination and autopsy finding is a skull fracture visible on the carbonized skull of a cremated corpse. Extensively burned bodies can show defects of the cranial bone. The question arises whether the fracture is caused by a gunshot wound. Reconstruction of the cranial remains with detached parts of the tabula externa can provide evidence that the suspicious defect can be classified as a heat-induced postmortem artifact.

Uncompleted cremations of bodies in fires are usually associated with fractures. In an intense fire, the external table of the cranium shows fissures or the sutures burst. Then the cranial vault is largely fractured, with the external table beginning to fragment: once the calvarium is burned away, a blackened brain is exposed. The facial bones are also calcined and disintegrate if the fire is still burning. Similarly, the skin of the anterior part of the trunk is fully burned and shows the anterior part of the ribs with the sternum and costal cartilage burned. The open thoracic and abdominal cavities expose blackened internal organs. After a longer delay, the exposed ribs are further calcined. In regard to the extremities, the forearms are generally reduced to their proximal portions at the same time as the cranium is fractured. Similar phenomena take place on the legs.

The diagnosis of fractures needs to be carefully evaluated since real traumatic injuries may also be encountered. They involve frightened people jumping from a height to escape fire and victims injured or killed by a falling wall or furniture in an accidental fire, but may also involve homicide victims whom their perpetrators wish to destroy in a fire lit after their death.

See Also

Anthropology: Cremated Bones; **Body Recovery**; **Fire Investigation, Evidence Recovery**; **Injury, Fatal and Nonfatal:** Blunt Injury

Further Reading

Barillo DJ, Goode R (1996) Fire fatality study: demographics of fire victims. *Burns* 22: 85–88.

Barillo DJ, Goode R (1996) Substance abuse in victims of fire. *Journal of Burn Care and Rehabilitation* 17: 71–76.

Baud FJ, Barriot P, Toffis V, et al. (1991) Elevated blood cyanide concentrations in victims of smoke inhalation. *New England Journal of Medicine* 325: 1761–1766.

Chaturvedi AK, Smith DR, Canfield DV (2001) Blood carbon monoxide and hydrogen cyanide concentrations in the fatalities of fire and non-fire associated civil aviation accidents, 1991–1998. *Forensic Science International* 121: 183–188.

DiGuiseppi C, Edwards P, Godward C, Roberts I, Wade A (2000) Urban residential fire and flame injuries: a population based study. *Injury Prevention* 6: 250–254.

Di Maio VJ, Di Maio D (2001) Fire deaths. In: *Forensic Pathology*, 2nd edn., pp. 367–387. Boca Raton, FL: CRC Press.

Istre GR, McCoy MA, Osborn L, Barnard JJ, Bolton A (2001) Deaths and injuries from house fires. *New England Journal of Medicine* 344: 1911–1916.

Iwasaki Y, Yashiki M, Kojima T, Miyazaki T (1998) Interpretation of accelerants in blood of cadavers found in the wreckage after fire. *American Journal of Forensic Medicine and Pathology* 19: 80–86.

Marc B, Blanchet P, Boniol L (2001) Domestic aerosol and flash fire: warning from a fatal case. *Burns* 27: 783–784.

McGwin G Jr, Chapman V, Rousculp M, Robison J, Fine P (2000) The epidemiology of fire-related deaths in Alabama, 1992–1997. *Journal of Burn Care and Rehabilitation* 21: 71–73; discussion 74.

Rogde S, Olving JH (1996) Characteristics of fire victims in different sorts of fires. *Forensic Science International* 77: 93–99.

Whitelock-Jones L, Bass DH, Millar AJ, Rode H (1999) Inhalation burns in children. *Pediatric Surgery International* 15: 50–55.

Drowning

D J Pounder, University of Dundee, Dundee, UK

Circumstances of Death

The majority of drowning victims are young adults and children who die accidentally. Among adults, males predominate, and there is a strong association with alcohol consumption. Homicidal drowning is uncommon and requires physical disparity between the assailant and the victim or a victim incapacitated by disease, drink, or drugs, or a victim taken by surprise. Disposal of a corpse in water may be attempted where the victim has already been killed by another means. In some cultures, drowning is a common method of suicide. In suicidal drowning, some clothing may be left in a neat pile close to the water, weights may be tied to the body, or the pockets filled with stones. The hands or feet are sometimes tied together, and an examination of the ligatures will establish whether they could have been tied by the deceased. There may be concurrent use of other suicide methods, such as alcohol or drug overdose or slashing of the wrists. Persons attempting suicide by jumping from a bridge or a cliff into water may suffer injuries from impact against rocks or the water itself. Impact with the water can produce severe injuries, including fractures of the ribs, sternum, and thoracic spine, and lacerations of the heart and lungs. Diving into shallow water may result in an impact of the forehead against the bottom with resultant hyperextension of the head and loss of consciousness. Common autopsy findings are hemorrhage into the deep muscles of the neck, with or without associated fracture of the cervical vertebrae and primary-impact bruises and abrasions on the face or forehead.

The investigation of a death in a domestic bath includes consideration of drowning. It is critical to establish the position of the body as found, the level of the water, and whether the nose and mouth were truly under the water. Unconscious persons can drown in quite shallow water as long as it is sufficiently deep to cover the nose and mouth. Unconsciousness following an epileptic seizure, a cardiac arrhythmia arising on the basis of coronary artery disease, the consumption of alcohol or drugs, or a minor head injury from a fall may lead to drowning in the bath. Suicide by drowning in the bath is uncommon; victims are often found face down and partly or fully clothed. Homicidal drowning in the bath is rare. The domestic bathroom presents hazards other than drowning, such as electrocution and carbon monoxide poisoning from faulty heaters.

Most diving fatalities are recreational scuba divers and snorkelers. Scuba is an acronym for a self-contained underwater breathing apparatus, which allows the diver to reach depths not usually attained by skin divers. The commonest causes of death are drowning and barotrauma. If drowning is the terminal event, it is important to identify potential underlying causes: natural disease, trauma, fatigue, panic, equipment problems; environmental factors, such as current instability; and causes of a decreased level of consciousness, such as nitrogen narcosis, intoxication, oxygen toxicity seizure, and hypercapnia. Amongst snorkelers, unconsciousness due to breath-holding following hyperventilation, sometimes loosely termed "shallow-water blackout," is a common cause of drowning. In divers using compressed gases, pulmonary barotrauma and cerebral air gas embolism (extraalveolar air syndrome) represent the next largest group of fatalities after drowning. In a diver who makes an uncontrolled ascent without exhaling, the volume of lung gas expands as the ambient pressure falls, and if the diver does not exhale, air is forced from the alveoli into the pulmonary circulation, to the heart, and then into the cerebral circulation. The characteristic history is of the diver coming to the surface rapidly, crying out, and then losing consciousness within minutes.

Pathophysiology of Immersion

The normal physiological effects during head-out immersion in thermoneutral water are a result of the hydrostatic pressure of the water on the body. Overall, there is a significant increase in the work of breathing, but from a practical viewpoint there is little evidence that these changes cause difficulty in a healthy individual. However, a sudden fall in skin temperature resulting from sudden immersion in cold water initiates a group of cardiorespiratory reflexes known as the "cold-shock" response. The respiratory response is an initial gasp of 2–3 l in an adult, followed by uncontrollable hyperventilation, and a sensation of breathlessness. This makes swimming very difficult and is thought to be a major causative factor in the failure to swim effectively in cold water. Additionally, the maximum breath-holding time is reduced to less than approximately 10 s. As a result, in choppy or turbulent water, there is a significant chance of aspiration of water. The cardiovascular response is an immediate increase in heart rate and cardiac output, which may induce a cardiac arrhythmia, particularly in middle-aged or elderly people with cardiovascular disease. These factors explain why drowning may occur at short distances from safe refuge, even among good swimmers.

A diving response characterized by apnea, generalized marked peripheral vasoconstriction, and bradycardia is initiated by immersion of the face in cold water. The diving response found in humans is similar to that found in diving mammals but quantitatively less marked, with the cold-shock response predominating in the majority of normally clothed adults. Nevertheless, about 15% of people do show a profound reaction, and this percentage increases with the use of protective clothing, which prevents rapid cooling of the majority of the body but leaves the face exposed to the cold stimulus. In these circumstances, the competing influences of the cold-shock and diving response reflexes cause a variety of cardiac arrhythmias. Swimming appears to be a common activity that triggers an arrhythmia in individuals with familial long QT syndrome. This may account for some otherwise unexplained drowning in children and young adults. Molecular testing for the genetic abnormality can be performed on autopsy tissues, whether fresh or archived.

Prolonged immersion in cold water carries the risk of hypothermia, defined as a deep body temperature less than 35 °C. During head-out immersion in laboratory conditions, the deep body temperature of the average adult wearing outdoor clothing falls to 35 °C after 1 h in water at 5 °C, after 2 h in water at 10 °C, and after 3–6 h in water at 15 °C. However, because of the rich supply of blood vessels to the scalp that do not vasoconstrict in the cold, heat loss from the unprotected head may be enhanced in open water by forced convection and evaporation, thus increasing the rate of body cooling considerably. As core temperature decreases to less than 34 °C, consciousness becomes impaired and aspiration of water is likely to occur. Cardiac arrest from ventricular fibrillation may occur at deep body temperatures less than 28 °C and asystole at 24–26 °C.

Pathophysiology of Drowning

Drowning was originally conceived as suffocation due to the mechanical obstruction of the airways by liquid. Animal models of drowning, studied during the 1930s, suggested that drowning induced significant fluid shifts and electrolyte abnormalities that were dependent on the osmolarity of the fluid that was aspirated. Subsequent studies of human drowning fatalities and survivors suggested that electrolyte abnormalities were not so great. Consequently, the relative importance of mechanical airways obstruction and fluid and electrolyte shifts in the pathophysiology of human drowning deaths is unclear.

After inhaled water enters the alveolar spaces of the lungs, fluid and electrolyte shifts should occur along osmotic and concentration gradients between the alveolar fluid and the blood. Fresh water is hypotonic and hyponatremic relative to blood, with the result that the inhalation of fresh water leads to movement of water from the alveoli into the blood and of sodium from the blood into the alveoli. The result is hemodilution, hypervolemia, hyponatremia, and hemolysis with associated hyperkalemia. By contrast, sea water, which is very hypertonic relative to blood, results in water movement from blood into the alveoli and movement of sodium, chloride, and magnesium from the alveoli into the blood. Consequently, there is hemoconcentration, hypovolemia, and hypernatremia.

Both fresh water and saltwater damage alveoli, destroy surfactant, and induce pulmonary edema with the transudation of protein-rich fluid into the alveolar spaces. There is decreased lung compliance and ventilation–perfusion mismatch so that blood flows through underventilated portions of the lung. The result is noncardiogenic pulmonary edema and hypoxia with secondary metabolic acidosis. It is these general effects of aspiration of water, rather than fluid and electrolyte shifts, that appear to dominate the pathophysiology of human drowning when contrasted with animal models.

The description of the various phases of drowning is based on animal experiments in which the animals were completely submerged and unable to break the surface. The initial submersion is followed by an immediate struggle and sometimes inhalation of water. Breath-holding lasts until carbon dioxide accumulation stimulates respiration, resulting in the inhalation of water, gulping of water, coughing, and vomiting. Loss of consciousness rapidly follows and is associated with involuntary respiratory movements with aspiration of water. Convulsions may occur. Death comes after some minutes. These phases of drowning observed in animal studies have been extrapolated to human fatalities generally but are probably only applicable to individuals who suddenly find themselves submerged and unable to break the surface of the water. Many humans drown when there is no eyewitness evidence of any struggle.

Bodies Recovered from Water

The investigation of presumed drowning is a challenge because the mechanism of death in drowning is neither simple nor uniform, and the circumstances of drowning introduce more variables. Furthermore, not every body recovered from water is a victim of drowning. In practice, these deaths present as a generic problem of a body recovered from water and give rise to a set of generic questions to be answered by the investigation. These questions are as follows:

1. Did death occur before or after entry into the water (i.e., was the victim alive or dead at the time of entry into the water)?
2. Is the cause of death drowning? If not, what is the cause of death?
3. Why did the victim enter the water?
4. Why was the victim unable to survive in the water?

In order to resolve these issues, it is necessary to correlate information about the circumstances preceding the death, including the past medical history of the decedent, the circumstances of recovery of the body from the water, and the autopsy and associated laboratory analyses. Unfortunately, there are no autopsy findings which are pathognomonic of drowning. Therefore, obtaining proof that the victim was alive on entering the water and excluding natural, traumatic, and toxicological causes of death are critically important. Although some autopsy findings are characteristic of drowning, the diagnosis is largely one of exclusion and depends highly on the quality of the broader investigation.

All bodies recovered from water show a spectrum of postmortem artifacts resulting from immersion. These changes will occur in any corpse immersed in water, irrespective of the cause of death. The most common immersion artifact is maceration of the skin, which becomes blanched, swollen, and wrinkled, as a result of increased hydration of the epidermis. Maceration is first apparent in the skin of the fingerpads and then appears on the palms, backs of the fingers, and back of the hand, in that order. When fully developed, it is most striking on the palms and soles. In warm water, the early changes can be seen within an hour. Generally, obvious changes occur within 24–48 h, but the process may be delayed for several days in very cold water. With the development of putrefaction, the epidermis, including the nails, peels off like a glove or a stocking. Fingerprints may be easily prepared from the glove of epidermis. The remaining exposed dermis will yield a reverse fingerprint, which is technically much more difficult to obtain. Scars and tattoos are readily seen in the exposed dermis. Occasionally, chromogenic bacteria (*Bacillus prodigiosus* and *B. violaceum*) invade the dermis after a period of at least 1–2 weeks' immersion and produce patterns of pigmentation, giving the impression of tattoos. Cutis anserina, or goose-skin, is another common immersion artifact seen in freshly recovered bodies. This appearance is a roughening or pimpling of the skin as a result of rigor mortis of the erector pilae muscles associated with the fine hairs of the skin. It is most prominently seen on the thighs. It is of no diagnostic significance, and no importance should be attached to it.

A body in water will usually sink. Some bodies float because the specific gravity of a corpse is close to that of water and small variations, such as from air trapped in clothing, have a considerable effect on buoyancy. Having once sunk to the bottom, the body will remain there until putrefactive gas formation decreases the specific gravity of the body sufficiently to create the buoyancy that allows it to rise to the surface and float. Heavy clothing and weights attached to the body may delay but will not usually prevent the body from rising. The principal determinant of the rate of putrefaction is the temperature of the water, so that in deep, very cold water the body may never resurface because there is no appreciable putrefaction. In the water, a body normally floats face-down with the head, arms, and legs lower than the torso. Consequently, livor mortis (hypostasis) is most prominent in the head, neck, and anterior chest. Putrefactive changes, when they develop, are most prominent within these areas of lividity.

Having sunk to the bottom, a body drifting along the water bed or being washed ashore will sustain a pattern of postmortem injuries, reflecting its head-down floating position. Postmortem abrasions are typically found over the forehead, the prominent points of the face, the anterior trunk, the backs of the hands, and the fronts of the lower legs. A wide range of other injuries may be produced by the body battering against rocks or by passing watercraft in navigable waters. The body may be attacked by sharks, small fish, and other fauna. The soft parts of the face are particularly vulnerable to fish and crustaceans. Postmortem injuries may be inadvertently inflicted during the recovery of the body using grappling irons, hooks, and ropes. Postmortem injuries in areas of dependent lividity, such as the face, ooze blood, mimicking antemortem wounds.

Pathology of Drowning

Some autopsy findings are typical of drowning but are nonspecific and not universally present. None are pathognomonic of drowning. The concurrent observation of foam around the nose and mouth, frothy fluid in the airways, and emphysema aquosum with overlap of the medial edges of the two lungs is very strongly supportive of a diagnosis of drowning but may be found in only 10% or so of cases. The frequency of these observations decreases significantly with an increasing time of postmortem immersion, as a consequence of developing putrefaction. The fine white froth or foam may be seen exuding from the mouth and nostrils and is found in the trachea and main bronchi. Sometimes it is tinged with blood, imparting a pink

color. The foam is a mixture of air, mucus, protein-rich pulmonary edema fluid, and, to a lesser extent, inhaled water, all whipped up by respiratory efforts. Thus, it is a vital phenomenon. However, it is not specific to drowning and is found in other instances of severe pulmonary edema, such as acute heroin overdose, congestive cardiac failure, and neurogenic pulmonary edema. In a body in water the foam persists until it is destroyed by putrefaction, which produces in turn pseudofoam of reddish-brown malodorous fluid containing bubbles of putrefactive gas, a finding of no diagnostic significance.

Emphysema aquosum (emphysème hydroaérique) is the second autopsy finding that is characteristic but not pathognomonic of drowning. Inhalation of the drowning medium, as well as reactive pulmonary edema and the struggling breaths of the victim, results in overinflation of the lungs and air trapping in the alveoli by fluid in the bronchial tree. The lungs appear ballooned, voluminous, and bulky. As a result, overlap of the medial edges of the two lungs is seen on removal of the breastplate at autopsy. The pleural surface of the lungs has a marbled appearance with gray-blue to dark-red areas that are interspersed with pink and yellow-gray zones of more aerated tissue. The lungs feel doughy and pit on pressure. On sectioning there is a flow of watery fluid. Although subpleural petechiae are rare, larger ecchymoses are sometimes seen, most often on the interlobar surfaces of the lower lobes. Subpleural bullae, which may be hemorrhagic, are occasionally found. These hemorrhages are a consequence of rupture of the alveolar walls, which is also the cause of blood tingeing of any foam in the airways. All of these findings in the lungs, although characteristic of drowning, may also be seen in cases of severe acute pulmonary edema from any cause. The microscopic appearance, reflecting the spectrum of macroscopic appearances, varies from being suggestive of drowning to entirely normal. Overdistension of the alveoli, thinning of the alveolar septa, and compression with narrowing of the capillary network are characteristic.

Contrary to expectations, lung weights in freshwater drowning are not statistically different from lung weights in saltwater drowning. The average combined weight of the two lungs in drowning in both media is approximately 1400 g with a standard deviation of approximately 400 g. These figures indicate that, in a minority of drowning deaths, perhaps amounting to 10–15%, the lungs are not heavy and waterlogged but rather are "dry." In the past, these cases were often characterized as "dry drowning," a confusing and misleading terminology that is not recommended. In the immediate postmortem period following drowning, there is transudation of fluid from the lungs into the pleural cavity so that there is a time-dependent decrease in the lung weight and a reciprocal increase in the pleural effusion volume. Following saltwater drowning and continued immersion of the corpse for more than 3 days postmortem, there is a decrease in the combined lung and pleural effusion weights, likely the result of fluid shifts induced postmortem by the osmotic effect of the saltwater. Lung weights in drowning fatalities are significantly influenced by the gender and age of the victim, likely reflecting differences in individual physical constitution and survival times.

Material, such as sand, silt, seashells, and weeds, may be found in the airways, lungs, stomach, and duodenum of bodies recovered from water. Foreign material may enter the pharynx, trachea, and larger airways during submersion postmortem, and it is possible that small quantities may enter the esophagus and stomach. It is unlikely that foreign material will reach the terminal bronchioles and alveoli to any significant extent, if the postmortem submersion is short. Therefore, the finding of abundant foreign material generally distributed within the alveoli provides strong evidence of immersion during life, as long as the body is recovered early (i.e., within 24 h). Finding large quantities of sand in the upper airways raises the possibility of inhalation of the thick suspension of sand in sea water produced by heavy surf; death is very rapid in these circumstances. The presence of large quantities of water and contaminating debris within the stomach strongly suggests immersion during life. After submersion, the victim may attempt to breath-hold for as long as possible, and it has been shown that voluntary breath-holding can be extended by movements of the respiratory muscles and swallowing against a closed glottis. Thus, ingestion of large amounts of water is only likely to be found in those who attempted to extend voluntary breath-holding. The absence of the drowning medium in the stomach suggests either a rapid death by drowning, or a death from some other cause, such as a heart attack, while in the water, or death prior to entry into the water. Rarely, weeds, branches, and other material may be found fixed in the hand of the victim by cadaveric spasm (instantaneous rigor). This observation provides good evidence that the victim was alive and conscious at the time of submersion.

Victims struggling violently to survive in the water bruise or rupture muscles, particularly those of the shoulder girdle, neck, and chest. The hemorrhages tend to follow the lines of the muscle bundles and may be unilateral or bilateral. When external blunt-force trauma can be excluded, by the absence of skin injury or subcutaneous hemorrhage, then these muscle hemorrhages are strong indicators that the victim was alive in the water. They are found in a minority of drowning deaths, but the frequency of their observation is directly related to the care with which they are sought through dissection of the appropriate muscles. Uneven putrefaction can cause reddish patches to develop in muscles, and this may be confused with hemorrhage.

Middle-ear and mastoid air cell hemorrhages are occasionally seen in bodies recovered from water. These hemorrhages produce a blue-purple discoloration of the bone of the roof of the mastoid air cells and middle ear, which are visible after stripping off the dura mater following removal of the brain. Microscopically, there is congestion of the vessels and associated hemorrhage into the tissues of the external auditory canal, mucosal layers of the middle ear, including the eardrum, ossicles, and mastoid air cells. The pathogenesis is unresolved and may be the result of barotrauma, the irritant effects of aspiration of fluid into the eustachian tubes, or extreme congestion. Identical hemorrhages are found in cases of head trauma, electrocution, and mechanical asphyxiation, so that their presence does not constitute evidence of death by drowning.

The absence of a pathognomonic autopsy sign of drowning has led to a search for a diagnostic laboratory test. Awareness of the fluid and electrolyte shifts that may occur in drowning suggested measurement of the specific gravity of blood, plasma chloride, and plasma magnesium as possible diagnostic tests. However, these testing methods are no longer considered reliable because unpredictable changes in blood electrolytes always occur after death; postmortem fluid and electrolyte shifts occur between the drowning medium, the lungs, and the heart blood; and the relative role of fluid and electrolyte shifts in the mechanism of human drowning is unclear. Currently, the only diagnostic laboratory test for drowning to have gained widespread acceptance is the diatom test. Diatoms, or bacillariophyceae, are a class of microscopic unicellular algae of which approximately 15 000 species are known, approximately half living in fresh water and the other half in sea water or brackish water. The cell structure of diatoms is unique in that they secrete a hard siliceous outer box-like skeleton called a frustule, which is chemically inert and almost indestructible, being resistant to strong acids. The classification of diatoms is based on the structure of their siliceous valves. During drowning, smaller diatoms present in the drowning medium enter the systemic circulation, having passed through the filter of the lungs, and become lodged in tissues, such as the bone marrow, where they can be demonstrated following acid digestion of the tissues. Lung tissue is not used for the tests since it can be readily contaminated postmortem by diatoms. The diatom test for drowning relies not only on the identification of diatoms in the bone marrow, but also the identification of the same species of diatoms as found in a sample of water obtained from the location of recovery of the body. Given adequate precautions to prevent contamination, the demonstration of diatoms of the appropriate species in organs, such as bone marrow, is strong corroborative evidence of death by drowning. This is true for decomposed bodies as well as fresh bodies, provided there is no gross mutilation of the corpse.

See Also

Autopsy: Procedures and Standards; **Injury, Recreational:** Water Sports

Sudden Infant Death Syndrome

R W Byard, Forensic Science Centre,
Adelaide, SA, Australia
T O Rognum, University of Oslo, Oslo, Norway

Introduction

There have been dramatic changes in the rates of sudden infant death syndrome (SIDS) since the 1990s due to public campaigns advising parents and child carers of risk factors such as sleeping facedown (prone), cigarette smoke exposure, and use of excessive bedding. At the same time developments in autopsy and death scene examinations and attempts to standardize procedures have resulted in improved accuracy of diagnosis in cases of unexpected infant deaths. This article deals with the approach to unexpected infant deaths and typical autopsy findings that may be found in cases of SIDS.

Definition

One of the major problems is that a number of definitions of SIDS have been applied with varying degrees of rigor over the years. This means that different research cohorts may have been defined quite differently from others and it may explain in part the great discrepancies that are sometimes found in the SIDS literature.

In 1991 the National Institute of Child Health and Human Development (NICHD) convened a meeting of experts who proposed that SIDS was "the sudden death of an infant under one year of age which remains unexplained after a thorough case investigation, including performance of a complete autopsy, examination of the death scene, and review of the clinical history." The significance of this definition was the emphasis on scene analysis and history review as integral parts of the investigation of possible cases. The definition is, however, one of exclusion and does not give weight to an association with sleep or to the findings of ancillary tests such as microbiological screening, skeletal survey, toxicological evaluation, and metabolic testing. Proposals have recently been made to stratify the definition so that cases with atypical features are more clearly identified.

Historical Background

SIDS has been documented as a cause of unexpected infant death for centuries: one of the first accounts is found in the judgment of Solomon in the Bible (1 Kings 3:16–28). Initially the cause of these infant deaths was thought to be accidental or deliberate suffocation of a sleeping infant by an adult who was sleeping or lying in the same bed. Wooden frames were devised to be placed over sleeping infants, and a mother or wet nurse who was found in bed with a dead infant without such a device could be excommunicated. Given the lack of autopsy examinations and formal investigations of these deaths in previous centuries it is not possible to have any accurate picture of death rates for specific conditions. Deaths due to sepsis and undernutrition were, however, common.

Developments occurred in the later part of the twentieth century whereby researchers started to look critically at possible causes of SIDS and interrelationships between endogenous and environmental factors.

Pathological Features

Unfortunately, there are no specific findings at autopsy that enable a conclusion of SIDS to be made based purely on the pathological features. Typically, an infant whose death is eventually attributed to SIDS shows no dysmorphic features, is well nourished, and has no significant underlying illnesses or injuries. However, the features of accidental or inflicted asphyxia may be identical in infancy to those routinely found at SIDS autopsies.

Features that are often present at autopsy include petechial hemorrhages of the thymus gland (**Figures 1** and **2**), epicardium and visceral pleura (**Figure 3**), blood-tinged oronasal secretions, pulmonary congestion, and edema. While nonpathologists often claim

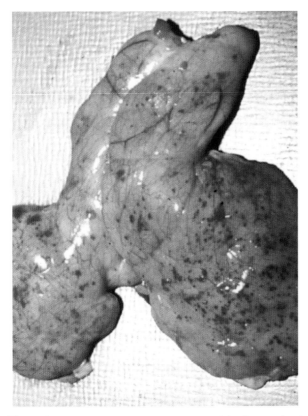

Figure 1 Scattered petechial hemorrhages of the thymus gland in a typical case of sudden infant death syndrome.

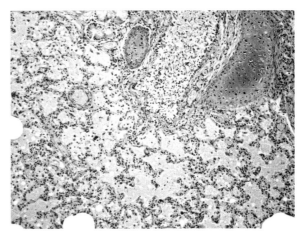

Figure 3 Photomicrograph of subpleural areas of lung demonstrating intraalveolar hemorrhage corresponding to petechiae noted macroscopically.

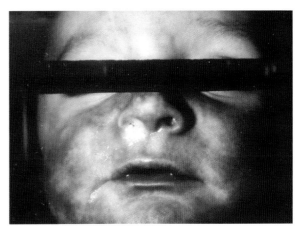

Figure 4 Foamy white pulmonary edema fluid in the nostril of a sudden infant death syndrome infant. Courtesy of WJ Klumann.

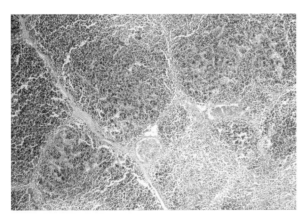

Figure 2 Interstitial hemorrhages within the thymus gland in a case of sudden infant death syndrome corresponding to petechiae noted macroscopically.

that the pathology findings are highly significant, experienced pathologists who perform autopsies on infants dying from an array of natural and unnatural conditions on a daily basis know that these findings are usually of minimal use in confirming or refuting different possible diagnoses.

Intrathoracic petechiae have been one of the most consistently described findings in infants who have died of SIDS, but are again in no way specific, as they are found in a variety of natural and unnatural deaths. They are demonstrated in 85–90% of SIDS cases and are most likely related to agonal gasping with increased negative intrathoracic pressure. The paucity of petechiae in the upper posterior portion of the thymus located in the neck above the innominate vein (Beckwith's sign) is in keeping with the effects of intrathoracic pressure changes, with protection of the cervical parts of the gland by the vein.

Oronasal secretions are usually present in SIDS infants and may fill the upper airway with frothy white pulmonary edema fluid (**Figure 4**), or may merely consist of a small amount of reddish fluid around the nostrils. The fluid derives from congested and edematous lungs and may be blood-tinged due to rupture of distal airway capillaries. Frank blood raises the possibility of an asphyxial event. Other possibilities include damage to the upper airway from attempts at resuscitation or local nasal lesions such as vascular malformations, or areas of infection.

The lungs in SIDS infants are usually quite congested and edematous due to agonal left ventricular failure. Although it has been suggested that the finding of intraalveolar hemorrhage on microscopy indicates an asphyxial event, this finding is also nonspecific and has been shown to be influenced by the time between death and the autopsy examination, attempts at resuscitation, the position of the body after death, and sampling from dependent congested areas of the lungs. Similarly, hemosiderin within the distal airways may indicate previous asphyxial episodes, but it may also occur in SIDS infants who have no significant histories and otherwise unremarkable autopsies. Hemosiderin may also not be present in infants who have asphyxiated if there have been no previous episodes. Laryngeal basement membrane thickening is not a marker for SIDS infants.

Minor inflammatory infiltrates within lung sections are not an uncommon finding in SIDS cases. While it has been suggested that these areas of inflammation are a subtle indicator of a cause of death from the interaction of the infecting organisms, toxins, and cytokines, a recent study has shown no difference in the occurrence of such foci in SIDS and control infants who had died of trauma. These inflammatory foci are, therefore, present in a range of infants. While this does not rule out an idiosyncratic response to minor infection, any possibility of a relationship to the cause of death must undoubtedly account for a complex interplay of individual, and as yet ill-understood, susceptibilities.

Unexplained or significant trauma or significant occult organic diseases preclude use of the term SIDS. If myocarditis is found, with established myocyte necrosis, the cause of death is myocarditis and not the self-contradictory "SIDS with myocarditis."

When multiple infant deaths have occurred within the same family the cases require extensive investigation. The circumstances of the deaths and a detailed family history must be obtained and meticulously reviewed as the possibilities include homicide from inflicted suffocation or poisoning, or an inherited cardiovascular or metabolic disorder.

Autopsy findings in certain inherited cardiovascular disorders such as Romano–Ward or Jervell and Lange–Nielsen syndrome may be minimal and so cause confusion with SIDS. Infants with either of these syndromes have prolonged QT intervals on electrocardiography and may develop arrhythmias and sudden death. The diagnosis depends on the demonstration of specific mutations that involve *KVLQT1(KCNQ1)*, *HERG*, and *SCN5A* genes,

and the *KVLQT1* and *minK (KCNE1)* loci on chromosomes 11p15.5 and 21q22 that are involved in potassium and sodium channels. If there is an underlying metabolic condition there may, however, be some autopsy evidence discernible. Cerebral edema with gyral flattening, and pallor of the liver, heart, and skeletal muscles may be present. Microscopically there may be storage material or fat within renal tubules, cardiac myocytes, or hepatocytes. The diagnosis usually requires intensive biochemical and molecular analyses.

Autopsy Approach

There has been an increasing awareness that the standard of autopsy examination in cases of unexpected infant deaths not only varies dramatically among countries but also within countries, and on occasion even between pathologists working within the same institution. The use of different definitions and dissection techniques with variable performance of ancillary testing has resulted in a confused picture emerging when cases have been reviewed. For this reason there have been strong moves internationally to standardize autopsy examinations for infants. Collaboration between researchers associated with SIDS International and the NICHD in the USA has led to the formulation of the International Standardized Autopsy Protocol (ISAP) (**Table 1**). This aimed at standardizing autopsy practices and improving diagnostic accuracy, providing additional information to supplement that obtained from the clinical history review and death scene examination, enhancing opportunities to reduce infant death rates, enabling more meaningful comparisons of infant death rates to be made between populations, and improving the quality of research into unexpected infant death. The ISAP has been endorsed by both the National Association of Medical Examiners (NAME) and the Society for Pediatric Pathology (SPP) in the USA. A number of other national autopsy protocols have also been developed in countries and regions such as the UK, Scandinavia, Germany, and Australia. Plans are developing for an update of the ISAP taking into consideration features that have been included or excluded from other protocols. A number of studies have validated the investigative steps that are specified in the ISAP and it has been clearly demonstrated that external examination, radiology, internal examination, histology, microbiology, toxicology, electrolyte and metabolic studies, and genetic studies have all contributed to significantly increased accuracy in diagnosis.

At around the time that the ISAP was produced there were also discussions about formalizing death

Table 1 International standardized autopsy protocol for sudden unexpected infant death

Decedent's name		Local accession number
Age/sex	Ethnicity	
Date of birth	Date/time of death	
Date/time of autopsy	Pathologist	
County/district	Country	

Final Anatomic Diagnoses

Microbiology results:
Toxicology results:
Chemistry results:

Pathologist_____

Decedent's name_____
Accession number_____
County and country_____
Pathologist_____

	Yes	No	
Microbiology Date/time:			
Done before autopsy			
Viruses: trachea, stool			
Bacteria: blood, CSF, fluids			
Fungi (discretionary)			
Mycobacteria (discretionary)			
Done during autopsy			
Bacteria: liver, lung, and myocardium			
Viruses: liver, lung, and myocardium			
Photographs, include:			
Name, case, number, county, country, date			
Measuring device color reference			
Consider front and back			
Gross abnormalities			
Radiographic studies, consider:			
Whole body			
Thorax and specific lesions			
External examination			
Date and time of autopsy			
Date and time of autopsy			
Sex (circle) male female			
Observed race (circle)			
White	Black		
Asian	Arab		
Pacific Islander	Gypsy		
Hispanic, other (specify)			

Table 1 Continued

	Yes	No	
Rigor mortis: describe distribution			
Livor mortis: describe distribution and if fixed			
Weights and measures			
Body weight			g
Crown–heel length			cm
Crown–rump length			cm
Occipitofrontal circumference			cm
Chest circumference at nipples			cm
Abdominal circumference at umbilicus			cm

Decedent's name_____
Accession number_____
County and country_____
Pathologist_____

General appearance/ development	Yes	No	No exam
Development normal			
Nutritional status			
Normal			
Poor			
Obese			
Hydration			
Normal			
Dehydrated			
Edematous			
Pallor			
Head			
Configuration normal			
Scalp and hair normal			
Bone consistency normal			
Other			
Trauma evidence			
Bruises			
Lacerations			
Abrasions			
Burns			
Other			
Past surgical intervention			
Scars			
Other			
Resuscitation evidence			
Facial mask marks			
Lip abrasions			
Chest ecchymoses			
ECG monitor pads			
Defibrillator marks			
Venepunctures			
Other			

Continued

Table 1   Continued

General appearance/ development	Yes	No	No exam
Congenital anomalies			
External			
Integument			
Jaundice			
Petechiae			
Rashes			
Birthmarks			
Other abnormalities			
Eyes (remove when indicated and legal)			
Color: (circle) brown blue green hazel			
Cataracts			
Position abnormal			
Jaundice			
Conjunctiva abnormal			
Petechiae			
Other abnormalities			
Ears			
Low-set			
Rotation abnormal			
Other abnormalities			
Nose			
Discharge (describe if present)			
Configuration abnormal			
Septal deviation			
Right choanal atresia			
Left choanal atresia			
Other abnormalities			
Mouth			
Discharge (describe if present)			
Labial frenulum abnormal			
Teeth present			
Number of upper			
Number of lower			
Tongue			
Abnormally large			
Frenulum abnormal			
Other abnormalities			
Palate			
Cleft			
High arched			
Other abnormalities			
Mandible			
Micrognathia			
Other abnormalities			
Neck			
Abnormal			
Chest			
Abnormal			

Table 1   Continued

General appearance/ development	Yes	No	No exam
Abdomen			
Distended			
Umbilicus abnormal			
Hernias			
Other abnormal			
External genitalia abnormal			
Anus abnormal			
Extremities abnormal			
Internal examination			
Subcutis thickness 1 cm below umbilicus			
Subcutaneous emphysema			
Situs inversus			
Pleural cavities abnormal			
Fluid: describe if present			
Right, ml			
Left, ml			
Pericardial cavity abnormal			
Fluid, describe if present, ml			
Other abnormalities			
Peritoneal cavity abnormal			
Fluid, describe if present, ml			
Retroperitoneum abnormal			
Petechiae (indicate if dorsal and/ or ventral)			
Parietal pleura			
Right			
Left			
Visceral pleura			
Right			
Left			
Pericardium			
Epicardium			
Thymus			
Parietal peritoneum			
Visceral peritoneum			
Upper-airway obstruction			
Foreign body			
Mucus plug			
Other			
Neck: soft-tissue hemorrhage			
Hyoid bone abnormal			
Thymus			
Weight, g			
Atrophy			
Other abnormalities			
Epiglottis abnormal			
Larynx abnormal			
Narrowed lumen			
Trachea abnormal			

Continued

Table 1   Continued

General appearance/ development	Yes	No	No exam
Stenosis			
Obstructive exudates			
Aspirated gastric contents			
Endotracheal tube tip location			
Mainstem bronchi abnormal			
Edema fluid			
Mucus plugs			
Gastric contents			
Inflammation			
Lungs	████	████	████
Weight			
Right			g
Left			g
Abnormal			
Congestion: describe location, severity			
Hemorrhage: describe location, severity			
Edema: describe location			
Severity (circle)			
Consolidation: describe location, severity			
Anomalies			
Pulmonary artery			
Thromboembolization			
Pleura abnormal			
Ribs abnormal			
Fractures			
with hemorrhages			
Callus formation			
Configuration abnormal			
Diaphragm abnormal			
Cardiovascular system			
Heart Weight			g
Left ventricular thickness			cm
Right ventricular thickness			cm
Septal thickness maximum			cm
Mitral valve circumference			cm
Aortic valve circumference			cm
Tricuspid valve circumference			cm
Pulmonary valve circumference			cm
Myocardium abnormal			
Ventricular inflow/outflow tracts narrow			
Valvular vegetations/thromboses			
Aortic coarctation			
Patent ductus arteriosus			
Chamber blood (circle) fluid clotted			
Congenital heart disease			

Table 1   Continued

General appearance/ development	Yes	No	No exam
Atrial septal defect			
Ventricular septal defect			
Abnormal pulmonary venous connection			
Other			
Location of vascular catheter tips			
Occlusive vascular thrombosis locations			
Other abnormalities			
Esophagus abnormal			
Stomach abnormal			
Describe contents and volume			
Small intestine abnormal			
Hemorrhage			
Volvulus			
Describe contents			
Colon abnormal			
Congestion			
Hemorrhage			
Describe contents			
Appendix abnormal			
Mesentery abnormal			
Liver abnormal			
Weight			g
Gallbladder abnormal			
Pancreas abnormal			
Spleen abnormal			
Weight			
Kidneys abnormal			
Weight	████	████	████
Right			g
Left			g
Ureters abnormal			
Bladder abnormal			
Contents, volume			
Prostate abnormal			
Uterus, fallopian tubes, and ovaries abnormal			
Thyroid abnormal			
Adrenals abnormal			
Right			g
Left			g
Combined			g
Pituitary abnormal			
Congenital anomalies, internal			
Central nervous system			
Whole brain weight	████	████	████
Fresh			g
Fixed			g

Continued

Table 1 Continued

General appearance/ development	Yes	No	No exam
Combined cerebellum/brainstem weight	███	███	███
Fresh			g
Fixed			g
Evidence of trauma			
Scalp abnormal			
Galea abnormal			
Fractures			
Anterior fontanel abnormal			
Dimensions			
Calvarium abnormal			
Cranial sutures abnormal			
Closed (fused)			
Overriding			
Widened			
Base of skull abnormal			
Configuration abnormal			
Middle ears abnormal			
Foramen magnum abnormal			
Hemorrhage, estimate volumes (ml)			
Epidural			
Dural			
Subdural			
Subarachnoid			
Intracerebral			
Cerebellum			
Brainstem			
Spinal cord			
Intraventricular			
Other			
Dural lacerations			
Dural sinus thrombosis			
Brain: if externally abnormal, fix before cutting			
Configuration abnormal			
Hydrocephalus			
Gyral pattern abnormal			
Cerebral edema			
Herniation			
Uncal			
Tonsillar			
Tonsillar necrosis			
Leptomeningeal exudates (culture)			
Cerebral contusions			
Malformations			
Cranial nerves abnormal			
Circle of Willis/basilar arteries abnormal			

Table 1 Continued

General appearance/ development	Yes	No	No exam
Ventricular contours abnormal			
Cerebral infarction			
Contusional tears			
Other abnormalities			
Spinal cord			
Inflammation			
Contusion(s)			
Anomalies: other abnormalities			

Decedent's name_____

Accession number_____

County and country_____

Pathologist_____

	Yes	No
Mandatory sections taken		
Skin, if lesions		
Thymus		
Lymph node		
Epiglottis, vertical		
Larynx, supraglottlc, transverse		
Larynx, true cords, transverse		
Trachea and thyroid, transverse		
Trachea at carina, transverse		
Lungs, all lobes		
Diaphragm		
Heart, septum, and ventricles		
Esophagus, distal 3 cm		
Terminal ileum		
Rectum		
Liver		
Pancreas with duodenum		
Spleen		
Kidney with capsule		
Adrenal		
Rib with costochondral junction		
Submandibular gland		
Cervical spinal cord		
Rostral medullar junction		
Pons		
Midbrain		
Hippocampus		
Frontal lobe cerebellum choroid plexus		
Oil red O stained sections, if indicated		
Heart		
Liver		
Muscle		
Discretionary microscopic sections		
Supraglottic soft tissue		

Continued

Table 1 Continued

	Yes	No
Lung hilum		
Pancreatic tail		
Mesentery		
Stomach		
Colon		
Appendix		
Testes or ovaries		
Urinary bladder		
Psoas muscle		
Palatine tonsils		
Basal ganglia		
Metabolic disorders		
Retain on filter paper in all cases		
Whole blood (1 drop) urine (1 drop)		
Hair (taped down)		
Toxicology and electrolytes		
Fuid and tissues saved for 1 year		
Whole blood and serum, save at $-70\,°C$ and $4\,°C$		
Liver, save 100 g at $-70\,°C$		
Frontal lobe, save at $-70\,°C$		
Urine, save at $-70\,°C$ Bile		
Vitreous humor		
Serum		
Gastric contents		
Analyses performed, but not limited to:		
Cocaine and metabolites		
Morphine and metabolites		
Amphetamine and metabolites		
Volatiles (ethanol, acetone, etc.)		
Other indicated by history and exam		
Frozen tissues, save at $-70\,°C$		
Lung		
Heart		
Liver		
Lymph node		

CSF, cerebrospinal fluid; ECG, electrocardiogram.

scene evaluations. This led to the sudden unexplained infant death investigation report form (SUIDIRF) prepared by the US Centers for Disease Control and Prevention.

The establishment of gold-standard protocols has been done with the full recognition that not all of the recommendations will be able to be implemented in every jurisdiction due to variations in local conditions, cultures, and resources. For those reasons protocols are designed to act as templates for local adaptation. The aim is to provide a pathologist with as much information from the scene, medical and family history, and autopsy assessment of an infant as is possible before formulating a cause of death.

An example of local adaptation of international protocols is detailed below. This describes the approach to unexpected infant and early childhood deaths that has been adopted by the pediatric forensic pathology service at the Forensic Science Centre in Adelaide, Australia, and describes the type of interaction with other agencies that may take place to facilitate understanding of the circumstances of death. Particular specimens that are taken for testing, such as for toxicology, will vary depending on local laboratory practices and so will require close collaboration with toxicologists and microbiologists.

The Investigation of Unexpected Infant and Early Childhood Death in South Australia

An Overtly Suspicious Case

Following discussion of the case with attending police officers by telephone, the pathologist usually attends the scene, unless death has been in hospital. At the scene the pathologist liaises with police officers, who will include physical evidence section, major crime, criminal investigation bureau, family violence unit, and uniformed officers. The body is then examined and preliminary assessments are made as to the presence and nature of injuries, and the possible cause and time of death.

All Other Cases

The pathologist will liaise with police officers, examining the body at the scene, or in the mortuary at the earliest possible convenience. Discussion also occurs with attending officers regarding the possible transfer of bedding, medication, feeding bottles, and scene videos to the mortuary for examination before the autopsy is performed.

In All Cases

Details are obtained for:

1. the circumstances of death and events over the preceding 24 h
2. the presenting, and any hospital, histories (particularly regarding methods of attempted resuscitation)
3. prescribed medications, and any medications or drugs at the scene
4. details of sleeping arrangements
5. the infant or child's developmental level
6. any significant or recent illnesses
7. community health center records
8. any specific police concerns.

Contact is made with the following:

1. the local child protection officer/physician for possible further background hospital and community health center information. The child protection officer/physician may also be invited to attend the autopsy to assist in the evaluation of injuries
2. the local child abuse report line for further background information and notification of the case if there are concerns for the safety of other children in the family
3. the local Sudden Infant Death Syndrome Association for additional information if SIDS support workers have attended the family
4. ambulance officers if additional information is required from the scene
5. local medical officer/nursing staff if additional medical information is required
6. local children's hospital pathologists for case discussion with possible attendance at the autopsy
7. the state coroner.

External Examination

The body is examined for external evidence of trauma and neglect. Limb deformities, swellings, bruises, lacerations, burns, abrasions, skin, and conjunctival petechiae are documented. The external auditory canals and nasal septum are examined by otoscope. Rectal/anogenital trauma is documented, or excluded, and the core temperature is taken. The palms and soles of feet are examined for burns or injuries.

Radiology

A full skeletal survey is performed at the local pediatric hospital Department of Radiology before the autopsy. A verbal report is obtained from the reporting radiologist and radiographs accompany the body back to the forensic science center mortuary if injuries have been found. (X-rays are routine for children under 2 years of age and discretionary after this, depending on history, circumstances, and external examination.)

Photography

Full external photographs are taken in addition to photographs during the autopsy (of positive or negative findings). Photographs include the front and back of the body, close-ups of the face, conjunctivae (using eyelid retractors if necessary), the inside of the lips and mouth, the dissected neck, chest, abdomen, back and buttocks, and the pleural, peritoneal, and cranial cavities (with organs *in situ* and removed).

Autopsy Protocol

The autopsy examination of the three body cavities, soft tissues, and limbs is undertaken according to a modified ISAP.

Routine Specimens (see Table 2 for checklist)

1. peripheral blood from iliac vessels, if possible, for blood toxicology. This includes common prescription and illicit drugs, and alcohol (blood will usually have to be taken from the heart in infants)
2. urine, if available, for toxicology
3. sample of liver for toxicology
4. heart blood, after searing the right atrium with a heated spatula or washing with isopropyl alcohol, for: (a) blood culture (anaerobic and aerobic) (b) storage for DNA analysis if required.

   Other specimens

1. cerebrospinal fluid for microbiology, by anterior lower spinal or posterior occipital approaches before removing the brain
2. lung and spleen swabs for microbiology
3. sample of heart for virology
4. blood spots on paper for metabolic screening
5. vitreous humor and liver for metabolic screening
6. liver, any spare blood (centrifuged for serum) and possibly gastric contents are stored in the freezer (liver and serum to be stored at −20 °C indefinitely)
7. hospital admission bloods and fluids are obtained by coronial warrant in suspicious cases for toxicological analyses.

Additional Steps to Usual Dissection and Organ Assessment

1. Measurements include crown–heel length, crown–rump length, head circumference, chest circumference, thickness of fat at anterior abdominal wall, and maximum width of anterior fontanels (normal values for age taken from standard charts are to be included in the autopsy report).
2. Skin and soft-tissue layer dissections of neck, anterior chest wall, abdomen, and back are performed. Buttocks (and possibly backs of legs) are incised for soft-tissue bruising (dissections are photographed).
3. Organs, in particular the heart with its venous and arterial connections, are examined *in situ* prior to evisceration of the body by the pathologist. The calvarium may be removed by the mortuary attendant but brain removal must be performed or supervised by the pathologist.
4. All organs are examined and weighed, including the thymus, adrenal glands, spleen, and pancreas (each lung and kidney is weighed separately)

Table 2 Checklist for cases of unexplained infant death

Case number:	**Date:**	
Attending personnel		
1. Police		[ ]
2. Physical evidence officers		[ ]
3. Child protection physician		[ ]
4. Pediatric pathologist		[ ]
5. Others (specify)		[ ]
Samples		
1. Blood/urine/liver for toxicology		[ ]
2. Blood/CSF for microbiological culture		[ ]
3. Lung/spleen swabs for microbiological culture		[ ]
4. Blood/vitreous/liver/skin for metabolic study		[ ]
5. Blood for DNA		[ ]
6. Heart tissue for virology		[ ]
7. Vitreous for electrolytes		[ ]
8. Liver/blood/gastric contents for storage (−70 °C)		[ ]
9. Filter paper storage	(a) blood spot	[ ]
	(b) urine spot (optional)	[ ]
	(c) hair (optional)	[ ]
Specimens		
1. Brain for neuropathology		[ ]
2. Cord for neuropathology		[ ]
3. Eyeballs		[ ]
Photographs		
1. Front, back, face		[ ]
2. Eyes, mouth		[ ]
3. Soft-tissue dissections		[ ]
4. Body cavities		[ ]
5. Other		[ ]
Phone numbers in cases of unexpected infant death		
Forensic technician		___
Police communications		___
Child protection pediatrician		___
Child abuse report line/crisis care		___
Pediatric pathologist		___
SIDS association		___
Ambulance officers		___

CSF, cerebrospinal fluid; SIDS, sudden infant death syndrome.

(normal weights for age taken from standard charts are to be included in the autopsy report).

5. In all cases of unexplained or suspicious infant and early childhood deaths, the brain is sent to the local Department of Neuropathology for formal examination and staining of sections for amyloid precursor protein. The spinal cord is removed and examined. If no abnormalities are detected macroscopically, routine biopsies (×3) are taken. If there is any evidence of possible inflicted injury, or unusual features in the history or presentation, the spinal cord is also referred for neuropathological assessment. In such cases the eyeballs are also removed and sections stained for hemosiderin.

6. Samples taken for histology (in addition to any abnormal tissues) include the heart (×2 sections), lungs (×5), kidneys (×2), adrenal glands (×2), pituitary gland, thymus gland, submandibular gland, tonsil, thyroid gland (including adjacent trachea and esophagus), rib (marrow and bone growth plate), liver, stomach, esophagus, small intestine, large intestine, appendix, spleen, pancreas, mesenteric fat and lymph nodes, bladder, gonad, and uterus. Brain sections include frontal lobe, centrum semiovale next to the angle of the lateral ventricle, corpus callosum and parasagittal white matter, basal ganglia, hippocampus, occipital lobe, midbrain, pons, cerebellum and dentate nucleus, and medulla. A representative lung section is also stained for hemosiderin.

7. Samples taken for microbiological assessment (following searing of organ surfaces with a heated spatula, or washing with isopropyl alcohol) include a lung swab, spleen swab, blood culture from the right atrium, and heart tissue for virological study. The middle ears are examined and swabbed if moist or obviously infected.

Organ Retention

Retention of whole organs such as the brain, spinal cord, eyes, or heart for further specialist examination requires specific permission and formal authorization by the coroner.

Special Circumstances

1. Inflicted injuries are described as follows.
   - Bite marks are swabbed for DNA, photographed and examined by a forensic odontologist.
   - Finger or hand pressure marks are swabbed for DNA.
   - Cases of possible/definite sexual assault are examined in conjunction with the local child protection officer, following the taking of radiographs. Colposcopic videos may be taken. Semen and microbiological swabs/smears of the anogenital region, mouth, and pharynx are performed.
   - Representative fracture sites detected at autopsy, or shown radiographically, are removed for decalcification and histological assessment.
   - Bruises, burns, and skin lesions are sampled for microscopy (routine histology plus staining for hemosiderin).
   - Fingernail cuttings/swabs and head hair samples are taken for future DNA analysis if required.

2. Metabolic disease: the local pediatric hospital metabolic physician is contacted as soon as possible for case discussion and receiving samples. The autopsy may need to be performed immediately if a metabolic disorder is suspected.
   Specimens taken include:
   - an alcohol-swabbed, sterile skin specimen for fibroblast culture (taken fresh and not frozen)

- fresh samples of liver, skeletal muscle, heart, and brain for snap freezing
- urine
- blood
- vitreous humor.

All specimens require immediate transfer to a metabolic laboratory for processing or optimal storage.

3. Gastroenteritis/heat deaths/dehydration: Specimens to be taken include: (1) fecal swabs for microbiology; and (2) vitreous humor for electrolyte assessment.

Conclusions

The adoption of safe sleeping recommendations has led to substantially reduced numbers of SIDS deaths in many communities. Unfortunately, despite these successes, it has become clear that not all infant deaths have been investigated to an appropriate level in the past. This has resulted in the term SIDS being used too readily for suspicious deaths, or not at all when it should have been, when basic autopsy findings have been misinterpreted. Researchers have continued to publish results based on SIDS cases that do not fulfill the basic requirements of the NICHD definition, and unwarranted significance has been placed on nonspecific pathological findings to bolster unproven hypotheses.

Agreement on a common definition of SIDS and adoption of unambiguous and comprehensive autopsy protocols are required to reduce the chances of miscategorizing infant deaths. The range of possible diseases that may be found at autopsy in infants must be appreciated by pathologists who undertake pediatric cases, and their significance must be understood so that conditions can be correctly regarded as causative, contributory, or completely coincidental to death.

See Also

Autopsy: Pediatric; **Children:** Physical Abuse; Sudden Natural Infant and Childhood Death; **Imaging:** Radiology, Pediatric, Scintigraphy and Child Abuse; **Sudden Infant Death Syndrome, Etiology and Epidemiology**

Further Reading

Arnestad M, Vege Å, Rognum TO (2002) Evaluation of diagnostic tools applied in the examination of sudden unexpected deaths in infancy and early childhood. *Forensic Science International* 125: 262–268.

Byard RW (2001) Inaccurate classification of infant deaths in Australia: a persistent and pervasive problem. *Medical Journal of Australia* 175: 5–7.

Byard RW (2003) Unexpected infant and childhood death. In: Payne-James J, Busuttil A, Smock W (eds.) *Forensic Medicine: Clinical and Pathological Aspects*, pp. 231–245. London: Greenwich Medical Media.

Byard RW (2004) *Sudden Death in Infancy, Childhood and Adolescence*, 2nd edn. Cambridge, UK: Cambridge University Press.

Byard RW, Krous HF (eds.) (2001) *Sudden Infant Death Syndrome. Problems, Progress and Possibilities.* London: Arnold.

Byard RW, Krous HF (2003) Sudden infant death syndrome – overview and update. *Pediatric and Developmental Pathology* 6: 112–127.

Byard RW, Krous HF (2004) Diagnostic and medico-legal problems with sudden infant death. In: Tsokos M (ed.) *Forensic Pathology Reviews*, vol. 1, pp. 189–198. USA: Humana Press.

Centers for Disease Control and Prevention (CDC) (1996) Guidelines for death scene investigation of sudden unexplained infant deaths: recommendations of the interagency panel on sudden infant death syndrome. *Morbidity and Mortality Weekly Report* 45: 1–22.

Fleming P, Blair P, Bacon C, Berry J (eds.) (2000) *The CESDI SUDI Studies 1993–1996*. London: The Stationery Office.

Krous HF, Beckwith JB, Byard RW, et al. (2004) Sudden infant death syndrome (SIDS) and unclassified sudden infant deaths (USID): a definitional and diagnostic approach. *Pediatrics* 114: 234–238.

Mitchell E, Krous HF, Donald T, Byard RW (2000) An analysis of the usefulness of specific stages in the pathological investigation of sudden infant death. *American Journal of Forensic Medicine and Pathology* 21: 395–400.

Rognum TO (ed.) (1995) *Sudden Infant Death Syndrome. New Trends in the Nineties.* Oslo: Scandinavian University Press.

Rognum TO, Arnestad M, Bajanowski T, et al. (2003) Consensus on diagnostic criteria for the exclusion of SIDS. *Scandinavian Journal of Forensic Medicine* 9: 62–73.

Autopsy, Findings, Adult Falls From Height *See* **Falls from Height, Physical Findings:** In Adults

Autopsy, Findings, Alcohol Use   *See* **Alcohol:** Acute and Chronic Use, Postmortem Findings

Autopsy, Findings, Asphyxia   *See* **Asphyxia**

Autopsy, Findings, Carbon Monoxide Poisoning   *See* **Carbon Monoxide Poisoning:** Incidence and Findings at Postmortem

Autopsy, Findings, Pediatric Falls From Height   *See* **Falls from Height, Physical Findings:** In Children

AVIATION ACCIDENTS, ROLE OF PATHOLOGIST

G Wagner, Medical Examiner's Office, San Diego, CA, USA

Definition

Aviation pathology is the application of traumatic pathology to flight safety. It has been defined by Mason as the comprehensive study of aviation fatalities, whereby the medical history of the casualty and the findings at autopsy can be correlated with the environmental factors, the structural or other damage to the aircraft, and the use or abuse of equipment, so that a complete picture of the accident may be formed. The objective of investigating fatal aircraft accidents is to find their causes and prevent similar accidents occurring in the future through thorough and complete investigations using a multidisciplinary team approach and multifactorial parameters.

History

The first documented application of aviation pathology in powered aircraft in the USA was the death of an army lieutenant in 1908 at Fort Myer, Virginia, during army testing of the Wright Flyer, with Orville Wright at the controls and Lt Thomas Selfridge as a passenger. The plane crashed at low altitude due to a faulty propeller. Orville survived with a simple fracture. Selfridge died of craniocerebral trauma from a skull fracture.

The German Air Force during the 1930s developed a basic scientific approach to the investigation of air crashes in World War II at the Aeromedical Research Institute in Berlin. They were also the first to incorporate protective headgear. In the USA during the 1940s, John Stapp contributed significant insight into human tolerance in short-term decelerations in a variety of sled experiments. A series of commercial air transport mishaps involving the British Comet in the 1950s and the role of the pathologist in determining causal factors led to the concept of "packaged crew and passengers" and the origins of aviation pathology as practiced today.

Principles

The pathologist is primarily concerned with the pathology and human factors in the mishap and is often able to implicate a contributory or proximal cause of the accident. This contribution to the mishap investigation occurs in seven main areas:

1. demonstration of disease in the pilot, which may be causative, contributory, or incidental to the mishap
2. circumstantial medical evidence, such as a history of psychiatric illness
3. toxicological evidence: alcohol, carbon monoxide, or drugs
4. mechanical defects manifesting as toxicological evidence, e.g., fumes in the cockpit
5. sequence of events in the mishap
6. whether the emergency was anticipated or occurred without warning
7. questions relating to survivability.

Aerospace pathology is a subset of forensic pathology and is typically practiced by forensic pathologists who also have operational qualifications such as in flight surgery or diving/undersea medicine. Operational experience and knowledge of the mission and operating procedures applied to the pathology findings and ancillary laboratory studies have enhanced our understanding of flight human factors. Following the Comet disasters, the Joint Committee on Aviation Pathology, involving the military safety centers and Armed Forces Institute of Pathology (AFIP) in the USA and Departments of Aviation Pathology in the military services of Canada and the UK was established in 1955 with the Secretariat located at the AFIP in Washington, DC, to serve as a forum for the exchange of information and ideas. Today, much of that effort is pursued in the forums of the Aerospace Medical Association and various North Atlantic Treaty Organization (NATO) working groups.

Concepts

Aircraft accidents are not random events but recurring themes with epidemiological patterns, often with specific pattern injuries identified with specific aircraft. There are unique characteristics of the flight environment that allow an investigation to focus on discoverable causes in engineering, human factors, and flight operations. In general, mishap investigation boards composed of multidisciplinary specialists pursue clues in the accident investigation to reconstruct the events based on comprehensive assessments of the aircraft and wreckage, flight operations, maintenance, crew and passengers, life support and protective equipment, and mission profile based on indepth coordinated inquiries. The format usually follows standards and recommended practices outlined in Annex 13 (Aircraft Accident Investigation)

of the International Civil Aviation Organization (ICAO), based in Montreal, Canada.

Organization of Mishap Investigation Boards

The US National Transportation Safety Board (NTSB) is responsible for investigating commercial aviation and transportation accidents in the USA and involving US carriers or aircraft overseas. The Federal Aviation Administration (FAA) has a similar responsibility in general aviation. The NTSB is an independent federal agency created in 1966 that serves as the overseer of US transportation safety with intermodal responsibilities, including railroad, highway, pipeline, marine, and civil aviation transportation. The mission of the NTSB is to determine the probable cause(s) of accidents through direct investigations and public hearings; and secondarily, through staff review and analysis of accident information, evaluations of operations, effectiveness, and performance of other agencies, special studies and safety investigations, and through published recommendations and reports to Congress. The Human Factors Group has a twofold responsibility. The first responsibility is to develop information that may assist in determining the probable cause(s) of the accident by assessing the psychological, physiological, and pathological aspects of crew performance. The second responsibility is to develop survivability factors, which include information on the crashworthiness of the aircraft's structures, seat, and restraint systems, operability of escape systems, emergency training of crew members and the effects of postcrash fire on the ability of occupants to escape from the aircraft. Similar agencies exist throughout the world. The US military has similar responsibilities relative to military aircraft mishaps. Each service has its own infrastructure, including a service safety center, to participate and review mishap investigation findings.

In mishap investigation boards (MIBs), the organization is focused on causal factors in a hazards management program involving 11 primary areas:

1. operations
2. structures
3. power plants
4. human factors
5. aircraft systems
6. witnesses
7. air traffic control
8. weather
9. flight data recorder
10. maintenance records
11. evacuation, search and rescue, firefighting.

The phases of the investigation are generally divided into five categories: (1) preliminary evaluation; (2) data collection; (3) data analysis; (4) conclusions; and (5) recommendations. Safety investigation concepts are based on a number of analytical systems: HW Heinrich's accident sequence influence, Bird and Loftus' updated domino sequence, management oversight risk tree (MORT), and multilinear events sequencing (MES). Heinrich's influence involves a domino principle of five factors: (1) ancestry and social environment; (2) fault of person; (3) unsafe act and/or mechanical or physical hazard; (4) accident; and (5) injury, each with underlying accident causes. Bird and Loftus' updated domino sequence expands on Heinrich's influence with more management parameters focused on people, equipment, material, and environment. Five factors are identified: (1) lack of control in management; (2) basic cause(s)/origins; (3) symptoms of immediate cause(s); (4) incident; and (5) people/property/loss. More recently, MORT and MES systems have been advocated as more effective analytic approaches. NTSB tends to use events and causal factor charting focused on identified systematic factors, contributing and direct factors. In these charting systems, events are occurrences, not a condition, and are precisely described, and quantified where possible and sequenced.

Litigation Focus

From a litigation perspective, aircraft accident investigation is divided between human and machine factors. Human factors include intoxication, cardiovascular pathology, carbon monoxide poisoning, hypoxia, depth perception in darkness and monocular vision, visual illusions, spatial disorientation and vertigo, operational errors, and design-induced crew error. Machine factors are focused on impact based on speed, direction of travel, angle of impact, and altitude and wreckage distribution based on scene documentation and momentum mechanics. Accident reconstruction is not equal to aircraft reconstruction but is based on the sequence of failure. Witness marks are probative evidence and include crush damage, wreckage capture position, primary and secondary impact marks, puncture and rotational marks, and smearing. Varieties of witness marks include paint transfers, paint scratches, bends, gouges and indentations, scratches and scoring, imprint transfers, and crushing. Explored airframe and system failures include propulsion, fuel system, control system, structural and mechanical failures, fatigue and corrosion, electrical systems, design, and complex automated flight controls. Identified human errors include: (1) pilot error; (2) inadequate planning; (3) failure

to plan before the flight; (4) inadequate use of checklists; (5) operations outside the norm (flight activities exceeding the safety specifications of that aircraft defined by airspeed, attitude, altitude, and G load tolerance); (6) operation with imperfect systems; (7) operation of a system incorrectly; (8) flying into bad weather; (9) operating when fatigued; (10) flying under the influence (both alcohol and drugs: illicit, prescribed and over-the-counter); (11) operating when not proficient; (12) flight crew errors; (13) air traffic controller errors; and (14) maintenance personnel errors.

Survivability Concepts that are Key to Analysis

Survivability is usually assessed by three parameters: (1) tolerable crash forces; (2) occupiable space; and (3) postcrash environment. Relative to these parameters the machine is evaluated according to the acronym CREEP, where C stands for container crashworthiness, R for restraints, E for environment, E for energy absorption, and P for postcrash environment. There are usually a number of concurrent investigations in a mishap investigation: the medical examiner/coronial inquiry, the safety investigation, and, if required, a criminal investigation. Each of these concurrent investigations has different goals and rules of discovery. The primary goals of the medical examiner or coroner are to determine the identification of the casualties, their cause of death and give an opinion on the manner of death. These are statutory death certificate requirements. As previously stated, the safety investigations are to determine the probable cause of the accident and identify correctable safety issues. A criminal investigation, usually pursued in the USA by the Federal Bureau of Investigation, is to identify culpability and pursue punitive measures.

Forensic Principles

For the pathologist, aviation accidents are often multiple-casualty incidents that require the seven basic questions in any forensic investigation to be addressed: (1) who? (2) what? (3) where? (4) when? (5) how? (6) by whom? and (7) why? In most cases, the most labor-intensive activity is the identification of the casualties for legal certification of death.

Identification

Casualty identification falls into three categories for legal certification: (1) positive; (2) presumptive; and (3) by exclusion. Positive identification is based on unique characteristics of the individual identified by pre- and postmortem comparisons of fingerprints, palm prints, footprints, dental comparisons, DNA profiling, and radiographic superimpositions. These methodologies are the preferred means of identification and in investigations usually involve two or more methodologies. Forensic odontology is the most available methodology since dentition often survives when there is otherwise significant biological degradation through decomposition, autolysis, fragmentation, and incineration. Computer dental identification databases have substantially improved the successful outcome of positive dental casualty identifications. However nuclear and mitochondrial DNA casualty identification is considered the "gold standard" for positive identifications and is frequently successful when other methodologies are inconclusive or not available. This is especially true with fragmented, commingled, and incinerated remains. In the absence of databases containing these DNA profiles or the specimens for such analysis, a presumptive template is necessary, either from personal effects such as toothbrushes and hair samples, or a family genealogical tree must be created based on DNA testing and profiling. This usually requires a conscious decision to DNA-test most, if not all, recovered individual specimens so that commingled remains can be separated and reassociated. In many aircraft mishaps there is considerable fragmentation, incineration and commingling of casualty remains. Recovery, separation, identification and reassociation of these remains usually involves a variety of disciplines. DNA profiling, now considered the gold standard for casualty identification provides the means to identify a single body from composite bodies where separated commingled remains are wrongly reassociated and assigned an identification. Comprehensive DNA testing of recovered specimens may be necessary to avoid misidentification. The expectation of success in this endeavor by the families of the deceased as well as the public makes this aspect of casualty identification expensive in time, labor, and cost. Presumptive identifications are based on class versus unique individual characteristics and include visual identification, personal effects, anthropometrics, serology, and medical conditions. Identification by exclusion requires a closed population in which all other variables have been eliminated.

Forensic Procedures and Resources

Following the identification process, which may involve an assembly-line multidisciplinary approach in mass casualties with significant coordination and information technology input, documentation of

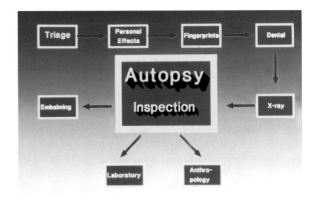

Figure 1 Diagram of medicolegal flow chart for mass-casualty incidents through autopsy and embalming.

the injuries and any preexisting medical conditions through comprehensive medical evaluation is pursued (**Figure 1**). This medical assessment involves radiographic, autopsy, and ancillary laboratory studies prior to the remains being released for embalming or cremation and final disposition to the next of kin. Resources for these mass-casualty medicolegal investigations often exceed those of the local jurisdiction and may require regional or national assets such as the temporary mortuary facilities of disaster mortuary operational response teams under Federal Emergency Management Agency or military resources such as the Dover (AFB; Air Force Base) Port Mortuary. Frequently, expertise is also available from resources such as the American Academy of Forensic Sciences (AAFS) or the National Association of Medical Examiners (NAME). Resources are often measured by the quality of appropriate facilities, including refrigeration units, radiographic capabilities, and adequate utilities and security. These are often deciding factors as to where this aspect of the investigation is completed relative to the crash site. Where possible, these two geographic requirements are colocated. The complexity of such activities requires the creation, practice, and use of a disaster plan with a coordinated command and control infrastructure.

The autopsy is a primary tool in developing the information for answering most of the forensic questions and must be supported by extensive photographic, histological, toxicological, radiographic, and diagrammatic representations of the findings, as well as the trace evidence analyses, DNA profiling, and physical anthropology studies that may be required. In general, the autopsy procedure follows that of any other forensic inquiry but usually requires additional procedures to document specific regional injuries. These procedures include a layerwise back-of-the-neck dissection (**Figure 2**), potential selective

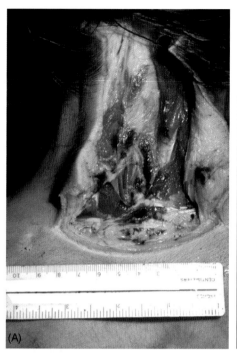
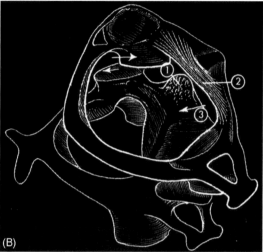

Figure 2 Back-of-neck layerwise dissection at autopsy to disclose cervical injuries. 1, lateral ligaments of the atlanto-occipital synovial membrane; 2, transverse ligament; 3, posterior atlanto-occipital membrane (a broad ligament).

angiography, examination of the spinal cord, and surgical exploration of select extremity injuries, especially those thought to be control surface-induced.

Injury Analysis and Reconstruction

Injury analysis is based on the documented gross and histological findings at autopsy supported by radiographic and toxicological evidence and is classified according to acceptable parameters into penetrating injuries, blunt-force trauma, thermal injuries, asphyxiation, drowning, hypothermia, gunshot wounds, and blast injuries. Injuries have characteristics that reflect applied force magnitude, direction, frequency, or interval, and are important in interpreting mechanism, instrumentality, time of injury, and time of death. In aviation accidents, this injury analysis is critical to reconstructing the sequence of events and human–machine interactions impacting on survivability. Crash force assessments include system trauma biodynamics and are usually characterized relative to applied force (G_z, G_x, G_y), system tolerance, and documented findings. The AFIP uses anatomical markers identified at autopsy to define likely tolerance parameters and compares that to physical evidence at the scene and crash force calculations to interpret survivability. These anatomical markers of quantifiable applied force have been developed over time and with experience and validated against data from

Table 1 Armed Forces Institute of Pathology (AFIP) morphological markers of crash forces

Observation	*g* force	Axis
Vertebral fractures	15–30	G_z, G_x
Pulmonary contusions	25–30	G_x, G_y
Rupture of atlantooccipital membrane	30–35	G_z, G_x
Laceration of aorta	50+	G_x, G_z
Transection of aorta	80+	G_x, G_z
Skull fractures	50+	G_x, G_z, G_y
Pelvic fractures	100+	G_z, G_x
Fragmentation	350+	G_x, G_z, G_y

completed mishap investigation reports (**Table 1**). These autopsy markers are force approximations and should be compared and validated against engineering data developed during the investigation and reflect the interdependent multidisciplinary requirements of such medicolegal death investigations. The most useful systems for evaluation include the vertebral column, cardiovascular system, and pelvis.

Reconstruction of the mishap sequence is possible through documented injury pattern comparisons linked to physical evidence at the scene, modeling, and "black box" data. Emphasis must be on injury patterns and specific injuries directly related to:

1. impact forces
2. time, duration, and direction of applied forces
3. cockpit or cabin configuration

4. nature of the accident and subsequent occurrences
5. occupant kinematics in the accident, particularly relating to restraint systems.

Each body portion has a tolerance, or a range of tolerances, to injury. In all, 70–80% of deaths and injuries in accidents result from head contact with structures. These kinds of statistics have driven the injury pattern analysis into two main categories: (1) diagnosis; and (2) injury prevention. In diagnosis, similarity and deviations in different accidents and in multiple casualties from the same incident become the sought-after pattern for analysis. In injury prevention, it is repetitive injury, for example, head injuries from cyclics, a control device in helicopters, in helicopter crashes, helmet loss or life support or restraint injuries; and modification of injury by environment and/or equipment.

Investigative Template

A series of questions often used by investigators to provide a basis for interpreting investigation results provides a useful template for analyses, conclusions, and if appropriate, recommendations:

1. Why did certain casualties die?
2. To what feature of the accident or of the aircraft can be attributed the escape of the survivors?
3. Would any modification of the aircraft or of its equipment have improved the chance of survival of those killed or reduce the severity of survivor injuries?
4. Would the incorporation of such modifications have a detrimental effect on any of the survivors' chances?
5. Is there any indication that the main or any subsidiary causes of the accident might have been medical in nature?

Patterned Injuries

Particular injury patterns deemed critical to this analysis include control surface injuries, restraint injuries, incapacitating injuries, penetrating injuries, such as those from intrusions, life support equipment injuries, flail injuries, and craniocervical injuries in ejections with or without helmet use. Radiographs of the casualty as recovered and while dressed as well as those obtained after undressing and cataloging of clothing, personal effects, gear, and equipment on the body may demonstrate possible causal interactions. Particular emphasis should be placed on the craniocervical segment, extremities, and the thoracoabdominal region.

Control surface injuries are specific skeletal and soft-tissue injuries of the hands, forearms, and distal lower extremities attributed to impact against aircraft control levers and pedals such as the stick, yoke, and rudder pedals (**Figure 3**). These injuries usually contain trace evidence supporting the interpretation. The importance of this series of injuries, assuming sufficient forces to create them, is to exclude in-flight crew incapacitation scenarios.

Restraint injuries reflect the type and configuration of restraints used, if any, and include abrasion/contusions of the shoulder girdle, abdomen, and pelvis. The presence of restraint injuries supports either an anticipated emergency or normal flight activities. The absence of restraint injuries in one or more persons in a multiple-casualty mishap where the majority of victims reflect these injuries suggests pursuing reasons for the "odd one out" injury pattern. The likelihood of flail injuries consisting of skeletal fractures and soft-tissue avulsions is defined by the safety norms (**Figure 4**). The margin of safety is determined by the characteristics of the aircraft design, the restraint system, and it is also determined by altitude, air speed, and attitude.

Incapacitation injuries are those that would either likely render the victim unconscious or prevent voluntary escape from the aircraft. This is particularly important in the postcrash environment if the aircraft mishap is otherwise considered survivable based on crash forces and occupiable space.

Thermal injuries are common and often complex, complicated by commingling and fragmentation. Evidence of survival is dependent on the documentation of all potentially fatal injuries and evidence of inhalation-soot in the airways, pulmonary congestion, positive toxicology findings for carbon monoxide and cyanide, as well as other potentially toxic substances. Full-body radiographs are critical. Artifacts commonly encountered include pugilistic body positions, extremity fracture/dislocations, heat amputations, epidural hemorrhages, and comminuted skull fractures. Fires are a common postcrash occurrence so injury analysis must be interpreted relative to survivability parameters. Evidence of life during the fire is dependent on the severity of documented trauma and extensive toxicology studies.

Drowning or water immersion is another relatively common postcrash environment circumstance and is a diagnosis of exclusion. The autopsy should be able to exclude other fatal injuries and perhaps explain why the occupant could not exit the aircraft because of incapitating injuries or entrapment. Hypothermia also plays an important role in immersion fatalities. Autopsy findings in drownings consist of pulmonary edema, hyperinflated lungs, pleural effusions and

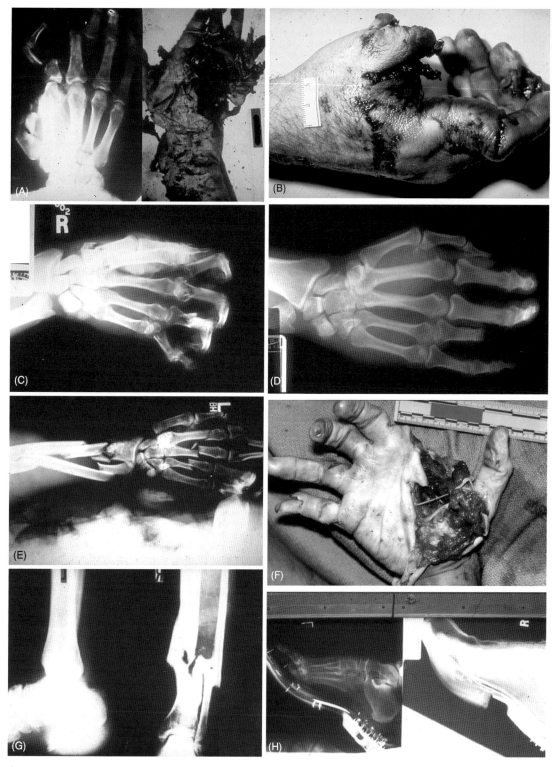

Figure 3 Hand and foot injuries including radiographs – control surface injuries. This series of photographs is of common soft tissue and skeletal injuries encountered on the hands and feet when they are in contact with aircraft controlling surfaces (rudders/pedals for the feet, yoke/control stick for the hands). The fractures are predominantly transverse rather than diagonal and are relatively uniformly spread across the bony structures. The pattern is consistent with the design of the aircraft's control surfaces. Those forces are also transmitted through the extremity to proximal joints/articulation. The most common soft tissue injuries are those to the soft tissues of the thumb and represent the thumb's usual apposition to the hand's other digits. The figures of the feet with boots on show bending of a longitudinal metal plate in the boot and separation of the sole. This finding is indicative of a force transmitted vertically through the foot. The significance of these findings are interpreted as proof of the pilot/aircrew member trying to control the aircraft at impact rather than being incapacitated (unconscious or not at the controls).

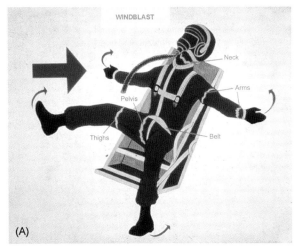

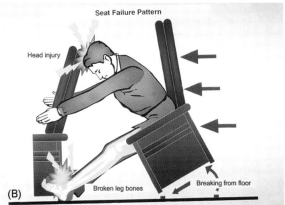

Figure 4 Classical pattern injuries. (A) Flail injuries common during high-speed ejection; (B) shows seated and restrained common injuries.

hemorrhages in the sinuses and middle ears, and possibly air embolism. Air embolism, excluding divers who fly shortly after a diving operation, is most likely found in water-immersed casualties recovered from the depths. In these cases, it is an artifact induced by the recovery ascent. Particularly in cold-water immersions, "dry drowning" may occur from laryngeal spasm.

Computer-assisted analysis of injuries has significantly improved injury analyses. A number of programs exist and allow the data to be tailored to the circumstance. This type of approach to injury epidemiology is being used with greater frequency and success. Studies done based on death certificate data indicate that, despite a reduction in the number of fatalities, the injury patterns were relatively stable. One such recent study showed that multiple injuries were listed as the immediate cause of death in 42% of fatalities, followed by head injury (22%), internal injury of thorax, abdomen, or pelvis (12%), burns (4%), and drowning (3%). Head injuries were most common amongst children. The majority (86%) died

at the scene or shortly thereafter on hospital arrival. Blunt-force trauma related to restraint and aircraft design remained the single greatest hazard identified. These kinds of study define persistent parameters of inquiry for injury reduction in design, engineering, and personal protective equipment.

Jurisdiction Issues

The documentation of injury and any preexisting disease is dependent on access to the casualty as well as to the scene and to the victim's medical and dental records. This requirement raises the issue of challenges to jurisdiction and possible conflicts between the NTSB, military services, and the local medical examiner or coroner. In the USA, there are three basic kinds of jurisdictions relative to fatal casualties: (1) exclusive federal; (2) concurrent; and (3) proprietary. In general, there are relatively few exclusive federal jurisdictions (i.e., Dover AFB, Delaware). Most investigations will fall into the concurrent jurisdiction arena where local authorities will have first right of refusal but there is concurrent federal or military interest and participation. In proprietary jurisdictions, the local authority retains control of fatalities regardless of federal or military interests (District of Columbia). Jurisdiction is also defined by the initial port of entry for deaths in international waters or air-space, and/or by treaty agreements such as those existing in NATO.

Preexisting Medical Conditions

Preexisting medical conditions are also an important aspect of the accident investigation and are classified as proximal, contributory, or incidental according to the severity of the documented condition and the overall sequence of events as defined by the safety investigation. In general, there are only three systems whose diseases can kill suddenly: (1) central nervous system (CNS); (2) cardiovascular; and (3) respiratory. These three systems deserve comprehensive pathological assessments. Histological microscopy studies supporting or expanding gross autopsy findings are important to document the presence and significance of these findings and to complement data developed from a review of available medical records, clinical laboratory, and toxicology studies. Radiographic data are particularly important in validating these conditions and should be used as appropriate in the documentation. Access to medical and dental records is mandatory in this aspect of the medicolegal investigation.

This pathology effort of the investigation is widely believed to be more subjective than most observers believe. There are three superimposable interpretative challenges: (1) mimicry; (2) superimposition; and (3) interruption. In mimicry, the results of trauma may closely mimic those of natural disease, for example, pulmonary congestion or intracranial hemorrhage. Superimposition of trauma on natural disease is problematic, especially in cardiovascular pathology and specifically in coronary artery disease. Trauma will also interrupt the course of natural disease so that the precursor condition rather than the endpoint of a disease must be defined. Much of this effort is focused on cardiovascular disease because, numerically, it appears to have a greater significance in relation to aircraft accidents. Aside from coronary artery disease, myocarditis is often identified as a causal factor. Other potentially dangerous conditions demonstrated only on microscopy include encephalitis, pneumonitis, sarcoidosis, and allergic states. Occult disease, such as epilepsy, that becomes discoverable through medical records, witnesses, and/or toxicological studies must also be considered. A more recent preexisting condition reported in passenger morbidity and mortality is pulmonary embolus from deep-vein thrombosis (DVT). Prolonged static positioning on long flights is the proposed contributing factor. Clinical molecular tests such as factor V Leiden may identify those predisposed to DVT.

Toxicology Analysis

Toxicology studies are an extremely important aspect of aircraft accident investigation. Materials from nonfatal mishaps (blood and urine) are routinely analyzed either at the FAA Civil Aeronautical Institute in Oklahoma City or for the US military at the Armed Forces Institute of Pathology in Washington, DC. Similar national reference laboratories exist in all countries. Tissues from fatal aircraft accidents are also analyzed at one of these two agencies and include blood, urine, bile, vitreous humor, gastric contents, and organ specimens. When necessary, similar studies can be carried out on muscle, bone, and hair as well as entomological specimens recovered on the remains. Blood and urine are screened for a variety of substances, including alcohol, carbon monoxide, and a spectrum of acid, basic, and neutral drugs. Confirmatory tests follow any positive blood or urine screening. These studies are then usually followed by specific organ tissue analysis to qualitate and quantitate any chemical substances present. The bulk of this analysis is done by advanced instrumentation, including gas chromatography, mass spectroscopy, high-pressure and capillary liquid chromatography, and a variety of immuno-based methodologies. Therapeutic drug screening may be crucial

in these chemical analyses either for identification purposes or for evidence of underlying preexisting medical conditions. In decomposition cases, a spectrum of alcohols, ketones, and aldehydes is present and may generally indicate that low levels of ethanol present could be an artifact. Vitreous humor analysis is useful in this circumstance since it is resistant to decomposition. Drinking and flying, while infrequent, appears to occur more often in general aviation than in commercial or military aircraft mishaps.

Fires are a common postcrash factor and in-flight fires are not unheard of, often resulting in aircraft structural damage contributing to mishap. In fatal crashes, and especially in casualties with thermal injuries, extensive toxicology studies are needed to evaluate the inhalation of fire products, particularly carbon monoxide, cyanide, and other pyrolytic chemicals. Carbon monoxide and cyanide are two substances that, when detected and linked to documented soot in the airways and thermal damage, are clear indications of a survival interval during or after the fire. Extensive chemical analysis for pyrolysis products may characterize a particular etiology or substance hazard. A high index of suspicion may be necessary to focus the chemical inquiry. Fire deaths in aircraft mishaps have not decreased in recent years despite engineering efforts to reduce risk. Fire remains a serious cause of morbidity and mortality in the air and on the ground. Heat, smoke, and toxic gases are potent causes of morbidity and mortality and continue to attract considerable interest in the aviation community. Recently, a number of investigators have questioned the importance of cyanide in fire deaths, especially since cyanide may be produced as well as metabolized in postmortem tissues. Additional future studies will hopefully clarify this issue.

Forensic Biochemistry

Biochemical postmortem analysis may be required to substantiate certain physiological conditions suspected beyond those addressed in toxicology studies. Many blood enzymes become unstable with an increased postmortem interval. Nonetheless, more expansive use of the clinical laboratory may be justified depending on the case and particular issue. Specimens used for evaluation include whole blood, serum, bile, urine, cerebrospinal fluid, and vitreous humor.

Scene Investigation

The scene investigation should be part of the pathologist's checklist and is particularly useful when linked to the assigned mishap board flight surgeon or aviation medical examiner, as well as

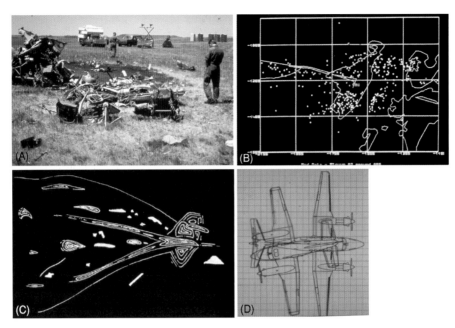

Figure 5 A typical crash site and charting.

other representatives from flight operations, maintenance, or engineering. This provides a broad-based multidisciplinary investigation platform. Furthermore, knowledge of the crash site characteristics is often useful in the subsequent injury interpretations resulting from the pathologist's findings. Recovered body location versus assigned seat locations and aircraft configuration provides insight into the crash sequence and may give clues to trauma etiology. The crash site, once secured, is typically divided into segments and coordinated recovery is correlated with segment and location for biological material, power plant, instrumentation and controls, ordnance, and aircraft structure (**Figure 5**). Ongoing security is critical as well as protection against hazardous materials. This risk appears greater today with the use of composite materials and is required by OSHA (Occupational Safety and Health Administration) or similar regulations. Access will not be permitted until the crash site and wreckage are rendered safe by explosive ordnance disposal, firefighters, and utility personnel. Heavy equipment is usually needed for wreckage recovery and transportation. This equipment and its operation provide additional hazards. Postcrash fires may delay the recovery of human remains and sifting through the wreckage, prolonging evidence retrieval.

Aerial photography, including infrared color photography, may provide valuable clues to wreckage distribution, witness marks, and impact parameters. Photographic and diagrammatic representations are essential and should be accurate, identified, and comprehensive. Success in these operations is often defined by the location and nature of the crash site and the availability of resources to exploit search-and-rescue and search-and-recovery efforts. In the Arrow Air crash in Gander, Newfoundland, Canada, in December 1985 that killed all 256 persons aboard, including 247 service members returning from the Sinai to Fort Campbell, Kentucky, the crash site on the side of a mountain needed to be excavated in February to recover all the remains and aircraft. This effort required the involvement of the people of Gander, the Royal Canadian Mounted Police, and the US Army with units from Fort Bragg, North Carolina and Fort Campbell, Kentucky, as well as the AFIP. Evaluation of the site also required the use of cadaver dogs, divers to explore Lake Gander, and Canadian military helicopters for surveillance, mapping, and wreckage transport. On-site pathology services proved critical to the successful recovery of all victims.

Summary

Aircraft accident investigations are studies in concurrent and multidisciplinary investigations where a successful outcome is based on cooperation, coordination, collaboration, and comprehensiveness. The medical findings at autopsy and its ancillary laboratory studies provide a critical perspective in the overall accident investigation as to probable cause, level of survivability based on crash forces, occupiable space, and the postcrash environment, and the role of any preexisting condition as a risk factor. A comprehensive medicolegal investigation will provide the data necessary to link those concurrent investigations.

See Also

Body Recovery; **Death Investigation Systems:** Japan; **Falls from Height, Physical Findings:** In Children; In Adults; **Fire Investigation, Evidence Recovery**; **Injury, Transportation:** Air Disasters

Further Reading

Armstrong JA, Fryer DI, Steward WK, Whittingham HE (1955) Interpretation of injuries in the Comet aircraft disasters. *Lancet* I: 1135–1144.

Balfour AJC (1988) Aviation pathology. In: Ernsting J, King P (eds.) *Aviation Medicine*, 2nd edn., pp. 703–709. London: Butterworths.

Fryer DI (1965) The medical investigation of accidents. In: Gillies JA (ed.) *A Textbook of Aviation Physiology*. 45: 1193–1201. London: Pergamon Press.

Hellerich U, Pollak S (1995) Airplane crash: traumatologic findings in cases of extreme body disintegration. *American Journal of Forensic Medicine and Pathology* 16: 320–344.

Hill IR (1986) The immediate problems of aircraft fires. *American Journal of Forensic Medicine and Pathology* 7: 271–277.

Hill IR (1986) Toxicological findings in fatal aircraft accidents. *American Journal of Forensic Medicine and Pathology* 7: 322–326.

Koelmeyer TD, Beer B, Mullin PR (1982) A computer-based analysis of injuries sustained by victims of a major air disaster. *American Journal of Forensic Medicine and Pathology* 3: 11–16.

Kreffts S (1973) Estimation of pilot control at the time of the crash. In: Mason JK, Reals WJ (eds.) *Aerospace Pathology*, pp. 96–104. Chicago, IL: American College of Pathologists Foundation.

Li G, Baker SP (1997) Injury patterns in aviation-related fatalities: implications for preventive strategies. *American Journal of Forensic Medicine and Pathology* 18: 265–270.

Mason JK (1973) Pre-existing disease and aircraft accidents. In: Mason JK, Reals WJ (eds.) *Aerospace Pathology*, pp. 76–85. Chicago, IL: American College of Pathologists Foundation.

McMeekin RR (1973) Patterns of injury in fatal aircraft accidents. In: Mason JK, Reals WJ (eds.) *Aerospace Pathology*, pp. 86–95. Chicago, IL: American College of Pathologists Foundation.

McMeekin RR (1985) Aircraft accident investigation. In: DeHart RL (ed.) *Fundamentals of Aerospace Medicine*, pp. 762–814. Philadelphia, PA: Lea & Febriger.

Moody GH, Busuttil A (1994) Identification in the Lockerbie air disaster. *American Journal of Forensic Medicine and Pathology* 15: 63–69.

Van den Bos A (1980) Mass identification: a multidisciplinary operation: the Dutch experience. *American Journal of Forensic Medicine and Pathology* 3: 265–270.

Wagner GN, Froede RC (1993) Medicolegal investigation of mass disasters. In: Spitz WU (ed.) *Spitz and Fisher's Medicolegal Investigation of Death*, 3rd edn., pp. 567–584. Springfield, IL: Charles C. Thomas.

AVIATION MEDICINE, ILLNESS AND LIMITATIONS FOR FLYING

K Blaho-Owens, University of Tennessee College of Medicine, Memphis, TN, USA

Introduction

The world has celebrated over 100 years of powered flight. In December 1903, on a very windy beach in North Carolina, USA, Wilbur and Orville Wright successfully designed, built, and flew the first powered aircraft. In the air for only seconds, it marked the beginning of modern aviation. In just a short time span, aviation has progressed to high-altitude flight, flight at supersonic speeds, and flight to space and back. Aviation is integrated into our modern world and has blurred the boundaries of countries, enhanced business and communication across the world, and become an integral part of military operations. Much has been learned in a century of flight, including the importance of aeromedical factors on the safety of flight.

While the medical regulations will differ between countries, there are some general guidelines that prevail over most aviation governing agencies. The most comprehensive source for international medical requirements is updated regularly and can be found on the International Civil Aviation Organization (ICAO) website or in its information sources. The ICAO compiles the medical regulations from over 180 contracting states, each with slightly different medical requirements. For specific medical requirements for a particular area, the chief medical officer, or, in the USA, a local flight surgeon or the Federal Aviation Regulations can provide current medical standards. Those requirements and factors that do not change are discussed in this article.

Fitness for Flight and Medical Certification

Pilots must have an overall fitness for flight. The ultimate safety and success of the flight depend on the pilot in command. An important component of any successful and safe flight is a healthy pilot who is "fit for flight." Fitness is a combination of physical and mental well-being, good preflight planning, and currency of training and, of course, an aircraft that is well maintained.

Most regulatory or licensing agencies will have their own specific medical and physical requirements for those who wish to obtain and maintain a pilot's license. Depending on the type of license (private versus commercial), the medical certification will differ in standards and is renewed at various time intervals. For example, in the USA, a commercial pilot must have a first-class medical certificate, which must be renewed twice yearly, while a private pilot who is less than 40 years of age must renew his/her medical certificate every 3 years. Most countries have

similar medical requirements to those in the USA. Using organ system class, some general requirements of US medical certification are listed in **Table 1**. **Table 2** provides a concise summary of two US general aviation accidents in which underlying pathologies and/or drug use were factors in the outcome.

Medication Use and Flight Performance

Table 1 describes conditions that pose a risk for the safety of flight because poor control or exacerbation of these disease states could adversely affect the pilot's performance of duties. For example, one of the well-known adverse effects of drugs used for the treatment of diabetes is hypoglycemia. Hypoglycemia may result in altered mental status, which can adversely impact a pilot's performance. In addition to the disease states listed in **Table 1**, other factors should be considered during preflight planning. Acute illness may also reduce pilot performance to an unsafe level. Infection, anemia, peptic ulcer, acute injury, or pain are examples of such conditions. Note that, even when some conditions are treated, the medications used may impair flight performance and cause undue risk. Use of certain medications may be precluded in pilots because they may alter memory, concentration, alertness, and coordination, or otherwise

Table 1 Summary of some of the requirements for medical certification for an airman certificate   US standards[a]

Organ/system	Standards
Eye	Distance visual acuity of 20/20, corrected or uncorrected
	Near vision of 20/40 or better, or Snellen equivalent at 16 in each eye separately with or without corrective lenses
	Ability to perceive those colors that are necessary for safe performance of airman duties
	Normal visual fields
	No underlying pathology that interferes with proper vision, or a condition that would progress to such, or one that is aggravated by flying
	Normal convergence
Ear, nose, throat, and equilibrium	Normal hearing by specific standards, no disease of the ear, nose, or throat that would interfere with duties as a pilot, absence of any disease or impairment that would interfere with speech communication
	No underlying condition that would cause vertigo or a disturbance in equilibrium
Mental	No history or diagnosis of a personality disorder severe enough to cause overt acts, psychosis, delusions, hallucinations, grossly bizarre or disorganized behavior. No history of substance abuse[b]
Neurologic	No medical history or clinical diagnosis of epilepsy, unexplained loss of consciousness, unexplained transient loss of control of nervous system functions, no other disorder that would render the pilot unable to perform the duties of an airman in a safe manner
Cardiovascular	No history or diagnosis of myocardial infarction, angina, coronary artery disease (requiring treatment or symptomatic), cardiac valve replacement, pacemaker implantation, heart transplant
Other	No history or diagnosis of diabetes mellitus requiring insulin or other hypoglycemic treatment, or other underlying disease, that at the medical judgment of the flight surgeon makes the safe performance of airman duties questionable

[a]The Federal Aviation Administration designates flight surgeons of the Armed Forces on specified military posts or designated aviation medical examiners on nonmilitary sites as those authorized to issue medical certification for flight.
[b]Those who have a history of substance abuse who have been abstinent for the preceding 2 years may be eligible at the discretion of the flight surgeon.

Table 2 Concise summary of National Transportation Safety Board investigations where underlying disease states or drug use were determined to be factors in the outcome

Case 1

In July 2003, a Piper PA28 was destroyed in daylight hours operating in visual flight conditions and without a flight plan. A witness described the airplane as flying over the airport at an altitude of 180–240 m (600–800 ft) above the ground. The witness reported that the aircraft suddenly turned to the left and flew straight into the ground. The pilot was fatally injured and the aircraft was destroyed. The pilot held a private certificate for single-engine aircraft and was instrument-rated. He had a valid third-class medical certificate and had a total flight time of 657 h, 442.5 of which were in that airplane. He reported on his application for a medical certificate that he did not take medication and he did not have a history of any illness.

Review of the pilot's medical records revealed that he had a 12-year history of depression. Two days before the accident he was admitted to an inpatient psychiatric facility for a suicide attempt in which he had ingested 8 Ambien tablets. He had been treated intermittently since 1991 with antidepressants. Because there were no inpatient beds available, the pilot was discharged home after several hours on citalopram (Celexa).

Postmortem toxicological analysis showed brain ethanol concentrations of 23 mg dl^{-1}, muscle ethanol 14 mg dl^{-1}, and trace amounts of diphenhydramine, citalopram, fluoxetine, and norfluoxetine in the liver and kidney.

Case 2

In August 2003, an experimental amateur-built Young Pietenpol Air Camper piloted by a recreational pilot was destroyed on impact with trees and terrain during a landing at a local airport. Visual flight conditions prevailed at the time of the accident and there was no flight plan on file. The pilot survived the accident only to die from his injuries during the following 24 h. The pilot had a recreational pilot certificate with a single-engine land airplane rating and a valid third-class medical certificate. He had 70 h total flight time, 15 of which were flown in the 6 months before the medical certificate was issued.

There were no witnesses to the accident, but it appeared from the wreckage that the aircraft may have impacted trees with its left wing. Postmortem toxicological analysis (more than 24 h after the accident) revealed that the pilot had ingested diphenhydramine around the time of his last flight.

Table 3 Drugs that may alter flight performance

Agent	Effect	Example
Sedating antihistamines	Sedation, dry mouth, mydriasis, cycloplegia	Diphenhydramine
Muscle relaxants	Sedation, impaired coordination	Cyclobenzaprene
Ethanol	Impaired judgment, increased reaction time, impaired coordination, visual disturbances, exacerbates the central nervous system depressant effect of other drugs, increased susceptibility to hypoxia, amnesia	
Sedatives	Sedation, impaired coordination, impaired judgment, amnesia, increased reaction time	Alprazolam
Antiemetics	Sedation, dry mouth, mydriasis, impaired judgment, increased reaction time	Promethazine
Antihypertensives	Risk of orthostatic hypotension, sedation	
Antidepressants	Sedation, impaired coordination, increased susceptibility to depressant effect of other central nervous system depressants	
Analgesics	Sedation, impaired coordination, increased reaction time	Hydrocodone, tramadol
Hypoglycemics	Hypoglycemia, change in mental status, loss of consciousness	Insulin, glipizide
Drugs of abuse	Impaired coordination, memory, judgment, and reaction time	Marijuana, phencyclidine, cocaine, ecstasy

compromise flight performance. Examples of these are listed in **Table 3**. Note that, in addition to affecting coordination, memory, judgment, and reaction time, central nervous system depressants predispose the pilot to the effects of hypoxia. Despite widespread knowledge of the effects of certain medications, postmortem toxicological analysis of samples from fatal accidents still indicates that these drugs are commonly used by pilots. A short review of National Transportation Safety Board (NTSB) cases shows that the drugs most commonly used by pilots involved in fatal accidents are diphenhydramine and ethanol. Use continues despite the well-known impairment of

driving performance by diphenhydramine. In a study published in 2000 in the *Annals of Internal Medicine*, 25 mg diphenhydramine was noted to cause more impairment in driving performance than a blood alcohol concentration of 0.10 mg dl^{-1}.

More examples of drug use and accident factors can be found on the NTSB database (www.ntsb.gov).

Flight performance is a combination of coordination, focus of attention, clarity of thought, judgment, training, and proficiency. Note that being "current" according to flight regulations does not necessarily ensure that a pilot is "proficient" to execute the flight safely. Fatigue, illness, stress, and emotional liability can degrade and detract from a pilot's ability to conduct a flight safely.

Summaries of aviation accidents and incidents from multiple sources consistently show that aviation accidents are rarely the result of one catastrophic event or cause. This is not to say that a single overwhelming cause does not exist; certainly, catastrophic events do occur. Data trending and analysis of aviation accidents show that the majority of accidents have multiple factors that contribute to unsafe flights. Surprisingly, many of these factors are easy to identify and to prevent by simply delaying or changing other aspects of the flight. In 1999, there were 1933 aircraft involved in 1906 accidents, 340 of which were fatal accidents. These numbers can be translated to 2.41 accidents per 100 000 h flown. Personal flights for recreational or business had a higher rate of fatal accidents, effectively double that of any other type of flying, such as commercial carriers and military flights. Seventy-four percent of personal/business flight accidents resulted in a fatality. Other notable factors associated with fatal aviation accidents include the failure to file a flight plan, flying in low-visibility conditions (either instrument meteorological conditions or at night), drug use, pilots with low flight time, and pilots flying in weather that exceeds their ability or training.

Other Factors and Flight Performance

Fatigue

Fatigue is one of the most indolent and difficult-to-recognize factors. The NTSB reviews general aviation accident data and summarizes the characteristics of each accident that degrade flight performance. Acute fatigue, flying after a long day of work, or lack of sleep can impair judgment, impair coordination, increase the work associated with flying, and negatively affect alertness. Lack of adequate rest can result in chronic fatigue. Commercial airlines have regulations on the number of hours a pilot is on duty per month, and the number of consecutive hours a pilot would be on duty without rest.

Stress

Stress can detract from alertness, concentration, and judgment, and can degrade the safety of any flight. Pressure to adhere to a time schedule, sometimes known as "get-thereitis," often promotes poor judgment and flights into weather conditions that are beyond the capability of either the aircraft and/or the pilot. Pressure from passengers or employers can often push pilots into making poor decisions that compromise the safety of the flight. Although pilots are trained and educated to dissociate from stressful factors, it is often impossible to identify and remove the causes of stress.

Emotional

Anger, depression, or other emotional trauma, like stress, can negatively impact the safety of flight by distracting the pilot, so that he/she executes poor judgment, and has decreased reaction time, and poor attention to detail. Case 1 in **Table 2** illustrates an extreme of this example.

A common acronym used in preflight planning includes not only an evaluation of the weather, the aircraft, and the route of flight, but also of the pilot. This personal checklist is taught to student pilots from their earliest lessons as part of the preflight checklist. "I am not impaired by" (I'M SAFE), where I is illness, M is medication, S is stress, A is alcohol, F is fatigue, and E is emotion.

Physiological Aspects of Flight

Effects of Altitude, Pressurization, and Depressurization

Hypoxia or relative lack of oxygen can occur in unpressurized aircraft or in aircraft that lose their pressurization systems. As altitude increases, the relative amount of oxygen decreases. Those organ systems that are particularly sensitive to hypoxia are the central nervous system, the heart, and the visual system. Because of the relative dependence of rhodopsin formation on the presence of oxygen, night vision begins to deteriorate at a mean sea level (MSL) altitude of 1500 m (5000 ft). This deterioration is more noticeable at night. If supplemental oxygen is not used, the effects of hypoxia progress as altitude increases. The danger in hypoxia is in its indolence. Judgment, memory, alertness, coordination, and ability to make calculations become progressively impaired. The pilot may feel drowsy or dizzy or euphoric and belligerent. These effects can also be produced by the presence of carbon monoxide in the cabin – also a cause of hypoxia in aviation. As hypoxia increases, peripheral vision decreases and tunnel vision can result. Extremities may become cyanotic and have a bluish hue. Lack of judgment and clarity of thought impairs the pilot from correcting the situation. Loss of consciousness can occur in as little as 20 min at an altitude of 5400 m (18 000 ft) MSL without oxygen supplementation, and in as little as 5 min without supplemental oxygen at an altitude of 6000 m (20 000 ft) MSL. At higher altitudes, seconds are available before hypoxia ensues, with rapid loss of pressurization of the aircraft. In the USA, the Federal Aviation Administration mandates that, at altitudes above 3750 m (12 500 ft) MSL, the flight crew must wear oxygen after 30 min. At altitudes of 4200 m (14 000 ft) MSL and above, all crew must wear supplemental oxygen, and at 4500 m (15 000 ft) MSL all passengers must be provided with supplemental oxygen. For pressurized aircraft, regulations stipulate that, at altitudes above 7500 m (25 000 ft) MSL, a minimum of 10 min of supplemental oxygen must be available for each occupant in the event of rapid decompression. At flights above 10 500 m (35 000 ft) MSL, a quick-donning type of oxygen masks must be worn.

Sinuses and Ears

As altitude increases, equalization of the pressure between each side of the tympanic membrane becomes unequal and can produce intense pain. This unequal pressure can be compounded by the presence of allergic inflammation or an upper respiratory infection can make equalization difficult. This results in ear pain and loss of hearing that can last for several hours after flight. Pain can be minimized by executing the Valsalva maneuver (pinching the nose and attempting to blow through it), by yawning, swallowing, or opening and closing the mouth. For very young passengers, often sucking on a pacifier, nursing, or swallowing can minimize ear discomfort. Tympanic membrane rupture can occur if the pressure difference is excessive. There are no data to indicate that topical nasal decongestants can reduce congestion around the eustachian tubes, but they may provide some palliative comfort.

Vision in Flight

US Federal Aviation regulations require that a pilot have or be corrected to 20/20 distance vision and no less than 20/40 near vision. It is understood that good visual cues and rapid interpretation are important for safe flight. Drugs that cause dry eye, mydriasis or cycloplegia, such as anticholinergics can impair vision. Changes in refractive error caused by underlying diseases such as diabetes can degrade a pilot's vision and have a negative impact on safe flight. The effects of hypoxia cause a loss of peripheral vision.

Illusions occurring in flight are well known. Orientation is maintained by a combination of systems; by the input of the visual system, the inner ear, or vestibular system, and sensory input from skin, muscles, and joints. With a decrease or lack of vision such as occurs in night flight or during instrument meteorological conditions (IMC), sensory input from the

inner ear and motion and position from gravitational (G) forces become more acute. The sensations of motion and position during various flight maneuvers are often misleading and may compel pilots to believe they are in straight and level flight when they are indeed in a bank or ascending or descending. In flight conditions where visibility is decreased, pilots are trained to ignore sensory input and focus on the information provided by the instruments of the airplane. During training, an instructor trains a student pilot by demonstrating the various forms of disorientation and methods used to prevent these illusions. In low-visibility conditions, failure to fly the airplane by the instruments and follow sensory input leads to disorientation and is one of the main causes of pilot error and accidents during low-visibility flight conditions. Illusions during flight are created when visual scenes and sensory input confuse the pilot. When this happens, pilots are spatially disoriented; they are unable to determine the attitude or motion of the aircraft accurately in relation to the earth's surface. Despite this widely known phenomenon of spatial disorientation, the Federal Aviation Administration Advisory Circular indicates that spatial disorientation as a result of continued visual flight into adverse weather conditions is a common cause or a factor in annual statistics on fatal aircraft accidents. It is not unusual for visibility to be above visual-flight-rule (VFR) minimums and a visible horizon to be absent. This is particularly common in night flight, flight in haze, flights over water, or over sparsely populated areas.

One of the most widely publicized aviation accidents in history that ended with three deaths was the last flight piloted by John F. Kennedy Jr in July 1999. Flying a Piper Saratoga, a high-performance aircraft, on a night flight in marginal night VFR conditions, this accident was like many others. It was not caused by one catastrophic mistake, but by a series of smaller, less severe errors, all leading to spatial disorientation and what is known as the "graveyard spiral" with impact into the Atlantic Ocean. The pilot, John F. Kennedy Jr, was a relatively low-time private pilot who was not instrument-rated. He had a total of 310 flight hours, 55 of which were at night; 3 h were solo in the aircraft he was flying at the time of the accident. The flight departed late, at night in marginal visual flight conditions after the pilot had worked a full day. There was no flight plan filed, and no contact with air traffic control. Review of radar tracings of his aircraft indicated that the aircraft entered a descent, then a right turn, then a left turn, followed by a descent that ended in the aircraft impacting the water at a descent rate of over 1410 m min^{-1} (4700 ft min^{-1}). Over water, where there were no lights or other horizon for visual reference, the pilot apparently became spatially disoriented and entered into a spiral downward attitude that ended with the aircraft impacting the water. Factors in this accident were determined to be haze, a dark night, and the pilot's failure to maintain control of the airplane.

Common illusions during low-visibility flight occur. One common illusion, known as "the leans," occurs when the airplane banks too slowly. When this happens, the fluid in the vestibular system does not move. Any abrupt correction of the bank angle can set the fluid in movement, and the pilot may sense a bank to the opposite side. The pilot may lean to the originally banked side until the fluid in the vestibular system is in concert with the bank.

The Coriolis illusion occurs when an aircraft is in a prolonged constant rate of a turn. If the pilot has an abrupt head movement the fluid in the vestibular system can create an illusion of turning or accelerating in an entirely different axis. The disoriented pilot may maneuver into a dangerous flight attitude in an attempt to correct this illusion.

The "graveyard spiral" occurs when the fluid in the vestibular system ceases movement while the aircraft is in a prolonged, constant-rate turn. The illusion created is an aircraft descent with the wings level. The disoriented pilot, in an effort to correct the perceived descent, may increase the pitch of the aircraft, tightening the spiral and increasing the loss of altitude.

A false horizon may occur when the pilot uses a sloping cloud formation for visual reference. An obscured horizon, a dark scene with ground lights, and stars can disorient pilots and cause the aircraft to be misaligned with the false horizon.

Autokinesis occurs when a pilot fixates his/her vision in the dark on a stationary light. When the pilot stares at a stationary light, it will appear to move, and the disoriented pilot may try to align the aircraft with the light.

During a rapid acceleration, like that occurring in the takeoff roll, spatial disorientation, also referred to as a somatogravic illusion, can create the illusion of the aircraft being in a nose-high attitude. The disoriented pilot may correct the aircraft into a nose-low or dive attitude.

The best mechanism for coping with spatial disorientation is thorough preflight planning, proficiency in instrument conditions, using visual references that are reliable fixed points, avoiding sudden head movements during critical flight times and ensuring that illness and medication use do not impair flight performance. If disorientation occurs, attention and focus should be on the flight instruments.

Other Considerations in Aviation

Night Flight

Under low light conditions, pilots should give themselves 20–30 min to adapt to night vision. Red lighting in the cockpit can maintain dark adaptation, but renders the colors on an aeronautical chart and small print difficult or impossible to read. Low lighting can exacerbate the effects of presbyopia, requiring some pilots to wear reading glasses for night flight. Dark adaptation can be impaired by some drugs such as Accutane (isotrenitoin), exposure to carbon monoxide through compromised engine exhaust, or smoking. Cabin pressures at greater than 1500 m (5000 ft) can also render the pilot less adaptive to low light conditions.

Motion Sickness

Motion sickness is intense nausea and/or vomiting. Symptoms of motion sickness are gradual and include salivation, anorexia, hyperhidrosis, dizziness, and disorientation. Nausea followed by vomiting can occur and it is possible that the pilot may become incapacitated. Classic antiemetic agents such as promethazine, although effective in preventing nausea and vomiting, have unacceptable side-effects for the pilot, including drowsiness, sluggish thought, mydriasis, and impaired visual accommodation. For acute motion sickness, minimal head movement, focusing vision on a point outside the airplane, and cool air directed at the face can provide some abatement. Termination of the flight should occur as soon as practicable if the symptoms do not improve or become severe.

Carbon Monoxide

Carbon monoxide is a colorless, odorless gas with an affinity to the oxygen-binding sites on hemoglobin that is 220 times that of oxygen. By binding to these sites, oxygen binding is prevented and hypoxia occurs. Sources of carbon monoxide in aircraft are limited to those with piston engines, and occur most commonly when airflow over the engine to the heating system becomes contaminated with exhaust fumes from manifold cracks and faulty engine seals. Signs of carbon monoxide exposure include headache, drowsiness, or dizziness, temporally related to the use of the aircraft heating system. A pilot who detects exhaust fumes in the cabin of the aircraft should shut any heating vents, open all vents to provide outside air into the cabin, and have the system examined with due haste. Cockpit carbon monoxide detectors are relatively inexpensive and can help detect faulty engine systems before they present a problem. If carbon monoxide exposure is suspected, it can be confirmed by measuring blood carboxyhemoglobin. Carboxyhemoglobin concentrations above 20% indicate exposure and are generally considered to be symptomatic. Treatment of carbon monoxide exposure includes removal from the source, oxygen administration, and, in severe cases, hyperbaric oxygen therapy that hastens the elimination of carbon monoxide.

Flying after Scuba Diving

During diving, there is an absorption of nitrogen into the blood. Flying too soon after diving, without allowing for the elimination of nitrogen, can result in decompression sickness, or the bends. The recommended wait time before flying above 2400 m (8000 ft) MSL is 24 h after the last dive that had a controlled ascent.

G-force

Gravitational force is the measure of the force of gravity. Normal gravitational force is 1, or 1 **g**. When an aircraft changes speed or direction, the magnitude of acceleration is measured by the G-force. With increasing positive G-forces, blood is forced downward and away from vital areas such as the brain and heart. Pooling blood in the legs and splanchnic circulation can result in loss of vision, and loss of consciousness. This is obviously more of a problem with high-powered aircraft or aerobatic flight than with a slower, less-powerful aircraft. The onset of G-induced hypoxia or loss of consciousness can occur gradually or can be nearly instantaneous, depending on the rate of change in G-force. Much has been published on the syndrome known to military pilots as "acceleration-induced near-loss of consciousness" or ALOC. The ALOC syndrome seems to be more common with rapid and short-lived changes in G-force. Short-term memory loss, degradation of vision characterized by light loss, loss of peripheral vision, sensory abnormalities, confusion, euphoria, dysphasia, and reduced auditory acuity are commonly encountered with short rapid changes in G-force. To combat G-force hypoxia and prevent loss of consciousness, early pilots were trained and taught to tense their legs and abdomen and to grunt, yell, or practice the Valsalva maneuver to keep blood in the brain. More sophisticated equipment was developed in the form of pressure suits, or clothing with air bladders that inflate automatically and help maintain blood flow to the brain during high-G-force maneuvers.

With vibration and rapid changes in acceleration, vertebral and cervical problems have been documented in pilots who fly both jet fighter and helicopter aircraft. With the development and implementation of helmet-mounted displays comes increased weight of head and neck musculoskeletal load. Helicopter pilots who wear heavy headgear are more likely to experience compression fractures – a complication that increases with age or with pilots who have osteoarthritic changes. Pilots with increased age and taller stature tend to be more at risk for vertebral problems.

Medical Risks Encountered with Commercial Flight

In patients with underlying risk factors for venous thromboembolism or pulmonary embolism, extended commercial flights increase the incidence of developing thrombus after air travel. One of the most significant modifiable risk factors is movement during flight. Complete immobility or limited movement is associated with a higher incidence of thrombus than in those patients with risk factors who have some type of activity during flight.

Communicable Infections and Commercial Flight

With the abolition of international boundaries by commercial aviation, and the relatively enclosed environment and air supply, there is a risk for person-to-person transmission of respiratory infections, including tuberculosis, influenza, and severe acute respiratory syndrome (SARS). Common-sense practices of hand-washing and the use of personal protective equipment can decrease the spread to illness.

See Also

Aviation Accidents, Role of Pathologist; **Injury, Transportation:** Air Disasters

Further Reading

Federal Aviation Administration. *Aeronautical Information Manual.*
International Civil Aviation Organization (ICAO): www.icao.int.
Kershner WK (1994) *The Advanced Pilot's Flight Manual*, 6th edn. Ames, IA: Iowa State University Press.
National Transportation and Safety Board (NTSB, US): www.ntsb.gov.
US Department of Transportation Federal Aviation Administration Flight Standards Services (1997) *Pilot's Handbook of Aeronautical Knowledge.* Oklahoma, OH.

B

BACK-TRACKING CALCULATIONS

R A Anderson, University of Glasgow, Glasgow, UK

Introduction

What is Backtracking?

Backtracking calculations ("back-calculations") are most commonly used to estimate previous concentrations of drugs, including alcohol (ethanol), in a biological fluid such as blood. Typically, a drug concentration is measured in a blood specimen taken some time after a critical event and it becomes necessary to establish what the concentration would have been at that earlier time. One example might be the estimation of blood alcohol concentration (BAC) at the time of a road traffic accident based on the analysis of a blood or breath specimen from the driver obtained some hours after the accident. It is clearly important to know if the driver was above the prescribed alcohol limit at the time of the accident. Another common example is the estimation of the maximum acetaminophen (paracetamol) concentration that might have been achieved in an overdose patient based on a blood sample taken on admission at the emergency room: the high-point concentration is critical in determining patient treatment and outcome.

The starting point for these calculations is the concentration of the drug in a sample of the biological fluid taken at a given time after the critical event. This is often measured in a forensic toxicology or clinical biochemistry laboratory but, with the advent of increasingly sophisticated and accurate on-site instruments, alternatives now include the police station and will potentially in future include the roadside or ambulance.

Backtracking calculations may also be used in completely different contexts within forensic medicine, for example, the estimation of the postmortem interval based on body temperature, but this article will be restricted to applications involving drugs, used here in its widest interpretation to include alcohol and other substances.

Pharmacokinetics and Pharmacodynamics

Back-calculation requires knowledge of the pharmacology of the relevant substance, particularly with respect to its pharmacokinetics, which is concerned with how the body handles the substance, i.e., the question: what does the body do to the substance? Pharmacokinetics relates to the rate of elimination of substances from the body and is critical for backward extrapolation. In contrast, the pharmacodynamics of the substance is more concerned with its effects, i.e., the question: what does the substance do to the body? Often these two questions are tied together when interpreting a forensic case, when an attempt is made to estimate a drug concentration in blood and relate it to its effects on the individual concerned.

Absorption, Distribution, Metabolism, and Elimination of Drugs

It is often easiest to consider drug concentrations versus time in a pictorial/graphical way and some common terminology is used to describe the different parts of the concentration-versus-time curve (**Figure 1**).

After administration, the concentration of drug in blood rises to a maximum (C_{max}) during the absorption phase and begins to decline in the distribution and elimination phase, following an exponential curve.

Concentration-versus-time Curves and Backtracking Calculations

The shape of the concentration-versus-time curve during the elimination phase is the basis of all backtracking calculations. Clearly, if the details of the curve are known, it will be possible to predict drug concentrations at any point on the curve. However, calculations are often restricted to the elimination phase unless details of dose and time of administration are known.

Some information is needed to allow the curve to be defined and difficulties arise if insufficient information is available. Typically, all that is known is the concentration of the drug of interest measured in a

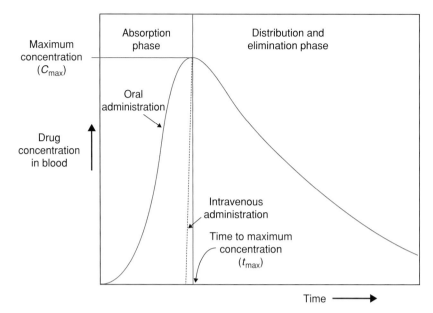

Figure 1 General graph showing concentration of drug in blood versus time after administration.

blood specimen taken at some stage after administration. To this must be added, usually from the literature, information on the peak blood levels obtained after administration of a known amount of the drug and the rate(s) of elimination of the drug. Additional factors need to be taken into account, for example, the weight of the subject, his/her build (tall, short, fat, thin), age, and experience/habituation to the drug. For most parameters of this type there is an average value for the population in general and an associated range of values encompassing the different values found in individual subjects. If the information is available in the literature, the population values used should relate to a population matched to the characteristics of the subject. As an example, the average rate of elimination of alcohol in a population of regular consumers of alcohol is higher than in a group of nondrinkers.

The shape of the curve in the elimination phase can adopt a variety of forms, depending on the dose of substance taken and its distribution and metabolism. For most drugs, the rate of elimination depends on the concentration of drug present – a constant proportion of the drug is eliminated in a given time interval and the curve is exponential. However, for a few drugs given in high doses, including alcohol and aspirin, a constant amount of drug is eliminated per unit of time and the curve is effectively linear. Alcohol will be considered separately below, then other drugs.

Alcohol

A typical concentration-versus-time curve for alcohol is given in **Figure 2** Alcohol is unique as a drug

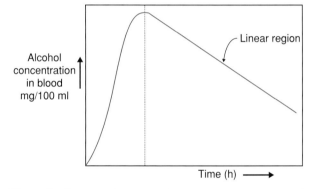

Figure 2 Concentration-versus-time curve for alcohol in blood.

because of the large doses that are administered (**Table 1**). No other drugs are administered in such large amounts. As a result, the concentration of alcohol in blood can be much higher than that obtained for any other drug and it saturates the metabolic capability of the liver (the main metabolic organ).

Units of concentration and dose of alcohol Concentrations of alcohol in beverages are given in terms of percentage alcohol by volume (vol%), which may be given on the bottle or packaging. Representative values are given in **Table 1**. When performing calculations it is advisable to establish the exact concentration of alcohol in the beverage consumed by the subject. The weight of alcohol in a measure of a beverage (equivalent to the "dose" of alcohol) can be obtained by multiplying the volume of alcohol it contains by the density of alcohol (0.791 at 20 °C).

Table 1 Representative alcohol concentrations in common beverages

Beverage	Alcohol (%vol)	Common measures (cl)	Weight of alcohol at 20°C (g)
Beer	3–6	Pint 56.8	15.7 (3.5% vol)
Strong beer	5–9	Pint 56.8	15.7 (3.5% vol)
		Bottle 33	10.4 (4%vol, 33 cl)
		Can 44	23.5 (9%vol, 33 cl)
Table wine	10–13	Bottle 75	71
		Glass 12.5	11.9
		Large glass 25	23.7
			(all based on 12%vol)
Fortified wines	15–20	Bottle 75	104
(sherry, port)		Glass 2.5	3.5
			(all based on 17.5%vol)
Spirits	35–40	Bottle 75	237
		"Single" 2.5	7.9
		"Double" 5	15.8
			(all based on 40%vol)

For example, 125 ml of wine (12 vol%) contains $125 \times 0.12 \times 0.791$ g alcohol at 20°C, i.e., 11.9 g alcohol.

Other units of relevance are those used to describe alcohol in biofluids – blood, urine, and breath. For blood and urine, the units most often used are milligrams per 100 milliliters (mg%) or grams per 100 milliliters (g%). The latter is obtained by dividing the former by 1000. For example:

Legal limit for driving in the UK is 80 mg%

$$= 0.08 \, g\%$$

Breath alcohol concentrations are much lower and are expressed as micrograms per 100 millilitres of breath (μg%). In other jurisdictions, for example the USA, the units are grams per 2100 liters of breath, because USA traffic legislation is based on a blood:breath ratio of 2100:1.

It is usually convenient to convert alcohol concentrations in breath or urine to the equivalent blood concentration, using the ratios specified by the prescribed limits in the relevant jurisdiction. After the calculations are carried out, the breath or urine concentrations can be obtained by reversing the conversion process.

Pharmacokinetics of Alcohol

Administration of alcohol is almost always by the oral route. It is absorbed from all parts of the alimentary tract but mostly enters the circulation from the small intestine. If the stomach is empty, the absorption can be rapid, within 30 min or less, but the presence of food can delay absorption for several hours. For the purpose of calculations, a period of 1 h after the last drink can be allowed for complete absorption of alcohol.

Ethanol is considered to be uniformly and rapidly distributed throughout the body water. The relative concentrations of alcohol in biological fluids or tissues therefore depend on their water contents.

Alcohol is also distributed into breath according to the partition ratio between blood and air in the lungs. The partition ratio used in UK legislation is blood:breath = 2300:1 and the prescribed limit for alcohol in breath when driving is 35 μg of alcohol per 100 ml of breath (note the different units: milligrams of alcohol in blood and micrograms in breath).

For the purposes of backtracking calculations, the elimination part of the blood alcohol curve is considered to be linear as long as the BAC is above 20 mg%, indicating that the rate of elimination is independent of the alcohol concentration ("zero-order" or "saturation" kinetics). When the alcohol concentration falls below 20 mg% the liver is no longer saturated and an exponential curve is followed. Many studies have been carried out in different populations to establish the average and range of elimination rates during the linear part of the curve. The average rate often used in backtracking calculations is 15 mg alcohol per 100 ml blood per hour (15 mg% h^{-1}). The range of elimination rates varies widely: 9–29 mg% h^{-1}. It has also been established that regular drinkers often have a higher elimination rate, averaging 18–20 mg% h^{-1}. An average elimination rate of 18 mg% h^{-1} is recommended by many workers in this field as the basis of backtracking calculations.

Calculations The simplest backtracking calculations relate to the linear portion of the blood alcohol curve (**Figure 3**). The starting point is usually a blood (or breath or urine) alcohol concentration in a specimen obtained at a known time. The aim of the calculation is to estimate the blood (or breath equivalent)

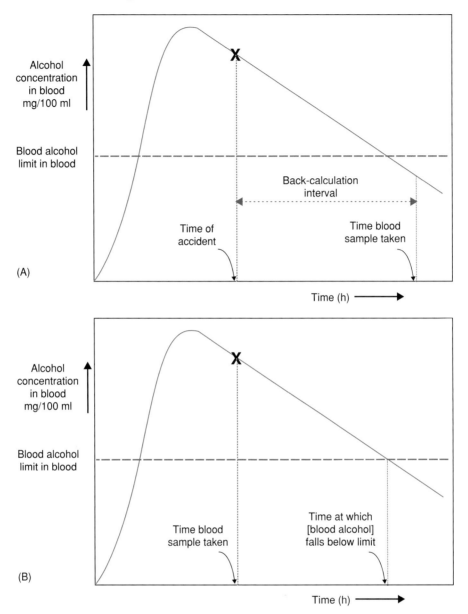

Figure 3 (A) Back-calculation; (B) no likelihood of driving.

concentration at an earlier time than when the specimen was obtained (back-calculation). Road traffic legislation in the UK permits this to be carried out for specimens obtained up to 18 h after an incident such as a road accident. A similar calculation can be used to determine when the blood (or equivalent) alcohol concentration would fall below the limit prescribed in the relevant jurisdiction. This is one of the two statutory defenses created within UK legislation – no likelihood of driving whilst unfit to drive through drink or drugs.

A more complex calculation is often requested as a result of postaccident consumption of alcohol – the other statutory defense allowed within the UK legislation. It concerns a defendant who consumes alcohol

after being involved in a road traffic incident, typically a road accident, and whose blood or breath alcohol is subsequently found to be above the prescribed limit. The defense seeks to establish that, at the time of the accident, the defendant's alcohol concentration was below the limit. It is important to recognize that calculations are based on the information supplied by the defendant, which may be incorrect either intentionally or unintentionally. The fact that a set of calculations supports a defendant's version of events does not mean that it is true.

Back-calculation Certain assumptions are made in this type of calculation and should be stated in a report prepared for court purposes:

- It is assumed that the BAC has been falling continuously and linearly during the time interval between the incident and obtaining the specimen from the defendant.
- It is assumed that no alcohol was consumed during this interval.

The back-calculation interval is the time between the incident/accident and the time at which the blood or other specimen was taken (**Figure 3A**). This is multiplied by the average rate of alcohol elimination to obtain the amount by which the BAC has fallen during the interval. The BAC at the time of the incident is then obtained by adding this value to the BAC measured in the specimen. A range of values can be calculated using the range of elimination rates given above.

This type of calculation is, arguably, acceptable over a short time interval of a few hours, but is likely to be inaccurate over a long period such as that permitted under UK legislation (18 h).

For example, a blood specimen was obtained from the defendant 4 h after a fatal road accident. The BAC was 60 mg%. Over a 4-h period the BAC would have fallen by $4 \times 18 = 72$ mg%, on average (range is 36–116 mg%, based on elimination rates of 9 and 29 mg% h^{-1}). The defendant's BAC at the time of the accident would have been 132 mg% (range 96–176 mg%).

Time to fall below prescribed limit Assumptions made in this calculation are:

- It is assumed that the defendant was in the elimination phase when the BAC was measured and that it would have continued to fall linearly until it fell below the prescribed limit.
- It is assumed that no additional alcohol would be consumed during this interval.

The difference between the measured BAC in the blood specimen and the prescribed limit for driving is obtained by subtraction. The clearance time (in hours) required for a decrease in BAC of this magnitude to occur is calculated by dividing this difference by the average elimination rate. The time of day when the defendant would have been entitled to drive can then be obtained by adding the clearance time to the time when the blood specimen was obtained. A range of times can be calculated using the range of elimination rates given above.

For example, a defendant was found sleeping in his car at 11.30 P.M. and his breath alcohol concentration was subsequently measured at midnight. This gave a reading of 55 µg of alcohol per 100 ml of breath. His defense is that he did not intend to drive until 8 A.M. the following morning.

In this example, the breath alcohol concentration can be converted into the equivalent blood concentration, using the blood:breath ratio incorporated into the legislation. In the UK this factor is 2300:1. Alternatively, the average elimination rates for blood can be converted into the equivalent values for breath.

The defendant's breath alcohol concentration needs to fall to 35 µg of alcohol per 100 ml of breath before he would be entitled to drive. This represents a fall of 20 µg of alcohol per 100 ml of breath. The equivalent fall in blood concentration can be obtained by multiplying by 2.3 (since the units for breath are 1000 times smaller than for blood), i.e., $20 \times 2.3 = 46$ mg per 100 ml blood.

Using the average clearance rate of 18 mg% h^{-1}, it would take $2\frac{1}{2}$ h for the defendant's BAC to fall by 46 mg%. The range of times obtained by using the fastest and slowest elimination rates is 1.6 h (1 h 36 min) to 5 h. Even with the slowest rate of elimination the defendant would have been below the prescribed limit at 8 A.M. the following morning.

Postaccident consumption of alcohol The defendant needs to provide the information listed in **Table 2**. This information can usually be obtained through the solicitor for the defense.

Table 2 Information required for postaccident drinking defense

- Details of alcohol consumption for the 24 h preceding the road traffic incident, i.e., the quantities and types of beverages and the time periods over which they were consumed. In many cases, the defendant has consumed alcohol before driving and being involved in the traffic incident. The aim is to establish that this would not have resulted in an alcohol concentration above the limit. It is also important to ensure that there is no residual alcohol from the previous day. The quantities of alcohol consumed by the defendant are often estimates made some time after the event. If the alcohol was consumed in a bar then bar measures are reasonably reliable with respect to volume. If the alcohol was consumed at home or elsewhere the defendant should be asked to mark on the original bottle or glass (if possible) how much was used
- The time of the traffic incident
- Details of postaccident consumption of alcohol (quantity, type, time period)
- Details of police involvement and subsequent breath or blood sample obtained. The defendant's recollection of the timescale may be inaccurate but police officers make a detailed and accurate note of their movements. Similarly, breath alcohol analysis instruments or attending physicians record the time of sample collection
- The result of the breath or blood analysis
- The defendant's height and weight at the time of the incident

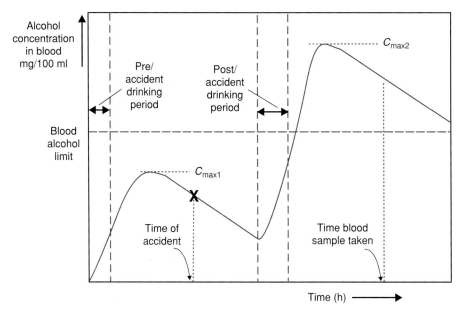

Figure 4 Blood alcohol-versus-time curve for a postincident drinking scenario.

The concentration-versus-time curve for this scenario is shown in **Figure 4**. The calculation breaks down into two parts corresponding to pre- and post-accident consumption of alcohol. Calculations shown below deal with BACs. Interconversion of breath and blood concentrations can be carried out using the blood:breath ratio accepted in the relevant jurisdiction.

Complete definition of the curve requires the information listed in **Table 2** on quantities and times of alcohol consumed. It is necessary to estimate C_{max1} and C_{max2}, i.e., to relate the BAC to the alcohol consumed.

Calculation of maximum alcohol concentration (C_{max}) after consumption of alcohol The number of grams of alcohol contained in the drink(s) consumed is calculated as described earlier. This alcohol is assumed to be completely and rapidly absorbed and evenly distributed throughout body water before any significant elimination has occurred.

The value of C_{max} can be obtained if the total volume of body water and the fraction of blood that is composed of water are known – this is relatively constant at 0.8 times the blood volume. The problem is now to estimate the total amount of water in the body. Several ways of doing this have been published in the literature (**Table 3**).

Perhaps the best known of these was published by Widmark in 1936. The factor r in **Table 3** is now usually called the "Widmark factor." Men and women, on average, have slightly different body compositions and Widmark's empirical values of r for men and women are 0.68 and 0.55, respectively.

Watson and coworkers in 1980 derived formulae for estimating total body water from anthropometric measurements (height, weight, and age) in men and women.

More recently, Forrest published in 1986 what might be considered the most reliable approach, based on the body mass index. The total body water can be calculated from the body's fat-free mass as the water content of fat-free tissue has been shown to be $724\,g\,kg^{-1}$ on average (standard deviation $34\,g\,kg^{-1}$). Body fat, in turn, can be calculated using the body mass index.

A rule-of-thumb method for C_{max} was derived by Smith and Oliver based on in-house measurements (personal communication). Each drink containing $9\,g$ of alcohol consumed by a 70-kg person increases the BAC by 20 mg%. The range on C_{max} is ±20%, which allows for differences in body composition. The C_{max} value is adjusted proportionately for body weight but no distinction is made between men and women.

Allowance for alcohol eliminated due to metabolism C_{max} is calculated on the assumption that alcohol is consumed and absorbed over a short time period, during which there is no significant loss of alcohol by metabolism. In reality, absorption may not be rapid and an allowance may be made for the absorption time – 1 h is reasonable for complete absorption of alcohol. C_{max} would therefore occur approximately 1 h after the last drink was consumed. In addition, more than one drink is often consumed and the period of consumption may well be a number of hours. In this situation, C_{max} is estimated as usual

Table 3 Methods of estimating maximum alcohol concentration (C_{max})

Author	Equations
Widmark	$a = c \times p \times r$ where: a = amount of alcohol consumed (g) c = blood alcohol concentration (g l^{-1}) p = the weight of the subject (kg) r = the ratio of water content of the whole body to that in blood i.e., r = (total body water/body weight) ÷ 0.8

Watson and coworkers	Total body water (men) = 2.45 + (0.107 × height) + (0.336 × weight) − (0.0952 × age)
	 Total body water (women) = 2.10 + (0.107 × height) + (0.247 × weight)
	 where total body water is in liters
	          height is in meters
	          weight is in kilograms

Forrest	Total body water = 0.724 × (body weight − body fat)
	 where total body water is in kilograms
	          (approximates to liters)
	          body weight is in kilograms
	          body fat is in kilograms
	 and
	 Fat as a percentage body weight (men) = 1.340 × body mass index − 12.469
	 Fat as a percentage body weight (women) = 1.371 × body mass index − 3.467
	 and
	 body mass index = (weight in kg) ÷ (height in meters)^2

Smith and Oliver (personal communication)	C_{max} in blood = 20 × (weight alcohol consumed/9) × (70/body weight)

but is then adjusted downwards to take account of metabolism during the consumption period. For example, if several drinks were consumed over 3 h, the C_{max} value would be adjusted by subtracting 3 × the elimination rate (average and range). An alternative approach advocated by some practitioners is based on the fact that metabolism begins as alcohol enters the blood circulation, i.e., immediately after drinking commences, so no allowance is made for the absorption time.

For example, a defendant's statement indicates that he went to his local bar and consumed four single measures of whisky (25 ml per measure, 40 vol%) and one pint of beer (3.5 vol%) between 8 and 10 P.M. He left the bar and later drove his car. He was involved in a road accident at midnight, in which his car skidded and ended up in a ditch. His car was badly damaged but no one was injured. He wandered away from the scene in a state of shock, arriving home at 12.15 A.M. He then consumed a further quantity of whisky to calm his nerves. The volume of whisky consumed was estimated from the glass used by the defendant as 150 ml. The police arrived at the defendant's house at 1 A.M. and subsequently a blood specimen was obtained at 2 A.M., which was found to contain 100 mg% alcohol, which is above the UK statutory limit of 80 mg%. The defendant's weight at the time was 11 stone (70 kg) and his height is 5 ft 8 in. (1.72 m). The defense wishes to show that

the defendant's BAC was below the limit at the time of the accident and that his postaccident drinking explains the alcohol found in his blood specimen.

This will be worked through using the method proposed by Forrest and also using the rule-of-thumb method of Smith and Oliver. For both calculations the quantities of alcohol consumed before and after the accident were:

- Alcohol consumed before driving:
  4 × 25 ml = 100 ml whisky = 31.6 g alcohol
  1 pint beer = 568 ml (3.5 vol%) = 15.7 g alcohol
  Total = 47.3 g alcohol
- Alcohol consumed after the accident:
  150 ml whisky = 47.5 g alcohol

Method of Forrest

- The defendant's body mass index (BMI)
  = (weight in kg) ÷ (height in m)^2
  = 70 × 1.72^2
  = 23.7
- Fat as a percentage of body weight
  = 1.340 × body mass index − 12.469
  = 19.3%
- Weight of body fat = 70 × 0.193 = 13.5 kg
- Total body water
  = 0.724 × (body weight − body fat)
  = 0.724 × (70 − 13.5)
  = 40.9 kg (= 40.9 l)

95% confidence interval based on ± 2 standard deviations is $\pm 3.8 l$
That is, 37.1–44.7 l
- Widmark factor r
= total body water $\div$ (total body weight $\times 0.8$)
= $40.9 \div (70 \times 0.8)$
= 0.73
    Range = 0.66–0.80
- Using the Widmark equation ($a = c \times p \times r$):
$47.3 = C_{max} \times 70 \times 0.73$
$C_{max} = 0.926\,g\,l^{-1}$ blood = 93 mg%
(rounded to nearest whole number)
Range = 0.845–$1.02\,g\,l^{-1}$
blood = 84.5–102 mg%
C_{max} will be obtained 1 h after the last drink, i.e., at 11 P.M.
- Adjusting C_{max} for metabolism between 9 and 11 P.M.:
Average rate of elimination
= 18 mg% h^{-1} (range 9–29 mg% h^{-1})
Loss of alcohol from 9 to 11 P.M.
= $2 \times 18 = 36$ mg% (range 18–58 mg%)
Adjusted C_{max} = 57 mg%
The range on this figure takes into account range on C_{max} and range in elimination rates:
Maximum range
= $(84.5 - 58)$ to $(102 - 18) = 26.5$–84 mg%
- At the time of the accident (midnight):
Additional loss of alcohol by metabolism from 11 P.M. to midnight is 18 mg% on average (range 9–29).
Net BAC = 39 mg% (range 0–75 mg%).
- Postaccident consumption of 150 ml whisky (47.5 g alcohol) between 12.15 and 1 A.M. would result in C_{max2} at about 2 A.M., when the blood specimen was obtained. Using the Widmark equation C_{max2} is 93 mg%. This value needs to be adjusted to allow for residual alcohol from the drinks consumed earlier and for metabolism between 12.10 and 2 A.M. Note that the defendant's blood alcohol never reaches zero at any time (referring to the average rate of metabolism) so metabolism continues without interruption. However, a fast metabolizer would achieve a zero BAC shortly after midnight.
Residual blood alcohol from preaccident consumption is 39 mg% (range 0–75 mg%) at midnight.
Blood alcohol increase from postaccident drinking is 93 mg% (range 85–103 mg%).
Total is 132 mg% (range 85–178 mg%).
C_{max2} is adjusted to take into account metabolism from midnight to 2 A.M. equivalent to 36 mg% (range 18–29* mg%) (asterisk represents fast metabolizers who would have achieved a zero blood alcohol shortly after midnight so a metabolism

period of 1 h is used).
Net result for C_{max2}
= 96 mg% on average (range 56–160 mg%).
- The alcohol concentration in the defendant's blood specimen was 100 mg%, which is in reasonable agreement with the average calculated value.

Method of Smith and Oliver (personal communication)

- Preaccident consumption of 47.3 g alcohol would give a BAC of $20 \times 47.3/9$ mg% on average = 105 mg% (range on this is $\pm 20\%$, i.e., 84–126 mg%). Adjusting C_{max1} for metabolism between 9 and 12 P.M. (an allowance of 1 h is made for the alcohol to be absorbed initially so the metabolism time begins at 9 P.M.):
Average rate of metabolism gives a decrease of $3 \times 18 = 54$ mg%.
Range: slow metabolism gives a decrease of $3 \times 9 = 27$ mg%; fast metabolism gives a decrease of $3 \times 29 = 87$ mg%.
Net BAC at the time of the accident:
Average: $105 - 54 = 51$ mg%
Maximum range is obtained by subtracting maximum and minimum decrease due to metabolism from the lower and upper end of the range on C_{max1}:
Low end of range: $84 - 87 = 0$ mg%.
Top end of range: $126 - 27 = 99$ mg%.
- On average, the defendant would have been below the limit at the time of the accident. However, note that the range is wide and extends above the limit. Values at the extremities of the range are theoretically possible but are unlikely to occur.
- Calculation of the BAC at 2 A.M. is based on the total alcohol consumed before and after the accident and the total metabolic time:
Total alcohol consumed = $47.3 + 47.5 = 94.8$ g.
This gives a C_{max} value of $20 \times 94.8/9 = 211$ mg% (range $\pm 20\% = 169$–253 mg%).
Total metabolism time = 9 P.M. – 2 A.M. = 5 h.
This gives a decrease in BAC = $5 \times 18 = 90$ mg%.
Range due to metabolism is: low end = $5 \times 9 = 45$ mg%; top end = $4 \times 29 = 116$ mg%* where asterisk represents metabolism period of only 4 h because the BAC would have been zero between midnight and 1 A.M. approximately.
Net BAC at 2 A.M.:
Average: $211 - 90 = 121$ mg%,
range: low end = $169 - 145 = 24$ mg%;
top end = $253 - 45 = 208$ mg%.
- The average calculated value is 121 mg%, which is somewhat higher than the alcohol concentration measured in the blood specimen. However, the range is very wide and it allows the defense to argue that the defendant's postaccident drinking would account for the blood test result.

Drugs Other than Alcohol

The curve shown in **Figure 1** applies to most drugs taken orally in a single dose. Obviously, administration of more than one dose would result in a more complex curve with multiple peaks and the following discussion is restricted to the part of the curve after the peak, i.e., the elimination phase.

The elimination phase is a sigmoidal, S-shaped curve, which can be represented mathematically by an exponential equation of the form:

$$C_t = C_0 e^{-kt} \qquad [1]$$

where C_t is the drug concentration at time t; C_0 is the theoretical drug concentration, which would be obtained if the drug had been administered at time t_0 and distributed immediately around the blood in circulation; and k is the elimination rate constant.

In practice, the elimination curve is more complex, and the equation contains two or more exponential terms rather than one, as in eqn [1]. These might be interpreted as the distribution (alpha) and excretion (beta) phases of the curve (**Figure 5**). Many data points are needed to define a multiexponential curve and backtracking calculations are necessarily restricted to the simpler single-exponential model. This, in turn, usually restricts the calculations to the terminal beta phase.

Eqn [1] is usually transformed to the following, which is easier to work with as it is the equation of a straight line (**Figure 6**):

$$\log_{10} C_t = \log_{10} C_0 - kt/2.3 \qquad [2]$$

An additional equation, the derivation of which is shown in all pharmacokinetic texts, relates the elimination rate constant to the half-life of the drug in plasma. This is the time it takes for the drug concentration to fall to half of its original value and it is available for most drugs in reference textbooks.

$$t_{1/2} = 0.693/k \qquad [3]$$

where $t_{1/2}$ is the plasma half-life and k is the elimination rate constant.

It is therefore possible to obtain k for most drugs using eqn [3] and as a result it is possible to solve eqn [2] to obtain drug concentrations at times prior to when the biological specimen was obtained. This is best illustrated with some typical examples.

Acetaminophen (paracetamol) The patient, Mrs Y, has been admitted to hospital after taking an overdose of acetaminophen tablets. This occurred at about 5–6 P.M. and it is now 10 P.M. The attending physician takes a blood sample from the patient

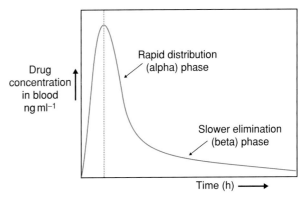

Figure 5 The elimination curve for most drugs contains at least two phases.

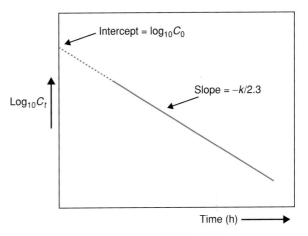

Figure 6 Semilogarithmic plot of elimination curve.

and sends it to the laboratory for acetaminophen measurement. The result from the lab is 50 mg acetaminophen per liter of plasma.

The course of treatment of an acetaminophen overdose depends on the amount of drug consumed and what the plasma concentration of the drug was at its highest. A threshold applies: if the peak concentration was below 150 mg l^{-1} plasma, then no intervention is necessary other than general support. However, if it was above this threshold, then severe liver damage is likely to occur and therapeutic intervention is indicated. This would entail the administration of a drug such as acetylcysteine, which protects the liver from damage caused by acetaminophen. It is therefore necessary to carry out a backtracking calculation to estimate the acetaminophen concentration in the patient's blood 4 h before admission to hospital. (In practice, standard graphs have been prepared and are used instead of calculations.)

Data required: the plasma half-life of acetaminophen is 2 ± 0.4 h.

The easiest way of doing this backtracking calculation is to divide the time elapsed by the half-life to get the number of half-lives which have passed since the peak drug concentration. In this example, the elapsed time is from 6 to 10 P.M., i.e., 4 h. The half-life is 2 h, therefore approximately two half-lives have passed since the drug concentration was at its highest and in each of these the concentration decreased by 50%. The concentration at 10 P.M. was $50 \, \text{mg} \, \text{l}^{-1}$. Two hours earlier (one half-life) it would have been twice this value, i.e., $2 \times 50 = 100 \, \text{mg} \, \text{l}^{-1}$ and 2 h before that it would have been $2 \times 100 = 200 \, \text{mg} \, \text{l}^{-1}$. This puts the patient above the threshold for therapeutic intervention.

Diamorphine (heroin) The deceased, Mr X, had a history of drug abuse. On the evening before his death, he was drinking in a bar with friends and purchased heroin before leaving. From statements obtained by the police, he injected the heroin intravenously shortly before midnight and lapsed into a semicoma. He was put to bed and his friends watched over him for about 2 h before they went to bed. His girlfriend looked in on him at 3 A.M. when she heard him snoring. Unable to sleep, she again looked in on him at 4 A.M. and found him unresponsive and not breathing. The paramedic team that arrived shortly thereafter found no trace of life and he was pronounced dead on arrival at the local hospital at 4.30 A.M. At autopsy, he was found to have significant pulmonary edema and congestion. A sample of blood taken at the autopsy had a blood morphine concentration of $0.15 \, \text{mg} \, \text{l}^{-1}$ of blood.

Data required: the half-life or morphine after administration of diamorphine (heroin) is 2.5 h.

When diamorphine is injected, it rapidly breaks down into morphine, which is measured in blood. The literature records many studies of heroin-related deaths in which the concentration of morphine is low and is not significantly above the therapeutic range. In this example, a blood concentration of morphine equal to $0.15 \, \text{mg} \, \text{l}^{-1}$ is about 50% higher than the usual therapeutically effective concentration range in patients who are not regularly treated with the drug (up to about $0.1 \, \text{mg} \, \text{l}^{-1}$) and does not indicate an obvious overdose concentration. However, during the period after intravenous injection, the blood concentration will decrease and the peak concentration can be estimated using the known half-life. The elapsed time is about 4 h between drug administration and death.

From eqn [3]:

$$t_{1/2} = 0.693/k$$

In this example, $t_{1/2} = 2.5$ h; therefore $k = 0.693/t_{1/2} = 0.28$.

From eqn [2]:

$$\log_{10} C_t = \log_{10} C_0 - kt/2.3$$

In this example, $C_t = 0.15 \, \text{mg} \, \text{l}^{-1}$, $t = 4$ h, and $k = 0.28$.

$$\log_{10} 0.15 = \log_{10} C_0 - (0.28 \times 4/2.3)$$

therefore $\log_{10} C_0 = -0.82 + 0.49 = -0.33$ and $C_0 = 0.47 \, \text{mg} \, \text{l}^{-1}$.

The peak concentration is well above the therapeutic range and incurs a significant risk of opiate overdose.

See Also

Autopsy, Findings: Drug Deaths; Postmortem Drug Measurements, Interpretation of; Postmortem Drug Sampling and Redistribution; **Pharmacology of Legal and Illicit Drugs**; **Road Traffic, Determination of Fitness To Drive:** Sobriety Tests and Drug Recognition; **Substance Misuse:** Substitution Drugs; Miscellaneous Drugs

Further Reading

Aselt RC (2002) *Disposition of Toxic Drugs and Chemicals in Man,* 6th edn. Foster City, CA: Biomedical.

Brody TM, Larner J, Minneman KP (1998) *Human Pharmacology: Molecular to Clinical.* St Louis, MO: Mosby.

Clark B, Smith DA (1986) *An Introduction to Pharmacokinetics.* Oxford, UK: Blackwell.

Drummer OH (2001) *The Forensic Pharmacology of Drugs of Abuse.* London: Arnold.

Emerson V (1998) Alcohol analysis. In: White P (ed.) *From Crime Scene to Court,* pp. 263–288. Cambridge, UK: Royal Society of Chemistry.

Ferner RE (1996) *Forensic Pharmacology.* Oxford, UK: Oxford University Press.

Forrest ARW (1986) The estimation of Widmark's factor. *Journal of the Forensic Science Society* 26: 249–252.

Hardman JG, Limbird LE, Gilman AG (eds.) (2003) *Goodman and Gilman's The Pharmacological Basis of Therapeutics,* 10th edn. London: McGraw Hill.

Jones AW (1991) Forensic science aspects of ethanol metabolism. In: Maehly A, Williams RL (eds.) *Forensic Science Progress,* pp. 31–89. Berlin: Springer-Verlag.

Moffat AC, Osselton MD, Widdop B (eds.) (2004) *Clarke's Analysis of Drugs and Poisons,* 3rd edn. London: Pharmaceutical Press.

Walls HJ, Brownlie AR (1985) *Drink, Drugs and Driving,* 2nd edn. London: Sweet and Maxwell.

Widmark EMP (1981) *Principles and Applications of Medicolegal Alcohol Determinations.* Davis, CA: Biomedical Publications.

BALLISTIC TRAUMA, OVERVIEW AND STATISTICS

S R Naidoo, University of KwaZulu Natal, Durban, South Africa

Introduction

Gunshot wounds are more destructive than most other injuries. An understanding of the biomechanics, together with the effects of the relationship between a high-speed penetrating missile and body tissues, is crucial to both forensic pathology diagnosis and optimal medical management of injuries. The nature of ballistic trauma presents surgeons with immense challenges, especially in regions where gunshot trauma remains prevalent.

The availability of firearms, especially those possessing considerable firepower and magazine capacity, is of great concern. In South Africa, it is estimated that a large proportion of firearms is illegally obtained. Globally, debate on strategies for improved control of gun ownership continues.

This article provides a broad overview of the general characteristics of ballistic trauma and related aspects.

Definitions

Certain terms, and gunshot wound appearances in particular, often confound interpretation because a term may mean different things to different people. The "burn" and even the "blackening" seen in a close-range wound are examples. To ensure unambiguous interpretation, the use of contentious definitions should be avoided.

Ballistics refers to the study of missiles and projectiles (objects in motion) and their effects. Internal ballistics refers to the dynamics of a bullet in motion between the ignition of the propellant and exiting from the firearm muzzle. External ballistics refers to the same during its flight in air. Terminal ballistics refers to the effects produced by a bullet when it strikes or penetrates any target, whereas wound ballistics is terminal ballistics where the body is the target.

History of Ballistic Injury

The origins of gunpowder manufacture are uncertain. Although it is historically recognized that the Chinese invented gunpowder in the thirteenth century, it is believed that the Muslims of Moorish Spain used combustible powder in the twelfth century. The use of gunpowder as a propellant for projectiles began in the early 1300s. Originally, black powder – a mixture of sulfur, charcoal, and saltpeter (potassium nitrate) – was used in cannons and then it was used in a crude type of hand cannon for more than five centuries until the mid-1800s, when smokeless powder was developed. Single-based propellant was developed in France in 1885, and double-based propellant was developed in England in 1889.

The earliest weapons were muzzle-loaders, in which powder and projectile were introduced through the muzzle by a ramrod. Spiral grooves cut on the inside of the gun barrel (rifling) imparted a spin to the emerging bullet and were first used in the early 1500s in sporting rifles only, not in military guns. The introduction of breech loading led to rapid progress in the development of weapons and ammunition. Over time, different types of firearms and ignition systems were developed (**Table 1**).

Firearms

Modern firearms are either rifled or smooth-bore, and are available in a range of brands and types.

Handgun

The handgun is a small rifled firearm that can be held and fired from one hand. The different types of handguns include single-shot firearms (derringers and air guns), revolvers, and semiautomatic self-loading pistols (**Figures 1** and **2**).

Rifle

The rifle is similar to the handgun, except that it is larger, has a longer bore, and is usually fired from the shoulder (**Figures 3** and **4**).

Shotgun

The shotgun is similar to the rifle, except that it is smooth-bore and usually fires a cluster of small

Table 1 Development of firearms and ammunitions

Year	Development
1450	Matchlock system
1517	Wheel-lock system
1575	First cartridge
1550	Flintlock firearm
1776	Breech-loading firearm
1807	Percussion systems
1814	Percussion cap
1835	Revolver
1836	Pinfire cartridge
1845	Rimfire cartridge
1858	Centerfire cartridge
1884	Machine gun
1892	Self-loading (semiautomatic) pistol

spherical lead balls (pellets) or a modified single projectile (rifle slug) (**Figure 5**).

Automatic Firearms

These are capable of automatic fire (continued firing of successive bullets with a single pull and continued pressure on the trigger).

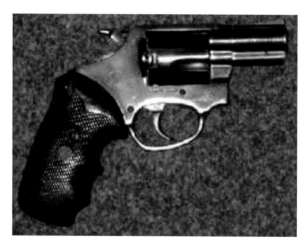

Figure 1 Typical revolver: a 0.38 special (Rossi model no. 27 snub-nose).

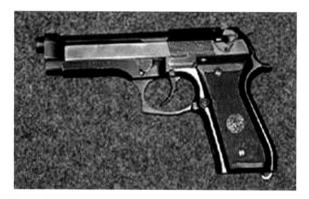

Figure 2 Typical pistol (semiautomatic): a 9-mm Parabellum Z88.

- Submachine guns (machine pistols) are held and discharged from the shoulder or hip, and use pistol ammunition fed by a magazine.
- Machine guns are larger, usually crew-operated, and fire rifle ammunition that is usually supplied on belts.

Other

- Homemade guns, country guns, and zip guns are terms used to describe firearms that are often crudely fashioned out of pieces of metal with a simple firing pin. In certain regions of Africa and Asia, where there is large-scale subversive violent activity or guerrilla warfare, "industries" may exist to meet the demand for firearms. They are also made and used by criminal youth and gang members, even in urban areas (**Figures 6** and **7**).
- Stud guns are industrial power tools used in the building industry that fire metal nails, studs, or fasteners into concrete or steel.
- Penetrating captive bolt instruments are used during the slaughter of animals. A bolt is fired and penetrates the head of the animal, causing a puncture wound several centimeters deep.

The ballistic dynamics are different for stud guns and captive bolt instruments because no free high-speed projectiles are used, and accidental and suicidal deaths have been reported.

The range of different types of ammunition produced today makes ballistic identification a skillful task, requiring extensive knowledge of modern weaponry and ammunition (**Figures 8** and **9**).

Statistics

Gunshot injuries impact greatly on both the criminal justice and the public healthcare systems, and globally they account for about 120 000 injuries and about 40 000 deaths per year. Statistics are vital in understanding socioeconomic burdens, and although many

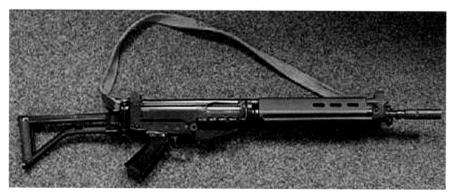

Figure 3 Typical (R1) rifle.

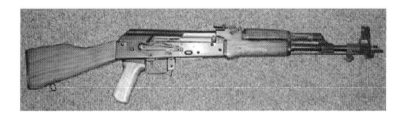

Figure 4 AK-47 rifle.

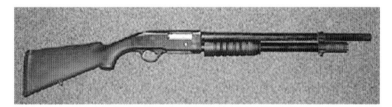

Figure 5 Typical shotgun (12-gauge).

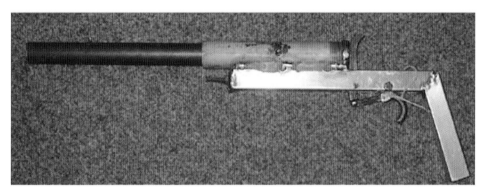

Figure 6 Homemade shotgun made of metal pipe and pieces. Note the simple trigger mechanism.

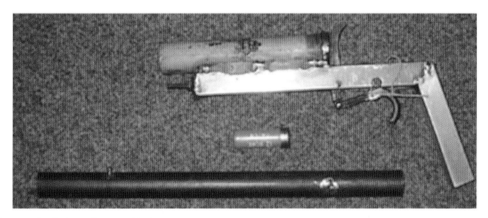

Figure 7 Homemade shotgun disassembled.

violence- and injury-monitoring systems are in place, a comprehensive universal database is lacking.

Although firearm-related injury and mortality may be declining in certain areas of the world, an increased incidence is noted in other regions, where the number of gunshot injuries from civilian strife has increased to the level seen in military conflicts (**Figure 10**). The USA has reported a decline in the number of gunshot incidents in recent years. The number of murders by firearm decreased by approximately 27%, from 18 300 in 1993 to 13 300 in 1997, and a similar trend has been seen for nonfatal gunshots. However, it is acknowledged that the rate of all firearm injuries and deaths is still unacceptably

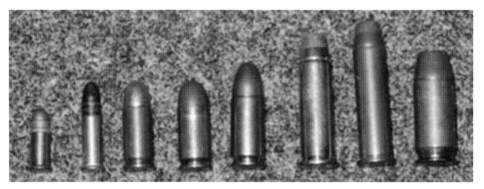

Figure 8 Handgun cartridges (from left to right): 0.22 short, 0.22 long rifle, 7.65 mm, 9 mm short, 9 mm Parabellum, 0.38 Special, 0.357, and 0.45.

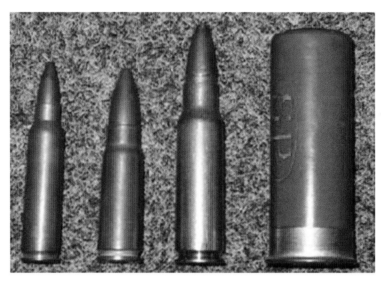

Figure 9 Rifle (and a shotgun) cartridges (from left to right): 5.56 × 45 (R4/R5/M16), 7.62 × 39 (AK-47), 7.62 × 51 (R1), and 12-gauge.

high in the USA – second only to traffic injuries as the leading cause of violent death.

In South Africa, there has been a disturbing accelerated incidence of injury and death from firearm use, a phenomenon that is seen in developing countries undergoing rapid sociopolitical and economic transformation. For a South African population in excess of 50 million, an estimated 70 000–80 000 unnatural deaths, mainly from injuries, were recorded in 2001. Most firearm homicides involve young adults (20–34 years of age) and are the leading cause of unnatural deaths in general for all groups between the ages of 15 and 64 years (**Figure 11**).

Changing trends in hospital admissions for penetrating torso trauma in one city (Durban) between 1988 and 1992 showed that stab wounds decreased by 30% while gunshot wounds increased by more than 800% (**Figure 12**). Interesting observations include a higher survival rate of victims with sharp (stabbing) wounds compared to gunshot wounds, reflecting the serious wounding capacity of firearms.

Characteristics of Missile Movement

Characteristics affecting missile movement include velocity, energy, mass, inertia, ballistics coefficient, spin, gravity, shape, air resistance, and other movement during flight.

During flight, a bullet spins on its longitudinal axis, providing stability and allowing for greater distance to be reached. Its velocity adds more to its kinetic energy than its mass. Its inertia will cause it to continue in motion, but it is affected by air resistance, which begins to slow it down progressively, and by gravity, which causes the projectile to assume a curved path (trajectory) in long flight.

The ballistics coefficient of a projectile depicts its capacity to maintain its velocity against air resistance. It is a relationship between mass (m), diameter (d), and a form factor (i) determined by the shape of the bullet, and it is represented by the following formula:

$$c = m/id^2$$

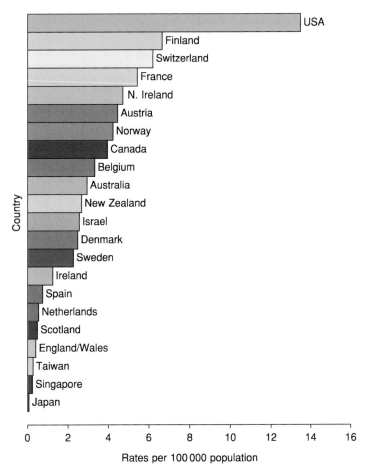

Figure 10 Global firearm death rates, 2001. The data represent combined suicide and homicide gun deaths. Many countries are not represented, largely due to unavailability of data. In South Africa, no crude national mortality rate for firearm deaths is available because mortality surveillance studies only reflect an urban focus.

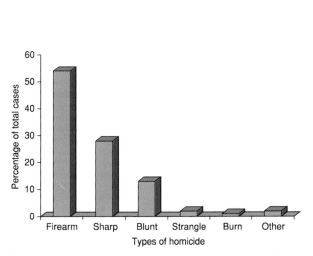

Figure 11 External causes of homicide, South Africa (2001). The data reflect prevailing trends in predominantly urban areas covered by the mortality surveillance system. Deaths by firearms account for more than half of all cases of homicide.

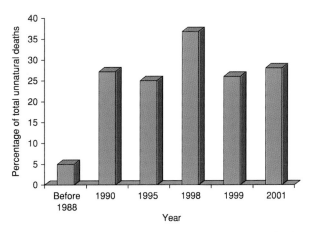

Figure 12 Trends in firearm deaths, Durban, South Africa (1988–2001). The figure shows the unprecedented surge in reported incidence of gunshot fatalities in Durban, a trend observed during the past two decades in metropolitan areas of South Africa. Deaths from gunshots increased from approximately 5% before 1988 to an average of 25–37% and have remained somewhat at a plateau since then.

Projectiles with a larger ballistics coefficient move more effectively and lose less velocity as they travel.

Bullets in motion are unstable because they are affected by many factors. Yaw is a divergence of the long axis of the bullet from a straight line as the tip bobs (wobbles) up and down during flight. This characteristic is important because a large angle of yaw will affect the presenting profile upon impact and contribute to greater kinetic energy loss and damage. Precession is a circular yaw around the bullet's center of gravity that takes the shape of a decreasing spiral as it moves away from the muzzle, and nutation describes a rotational movement in a small circle that forms a rosette pattern like a spinning top, but these have less effect on wounding.

Shotgun pellets are spherical lead balls that have a poor ballistics coefficient and unfavorable aerodynamics. They do not have the penetrating ability of bullets.

High- and Low-Velocity Injuries

Wounds can be classified according to effects due to missile velocity (**Table 2**).

Wounding Capacity of a Bullet

The capacity to injure depends on the amount of energy dissipated to the tissues as the bullet impacts and passes into the body. This depends on the velocity of the hurtling projectile and on other variables, such as its mass, shape, physical structure, behavior upon impact and entry, and the physical characteristics of the tissues penetrated. The velocity mainly determines the amount of kinetic energy possessed by the bullet, as reflected in the formula for the energy of an object by virtue of its motion:

$$E = 1/2m \times v^2$$

where E is kinetic energy, m is mass, and v is velocity.

Table 2 High- and low-velocity firearms[a]

Type	Velocity ($m\,s^{-1}$)
Low-velocity	Less than 366 $m\,s^{-1}$
Medium-velocity	Between 366 and 762 $m\,s^{-1}$
High-velocity	Between 762 and 1260 $m\,s^{-1}$
Very-high-velocity	Greater than 1260 $m\,s^{-1}$

[a]For all practical purposes, despite the above, pathologists usually categorize wounds as either low- or high-velocity on the basis of distinctive and recognizable appearances at autopsy: the breakpoint between these is about 700 $m\,s^{-1}$. Most handguns are low-velocity, whilst rifles are high-velocity firearms, but a few large handguns do edge on to the high-velocity range.

Because bullets possess most velocity at the point of leaving the firearm muzzle, one would expect a greater degree of injury with impacts at closer ranges of fire. Also, a larger, heavier projectile should produce more injury than a smaller one, all other factors being equal. However, these distinctions, when evaluating wounds, tend to be overshadowed by the other significant variables.

Upon puncturing skin and passing into tissues, a rapidly spinning bullet creates a direct path by crushing and tearing the tissue directly ahead. For low-velocity bullets, this is the most significant mechanism of injury.

At the same time, and conspicuously with high-velocity injury, the tissue on either side of the perforating path is violently hurled outward at right angles by forces generated by energy transfer. This produces, directly behind the missile, a large and often spindle-shaped temporary cavity that pulsates vigorously outward back and forth for several milliseconds until it finally settles around the bullet path, forming the permanent visible wound track. Pathologists also refer to a related phenomenon in which shock waves generated ahead of the speeding missile may produce distant injury by propagation of the wave along fluid-filled vessels and organs such as blood vessels, heart, bladder, bowel, and the brain-filled cranial cavity.

It is the extent of the temporary cavity that defines the real amount of the tissue damage, not just the permanent track. The greater the energy dissipated by the bullet, the larger the size of the temporary cavity (and injury), all other factors being equal. The devastating effects of a temporary cavity are seen in high-velocity gunshot wounds, where the cavitation does not regress completely but remains as a larger permanent cavity (**Figure 13**). Bone fracture from cavitation, however, is very rare. For most practical purposes, cavitation is only of significance in high-velocity injuries (rifles) and it is much less of a factor in low-velocity (most handgun) injuries.

As a general principle, if a bullet exits the body, its energy is only partially lost in the tissues. If a bullet lodges in the body, its total kinetic energy is imparted, and therefore a greater degree of injury is sustained.

The other factors that tend to enlarge the size of the temporary cavity by increasing the energy lost include yaw or tumbling of bullet, bullet deformation and fragmentation, and the density/consistency of the tissues. Although stabilized by its spin after leaving the barrel, a bullet still possesses some instability due to initial yaw or wag and, if striking tissue at this point, will be more destructive; this partially explains the tendency for greater destruction at closer ranges of fire. The yaw is soon reduced in flight, but it begins to increase later when losing velocity. Yaw is also greatly increased after the bullet passes through tissue: its

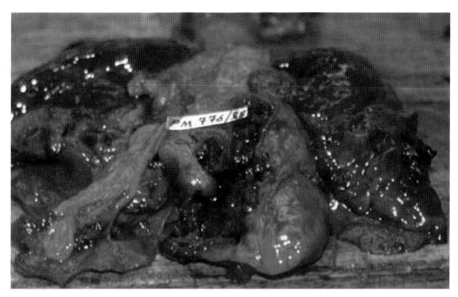

Figure 13   Mutilated heart from a high-velocity gunshot injury.

entrance profile widens, the drag on it increases, and it may also tumble.

The tendency for bullet deformation and fragmentation is an intended feature of the bullet by virtue of its physical makeup, and the bullet is fashioned for this effect by the manufacturers of ammunition. Bullets with a rounded or blunt configuration of nose will have a greater amount of drag and impart more energy and damage to tissue than bullets with a pointed nose. Bullets that distort at the nose, such as soft-point or hollow-point ammunition, creating a "mushroom" effect of deformation, also cause greater damage than pointed-nose projectiles. With increased velocity, bullets also tend to break up. This applies to soft-point and hollow-point rifle bullets especially, and it is generally not seen with handgun velocities. Shrapnel fragments will then be secondary missiles that create their own tracks and increase damage. In addition, certain types of pointed, full-metal-jacketed (military) rifle bullets are also designed to fragment extensively. For example, the 5.56-mm round fired by the R4 and R5 rifles in South Africa causes exceptionally severe wounds due to its velocity and tendency, due to yaw, to break up from the base, extruding and dispersing its lead core, as it compresses out along its length and bends at the cannula, with the pointed tip remaining intact with lodgment or exit (**Figure 14**).

Density, elastic cohesiveness, and recoil to injury of different tissues vary and affect the extent of wounding. Generally, physical disruption of tissue occurs when the limits of elastic accommodation to deformation are exceeded. Skin has great elastic ability but is easily punctured by a bullet, leaving a small perforation. Muscle is of good density and also has remarkable elastic recoil and cohesion, and the

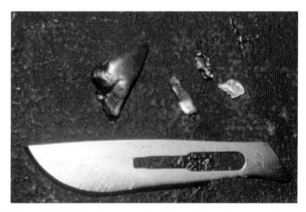

Figure 14   Bullet fragments of a 5.56 × 45 round extracted from a body.

permanent wound track remains small. Lung tissue has low density and is exceedingly elastic, suffering less permanent destruction of tissue. Liver and kidney, on the other hand, are dense tissues, but with less tissue suppleness and cohesiveness, and suffer the consequences of wider and greater damage.

Effects of Intermediary Obstructions

Bullets may strike solid intervening structures or surfaces and then enter a body, either having passed through the structure or deflected off it. A bullet ricochets (bounces) upon impact on a surface at certain critical small angles of approach, with the outcome determined by velocity and physical characteristics of the bullet and also the nature of the surface struck.

Ricocheting bullets are unstable, erratic, and unpredictable, and they may tumble, producing irregular and atypical entrance wounds, tending to lodge in the body. A bullet may also show a flattened side from first impact. Portions of the body surface adjacent to or on the surface struck by the bullet may show a shower of punctate abrasions due to fine fragments of surface and missile; examples of these may be seen with a ceramic tiled surface, or tarred or concrete pavement surface. This appearance may be mistaken for gunpowder "tattooing" abrasions, but they are usually larger, irregular, and coarser than true tattooing. Intermediate targets may also include glass, wood, and clothing/fabric.

Path through the Body

A bullet passing through the body tends to retain its original direction, except when at sufficiently low velocity to ricochet off bone. In the cranium, for example, a bullet may ricochet off the base of the skull, deflecting upward into the brain at another angle.

Wounds from Shotguns

Shotguns differ from rifled weapons in that they discharge a cluster of pellets, which begin to disperse after a short distance and fan out as multiple single projectiles. At close distances, injuries can be devastating due to the effects of multiple pellets. Because of poor aerodynamics, the pellets do not reach the distances that bullets do and lose velocity rapidly, being much less effective at longer ranges. In addition to the constituents of a conventional rifled gun discharge, wadding (plastic, cardboard, or felt "spacers" between propellant and pellets in the cartridge) and sometimes fragments of the cartridge case may also emerge from the muzzle, causing injury at close range. The appearance of the cluster of pellet wounds varies greatly with firing distance and helps to establish such range of fire. Rare usage of shotgun slugs may produce severe wounds due to missile size.

Consequences of Gunshot Injury

The course and extent of the missile track and whether or not vital structures are hit are very significant factors that determine the degree of injury, apart from the quantity of energy transfer. Serious wounds may still occur with low-velocity bullets, which can injure vital organs. The manifestations of wounds also depend on the type of projectile (deforming or nondeforming types, small pellets, large slugs) and the type of tissue. With shotguns, the severity of wounds depends mainly on the distance from the shooter. Gunshots are also likely to be contaminated.

Effects on Skin

Skin is tough because it is resilient and elastic, and it is more resistant than muscle to injury and perforation. The minimum velocity required by the projectile to perforate the skin ranges from $58 \, \mathrm{m \, s^{-1}}$ for a .38-caliber lead handgun bullet to $101 \, \mathrm{m \, s^{-1}}$ for a small lead airgun pellet. Lighter projectiles need higher velocity for penetration. Velocity lost in perforating skin alone is less than that required to pass through muscle tissue bulk.

Effects on Bone

Bullets cause fractures and often fragmentation, thrusting bony fragments forward in the direction of the track, that then act as secondary missiles. The appearance of a fracture may help to establish the direction of the track because the bullet levers (bevels) out the edges of the bony shelf around the perforation on the exit side, creating a cone-shaped excavated appearance and a neat "punched-out" hole on the entry side. This is best seen in the skull, due to its double layer of compact bone with a sandwiched inner spongy layer of diploe. Skull bone defect characteristics also help to establish the nature of oblique and tangential shots (keyhole and gutter types). Another phenomenon seen with high-energy gunshots of the skull vault (particularly with contact wounds) is remote fractures of the base, especially at the orbital plates, due to cavitational and expansile pressure waves in the rigid cranium (**Figure 15**).

Effects on Internal Tissues

With low-velocity wounds, wounding is caused by laceration of tissues along a wound track. The seriousness of wounding depends on the importance of the damaged structure to sustaining life (e.g., the heart and great vessels, major air passages, and vital brain centers) and on the rate and degree of bleeding. High-velocity wounds are accompanied by widespread damage due to cavitation, especially in solid organs such as liver and brain.

The wound track through the brain may be wide, with surrounding tissue contusion at both entry and exit sites and along the track. Contusions may also be seen on the entire basal brain surface overlying basal skull bone irregularities and prominences. Fine bone splinters dispersed along the brain track adjacent to the entry wound may also help establish the direction of the track in uncertain cases. Deaths from gunshot to the brain are usually due either to vital center injury or, if the individually briefly survives, to complications of increased intracranial pressure and other extracranial sequelae (**Figure 16**).

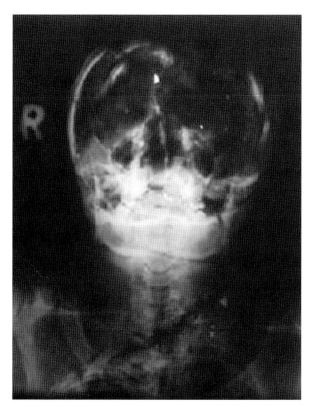

Figure 15 X-ray showing high-velocity gunshot of the head with explosive effect and another wound obliquely across the cervicothoracic spine.

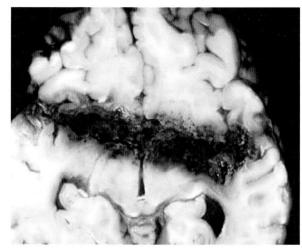

Figure 16 Gunshot wound track through the brain.

Morbidity and mortality from delayed complications of abdominal gunshot wounds, especially those involving the bowel, are high, due to rapid contamination and blood stream dissemination of sepsis.

Ability to Act after Rapidly Fatal Injury

It is often relevant in legal proceedings to know if someone who died from injuries was immediately killed or incapacitated; if not, what type of activity was possible, and for how long? The period of survival and ability to act are not the same. The subject is fraught with difficulty due to unreliability of reported time periods and physiological variability between individuals. Any two people suffering identical injuries may differ in their capabilities to act and survive.

Aside from age, fitness, and preexisting disease, the nature of injury is relevant. Reported cases show that individuals sustaining serious gunshot wounds are capable of extraordinary actions in the several seconds before they collapse and die. With an extensively lacerated heart or severed large artery, an individual can retain consciousness for at least 10–15 s before oxygen remaining in the cerebral capillaries is depleted. In addition, with gunshots of the brain, victims with severe frontal lobe wounds may have prolonged survival periods, while wounds of the basal ganglia may result in immediate unconsciousness and incapacity. Although severe brainstem wounds usually result in immediate unconsciousness, incapacitation, and death, there have been a few reported cases of short survival in a vegetative state.

The issue of "stopping power" of a bullet is also relevant. It is believed that deforming and expanding bullets are more able to incapacitate. Although they may theoretically produce worse internal injuries than nondeforming ones, trauma surgeons and pathologists are unable to distinguish between these appearances. Stopping power is more likely a characteristic of the type of vital organ or structure injured than the degree of damage sustained.

Firearm Discharge Residue

Discharge of a firearm is accompanied by heated gases and flame for a very short distance, soot, unburnt or burning powder particles, primer residue, fine vaporized metal from the bullet or cartridge case, and fine metal particles stripped from the bullet. Soot and powder particles carry for slightly longer distances than the other constituents. Determining the range of fire from the varying configurations in wounds of these types of residue is a critical part of wound evaluation.

The detection of gunshot residue from wounds, clothing, hands of the victim, and suspected shooter is a specialized forensic ballistic examination. Meticulous and timely collection of evidentiary material is important (**Table 3**).

Table 3 Firearm discharge residue

Source	Major constituents
Primer	Lead, antimony, barium
Powder	Nitrocellulose, nitroglycerine
Bullet	Lead, copper, iron
Cartridge	Copper, zinc, nickel
Barrel	Iron, oil

Modern methods of laboratory analysis of primer residue (barium, antimony, and lead) include flameless atomic absorption spectrometry and scanning microscope–energy dispersive X-ray spectrometry. Trace metal detection techniques are used to link the use of a particular weapon with an individual, and they rely on trace metal residue remaining on the palms after gripping a gun. Soot and powder deposits seen on clothing or wounds with the naked eye, magnification lens, or microscope by an experienced pathologist are usually sufficient to make a finding of range of fire. Laboratory analytical tests for nitrites produced by the burning of smokeless powder (cellulose nitrate) and for the detection of lead residues are available.

Value of the Scene Examination

As with all suspected homicides and other cases in which uncertainty and/or suspicion prevail, a visit to the scene by the pathologist or forensic practitioner is particularly important in the case of gunshot fatalities.

The scenario is often critically dissected out in subsequent court hearings in which range of fire, intermediary obstructions, disturbances of the scene, direction of fire, patterns of blood splatters, and amount of physical activity following injury relating to the degree and position of significant lost blood are considered. In addition, positions of the firearm and cartridge cases ejected (particularly in suspected suicidal gunshots of the head) in relation to the body and the number of shots fired, among other issues, may be debated. A scene examination places the medical examiner in a far superior position to express critical opinion.

Autopsy on the Gunshot Victim

The postmortem examination on the gunshot victim should be as meticulous as any standard forensic autopsy examination. Prerequisites include a good circumstantial history of the case up to and near the time of the death and a scene examination where possible. Particularly important is the careful examination of clothing, radiography, photography, and skillful collection of gunshot residue (in correct receptacles). For optimal evaluation of wound detail, good light, preferably natural, is crucial.

Value of Radiography

Radiography is an invaluable tool in gunshot autopsies, and it should be mandatory. It indicates not only the location of lodged missiles but also the nature of the dispersion of bullets and shrapnel fragments, where fragmentation and deflection occur, and the pattern of the bony injuries sustained. Imaging may either be by plain film radiography or by fluoroscopy, and a permanent record may be obtained either by plain films or by thermal-type prints for legal purposes. Two film views at right angles to each other are necessary for precise location of a missile. Radiography is equally important when an exit wound is present, contrary to some common perceptions, because an exit wound may lead one to believe that the entire missile has passed through, whereas a bone or bullet fragment may have exited and the evidence-bearing bullet or fragment may still be lodged internally. This may be easily missed at autopsy if X-ray examination is not done beforehand (**Figure 17**).

Unusual consequences, such as bullet embolism, may require radiographs of peripheral and remote regions.

Miscellaneous Considerations

Manner of Death

The distinction between murder, suicide, and accident is of prime importance in any firearm death and may be complex. It requires consideration of complete circumstantial history, witness statements, scene examination, and autopsy, ballistic, and other laboratory evidence. There is no known distinguishing manifestation of a gunshot wound that proves a specific manner of death.

Suicide by Firearm

Most suicides occur with handguns, and in males, and most are of a contact nature. These are usually inflicted into the head (80%) but may also involve the chest (17%) or abdomen (2%). Wounds of the head may be bitemporal or intraoral, but they may vary with regard to position. Appearances may also vary with sex or handedness of the deceased. Although suicide patterns of wounds are recognizable, there are no absolutes and many variations occur. Victims have shot themselves at intermediate and greater ranges and in uncommon places on the body, including the back of the head, and even multiple gunshots are seen. Some cases may be difficult to distinguish from accident and homicide. Discovery of a body may reveal a gun still held in the hand or otherwise close to the body. The firing hand (and

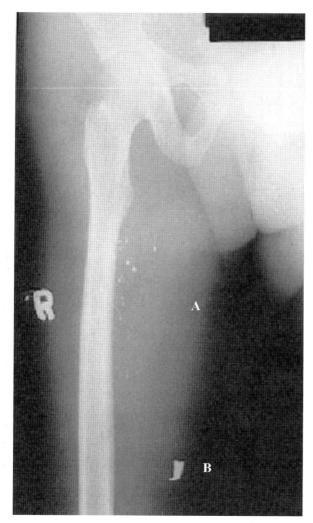

Figure 17 X-ray, high-velocity missile. The X-ray shows the appearance of a high-velocity gunshot wound of the right thigh with only soft-tissue injury caused by the 5.56 × 45 military round (M16 or R4/R5 rifle). The typical fine shrapnel fragments of the lead core of the bullet provide the "snowstorm" appearance and crimping of the bullet with the characteristic "bent triangle" of the bullet tip. A, fine shrapnel fragments; B, bullet head.

even the firearm muzzle) may show a "backsplatter" of fine blood droplets, which occurs more often with higher-caliber gunfire. This may also be seen on the other hand if it was used to support the barrel. The absence of such blood splatter does not preclude a contact wound.

Wounds from Homemade Firearms

Characteristics of homemade gun wounds include extensive soot deposits and burns in very close and contact wounds, atypical muzzle imprints, and lacerations of the firing hand. In addition, there is reduced depth of incursion into the body by the bullet, which shows the absence of typical rifling marks.

Accidents by Firearm

In addition to a pathologist's consideration of the nature and positions of wounds and information from reconstruction of scenes, the evaluation of the functional state and safety characteristics of a firearm (including its capability to discharge when dropped or with very light trigger pressure) is a technical matter within the ambit of a firearms examiner.

Gunshots Involving the Gravid Uterus

These are not uncommon, and effects include miscarriage, premature delivery, or intrauterine death, although maternal deaths are rare.

Hunting Accidents

Hunting accidents are frequently associated with negligent handling, careless behavior with weapons, and disregard for basic issues of safety.

Armed Conflicts and Civilian Shootings

In armed conflict, the number of people wounded is normally at least twice the number killed. In situations in which international codes governing warfare are not adhered to, as in extrajudicial executions of prisoners or civilians, the number killed may be greater than the number wounded when shots are fired against persons or a group who are immobilized, in a restricted space, or incapable of defending themselves. Victims may be shot from closer distances and sustain multiple shots in vital regions from automatic weapons, increasing the probability of fatal injury. This distinction may have significance for the recognition of war crimes.

Lead Poisoning from Retained Bullets

This is a rare complication, occurring mainly when a bullet lodges in a joint space, with the synovial fluid appearing to promote the dissolution of lead and entry into tissues.

Embolism of Projectiles

This is an occasional phenomenon, usually suspected when there is no exit wound and no bullet visible on X-ray, or none is retrieved during exhaustive examination of the region expected to contain the lodged missile. Cases usually involve gunshot entry wounds of the chest and abdomen. The bullet is usually of smaller caliber and of low velocity, having insufficient penetrating ability. If entering the left side of the heart, thoracic aorta, or abdominal aorta, it usually embolizes into the femoral and popliteal arteries of the lower limbs; occasionally, pellets have embolized to the brain. In the case of less frequent venous embolism, bullets may enter the right side of the heart, inferior vena cava, or iliac veins, with retrograde passage either to veins of the lower limbs or upward to the heart. Nonvascular "embolization" or migration of bullets along tissue planes, body cavities, flat and curved bone surfaces, air passages, and sinuses has occasionally been reported.

Pistol Whipping

This refers to blunt assault using the butt of a firearm, usually to the head or face but also to the body.

Bullets in Free Fall

Injuries, including penetrating wounds of the head, have been caused by bullets falling downward to the ground after having been shot into the air, particularly in festive times and at celebratory events, such as on the eve of a new year. The velocity of the free-falling bullet may increase to beyond the minimum level for skin penetration.

Rubber and Plastic Bullet Injuries

Developed within the past three decades for police riot-control purposes, rubber and plastic bullets are intended for firing distances of not less than 20–30 m and to cause pain and minor incapacitating injury only. Many injuries, and a number of deaths, have since been reported.

Blank Cartridge Injuries

Used in starter pistols for athletic races, blank cartridges are intended for audible detonation only and do not fire a bullet or pellet because the cartridge contains only detonating powder. However, if discharged with the muzzle in contact with the body, especially at the chest and abdomen, fatal injuries may ensue.

Ballistic Identification

Ballistic identification is another function of the ballistic examiner or firearm identification expert. Ballistic identification deals mainly with the comparison of fired bullets and/or cartridge cases with firearms to ascertain whether a bullet or cartridge case was fired from a particular gun. To do this, the rifling marks on fired bullets found at a crime scene are evaluated by microscopy in comparison with those on control bullets fired in the laboratory from the firearm in question. Cartridge cases are compared to fired control cases by firing pin impressions on the base and other various ejector, extractor, magazine, and breechblock markings. It is important to use the same brand and type of ammunition in the testing. Other related examinations include comparison between fired bullets and between fired cartridge cases. Bullets are compared according to their class (type, caliber, and rifling marks) and individual characteristics (scored on the bullet shoulder as it passes through the barrel).

Fingerprints may sometimes be obtained from a gun, and often they can also be obtained from fired cartridge cases. Tissue and blood trapped on a bullet or bullet fragment, having passed through a body, may be subjected to histological or cytological examination to establish the tissue or organ perforated and for DNA "fingerprint" analysis to identify the victim.

Chain of Custody of Specimens

Ensuring the continuity and legal acceptability of all evidence is a critical aspect of forensic and ballistic examinations, and it includes the correct handling of bullets so as not to deface or mark them in a manner that spoils evidence.

Surgical Management of Soft-Tissue Gunshot Wounds

Low-velocity soft-tissue injuries are amenable to conservative, local treatment. Contamination is not severe, and fractures are treated conventionally, dictated by the nature of bony injury. In high-velocity and other severe injuries, extensive tissue destruction, devitalization, and gross contamination necessitate open surgical management, debridement, irrigation, and antibiotic cover.

See Also

Imaging: Photography; **Injury, Fatal and Nonfatal:** Firearm Injuries; **Injuries and Deaths During Police Operations:** Shootings During Police Stops and Arrests; **War Crimes:** Pathological Investigation

Further Reading

Bartlett CS (2003) Clinical update: Gunshot wound ballistics. *Clinical Orthopedics* 408: 28–57.

Centers for Disease Control and Prevention, National Center for Health Statistics (2001, September 21) National vital statistics reports, deaths: final data for 1999, vol. 49, no. 8. Available online at www.cdc.gov/nchs/fastats/firearms.htm.

Dada MA, McQuoid-Mason DJ (eds.) (2001) *Introduction to Medico-Legal Practice*, pp. 205–222. Durban, South Africa: Butterworths.

Di Maio VJM (1999) *Gunshot Wounds: Practical Aspects of Firearms, Ballistics and Forensic Techniques*, 2nd edn. Boca Raton, FL: CRC Press.

Fackler ML (1996) Gunshot wound review. *Annals of Emergency Medicine* 28(2): 194–203.

Knight B (1996) *Forensic Pathology*, 2nd edn. London: Arnold.

Krug EG, Dahlberg LL, Mercy JA, Zwai AB, Lozana R (eds.) (2002) *World Report on Violence and Health.* Geneva: World Health Organization.

Matzopoulos R (ed.) (2002) *A Profile of Fatal Injuries in South Africa, 2001.* Third annual report of the National Injury Mortality Surveillance System. Cape Town, South Africa: Medical Research Council.

Peden M, Meumann C, Dada M (1998) Homicide in Durban. *Trauma Review* 6(2): 7–8.

World Health Organization (2001) *Small Arms and Global Health.* Contribution to the United Nations Conference on Illicit Trade in Small Arms and Light Weapons, July 9–20. Geneva, Switzerland: WHO.

Ballistic Trauma, Injuries *See* **Injury, Fatal and Nonfatal:** Explosive Injury; Firearm Injuries; **Tactical Medicine**; **Terrorism:** Suicide Bombing, Investigation; **War Injuries**

Bioterrorism *See* **Terrorism:** Nuclear and Biological

BLOOD GROUPING

G S Williams, Northern Illinois University, DeKalb, IL, USA

Introduction

Standard blood grouping involves typing for antigens found on the surface of blood cells using serology. These blood cell antigens are also found on other body tissues and in body fluids of secretors. A broad range of antigen systems on red blood cells (RBCs) and white blood cells (WBCs) are stable, polymorphic markers for a wide variety of uses. Blood grouping has been performed for medicolegal purposes since the 1920s. Although it is not used at all in many forensic laboratories, due to the availability and convenience of automation of DNA profiling methods, it is still used for parentage testing in some areas in order to decrease cost. Parentage testing by blood grouping can be applied to inheritance issues, immigration of relatives, kidnapping cases, baby mix-ups, and traditional paternity cases. In addition, blood grouping is critical for transfusion medicine and transplantation medicine.

Blood grouping is performed by directly typing fresh blood samples or fresh stains collected in normal saline (0.85% NaCl). Methods for typing dried blood stains include absorption–inhibition, absorption–elution, or microagglutination methods. Other body fluids of secretors are typed for ABH substances and Lewis antigens. Although most tissues of the body also have ABH and Duffy antigens on them, most RBC antigens are only on RBCs.

WBCs may also be typed for human leukocyte antigens (HLAs). These antigens are on all nucleated cells in large amounts, and reduced amounts on nonnucleated cells such as RBCs and platelets. The traditional microlymphocytotoxicity method is cumbersome and technically challenging. Newer nucleic acid testing has replaced much of the serological HLA testing. Platelets have polymorphic antigens as well, but the typing of them is challenging and is not routinely performed in medicolegal laboratories.

The purpose of this article is to cover key blood groups useful for identity and parentage testing, and the methods used to detect them in fresh and dried samples.

Major RBC Systems

ABO, Secretor, and Lewis

The ABO system has been used the longest and is very useful for excluding a wrongfully accused person. The reagents are readily available and the testing is easy to perform and read. Gene frequencies have been established for almost every regional and ethnic population and the frequencies have been stable over time. Refer to **Table 1** for a sample of phenotype frequencies in diverse populations. Mutations resulting in a new viable phenotype are rare. The full expression of the ABO antigens encoded on chromosome 9 is dependent upon genes at the *Hh* and *Se* loci closely linked on chromosome 19 as well. Lewis antigen expression is also related to *Hh* and *Se* loci.

ABO, H, and Lewis antigens are carbohydrates. They are added to type 1 or type 2 precursor molecules composed of chains of sugars with different linkages. The H glycosyl-transferase prefers type 2 chains present on cell membranes. The precursor substance attached to type 2 chains is H (fucose) and a person must inherit *Hh* or *HH* to express H substance. Glycosyl-transferases add H to soluble glycoproteins, sphingolipids, lipids, or to glycoproteins or glycopingolipids embedded in the RBC membrane and other tissue cell membranes. H is then enzymatically changed to A (terminal N-acetyl-glucosamine) or B (terminal β-D-galactose) or both by glycosyl-transferases. These are the gene products of group A, B, or AB blood types. The O allele codes for a nonfunctional gene product. H is expressed for nearly 100% of group Os. When individuals are *hh*, they do not express H substance. Even though they may inherit A or B glycosyl-transferases, they will not express it on cells; although a few people with *hh* genotypes inherit Se and have converted type 2 chains to A, B, and/or H. The RBCs will type like an O by standard typing methods. This is called the Bombay phenotype and is extremely rare. All Bombays produce anti-H that reacts with all normal O cells strongly, thus they are easy to differentiate from a true O. Bombay and rare subgroups must be considered when typing discrepancies occur.

For ABH to be present in secretions another locus is required. *Se* is the secretor gene. People who inherit *SeSe* or *Sese* express ABH antigens in their secretions and people who inherit *sese* do not. Type 1 chains present in secretory glands are preferred. The ABH antigens in secretions match those on RBCs. Rare exceptions exist and will be discussed later. ABH is found in easily measurable amounts on all tissues except eye lens, cartilage, hair, and nails. For secretors it is found in saliva, sputum, sweat, semen, tears, pus, nasal and bronchial secretions, gastric juice, urine, and other tissue fluids except cerebrospinal fluid.

Common blood types for the ABO system include: O, A_1, A_2, B, A_1B, and A_2B. The alleles A_1, A_2, B, and O are codominant alleles; each person has only two, one from each parent. A group O is genetically *OO*. A group A could be A_1A_2, A_1O, A_1A_1, A_2A_2, or A_2O. A group B genotype could be *BB* or *BO*. People with blood type AB are either A_1B or A_2B.

Secretors are Le(a–b+) and nonsecretors are Le(a+). *Le* encodes for a glycosyl-transferase also but only acts on type 1 chains in secretory glands. The resulting substance is a glycosphingolipid. Lewis is, therefore, adsorbed on to RBCs, not an integral part of the membrane. Lewis typing is not commonly done for parentage testing due to complex inheritance patterns and delayed full expression until about age 6. It can be useful for determining secretor status of older children and adults by testing blood, saliva, or stains. Le^a will be found in the saliva of an Le(a–b+) person because Lewis substance is not completely converted. An extremely rare phenotype, Le(a+b+), found in Asians and Australian Aborigines, has been described; Le(a+b+) may be secretors or nonsecretors. Le(a–b–) is also a less common phenotype; most secretors have ABH in their secretions but, rarely, someone who secretes B and no H, or A and no H is found. The antigens that would be expected on RBCs and in secretions depending upon expression of Hh, Se, and Le phenotypes are listed in **Table 2**.

RH System

The RH system was first recognized in 1939 and defined as D in 1940. RH is short for Rhesus. The antibody produced by guinea pigs and rabbits in response to Rhesus monkey cells agglutinated 85% of human RBCs. This was called anti-Rhesus and the corresponding human antigen was called Rhesus. It is now known that RH is not identical to D. The

Table 1 ABO phenotype percentages in selected populations

Population	O	A1	A2	B	A1B	A2B
Vietnamese	45	21	0	29	5	0
Bengalese	22	22	2	38	15	1
South American Indians	100	0	0	0	0	0
Australian Aborigines	44	56	0	0	0	0
Lapps	18	36	19	5	6	6

Data from Mourant AE, Kopec AC, and Domaniewska-Sobczak K (1976) *The Distribution of the Human Blood Groups and Other Biochemical Polymorphisms*, 2nd edn. Oxford, UK: Oxford University Press.

Table 2 ABH and Lewis antigens in secretions and on blood cells based on phenotype

Phenotype	Antigens on red cells	Antigens in secretions
Le, Se, H, ABO	Le^b, ABH	Le^a, Le^b, ABH
le, Se, H, ABO	ABH	ABH
le, se, H, ABO	ABH	None
Le, Se, h, ABO	Le^a	Le^a
Le, se, h, ABO	Le^a	Le^a
le, Se, h, ABO	None	None

"RH" antigen on human RBCs is actually LW. Now that the molecular biology of the Rh system has been worked out, two types of nomenclature are accepted for current use in documents: numerical and CDE. The Weiner nomenclature Rh-Hr based on a one-locus hypothesis is no longer used except in verbal communication about phenotypes. The Rh-Hr nomenclature is an easy shorthand method for the most common phenotypes and haplotypes. It is easier to say R^1 rather than DCe (verbally: big D, big C, little e). Similarly, the numerical system works well for computerization, but is too cumbersome for verbal communication. There are 46 alleles associated with the Rh system but only a few have readily available monospecific antisera and useful polymorphism. The RH system has its greatest usefulness in parentage testing. RH antigens are well developed at birth and are inherited as autosomal dominant genes. Testing for DCEce does not provide genotype information that is critical to excluding alleged fathers unless a family study can be done with his parents, siblings, or multiple children. However, when race is known, an educated guess of probable genotypes from the phenotypes may be made. Additional testing for combination antigens Ce and ce helps to establish genotypes even when only the alleged father and child are available. Blood stains that are fresh and intact RBCs can be RH-typed; older stains are tested in only a few laboratories. **Table 3** shows frequencies of Rh haplotypes.

RH genes are on chromosome 1 and are closely linked. RHD and RHCE are closely linked loci. The alleles for RHD are either RHD (D+ or Rh+ or RH:1) or deleted (D– or Rh– or RH:–1) for Caucasians, and RHD (D+ or Rh+ or RH:1) or inactive (D– or Rh– or RH:–1) for Blacks, Japanese, or Chinese. The alleles for RHCE are $RHCe$, $RHcE$, $RHCE$, and $RHce$.

RHD and $RHCE$ genes code for proteins with no carbohydrates. These proteins are integral membrane proteins that are also required for full expression of other gene products: LW, Duffy (Fy5), and SsU. Another gene product, RHAG, a glycoprotein encoded on chromosome 6, is also required for RH expression. Most RH null RBCs do not express any RH even though they have the genes for RHD and RHCE because they lack RHAG. Other RH null RBCs result from a deletion of RHCE and already have the deleted RHD. Complete or partial deletion of RHCE and increased expression of RHD is also a rare finding.

MNS

Glycophorin A and B contain MNSs antigens and are well developed at birth. Now over 40 antigens have been found in the MNS system. Of these, only MNSs and U are routinely typed. In laboratories doing DNA testing, the results for glycophorin A and B closely linked on chromosome 4 would overlap the RBC antigen studies for this system. Glycophorin A has M and N antigens and glycophorin B has S, s, and U. These genes are closely linked and viewed as haplotypes *MS*, *NS*, *Ms*, and *Ns* for parentage studies. One precaution: anti-N commercial antisera may cross-react with M+ cells.

Duffy

Duffy antigens that are routinely typed are well developed at birth. Duffy antigens are glycoproteins encoded on chromosome 1 but not linked to the RH system. This glycoprotein is the receptor for entry of *Plasmodium vivax* into RBCs; therefore, the distribution of the antigens is profoundly different for countries with endemic malaria. It is a selective advantage to be Fy(a–b–) where exposure to malaria is high. There are six possible alleles: Fy^a, Fy^b, Fy, $Fy3$, $Fy4$, and $Fy5$. Fy^a and Fy^b are the most frequently tested antigens in the system.

Duffy is present in other tissues besides RBCs. Brain, kidney, spleen, heart, and lung tissue cells also express Duffy antigens. Blacks who are Fy(a–b–) negative on RBCs may express Duffy antigens on solid tissue cells. Fy(a–b–) is rare in whites and common in African-Americans (68%).

Kidd

Kidd antigens are only on RBCs as urea transport molecules. Jk^a, Jk^b, $Jk3$, and Jk are alleles. Jk, an amorph, is extremely rare and found in Polynesians and other Pacific Islanders of Chinese descent with an even rarer occurrence in North Europeans by a different mechanism (suppressed by the Lutheran antigen inhibitor). Kidd antigens are enhanced by enzymes. Antisera to Jk^a is scarce and antisera to Jk^b is even scarcer, thus typing for this antigen is

Table 3 Rh system phenotype incidence using DCcEe nomenclature

Haplotypes	Blacks	Whites	Asians	Native American
DCe	17	42	70	44
DCE	<1	<1	1	6
DcE	11	14	21	34
Dce	44	4	3	2
Ce	2	2	2	2
CE	<1	<1	<1	<1
cE	<1	1	<1	6
ce	26	37	3	11

not routine. In addition, Kidd antibodies are fragile. Kidd antibodies often disappear rapidly from people who produce them. In addition, a few days after putting a clotted specimen in the refrigerator, the antibodies lose potency. Freeze-dried antisera appear to retain their activity. This system shows useful polymorphism and adequate expression on fresh samples; thus, Kidd system typing can give extra information in parentage testing where antisera are available.

Kell

Kell antigens are proteins bearing homology with neutral endopeptidases. These proteins contain a large number of cysteine residues forming disulfide bonds required for tertiary structure and thus intact antigenic expression. Kell antigens are destroyed by acid or reducing agents such as dithiothreitol or 2-mercapto-ethanol and structure disruptor ethylenediaminetetraacetic acid-glycine. There are 11 alleles, all rare except K (K1) and k (K2). Other allelic antigens in the Kell system include Kp^a, Kp^b, Js^a, Js^b, and Ko. A person homozygous for *Ko* expresses no Kell antigens.

Lutheran

Lutheran (Lu) antigens are found on a RBC glycoprotein with adhesion properties. The genes encoding *Lu* are linked to *Hh* and *Se* genes found on chromosome 19. These antigens are poorly expressed at birth, in low density in adults, and the antisera scarce; therefore, these are not routinely used for parentage studies.

The common antigens are Lu^a (Lu1) and Lu^b (Lu2). In whites, the frequency of Lu(a+b−) is 0.15%, Lu(a+b+) is 7.5% and Lu(a−b+) is 92.35%. Lu(a−b−) is extremely rare. Twenty other antigens are in the Lu system, but only Au^a (Lu18; 80% of whites) and Au^b (Lu19; 50% of whites) might be of use for parentage studies. The other antigens are high-incidence or low-incidence antigens. The inheritance of one dose of the inhibitor of Lu antigen (In(Lu)) gene suppresses the expression of Lu on RBCs and must be considered when analyzing data.

Xg

Xg^a is an antigen found with higher frequency in females than males. It is located on the X chromosome. The frequency in whites of Xg^a in females is 88.7% and 65.6% in males. It is most useful for parentage studies involving alleged fathers who are Xg(a+) and mothers who are Xg(a−). All sons would be Xg(a−) and all daughters would be Xg(a+) if he is the biological father.

Standard Methods with Intact Blood

Blood group antigens are detected with antibodies to each specific antigen. Each antibody–antigen reaction is optimized by modifying the ratio of antigen to antibody, time, temperature, and additives. Many of the blood group antigens can be tested by slide, tube, or microplate methods and require no incubation. Agglutination (clumping) or hemolysis (breakdown of the RBCs) is traditionally observed for positive reactions. Certain antibody–antigen reactions require incubation at room temperature or 37 °C for 20 min to 2 h. For reactions at 37 °C, an antiglobulin test (Coomb's test) involves washing excess unbound antibody from the sample, antihuman globulin is mixed with the RBCs to detect bound antibody, and the tube or microplate is centrifuged and read for agglutination. Additives that enhance or modify reactivity include low-ionic-strength solutions, polyethylene glycol, enzymes (ficin, bromelain, papain, or trypsin), albumin, and positively charged polymers (hexadimethrine bromide, protamine sulfate, poly-L-lysine). Newer methods use enzyme immunoassays or solid-phase RBC adherence to view positive reactions. In addition, fluorescent and ferritin-bound antibodies can be used to distinguish homozygosity from heterozygosity. Currently, DNA sequencing is available for detecting heterozygotes and blood group DNA microarrays are available to determine complete genotypes.

Systems that react rapidly and best at room temperature or cooler temperatures include ABO, MN, P, Lewis, and Lu(a+). The P system is not useful for forensics because the antisera are unreliable and the expression quite variable. Antigens that are best typed at body temperature (37 °C) and incubated include most of the CcEe and some weak expressions of D, Kell, Duffy, Kidd, Ss, and Lu(b+). RH system antigens react best with antisera containing extra protein or enzymes. Proper controls of antisera to rule out nonspecific binding must be done whenever enhancement materials are present. These controls contain the same contents as the antisera but lack the antibody.

Standard ABO slide testing involves mixing a drop of antisera (anti-A, anti-B) with a drop of whole blood and viewing for agglutination (clumping of RBCs and antisera). The reverse typing for ABO involves taking RBCs of known type A$_1$ and B and sometimes O and reacting these against the plasma or serum of the test case. For ABO tube or microplate grouping, the RBCs of the individual are diluted to 2–4% in normal saline (0.85% NaCl) and mixed with antibodies to A and B (anti-A,B, or anti-H may be used to clear up discrepancies). These are centrifuged briefly and then read for agglutination. A reverse type would also be set up. For detection of the two common subgroups of A, *Dolichos biflorus* lectin is used. A_1 cells are positive and A_2 cells are negative.

RH typing for parentage testing is usually limited to mixing RBCs with anti-D, C, c, and E. Antisera are not always monospecific and care must be used when dual specificity is found, such as with anti-Ce; e-negative RBCs would not react well with this antisera. It is so rare to be e-negative in most populations that anti-e is not used routinely. Exceptions include Mexicans, Native Americans, and Asians (**Table 3**).

Testing for M and N is performed by mixing RBCs with anti-M and anti-N, centrifuging, and observing for agglutination. Testing for S and s, Duffy (Fy^a, Fy^b), Kidd (Jk^a, Jk^b), and Kell (K, k) involves incubation at $37\,^\circ$C and antihuman globulin. Special controls of test RBCs without reagent antibody must be included to ensure that they are not already coated with antibody. These Coomb's-positive cells would test positive for every marker requiring antihuman globulin as part of the procedure.

Not all antigens are expressed well at birth; system antigens with nil to moderate expression include Lewis, P, Lutheran, and Kx. In addition, reverse typing for ABO will not be reliable in newborns up to 6 months of age because they have circulating maternal antibodies and do not produce their own ABO antibodies until their immune system is mature. They need effective exposure to the environmental antigens that are ubiquitous in nature to stimulate production of anti-A, anti-B, and/or anti-A,B. Elderly individuals also have waning expression of the ABO antibodies. Other considerations include transfusion history, chimeras, transplantation, dispermy, and cancer (especially leukemia and colon cancer with known alterations in ABO expression).

Testing Blood Stains

In selecting antigens for testing blood stains, stability of the antigen in diverse conditions is an important consideration. For instance, ABO is very stable whereas Kidd antigens are not. The availability of highly specific antisera is also an important consideration. Anti-C without anti-G is hard to find; anti-Jk^b is extremely rare; anti-N that does not cross-react with M is uncommon. Anti-Lutheran antibodies are also not easily obtained. Testing RH, Fy, K, MNSs, and Jk^a (in fresher stains) are plausible choices. ABO, RH, and MN are most likely to be successful on blood stains, and are the most widely used by crime laboratories.

Methods to test for RBC antigens in stains include absorption–inhibition, absorption–elution (100 times more sensitive than absorption–inhibition), mixed agglutination, fluorescent and ferritin-labeled antibody, formalin-treated RBCs (not widely used), and reversible agglomeration (used to retrieve RBCs from putrefied blood clots, not for typing itself).

The absorption–inhibition test has been used since the early 1920s and was the only one until 1960. It requires large amounts of sample compared to the newer methods. Basically, biological fluids, RBCs, or stroma from a stain are tested or scraped into a tube with saline (0.85%), anti-A, anti-B, and *Ulex europaeus* anti-H lectin are incubated with the sample. The serum is removed and tested for its ability to agglutinate A cells, B cells, or O cells compared to a saline (no RBC control). A significant reduction in the ability of the test sera to agglutinate cells indicates that the original sample was that blood type. For instance, anti-A after incubation with group A sample will not agglutinate group A RBCs well because the anti-A was absorbed by the sample.

The absorption–elution technique is widely used and requires 100 times less RBC sample. First, an optional RBC fixation can be achieved by heating blood-stained samples to near boiling for 30 s in a buffer. Then anti-A, anti-B, and/or anti-H are absorbed on to the fixed or unfixed extracted sample; excess antisera are washed off at cool temperatures. The absorbed antibody is then eluted off the sample. Test the eluates from the sample as follows: anti-A eluate with A_1 cells and A_2 cells, anti-B eluate with B cells, and anti-H eluate with O cells. All main blood types have been successfully typed by this method.

Microagglutination also requires only minute samples. The sample is treated with antisera, washed, and mixed with the same blood type as the antisera used. It is viewed under a microscope for RBCs attached to the fibers of blood-stained cloth or materials.

Testing Other Body Fluid Stains for Blood Groups

Some antigens are only on RBCs (RH, Kidd, Kell, MNS, Lutheran). Testing of body fluid stains requires careful collection of the stain and an adjacent area with everything but the stain to be sure the typing is not from the environmental source rather than the specimen of human body fluid. ABH antigens are found on bacteria, wood, soil, other mammals, dust, and other places. Therefore, careful collection is a must. In addition, organisms in the environment may enzymatically alter blood group antigens. *Clostridium* spp., *Bacillus* spp., and *Aspergillus niger* as well as coffee beans can change or eliminate certain blood group substances. In addition, it is advised to test for A or B when the test for H is negative. Testing for anti-A and anti-B in stains or fresh body fluids besides blood is also possible; awareness of false negatives and positives is important.

Testing for Secretor Status

Testing for secretor status may be accomplished by two different methods: testing blood for Lewis antigens or secretions for ABH substances. The concentration of ABH is high in saliva, semen, gastric juice, breast milk, and amniotic fluid and low in tears and urine. When testing body fluids, special precautions and procedures must be followed. For instance, saliva has enzymes that degrade the ABH so it must be either dried immediately or heat-treated to inactivate the enzymes. Urine requires concentration; semen is fragile.

Testing blood for adhered Lewis antigens is one way to predict secretor status. Le(b+) people are secretors and Le(a+) are nonsecretors of ABH substance. Alternatively, and more specifically, test saliva or other body fluids for H substance using *Ulex europaeus* anti-H lectin to absorb on to the H in the sample. The supernatant will not be able to agglutinate O cells if there is H substance in the sample. If the individual is a nonsecretor, no anti-H will be absorbed, and the O RBCs will agglutinate with equal strength compared to the saline control. If the test is negative for H, test for A or B to detect secretions that express A or B, and not H.

Blood Groups on White Cells and Platelets

HLA is on all nucleated cells of the body in large amounts and reduced amounts on nonnucleated cells. Until DNA testing became widely used for typing purposes, HLA testing was done by microlymphocytotoxicity assays. Trays with multiple wells are filled with antisera from multiparous women and overlayed with oil, then frozen until needed. Each antigen is represented by at least three different sources of antisera as a control check. Typed cells are T lymphocytes or B lymphocytes from fresh ACD anticoagulated blood. The T lymphocytes are used for the HLA-A, B, C antigen plates and the B lymphocytes are used for the HLA-DR, DP, DQ antigen typing. The cells are added to an entire plate of antisera, incubated, and then rabbit complement is added. An indicator dye helps differentiate dead from living cells using phase contrast. Brightly refractile cells are alive. The dark cells are dead and therefore

had antibody plus complement to kill them. The grading system is from 0 to 8 where 0 = no dead cells and 8 = 100% dead cells. Most procedures resulted in lots of scores of 6 or 4 and require very experienced people to interpret results.

HLA typing using DNA probes is also cumbersome and time-consuming, requiring experienced personnel for interpretation. Systems are now available using DNA testing with allele-specific primers for HLA-A, B, and DR and are interpreted by the computer.

Conclusion

Blood grouping has been replaced by DNA methods in most forensic laboratories throughout the world. Classic blood grouping is still performed for parentage testing and for transfusion and transplantation medicine.

See Also

Crime-scene Investigation and Examination: Collection and Chain of Evidence; **Immunoassays, Forensic Applications**; **Mass Disasters:** Principles of Identification; **Postmortem Changes:** Overview; **Serology:** Overview; Blood Identification

Further Reading

Brecher ME (ed.) (2002) *AABB Technical Manual*, 14th edn. Bethesda MD: American Association of Blood Banks.

Gaensslen RE (1983) *Sourcebook in Forensic Serology, Immunology, and Biochemistry*. Washington, DC: US Government Printing Office.

Gaensslen RE (1983) *Sourcebook in Forensic Serology, Immunology, and Biochemistry. Unit IX: Translations of Selected Contributions to the Original Literature of Medicolegal Examinations of Blood and Body Fluids*. Washington, DC: US Government Printing Office.

Harmening DM (1999) *Modern Blood Banking and Transfusion Practices*, 4th edn. Philadelphia, PA: FA Davis.

Issitt PD, Anstee DJ (1998) *Applied Blood Group Serology*, 4th edn. Durham, NC: Montgomery Scientific.

Mollison PL, Engelfriet CP, Contreras M (1997) *Blood Transfusion in Clinical Medicine*, 10th edn. Oxford, UK: Blackwell Scientific.

Mourant AE, Kopec AC, Domaniewska-Sobczak K (1976) *The Distribution of the Human Blood Groups and Other Biochemical Polymorphisms*, 2nd edn. Oxford, UK: Oxford University Press.

Race RR, Sanger R (1975) *Blood Groups in Man*, 6th edn. London: Blackwell Scientific.

Sussman LN (1976) *Paternity Testing by Blood Grouping*, 2nd edn. Springfield, IL: Charles C. Thomas.

BODY CAVITY SEARCHES, PRACTICAL ISSUES AND CONSENT

M M Stark, St. George's Hospital Medical School, London, UK

Introduction

Searches of body cavities may be requested by police or customs and excise and other governmental authorities because of the suspicion that an individual may smuggle drugs, or has a weapon concealed.

Doctors or other appropriately qualified healthcare professionals may be asked to search intimately for such articles. There is an overriding duty of care to the individual in these cases.

Doctors working near ports of entry need to be aware of the various presentations of drug smuggling as early detection of intoxication will reduce mortality. This article will outline relevant definitions in the area, discuss the importance of consent, give a detailed example of legal provisions that exist in England and Wales, and outline the practical aspects of body cavity searches.

Definitions

Intimate Search

An intimate search is defined in law in England and Wales as 'a search that consists of a physical examination of a person's body orifices other than the mouth.'

Safety Search

A safety search may be authorized when a person who has been arrested and is in police detention is thought to have concealed on him/her anything which could be used to cause physical injury to him/herself or others and it is thought that he/she might use it while he/she is in police detention or in the custody of a court.

Drug Offense Search

A drug offense search may be authorized when it is believed that an individual has a class A drug concealed on him/her and he/she was in possession of it with criminal intent before his/her arrest. Class A drugs include major natural and synthetic opiates (heroin and methadone), lysergic acid diethylamide (LSD), cocaine, ecstasy, and injectable amphetamines.

Appropriate criminal intent would be an intent to commit an offense of possession of a controlled drug with intent to supply, or export with intent to evade a prohibition or restriction.

Body Packer

Body packers are those who deliberately ingest packages of drugs in order to avoid detection by authorities. The term "surgical mules" may also be used.

The drugs are normally packed in layers of tightly wrapped cellophane, or in condoms, and swallowed. Constipating agents, such as loperamide or diphenoxylate hydrochloride with atropine (Lomotil®) may be taken to prevent the passage of the packages on a long-distance flight, before the end of the journey ("stoppers").

Drugs such as cocaine, heroin, amphetamine, and cannabis may be packed in variable amounts. For example, packages containing between 1 and 15 g of cocaine have been reported.

Body-packer syndrome consists of intestinal rupture or potentially lethal intoxication caused by rupture of the packets.

Body packing has rarely been reported in children, but two boys aged 12 and 16 years who had concealed heroin and who survived were reported in 2003.

Body Stuffer

Body stuffers may take drugs orally ("swallowers") just prior to arrest by police in an attempt to avoid being found in possession of illicit substances, or alternatively they may put drugs in the rectum or vagina – "body pushers." These drugs may not be so well wrapped as those taken orally by body packers and so may result in symptoms and signs within a couple of hours.

Good practice suggests that if a recently detained prisoner has or is suspected of having swallowed drugs, he/she must be treated as having taken an overdose and an ambulance should be called for immediate transfer to an accident and emergency facility. If the prisoner refuses to go to hospital and declines any medical assistance the refusal should be noted on the custody record and his/her condition closely monitored for signs of deterioration.

Medical assistance should be summoned immediately, and on arrival a full assessment should be performed by the doctor to consider whether hospital transfer is required. If so, the doctor should explain to the prisoner why such transfer is in his/her best interests.

Dumping

The term dumping is used for the removal of a corpse after a drug-related death, usually to public places not far from where the death occurred, after the individual passed away in the presence of others, or in someone else's home. Postmortem celiotomy may be performed to recover unpassed packets.

Consent

Ethically no medical practitioner should take part in an intimate body search of an individual without that individual's consent even though there may be no legal requirement to obtain the individual's consent to the search.

Healthcare professionals should remember that for consent to be valid the individual must be given sufficient, accurate, and relevant information and have the competence to consider the issues and reach a voluntary decision. The effects of ingestion and absorption of any suspected substances or the effects of ingestion and concealment of a weapon should be fully explained to the prisoner. The possibility of a package splitting and resulting in overdose should be discussed as this may be a problem even with an individual who is dependent on the suspected concealed drug.

It should be remembered that an individual's competence to make a decision might be affected by the effects of drugs or alcohol, and any lack of privacy during the discussion, e.g., with the presence of a police chaperone, may affect the individual's willingness to ask questions. In some circumstances the individual has no choice about whether the search will proceed, only the choice of whether it is carried out by a medical practitioner or by a police officer.

In some cases it may be possible to seek consent for a noninvasive method of searching such as an ultrasound examination and this approach should be discussed with the prisoner and hospital colleagues.

In an emergency, for example, if a detainee collapses and there are reasonable grounds for suspecting that he/she has something concealed that has led to this collapse, an intimate search may be justified to save the life of the individual. An intimate search might, exceptionally, be conducted by a doctor if he/she believes it is necessary to remove a concealed object that is of immediate danger to the life or personal safety of those responsible for the detainee's supervision.

It is reasonable to assume that young people aged 16 or 17 have the capacity to consent to an intimate search. However, in addition to gaining consent from the juvenile, when an intimate search is going to be carried out on a child younger than 16, it is good practice to inform and obtain the consent of the person with parental responsibility whenever reasonably practicable.

Legal Provisions

The legal provisions regarding authorization of body cavity searches will vary between jurisdictions. In England and Wales section 55 of the Police and Criminal Evidence Act 1984 provides that an intimate search of an individual may be conducted on the authority of a police officer of at least the rank of inspector only if there are grounds for suspecting that an individual has secreted about him/her either an object that might be used to cause physical injury while he/she is detained or has a class A controlled drug.

The authorizing police officer is responsible for determining which grounds exist and that an intimate search (either a safety search or a drug offense search) is the only practicable means of removing the dangerous items or drugs.

In England and Wales over 2002–2003, 172 intimate searches, mostly for drugs, were carried out, an increase of 70 over 2001–2002. Searches made for drugs (91% of all searches made) showed a 5% rise in 2001–2002. In 2002–2003 class A drugs (mainly heroin, other opiate drugs, LSD, and cocaine) were found during one in three of the searches made for drugs. In nine searches for harmful articles, only two articles were found.

In Scotland where an intimate search is considered necessary in the interests of justice and in order to obtain evidence, this may be lawfully carried out under the authority of a sheriff's warrant.

If, in the USA, after arresting a person, an officer believes that there is evidence of a crime in a body cavity, a search warrant should be obtained to enable a qualified person to conduct any search in a reasonable manner.

Specific Drugs

Individuals may present with the acute effects of the drugs ingested; for example, "drug-smuggler's delirium" may be a presentation of acute cocaine toxicity.

Clinical effects of cocaine and amphetamine are similar, with stimulation of the sympathetic nervous system. Intoxication results in euphoria, sweating, hyperthermia, dilated pupils, tachycardia, increased blood pressure, dysrhythmia, seizures, and excited delirium.

Symptoms and signs of severe intoxication with heroin include pinpoint pupils, respiratory depression, central nervous system depression, hypotension, hypothermia, and coma.

If there is coma or bradypnea, naloxone is indicated in a dose of 0.8–2 mg intravenously repeated at intervals of 2–3 min to a maximum of 10 mg. If respiratory function does not improve, then the diagnosis should be questioned. Since naloxone has a shorter duration of action (less than 1 h) than many opioids, close monitoring and repeated injections are often necessary and the detainee should be kept in hospital.

Practical Aspects

Any healthcare professional who agrees to undertake an intimate search should have the required skills and a comprehensive understanding of the risks involved and their management. There is a real danger that a drug package could leak or a weapon could cause injury (to either the practitioner or the prisoner) during attempts to remove them.

A safety search could be performed at a police station, a hospital, or other medical premises. The doctor should decide the appropriate venue depending on the circumstances of the search. Drug offense searches should be at a venue with full resuscitation facilities – ideally at an accident and emergency facility.

When asked by the relevant authorities to conduct an intimate search the doctor should speak directly with the officer involved in order to determine if the person is fit to remain in custody or if he/she should be transferred urgently to hospital in an ambulance.

The doctor should ensure that any legal provisions, including proper authorization, has been obtained and document who has given authority for the search and under what grounds the search is being carried out.

The doctor may arrange to meet the police and the prisoner at the local accident and emergency department. The police or customs authorities can be asked to contact the nurse in charge to arrange a suitable room.

On arrival the doctor should be fully briefed by the officers involved as to the condition of the prisoner when arrested, any change whilst in custody in particular, and whether there has been any deterioration in the state of the person. Any other relevant information regarding past medical history, current medication, substance misuse, including alcohol, and previous police warnings should be available to the doctor.

Urgent hospital transfer of any individual in the custodial environment should be considered if there is a deterioration in the clinical condition of the prisoner, if a weapon is identified but cannot be removed by the doctor, and/or if the prisoner refuses to consent to a drugs search.

Although in the case of the latter it may be possible to observe a detainee in the custodial situation for a short period, it is not appropriate for nonmedical personnel, who may have insufficient knowledge of the symptoms and signs of toxicity, to conduct observations of a prisoner over a prolonged period.

The healthcare professional should always attend and assess a prisoner whenever a request has been made by the police/custom authorities to conduct an intimate search.

On arrival at an accident and emergency department the doctor should explain to the emergency staff the risks of performing an intimate search and ensure that there will be immediate assistance should an emergency arise. At hospital the responsibility for performing an examination lies with the doctor performing the search as opposed to any hospital staff.

The doctor will need close-fitting disposable gloves and access to an auroscope, a proctoscope, a speculum, lubricating jelly, sponge forceps, and a free-standing or wall-mounted light.

No person of the opposite sex who is not a medical practitioner or nurse should be present. A minimum of two people other than the person searched should be present. Preferably an officer of same sex as the prisoner should be present during the examination and anything found should be given to him/her.

The doctor will be guided by the authorities as to which orifice(s) to search. Any of the following orifices may be used to conceal drugs/weapons and should be examined in the following manner:

- mouth: visual inspection with light source
- nostrils: visual inspection with auroscope
- ears: visual inspection with auroscope
- umbilicus: visual inspection with light source
- foreskin: visual inspection with light source
- rectum: gentle digital exploration followed, if necessary, by proctoscopy
- vagina: gentle digital exploration followed, if necessary, by insertion of speculum and inspection of the vaginal fornices.

A full contemporaneous note should be made in the doctor's original notes as regards the procedure, including the relevant history taken and examination performed.

If a drug package has been swallowed or concealed in the rectum, given time, it may pass or dislodge naturally. In these cases the doctor should discuss the proposed admission with hospital colleagues. Depending on legal restrictions the custodians may be able to detain suspects for longer periods and repeated urinalysis may be performed where presence of drug metabolites in the urine can be detected by enzyme immunoassay. Rarely urinalysis may be negative due to good packaging.

Packages may be visible on standard abdominal X-ray (if consent is given for such a procedure), e.g., a supine and upright abdominal radiograph with or without contrast. Diagnostic radiographic features include the "double condom" (air trapped between layers of condoms), and "rosette" sign (air trapped in the outer package at the end where the knot has been tied).

Management in Hospital

Detainees admitted to hospital should be closely monitored with pulse, blood pressure, temperature, and electrocardiogram recording. The main complications are intestinal obstruction or massive intoxication by cocaine, which is usually of rapid onset and is frequently fatal. Early specialist advice should be sought for any complications such as hyperthermia or intestinal obstruction.

Often packages pass spontaneously and conservative management may be appropriate, such as mild laxatives with a liquid diet, keeping the individual under close observation. Surgery may be required to retrieve packages if signs of obstruction or intoxication develop. If there is evidence of packet degradation with pieces of packet wrappings or actual packets with deteriorating packaging being passed, then emergency surgery may be required.

It is difficult to give definitive advice regarding the period of observation in hospital. Although the body packer should know the exact number of packets ingested, it would be unwise to rely on inaccurate information. Obviously an accurate history should be obtained, all packages should be passed, and there should be no evidence of intestinal obstruction; the patient should be asymptomatic with normal X-rays and a negative drug screen.

Options such as X-ray and computed tomography scanning both involve irradiating the patient and may not be suitable for female detainees who may be potentially pregnant. Ultrasound may be used for noncontact searching but requires an individual's cooperation.

Risk of Death

Smuggling packets of drugs by ingestion can result in the death of the courier by various causes. The most common cause is acute intoxication due to partial or complete rupture of the package(s) and absorption of the drugs. Deaths may also occur from bowel obstruction or perforation. The most common drugs implicated in deaths of body packers are heroin and cocaine. It appears that heroin deaths are becoming more common and that intestinal obstruction and/or perforation is more common with heroin. Opiates do slow intestinal motility and so may contribute physiologically to intestinal obstruction.

Suicide by reingestion of passed packages has been reported and detention personnel should be aware of this possibility.

See Also

Custody: Death in, United Kingdom and Continental Europe; Death in, United States of America; **Drug-Induced Injury, Accidental and Iatrogenic**; **Forensic Psychiatry and Forensic Psychology:** Drug and Alcohol Addiction; **Substance Misuse:** Medical Effects; Miscellaneous Drugs

Further Reading

Association of Forensic Physicians and British Medical Association (2003) *Guidelines for Doctors Asked to Perform Intimate Body Searches.* London: BMA/AFP.

Association of Police Surgeons and Royal College of Psychiatrists (2000) *Substance Misuse Detainees in Police Custody. Guidelines for Clinical Management*, 2nd edn. Report of a Medical Working Group. Council Report CR81. London: Royal College of Psychiatrists.

British Medical Association Ethics Department (2004) *Medical Ethics Today. The BMA's Handbook of Ethics and Law.* London: BMJ Publishing.

Payne-James JJ, Busuttil A, Smock W (eds.) (2003) *Forensic Medicine: Clinical and Pathological Aspects.* London: Greenwich Medical Media.

Stark MM (ed.) (2000) *A Physician's Guide to Clinical Forensic Medicine.* Totowa, NJ: Humana Press.

Stark MM, Payne-James JJ (2003) *Symptoms and Signs of Substance Misuse.* London: Greenwich Medical Media.

Stark MM, Rogers DJ, Norfolk GA (eds.) (2001) *Good Practice Guidelines for Forensic Medical Examiners.* London: Metropolitan Police.

BODY RECOVERY

R L Ellen and M J Lynch, Monash University, Southbank, VIC, Australia

Introduction

The appearance of a deceased person, and the subsequent evaluation of evidence or injuries present may be influenced by the manner in which a body is retrieved, preserved, and transported from a crime scene to the mortuary. It is vital that the officer in charge of the crime scene, the forensic pathologist, and the body transporters work together to ensure the body is handled and transported in such a way that postmortem artifacts are minimized and evidence is not lost. Any clothing, property, or evidence noted on the body at the scene should remain in its original position, for example, a ligature in a case of hanging. The position of all extracorporeal material should be protected whilst in transit to the mortuary. Furthermore, any interference with the deceased, including precautions taken to prevent evidence being destroyed, should be documented.

Personnel recovering and transporting bodies need to be aware of various procedures used to maintain the continuity of the property and evidence. All staff must wear appropriate personal protective equipment and be trained in procedures to minimize infectious risks as well as those associated with physical strain. It is essential that all staff are familiar with crime-scene procedures and appropriate hierarchy of command and are well versed with necessary protocols for dealing with media and public attention. Staff should be alert and observant and at all times prepared to maintain the necessary evidentiary chain and to minimize interference with the integrity of the deceased. In addition, staff dealing with deceased persons should at all times treat the deceased with dignity.

This article will outline the techniques necessary for preserving the body and associated evidence during transport, including specific considerations for different types of cases.

Preservation of the Body Prior to Removal

Prior to the deceased being removed from the scene the following procedures should be implemented to maintain integrity of the deceased:

- The body is allocated a unique identifying number and labeled as such.

- The body is wrapped in clean plastic or linen sheeting and/or placed in a body bag.
- Where indicated, the body and scene are photographed and examined for trace evidence.
- Where appropriate, the body is searched, and clothing and property are removed.

The way in which a body is preserved prior to its removal from the scene of death will depend significantly on the circumstances of the death. In some cases crucial forensic evidence may be lost if precautions to guard against this are not taken. In many cases protecting the clothing, body, and hands of the deceased will assist with the preservation of this evidence. A number of methods for this are routinely used:

- The hands are covered with paper bags and secured about the wrists with tape, ensuring the presence of injury or evidence is not obscured nor altered.
- A clean plastic body pouch or plastic sheet may be enough to ensure evidence is not lost. The deceased is carefully placed on plastic then wrapped securely before transit.

In some cases, additional measures may need to be taken to assist with the preservation of evidence. These include protecting the body parts themselves from being damaged. In cases where significant incineration or decomposition has occurred, parts of the body may be wrapped individually to prevent them from becoming detached. Any precautions such as these must always be clearly noted, performed in the presence of the pathologist or homicide detective, and commenced only after the police, pathologist, and crime-scene examiners have completed their examination.

Body Lifting and Moving

There are a number of different techniques employed in moving a body; however, in the majority of cases a standard procedure can be applied. After being identified and labeled, the deceased may simply be carefully lifted and placed on to a bed sheet, length of plastic, or body bag and wrapped for transport. With particularly heavy bodies, decomposed, or fragile remains, rather than lifting, it is recommended to roll the deceased one way, placing the body bag beneath, and then roll the body the other way, pulling the body bag across. It is important for the body not to be dragged or forcibly lifted, as this may cause artifactual injuries.

Being mindful of the risk of physical injury, standard lifting techniques should be used, that is, bending the knees and keeping the back straight.

Equipment

All equipment used should be of good quality, easily obtainable, and in adequate supply:

1. Plastic zip-lock bags – to seal and transfer property, clothing, or evidence not attached to the deceased.
2. Labels – to label property and evidence bags. They should be appropriate for use with permanent marker, waterproof, and freezer grade, suitable for long-term storage.
3. Gloves – multiple sizes and types, thin disposable gloves for ease of use, heavier duty for infectious cases or chain-mail gloves for bodies with sharp edges such as incinerated remains, and specialized gloves for use with chemically hazardous cases.
4. Body tags – it is of utmost importance that body tags are appropriately selected based on case type. They must be strong, waterproof, and easy to label. They must be attachable to the deceased in such a way that will not interfere with the integrity of the deceased or alter the appearance of injuries or clothing. To minimize confusion it is wise to label the deceased twice, that is, one tag securely attached to the person, e.g., wrist or ankle, and another tag on the outer bag area.
5. Plastic skeds – to enable lifting and transfer of heavy or awkward bodies. These tools are also used in the exhumation of buried remains or the lifting of fragile skeletal cases, to prevent the body from disintegrating.
6. Body bags – all bags should exhibit the following characteristics:
   a. constructed of tough waterproof material
   b. have strong zips with covers to prevent leakage
   c. be generous in size to allow for bodies in rigor mortis, or showing extensive decomposition
   d. have at least four (ideally six) sturdy handles.
7. Additional equipment may include plastic and linen sheeting and towels; various types of indelible markers; heavy-duty tape for sealing and securing bags; cotton wool and superglue; disinfectant spray and cleaning equipment; plastic aprons and safety equipment such as respirators, face masks, and protective eyewear; and a change of clothes and/or protective footwear.

Property and Clothing

It is vital that all property and clothing are handled according to strict protocols. While systems for handling such extracorporeal material will vary between jurisdictions, for the most part it is preferred for routine cases that all clothing and property is left at the home of the deceased. In such instances, once the police and forensic pathologist are satisfied the case is routine in nature, the clothing and property are removed and clearly recorded. In the description of such items, generic terms should be used at all times; for example, a gold ring with rubies should be described as a gold-colored ring with red-colored stones. It is recommended that the removal of clothing and property be done in the presence of two independent parties such as a police officer and the body transporter. Both parties will then sign the accompanying documentation in order to maintain a clear chain of custody of the items.

On occasion it is inappropriate to remove the clothing and property at the scene, for example, when the death occurs somewhere other than at the person's home, such as in the street, or for cases that are nonroutine in nature. In this instance any clothing, property, and extracorporeal material will be removed on arrival at the mortuary or after examination by the pathologist. Again an independent person should witness the forensic technician removing the clothing and property and sign the appropriate property sheets.

It should always be assumed that the family would like the clothing and property returned, regardless of the state. When this occurs, whether it is via the funeral director or the family directly, custody details should be recorded on the property sheet and co-signed by the two parties.

Suspicious Deaths

The preservation of evidence during victim recovery is of utmost importance for suspicious deaths. The body should only be touched or moved in consultation with the police, forensic scientists, and/or forensic pathologist. Prior to removal, the body should be carefully placed on a sheet of plastic and then into a body bag, which is sealed in the presence of investigating police members. The reasons for this process are twofold: (1) to ensure no fibers or trace evidence are lost; and (2) to maintain an appropriate chain of custody of the deceased, all clothing and property, and any evidentiary material present. In the majority of these cases, it is important that the deceased remains absolutely undisturbed before examination by the forensic pathologist. This ensures accurate interpretation of evident disturbances to the deceased, his/her clothing, and property. For example, in cases of sexual assault the disarray of clothing may provide the pathologist with an indication of such an assault, and might highlight the possibility of injury. In addition, the clothing folds may contain evidence such as semen, hairs, or fibers that would otherwise be disturbed in removing the clothing or transporting the body. Alternatively, folds or patterns in clothing where it is bunched about the deceased may be causative of certain injuries, the interpretation of which is best performed in conjunction with viewing the clothing *in situ*.

In certain circumstances it may be advantageous to remove clothing or evidence at the scene, for example, to preserve blood-spatter evidence. This should only occur at the direction of the investigating police members and after specific consultation with the forensic pathologist. All personnel involved with a suspicious death should be trained in dealing with continuity of evidence and associated procedures. In such cases, a police officer should accompany the deceased to the mortuary and oversee the transfer of the body.

Specialized Cases

Hospital Deaths

The training of staff in these procedures, and specific advice regarding requirements given to nursing/hospital staff, ensures there is consistency between cases. In some cases, funeral directors and hospital staff may have "packed and prepared" the body before its removal from the ward to the mortuary. This preparation includes the body being laid in the anatomical position with the hands and feet tied and cotton wool being placed in all body orifices. These procedures should not occur in forensic cases as they may produce postmortem artifact or injury, which is sometimes difficult to interpret at a later stage. Occasionally, a case which initially seems straightforward and does not warrant further investigation turns out to be something more complex and as such may require more detailed forensic examination. Hence these procedures are important in every case. All treatment and resuscitation equipment such as intravenous lines or tubes, cardiac resuscitation pads, or wound dressings must be left *in situ* to be assessed as part of the autopsy examination.

Incinerated Cases

The peripheral parts of severely incinerated bodies, particularly small bones and teeth of the deceased, may be brittle, fragile, and at risk of being damaged or lost. Care should be taken both in transport and in preparation for transport. When stabilizing stretchers and bodies in bags or in vehicles care must be taken not to crush the fragile tissue. Elastic ties or "seatbelts" may be used in place of more rigid-type stabilizers.

In any case where the deceased is unrecognizable visually, establishing identity will be an important part of the investigation, and incineration of bodies makes the identification very difficult. A commonly used method is for a forensic odontologist to compare the antemortem dental records with the teeth of the deceased person. The teeth and bones are often very brittle and fragile and teeth may be broken or lost during transportation to the mortuary. To prevent losing fragile teeth and bones, the head may be photographed *in situ* and then wrapped in cotton wool and/or bubble wrap, and supported by a plastic bag or container which is secured about the neck of the deceased. Thus if the teeth are dislodged they remain contained within the bag.

It is important that any body part found at the scene and not attached to the deceased is not assumed to belong to the deceased, and as such is bagged separately from the body and clearly labeled both in regards to its physical description and the specific location in which it was found, e.g., "tooth found in the vicinity of body X."

After the body is moved, the ash and debris on the floor or ground in the immediate vicinity should be carefully searched and sifted to screen for teeth, small bones, or other matter important to the case. This sifting is most appropriately done at the mortuary where lighting is optimal and suitable equipment readily available. The debris should be bagged and labeled according to the section of body immediately above it, and should be transferred to the mortuary with the deceased.

Suicides

In many cases of suspected suicide, items contributing to the death are found on or near the body. In some cases this evidence may be the only indication of what may have occurred. It is thus important that anything attached to the body remains as such and its position is preserved as best as possible. This is to ensure the items can be examined with specific relation to their position on the deceased, in connection to additional devices, and any injury it/they may have caused. In rare cases this technique can help rule out the involvement of any other person in the death. In addition, as mentioned previously, if the evidence is removed before the pathologist's examination the mode of death may be unclear. On occasion the item may have been removed on discovery of the deceased to assist with resuscitation. In this instance, care should be taken to ensure the items are bagged individually and clearly labeled for transportation.

For example, in a case of hanging, the ligature should remain intact and *in situ*. Where the deceased is suspended, the rope should be cut away from the suspension point, leaving the knots/attachments intact. If the ligature has been removed from the neck to facilitate resuscitation, the section of the ligature originally in contact with the deceased should be reconstructed, the ends tied together with string, then bagged, labeled, and transported with the body. Where there is evidence that has legal requirements for transport, such as firearms, drugs, or volatile substances, the chain of custody of these items should be documented clearly and completely. The police or ballistics expert experienced in safe handling procedures usually transports or may offer advice in the handling of firearms and other dangerous weapons.

Case study 1 Police attended the premises of a residential unit and observed an 82-year-old female deceased in her bed. Her family had discovered she had passed away and phoned emergency services. Resuscitation was not attempted. On further investigation, it was discovered the female had no relevant medical history and death was not expected. She had been treated for depression following the death of her husband some five years previously. On learning of the necessity for autopsy, the next of kin informed police members that the deceased had initially been found with a plastic bag covering her head. This had been removed and concealed prior to their attendance.

Firearm Deaths

When a gun is fired, gunshot residues (GSR) are ejected from the weapon on to the hands and clothing of the person firing the weapon and, to a lesser degree, any persons in the immediate vicinity. Assessment of the presence and distribution of GSR on the individuals present at the scene of death can assist police with the inclusion and/or exclusion of suspects and assist them in determining the approximate position of other people present at the time of the event. Ideally, this assessment should be performed as soon as possible after the incident and before the transport of the deceased. In some instances this is neither practical nor timely, and it is recommended this procedure be done after the deceased is transported to the mortuary. In this situation any GSR on the deceased person must be preserved during transit. To do this, the deceased is transported in a sealed body bag, and the clothing of the deceased should remain undisturbed. In addition, paper bags are placed securely over the hands. It is essential that paper bags be used rather than plastic as the hands may sweat if contained in plastic, which can alter the presence of the GSR.

After the deceased is transferred on to a stretcher and removed from the scene, the immediate vicinity of the deceased is searched carefully for projectiles or spent cartridges. The body transporters must be aware of this as a projectile may be on the surface of the skin or in the clothing and as such there is a risk of disturbance when the body is initially moved.

Case study 2 A deceased man argued with his wife of many years. He had a well-documented social history of violent, abusive behavior, and a familiarity with guns. He locked himself in a spare bedroom when his wife stormed out after a particularly heated argument. She returned home some hours later to find him deceased on the bed with a gunshot wound to the head. The body was described and photographed. Two weapons were found in the immediate vicinity of the deceased and he had many additional weapons within the household. The case was reported to the coroner/medical examiner as suspected suicidal gunshot wound to the head. On admission to the Forensic Institute, four gunshot wounds were noted. The case was radiographed and found to contain no projectiles. The projectiles were later found, one having entered the neck, exited through the top of the head, and embedded in the ceiling. The other dislodged in transit and was found amongst the clothing of the deceased. On the basis of this information, the location and track of the two wounds, and the results of samples taken from the hands of the deceased for analysis of GSR, the pathologist was satisfied that this was a rare case of gunshot suicide involving two weapons fired simultaneously.

A number of precautions were taken at the scene prior to transport of the deceased, which may have impacted on the outcome of the case. These included:

- wrapping the head of the deceased in cotton wool to preserve the presence and situation of projectiles
- securing the hands of the deceased in paper bags to promote sampling for GSR
- photographing the deceased *in situ* with the two weapons in the immediate vicinity, demonstrating the patterns of blood spatter on the wall behind the deceased and a defect in the ceiling from one of the projectiles.

Decomposed Bodies

Dealing with a decomposed body involves a number of associated risks. Flies and maggots are often present, as are spiders, beetles, and other insects. The decomposing body presents a difficult situation, in terms of body removal, which may be dealt with in a number of ways. The body may be very bloated or fragile, and sometimes beginning to break apart. Moving a severely decomposed body can complicate this process further and if care is not taken, may result in the removal of skin and/or the detachment of limbs. To overcome this, rather than lifting the body on to plastic, it should be carefully rolled on to its side, and the plastic tucked underneath the deceased. The body can then be lifted using the plastic to hold the remains intact and gently placed into a body bag. Care should be taken to avoid being bitten or stung; however, fly spray or deodorizer should not be used on the body as it may interfere with toxicological and/ or microbiological testing. Fluid-filled blisters, called buboes, may rupture and splash body transporters, and appropriate safety attire should be worn.

Skeletal Remains

The process of recovering skeletal remains is slow and meticulous as the soil and vegetation deposited after the death are removed layer by layer without disturbing the skeleton. The bones are packed in paper bags either grouped or separately depending on the case. It is recommended that the skull is wrapped in cotton wool and supported by a box or container, similar to the procedure used when recovering incinerated remains. In some circumstances where some tissue is still attached to the bones, and the deceased is not completely skeletonized, it may be more beneficial to slide a large board underneath the deceased and lift the remains with the board, keeping it intact for transportation. As with incinerated bodies, the soil around the deceased should be bagged, labeled, and sifted later to search for teeth, small bones, and other evidence.

Diving Fatalities

The recovery of diving fatalities presents one of the more difficult situations in body removal. The equipment may provide vital information as to the cause of death or the circumstances immediately before death and thus it must all remain intact and accompany the deceased. This procedure makes for a bulky and awkward body transfer. Ideally an expert should be present at the scene to examine the equipment, ensuring all valves are turned off, and settings are secure so as not to be accidentally altered during transit. In diving fatalities, radiography for air embolism should be performed as soon as possible. In light of this, it is crucial that the body be transported as quickly as possible to the mortuary.

Biohazard Cases

Universal precautions to minimize the spread of infectious disease should be employed with every body removal regardless of its infectious state, and all bodies treated as potentially infectious; personal protective equipment should always be worn. However, certain cases are deemed high risk purely due to their nature. These high-risk cases include intravenous drug users, prostitutes, homosexuals, or persons recently imprisoned. If this is the situation, extra care should be taken to avoid contact with body fluids,

and safety glasses, surgical masks, and double gloves may be worn. Staff should always be observant for sharps and other foreign objects. To prevent splashes, a towel or absorbent material can be placed over any open wounds, or the face of the deceased person. In cases where there is identified a risk for airborne biohazard such as tuberculosis or severe acute respiratory syndrome (SARS), a towel should be placed over the face to prevent the escape of sputum or other fluids, and an appropriate face mask or respirator worn by the body transporters.

Chemical, Biological, and Radiological Hazards

Before a chemically contaminated body is recovered and transported, the chemical must be identified and assessed to ensure the appropriate precautions are taken to maintain a safe work environment. In many instances, once the body is removed from the scene the level of contamination is low. However, each situation needs to be separately and fully assessed on an individual basis. Representatives from Environmental Protection Agency (EPA) and/or Work Safe or similar occupational health and safety authorities may be able to offer advice on specific risks.

If the chemical cannot be identified, the case should be treated as highly toxic and maximum protection should be worn by workers. In extreme cases the body is decontaminated prior to removal. To do this, it is recommended the body be photographed *in situ*, and then the clothing and property removed, bagged, and labeled. Scene workers wearing self-contained breathing apparatus should then repeatedly hose the deceased. Generally, the fire brigade controls the scene, and only personnel trained in decontamination procedures should enter. In any case where there is suspicion of chemical contamination, a safety officer should be assigned to monitor the level of toxic fumes continually and ensure that the safety of the staff is adequate.

Disaster Victim Identification

In the event of a mass disaster, body recovery can be crucial in assisting in both the final identification of the deceased person, and the reconstruction of the events just prior to the incident. The international disaster victim identification (DVI) forms published by Interpol are well recognized as the preferred method for documenting body recovery and identification in the event of a disaster. Systematic recording and accurate descriptions of deceased persons involved in a mass fatality incident are essential to facilitate adequate reconstruction of the event. The likelihood of some element of criminality being associated with the event is high. In light of this, all deceased persons should be treated as suspicious deaths irrespective of the size, location, or type of disaster.

The DVI protocol consists of five phases:

- phase 1 – the scene
- phase 2 – the mortuary
- phase 3 – antemortem retrieval
- phase 4 – reconciliation
- phase 5 – debriefing.

Phase 1

Once the injured have been triaged and removed from the scene, the scene should be secured. DVI scene teams are formed. These teams consist of a crime-scene examiner, a photographer, and a recorder. A pathologist and a forensic odontologist support each team.

The location of each body or specimen is recorded such that it is related to a known reference point, usually a grid reference. A unique DVI number is given to each body or body part. Property not attached to a body is also recorded with reference to its location and handed to a property officer.

The Interpol DVI form B is completed and the body or body part is moved to an appointed holding area. During phase 1 the pathologist certifies death and assists with the identification of body parts.

Phase 2

The body is transported to the mortuary in a body bag. Once at the mortuary, the body is radiographed and autopsied. The autopsy involves the assistance of DVI autopsy teams. These teams consist of a recorder, an examiner, and a photographer.

With the assistance of a pathologist and a forensic technician, the DVI teams record and photograph all the clothing and property. Once the body has been photographed, identifying features such as hair color, eye color, scars, and tattoos are recorded.

The autopsy is performed and the recorder again documents all details that may be utilized during the identification, such as the presence of an appendix, gallbladder, foreskin.

A forensic odontologist examines the teeth of the body, and fingerprint personnel take fingerprints where appropriate. During the autopsy examination a sample of blood or tissue is retained for DNA analysis and comparison.

These details are all recorded on DVI Interpol forms C1 to G.

Phase 3

Trained police personnel interview family members of missing persons (presumed to have died in the mass disaster) to gather information regarding all identifying features of that person. This includes the color and type of clothes that the person may have worn and other identifying features such as hair color, eye color, scars, and tattoos. They are also responsible for gathering the dental and medical records, and where relevant the collection of antemortem samples for DNA comparison.

Phase 4

Antemortem forms and postmortem forms completed during phases 1 and 2 are compared during the reconciliation phase. This comparison is achieved systematically using a reconciliation chart and grouping each set into male and female, black and white, and ages 0–15, 15–75, 75 plus. If in doubt, the deceased is placed in the 15–75 group. The final identification of each case is presented to the coroner along with an appointed identification panel for the final decision and authority to confirm identity.

Phase 5

It is essential for all staff involved in the body recovery of a mass disaster to undergo debriefing. This process could involve a "hot" debriefing immediately after the event and at the end of each working day, and could also involve a later debriefing which also examines the procedures utilized and ways of improving these processes.

Summary

All personnel should be aware that any action in handling a deceased person prior to examination at a mortuary may impact the manner in which the case is treated in ongoing investigations. It is vital that suitably qualified medical personnel, e.g., forensic pathologists, are consulted before any steps are taken to retrieve, secure, and transport the deceased.

This article is designed to offer some instruction to those persons performing body retrieval from a scene of death. It is in no way suggesting that these persons should replace the role of the forensic pathologist. It should be emphasized that all steps taken to secure the body that may interfere with the deceased in any way should occur only after examination or observation of the deceased by a forensic pathologist and should always be appropriately documented.

See Also

Crime-scene Investigation and Examination: Major Incident Scene Management; Recovery of Human Remains; **Crime-scene Management, Systems:** Continental Europe; United Kingdom; United States of America

Further Reading

Clark SC, Ernst MF, Haglund WD, Jentzen JM (1996) *The Medicolegal Death Investigator.* Occupational Research and Assessment.

Geberth VJ (1996) *Practical Homicide Investigation.* CRC Press.

Kendall RE (ed.) (1992) Disaster victim identification. *International Criminal Police Review.* Oct: 437–438.

Knight B (2003) *Forensic Pathology,* 3rd edn. Edward Arnold.

Krogman WM, Iscan MY (1986) *The Human Skeleton in Forensic Medicine,* 2nd edn. Charles C Thomas.

Brain Death *See* **Medical Definitions of Death**

CARBON MONOXIDE POISONING

Contents

Clinical Findings, Sequelae In Survivors

J Payne-James, Forensic Healthcare Services Ltd, London, UK
S Robinson, Altrincham, UK

Introduction

Intoxication from carbon monoxide (CO) is a phenomenon that occurs in a wide variety of settings worldwide. CO is a major environmental toxic agent whose effects were described over a century ago by Haldane. The effects cover a range of physical and neurological signs and symptoms ranging from none to death.

Exposure occurs in two main ways – (1) acute exposure for varying lengths of time, where the effects are generally immediately obvious, and (2) delayed or chronic exposure, where the effects may be unrecognized for days, months, or years. The diagnosis of CO exposure may be one of exclusion. The problems of recognizing low-grade exposure to CO may result in a considerable underestimation of the problem.

It has been estimated that there are up to 6000 deaths per annum in the USA from CO poisoning, with up to 40 000 emergency department attendances for nonfatal exposure.

Pathophysiology

Incomplete combustion of hydrocarbons results in the formation of colorless, odorless, and nonirritant CO. CO dissolves in plasma and binds to oxygen-transporting proteins – hemoglobin (in plasma), myoglobin, and the cytochrome system in tissues. The most significant affinity is for hemoglobin (Hb). CO is absorbed through the lungs and binds to Hb, forming carboxyhemoglobin (COHb). This a reversible reaction which can be described as follows:

$$HbO_2 + CO \rightarrow COHb + O_2$$

The affinity of Hb for CO is up to 250 times greater than that for oxygen, and the presence of CO results in a shift of the oxygen–hemoglobin dissociation curve to the left, causing decreased oxygen-carrying capacity and impaired delivery of oxygen to the tissues. Cellular hypoxia results in this setting from the presence of CO and impaired (hypoxic) cardiac function. The link between levels of CO and effects is not direct. The amount of uptake is governed by a number of variables, all of which interrelate and include relative concentrations of CO and oxygen, alveolar ventilation, duration, and intensity of exposure. However, high levels of CO and chronic exposure lead to CO binding to those proteins with less affinity than hemoglobin, myoglobin, and cytochromes a3 and P450, and these may also account for some of the variations in response to exposure. Hypoxic stress caused by CO exposure alone would not seem to account for some of the longer-term effects and it is believed that CO also affects via a cascade of events, resulting in oxidative stress.

Atmospheric CO concentrations are generally less than 0.001%, although levels in urban areas will be more than in rural areas. Normal individuals who are nonsmokers have a base COHb level of about 0.5%, although normal ranges of 1–3% are described in some studies. These levels originate from endogenous CO, which is produced within the body from the breakdown of heme-containing proteins and in addition the atmospheric levels of

Table 1 World Health Organization maximum levels of carbon monoxide in air (to prevent carboxyhemoglobin rising above 2.5%)

100 mg m^{-3} (87.1 ppm) for 15 min
60 mg m^{-3} (52.3 ppm) for 30 min
30 mg m^{-3} (26.1 ppm) for 60 min
10 mg m^{-3} (8.7 ppm) for 8 h

Table 2 Examples of sources of carbon monoxide exposure

Paint stripping/varnish removal/certain paints
Barbecues
Wood stoves
Coal, oil, or gas boiler
Gas refrigerator
Leaking chimneys
Fireplaces
Cars in garages (domestic and work)
Warehouses with forklifts
Smoking
Cars
Building fires

CO. Endogenous sources are believed to contribute approximately 75% of the overall levels. These levels increase in smokers and are secondary to environmental CO.

Blood COHb levels of 2.5–4% have been shown to be associated with decreased short-term maximal exercise duration in healthy volunteers; levels from 2.7 to 5.1% decreased exercise tolerance in patients with angina; levels between 2 and 20% have been described by an Expert Panel on Air Quality Standards (in the UK) as leading to "equivocal effects on [amongst others] visual perception, motor and sensorimotor performance, vigilance, etc."

The World Health Organization has issued guidelines for the level of CO in the air which will prevent blood COHb levels from rising above 2.5%. These are shown in **Table 1**. Some countries identify their own levels, which are generally of similar orders of magnitude.

The significance of these different values is that low levels of CO may not result in clinically obvious effects, and that those exposed to low levels for prolonged periods may suffer marked effects that are not readily diagnosed.

Methods of Exposure

Exposure to CO may be difficult to detect. **Table 2** lists a number of situations that have resulted in CO exposure. Many locations are fine with adequate ventilation. However, with no air movement or stagnant air, risks of exposure and adverse effects increase. Work, domestic, and leisure settings may all

account for exposure. If exposure is suspected it is appropriate to use a system such as the CH^{2}OPD^2 mnemonic to try to explore the source of environmental exposure – enquiring about community, home, hobbies, occupation, personal habits, diet, and drug issues. Systematic enquiry is the most efficient way of establishing a cause and a source.

Clinical Findings

A vast range of symptoms of CO exposure have been described, hence the description of CO poisoning as a "disease with a thousand faces." Classically, acute CO intoxication is said to cause the triad of cherry-red lips, cyanosis, and retinal hemorrhages, but this type of presentation is rare. In many cases a more insidious presentation develops, with the only indicator a general malaise or suspicion of a viral-type illness. The group of illnesses broadly described as chronic fatigue syndromes may have features that are attributable at least in part to CO exposure.

It appears that CO particularly damages those organs that have high oxygen utilization, including the cardiovascular system and central nervous system. Specific symptoms include headache, dizziness, nausea, shortness of breath, altered vision, altered hearing, chest pain, palpitations, poor concentration, muscle aches and cramps, and abdominal pain. Sometimes these may occur in clusters and sometimes in isolation. More serious effects may be noted predominantly as a result of tissue hypoxia and include loss of consciousness, myocardial ischemia, hypotension, congestive cardiac failure, arrhythmias, mental confusion, and lability of mood. These symptoms and signs may be present during acute exposure at higher levels in nonfatal cases, but also in the more chronic or prolonged case.

Acute poisoning can cause ventilatory disturbances in almost two-thirds of those exposed, even if they have not previously suffered from respiratory disease. Rhabdomyolysis can result in renal failure, and this may be due to direct toxic effects of CO. Diabetes insipidus is also a rare complication. Postpartum hemorrhage has also been documented and this has been attributed to CO, via activation of guanylate cyclase causing arterial vascular smooth-muscle relaxation with subsequent vasodilation. Additionally CO inhibits platelet aggregation.

In addition to the symptoms and signs discussed above there are a variety of neurological, psychiatric, and psychological sequelae that may develop days, months, or years after initial exposure. These delayed sequelae are grouped together as the "neuropsychiatric syndrome." It has been suggested that the syndrome occurs in up to 30% of CO poisonings,

Table 3 Examples of specific carbon monoxide exposure-related sequelae

Source	Exposure/circumstances	Sequelae	Treatment
Kim JS et al. (1987) Mycoclonus, delayed sequelae of CO poisoning, piracetam trial. Yonsei Medical Journal 28: 231–233	Found in a comatose state in a room with a heater	One month after: uneven gait, incontinence, memory loss, disorientation, emotional instability. Myoclonic jerks of neck and lower limbs occurred spontaneously 8 weeks after poisoning	Piracetam administered for 11 days – myoclonic jerks ceased
Gillespie ND et al. (1999) Severe parkinsonism secondary to CO poisoning. Journal of the Royal Society of Medicine 92: 5–6	Found collapsed in house with gas fire switched on but unlit; COHb 42%	Discharged after 10 days. Six days later: deterioration – bradykinetic, marked rigidity, poverty of facial expression. CT scan showed mild atrophy. MRI showed increased signal in periventricular white matter; basal ganglia unaffected	Levodopa/benserazide and pergolide – no effect. Some temporary improvement with hyperbaric oxygen
Benaissa ML et al. (1999) Delayed transient loss of consciousness in acute CO intoxication. Human and Experimental Toxicology 18: 642–643	Malfunction of heater in a church resulted in multiple CO poisonings	Arrived in hospital 3.5 h after the incident fully conscious, with headache, nausea, vertigo and weakness. Loss of consciousness observed 1 h after incident. COHb 5.8%	Given hyperbaric oxygen due to loss of consciousness. No known sequelae
Simmons IG, Good PA (1998) CO poisoning causes optic neuropathy. Eye 12: 809–814	Three cases of visual loss following CO poisoning: (1) car exhaust: attempted suicide; (2) car exhaust: attempted suicide; (3) exposed to exhaust fumes after road traffic accident	(1) presented 3 weeks after with loss of central vision; (2) presented 10 years after suicide attempt; (3) comatose for 6 weeks; awoke complaining of visual loss	Findings suggest CO poisoning can cause a toxic optic neuropathy. Treatment with hydroxycobalamine may be of some benefit
Kelafant GA (1996) Encephalopathy and peripheral neuropathy following CO poisoning from a propane-fueled vehicle. American Journal of Industrial Medicine 30: 765–768	Presented 6 years after exposure as driver of propane fueled vehicle	At time of presentation had numbness in hands, feet and lips, loss of balance, slurred speech, inability to express thoughts, forgetfulness. Physical examination showed diffuse hyporeflexia	None
Mascalchi M et al. (1996) MRI of cerebellar white matter damage due to CO poisoning. Neuroradiology 38: S73–S74	12-year-old referred for MRI because of a generalized tonic–clonic seizure. Six years previously, he had been admitted to hospital following 1 h exposure to CO from gas stove. COHb 18.5%. Discharged without sequelae	MRI 6 years after exposure showed bilateral loss of tissue in parietooccipital regions with small areas of abnormal signal in overlying cortex and almost symmetrical altered signal in posterior cerebellar white matter	None
Balzan M et al. (1993) Intestinal infarction following CO poisoning. Postgraduate Medical Journal 69: 302–303	65-year-old male found unconscious in bathroom. Butane heater found to have blocked flue. COHb 90 min after removal was 45%.	Given hyperbaric oxygen. Deteriorated over 36 h. At autopsy was found to have ischemic necrosis of all abdominal organs with no evidence of significant atheroma or thrombotic or embolic occlusion	None
Florkowski CM et al. (1992) Rhabdomyolysis and acute renal failure following CO poisoning. Clinical Toxicology 30: 443–454	Two cases of rhabdomyolysis with acute renal failure: (1) attempted suicide in bathroom with petrol-driven lawnmower: COHb 7.5% some hours after; (2) rescued unconscious from smoke-filled room: COHb 13.8%	Both patients showed enzymatic and muscle biopsy evidence of muscle necrosis. Rhabdomyolysis and acute renal failure subsequently developed	(1) survived after hemodialysis and hemofiltration; (2) developed anuric renal failure together with acute respiratory distress syndrome and died

Continued

Table 3 Continued

Source	Exposure/circumstances	Sequelae	Treatment
Yanir Y et al. (2002) Cardiogenic shock complicating acute CO poisoning despite neurologic and metabolic recovery. Annals of Emergency Medicine 40: 420–424	Two cases, both from the same incident: (1) 29-year-old female: COHb 22.6%; disoriented after 1 h, comatose at 3 h; (2) 8-year-old female: unconscious: COHb 20.4%	(1) cardiogenic shock with recovery after 11 days; (2) cardiogenic shock: recovery after 24 days	Hyperbaric oxygen and full supportive intensive care
Chang M-Y, Lin J-L (2001) Central diabetes insipidus following CO poisoning. American Journal of Nephrology 21: 145–149	Two cases, both from the same incident: (1) 20-year-old female: exposure to CO in unventilated bathroom. Found unconscious. COHb 18.6% 90 min after exposure; (2) 9-month-old child: COHb 100 min after exposure: 4%	Both developed diabetes insipidus, with subsequent hypernatremia, subarachnoid hemorrhage, brain edema and permanent brain injury	ADH and desmopressin. Mother remained comatose in PVS. Child died of nosocomial pneumonia. Full supportive measures
Ramsey PS et al. (2001) Delayed post-partum hemorrhage: rare presentation of CO poisoning. American Journal of Obstetrics and Gynecology 184: 243–244	41-year-old female admitted to hospital. Later found to have faulty gas heater; COHb 17%	Presented with profuse vaginal bleeding 2 weeks after uncomplicated delivery. No problems until 2–3 h before presentation. Also reported light-headedness, nausea, blurred vision, headache, and chills	100% oxygen given and over 4 h bleeding resolved and mental status normalized

COHb, carboxyhemoglobin; CT, computed tomography; MRI, magnetic resonance imaging; CO, carbon monoxide.

although the true incidence may be more, but remains undiagnosed. A substantial minority of survivors will develop full neurological impairment such as dementia, psychosis, or Parkinsonism, whilst others will develop less florid subtle neurological and psychiatric disorders including cognitive deficit and personality change.

Cognitive deficits that have been observed include impaired memory, attention, visuospatial skills and executive function, with apraxia, and mood disturbances including psychosis. Aggressive behavior is not a common feature. Memory deficits appear to be due to damage to the hippocampus which is particularly vulnerable to anoxia and ischemia.

Table 3 lists specific cases of the less common complications of CO poisoning mentioned above but which were found to be directly related to exposure.

Diagnosis and Investigation

Diagnosis is made by measuring venous COHb levels; however, there is no absolute level which can confirm the presence or absence of poisoning, but a level above 10% is generally considered to confirm the diagnosis, unless the individual is a heavy smoker. COHb levels in arterial blood are not significantly different from venous levels and so an arterial sample is not required for diagnosis. Arterial blood-gas measurements can show a mixed picture of normal partial pressure of oxygen, variable partial pressure of carbon dioxide and decreased oxygen saturation in the presence of a metabolic acidosis. Problems arise particularly due to chronic, lower-dose exposure, because the COHb levels will revert to "normal" values once removed from the exposure, depending on the half-life of COHb in the particular setting. Normal COHb does not necessarily rule out CO poisoning.

Imaging techniques such as magnetic resonance imaging (MRI) and computed tomography (CT) scans show a number of specific lesions following CO exposure, including in both cerebral white and gray matter and the basal ganglia. Low-density whitematter lesions have been seen in the frontal lobes and globus pallidus on CT and bilateral symmetric hyperintensities of the periventricular white matter and centrum semiovale, with iron deposition in the thalamus and necrosis of the basal ganglia on MRI. Positron emission tomography (PET) and single-photon emission computed tomography (SPECT) have shown evidence of cerebral hypoperfusion following CO poisoning, with some indication of reduced regional cerebral blood flow in frontal and temporal cortices.

Studies indicate significant links between neurobehavioral disorder and abnormalities seen using imaging techniques.

Management

Acute CO exposure should be treated immediately as a medical emergency with attention to the basics of airway, breathing, and circulation. Higher levels of exposure can result in reduced consciousness and cardiorespiratory compromise to a degree requiring intubation, ventilation, and circulatory support within an intensive care setting. The antidote to CO poisoning is the administration of oxygen. COHb half-life varies according to the amount of available oxygen. A mean $t_{1/2}$ of 320 min (range 128–409) has been reported in normal healthy volunteers in room air, down to 23 min in those breathing 100% oxygen at 3 atm. Thus, the administration of 100% oxygen via a tight-fitting face mask with a nonrebreather reservoir bag should be commenced and continued for several hours. Hyperbaric oxygen may have a role in the management of certain cases, particularly those with a history of unconsciousness, neurological signs, cardiovascular compromise, or a severe metabolic acidosis, but the evidence for improved outcome is not strong. It has also been recommended as treatment when CO exposure occurs during pregnancy if the conscious state is altered or if COHb reaches a level of 20%.

Summary

CO poisoning is a cause of great morbidity worldwide. It can give rise to a profuse number of complications – some that occur early and are reversible and some that occur very late and are irreversible. The vagueness of many of the signs and symptoms means that the diagnosis is often missed. A low threshold for consideration of the diagnosis should be held for any individual brought into hospital or found in a state of altered consciousness, and detailed histories should be taken from those whose symptoms might be accounted for by exposure to CO.

See Also

Carbon Monoxide Poisoning: Incidence and Findings at Postmortem

Further Reading

Abelsohn A, Sanborn MD, Jessiman BJ, Weir E (2002) Identifying and managing adverse environmental health effects: carbon monoxide poisoning. *Canadian Medical Association Journal* 166: 1685–1690.

Aubard Y, Magne I (2000) Carbon monoxide poisoning in pregnancy. *British Journal of Obstetrics and Gynaecology* 107: 833–838.

Fisher J (1999) Carbon monoxide poisoning: a disease of a thousand faces. *Chest* 115: 322–332.

Gale SD, Hopkins RO, Weaver LK, *et al.* (1999) MRI, quantitative MRI, SPECT and neuropsychological findings following carbon monoxide poisoning. *Brain Injury* 13: 229–243.

Hawkins M (1999) Carbon monoxide poisoning. *European Journal of Anaesthesiology* 16: 585–589.

Juurlink DN, Stanbrook MB, McGuigan MA (2000) Hyperbaric oxygen for carbon monoxide poisoning. *Cochrane Database Systematic Review* 84: 584–586.

Marshall L, Weir E, Abelsohn A, Sanborn MD (2002) Identifying and managing adverse environmental health effects: taking an exposure history. *Canadian Medical Association Journal* 166(8): 1049–1055.

Petersen J, Stewart R (1970) Absorption and elimination of carbon monoxide by active young men. *Archives of Environmental Health* 21: 165–171.

Simini B (1999) Cherry red discoloration in carbon monoxide poisoning. *Lancet* 352: 1154.

Townsend CL, Maynard RL (2002) Effects on health of prolonged exposure to low concentrations of carbon monoxide. *Occupational and Environmental Medicine* 59: 708–711.

WHO (1999) *Environmental Health Criteria 213: Carbon Monoxide,* 2nd edn. Finland: World Health Organization.

Incidence and Findings at Postmortem

J C U Downs, Georgia Bureau of Investigation, Savannah, GA, USA

Introduction

Carbon monoxide (CO) is a ubiquitous gas, primarily encountered forensically as the product of incomplete combustion (oxidation) of reduced carbonaceous compounds. It constitutes one of the major pollutants in the lower atmosphere. Naturally occurring CO averages 1–2% in the blood of nonsmokers. Because it is odorless, colorless, and tasteless, CO may become an undetected "silent killer" even if only slightly elevated.

Recent studies of the frequency of CO intoxications extrapolate to some 40 000 cases annually in the USA. The actual number is likely significantly higher due to the lack of recognition of cases. In excess of 5000 deaths, over two-thirds of which are suicides, are directly attributed to CO inhalation each year. Recent declines in accidental CO fatalities have coincided with an increased suicide rate. In addition, the vast majority of the estimated 3350 annual fire-related fatalities are due to CO inhalation in whole or in part. Most documented CO-related deaths occur at the scene of exposure, prior to receiving medical therapy. The most cited gross finding with significant CO exposure is bright-red or "cherry-red" coloration of the blood and tissues (**Figures 1** and **2**).

Ambient Concentrations

Relevant features in a CO exposure include a confined space, a CO source, and time. The major factors affecting carboxyhemoglobin (COHb) levels, and thus morbidity and mortality, are the dose and duration of exposure. **Figure 3** provides a general range of concentrations and corresponding symptoms.

In addition to the primary source of vehicular exhaust, CO may be produced by any internal combustion engine, fires, malfunctioning furnaces/heating systems, dihalomethane (methylene chloride, dibromomethane, and bromochloromethane) metabolism, acetylene gas, carbonyl iron, coal gas, illuminating gas, and marsh gas. A small quantity of CO is produced endogenously at the rate of $0.4–0.7 \, ml \, h^{-1}$, during the degradation of the heme protoporphyrin ring of hemoglobin (Hb). Cigarette smoking is a significant source of CO. Smokers can have up to 10% COHb compared to a nonsmoker's maximum of 5%. Pipes and cigars burn longer and at lower temperatures; thus may result in COHb concentrations of up to 20%. These levels are reached only rarely, as typically the user does not inhale pipe/cigar smoke as deeply. **Figure 4** summarizes typical reference ranges for several "normal" populations. Individual baselines should be considered when interpreting deaths with low-level CO exposure.

Location and environmental conditions significantly impact ambient CO levels. The established occupational threshold is 25 ppm. Ambient air may reach up to 50 ppm in a smoke-filled room or along a highway. Temperature inversions, especially with urban traffic, may escalate the level to 100 ppm. Further, tree-lined major thoroughfares may trap ambient CO, which may then affect drivers as well as pedestrians. Equilibrium COHb concentrations are 8% at 50 ppm and 16% at 100 ppm. Under such conditions, neuropsychiatric effects of poisoning could be contributory in motor vehicle collisions and even in pedestrian deaths.

Physiology

CO is a normal physiologic metabolite and may act directly as a neurotransmitter. The primary *in vivo* effect of exogenously introduced CO is to bind to the Hb molecule, which normally functions to transport

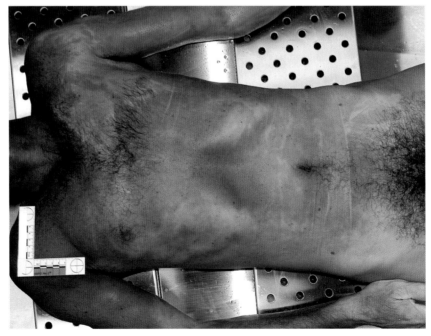

Figure 1 Cherry-red lividity. The most recognizable and cited gross correlate to elevated carboxyhemoglobin is a bright-red or "cherry-red" color to blood and other tissues. This is most likely to be recognized with carboxyhemoglobin ≥30%. In lightly pigmented individuals, the color may be easily appreciated in the livor mortis. Other sites that may be assessed, particularly in darkly pigmented bodies, are in the mucosae of the eyes and mouth.

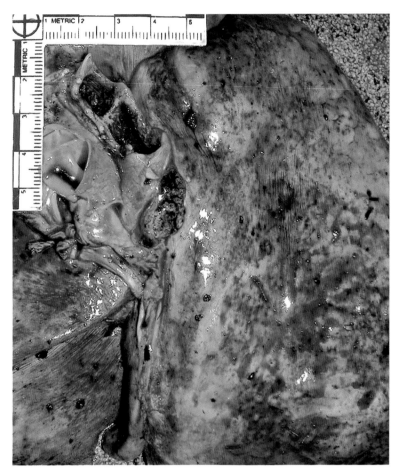

Figure 2 Cherry-red lung tissue and soot within airway. In addition to the classic "cherry-red" livor pattern, the soft tissues and organs exhibit the same hue. Here the lung tissue demonstrates the same bright-red color as is evident elsewhere. The carboxyhemoglobin in this fire fatality was 75%. Black foreign material is evident lining the bronchial tree, confirming smoke inhalation in a typical sooty blaze.

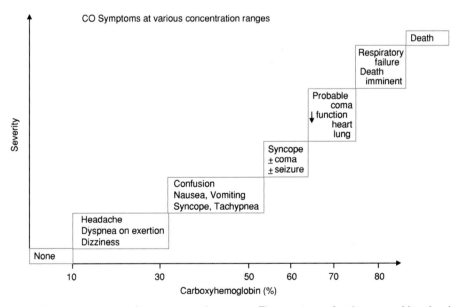

Figure 3 Carbon monoxide symptoms at various concentration ranges. The symptoms of carbon monoxide poisoning are myriad and overlap. In general, subjects are asymptomatic at carboxyhemoglobin of ≤10%. Symptoms are primarily dependent on ambient carbon monoxide concentration and duration of exposure. Gradually, blood carboxyhemoglobin levels climb, resulting in progressively worsening symptoms. Levels of ≥50% are generally considered lethal; however, with existing disease and/or other stressors impairing oxygen exchange, levels as low as 15–20% may be fatal.

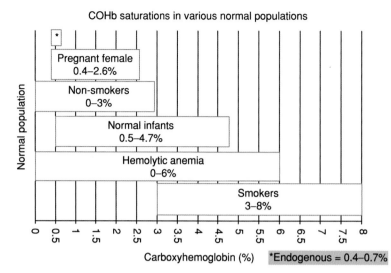

Figure 4 Carboxyhemoglobin (COHb) saturations in various normal populations. A trace of COHb is present (0.4–0.7%) due to endogenous metabolism from the degradation of the heme protoporphyrin ring; however, this is slightly higher in pregnant females (up to 2.6%). Nonsmokers usually have <3%, but may have up to 5% depending on environmental conditions and exposure. In conditions where the erythrocytes break down at an increased rate, the baseline COHb will be elevated. Smokers typically have twice the carbon monoxide content of nonsmokers, but may have even higher baseline concentrations, depending upon the type of tobacco used and the extent of inhalation. Second-hand smoke in a confined environment can also increase COHb in nonsmokers.

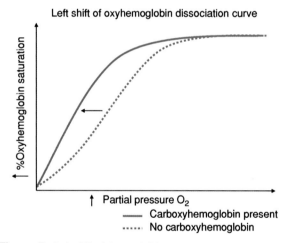

Figure 5 Left-shifted hemoglobin oxygen dissociation curve with carbon monoxide. At any given concentration of blood oxyhemoglobin (ordinate), if carboxyhemoglobin (COHb) is present (solid line) the hemoglobin molecule holds on to bound oxygen more tenaciously than if COHb is absent (dashed line). Thus, at any given partial pressure of oxygen (abscissa), the oxyhemoglobin level will be increased if COHb is present (solid line) in comparison to if COHb is absent. This occurs in skeletal muscle (myoglobin) where the partial pressure of O_2 is normally lower than in the blood; thus the oxyhemoglobin would normally tend to dissociate the O_2 in muscle. If COHb is present, more oxyhemoglobin remains bound, resulting in a net oxygen deficit in skeletal muscle.

oxygen in the blood. In addition to binding to Hb, forming COHb, CO can also bind to myoglobin (Mb) to form the muscle oxygen-storing protein carboxymyoglobin (COMb). CO binds to both Hb and Mb with an affinity ~250 times that of oxygen. Isolated in solution, a single heme molecule binds CO in a tight linear iron–carbon–oxygen array up to 25 000 times as tightly as it does pure oxygen (O_2). Biologically, this tenacious binding is tempered by an angled arrangement of the globin portion of the Hb molecule, such that the *in vivo* binding of CO is significantly decreased. The net result is that, under normal conditions, approximately 1% of all body Hb is bound to CO. Body Mb is a potential large reservoir for CO due to its high binding affinity and left-shifted dissociation curve (**Figure 5**).

The absolute amount of "bioavailable" O_2 is lessened, and this is directly proportional to the COHb level due to competitive binding. Hb transports oxygen from lungs to tissues where it then delivers (dissociates) the oxygen molecule from the Hb. This mass-action phenomenon follows a sigmoidal relationship (**Figure 5**, dashed line) with the percentage of oxygen saturation varying directly with the partial pressure of inspired O_2. When COHb is present, however, the dissociation curve shifts to the left (**Figure 5**, solid line). The net effect is that, for any given partial pressure of O_2, it is harder for the oxyHb to deoxygenate with COHb present, resulting in a higher percentage of circulating blood oxyHb than would normally be present while the tissues remain hypoxic.

In addition to blocking oxygen delivery to tissues, CO is a direct intracellular toxin, blocking cell respiration via the electron transport chain (P450 system and cytochromes a and a_3 are blocked by CO binding to ferrous (2^+) iron).

With normal lung function, exchanging 6 l of air per minute, a 50% COHb can be reached in 8 min with a 1% ambient CO level. An estimated expected COHb concentration can be calculated by the formula:

$$[\%COHb] = (6\,l\,min^{-1})(\%ambient\,air\,CO)(min\,exposure)$$

There is no significant metabolism of inspired CO. Pulmonary elimination is the primary pathway, with only 1% of body CO metabolized to CO_2 *in vivo*. The half-life $(t_{1/2})$ of CO in the body is also affected by competitive binding of O_2 to Hb. The latter is exploited therapeutically to cause a CO-poisoned patient to "blow off" CO. The usual $t_{1/2}$ of COHb in ambient air (21% O_2) is 4.5–6 h. The $t_{1/2}$ can be reduced to 0.5–1.5 h with 100% ambient oxygen and to 23–30 min with 200% (2 atm – hyperbaric oxygen).

Normal pulmonary CO elimination may pose difficulty for the treating physician as well as the forensic pathologist. Once the patient is removed from the CO source (e.g., removed from the smoldering building, taken out of the car, intubated by the ambulance, etc.) the victim begins to eliminate Hb-bound CO. Any subsequent analysis will report a blood COHb concentration "at the point in time when the sample was drawn." This may not be at all reflective of the true CO level. To make matters worse, in subtle poisonings, the possibility of CO may not be suggested for hours or even days, depending on the clinical picture. By his time, the COHb could have fallen into a normal range, mandating a retrospective, circumstantial diagnosis.

Therapy with O_2, especially combined with CO_2, can allow CO levels to dissipate 10–20 times more rapidly. This is critical in preventing deaths, as hyperbaric oxygen (HBO) given at ≥ 6 h postexposure has an almost one-third fatality rate while early HBO can cut the rate to less than 15%.

Testing

The optimal sample for postmortem forensic COHb analysis is ethylenediaminetetraacetic acid (purple-top tube) or sodium fluoride (gray-top tube) preserved whole blood. The tube should be as completely filled as possible, to minimize the empty headspace over the sample in the tube. With exposure of blood to air, bound CO can equilibrate with the headspace, artificially lowering the test result on the sample. Samples are best held frozen, but may be refrigerated. Improperly stored toxicology blood samples can artifactually lose 60% of the bound CO.

Spleen and other high-Hb fluid-containing tissues are also acceptable specimens. Spleen COHb is interpreted broadly as a significant or insignificant concentration. In general, spleen levels <10% are seen with blood COHb <10%, while >30% spleen COHb corresponds to blood toxic and lethal concentrations. Cases with spleen COHb between 10% and 30% COHb are indeterminate.

There are a few caveats regarding nonblood tissue CO samples. Severely charred tissues are unsuitable, as they tend to desiccate and thus contain little blood (Hb). In decomposed bodies, low-Hb-content serosanguineous fluid collects in the chest cavity. Spectrophotometric and other analyses reliant on an intact Hb molecule are compromised; however, quantitation is possible by direct analysis for CO independent of Hb.

The characteristic red color associated with CO exposure is based on the light absorbance of the COHb molecule as compared to that of oxyHb and other Hb moieties. The quantitation of CO can be performed toxicologically using co-oximetry and/or spectrophotometry. Because CO is a frequently encountered toxin and because of the potential for additional loss of life if CO poisoning goes undetected, several screening tests are available to the pathologist if immediate testing capacity is otherwise unavailable. A suggestive pink color results from the combination of 1 part 0.01 mol l^{-1} ammonia with 20 parts CO-positive blood. An easier screening test involves the reexamination of tissue sections retained in formaldehyde from the autopsy (the so-called "stock" or "save" container). Normally, non-CO-containing viscera will take on a brown tone after several hours in formaldehyde, as the proteins denature. CO-containing tissues retain their characteristic bright-red hue for days to weeks following formalin denaturation (**Figure 6**).

CO is not formed within the body to a significant extent postmortem, unlike cyanide (CN) – an important consideration in handling toxicology samples for quantitation. The characteristic CO color may persist for weeks in an unembalmed body and for at least several days following embalming. The embalming process interferes with CO analysis and may result in unreliable quantitative results. With time, CO livor color progresses from bright-red to dark-green to brown.

Scene Investigation

The physical performance of an autopsy is one test which must be integrated and interpreted in light of all other available data pertinent to a specific case. This includes medical records, symptoms expressed,

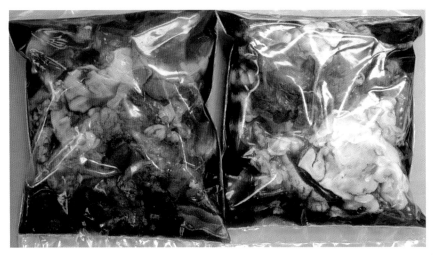

Figure 6 Persistence of cherry-red color in formaldehyde-fixed tissues with CO. A quick screen for the presence of COHb is a reexamination of tissue portions retained in formaldehyde. If examined within several days of autopsy, the COHb-positive tissues and fluid in the "save" container stay bright-red (left) while CO-negative tissues quickly turn brown (right).

signs observed, and investigative information. One of the most critical elements in the practice of forensic pathology is scene investigation. In many deaths, the definitive and even sole clues to the actual cause and manner of death are scene-derived. CO deaths, especially subtle ones, are prime examples. A (relatively) confined environment is one of the investigative clues to a potential CO fatality. Even something as apparently innocuous as smoking in the confined space of an automobile cabin or a submarine may produce potentially hazardous CO levels.

Location within a scene is also important, as CO has a density 97% that of ambient air and as a result, tends to accumulate at a height of 1.5–2 m (5–6 ft), which would enhance its potential action as a human intoxicant by concentrating the ambient CO at the level of the face.

Most often CO deaths affect one person; however, because the environment is actually poisoned, any and all living creatures in the area are potentially at risk. This includes pets and children who are at increased risk due to their higher basal metabolic rates. Thus, they may succumb at a lower %COHb than adults in the same environment.

An uncommon scenario would be a child sleeping in the back of an auto on a long trip. A defective exhaust may allow CO to build up in the rear of the cabin but not in the more adequately vented front. The net result is that the child, who had been thought to be sleeping, is discovered dead and those in the front are asymptomatic. In ambient asphyxiation cases, environmental testing may prove beneficial in determining the exact sequence of events and prevent additional deaths.

Based on the CO source as determined by scene investigation, most CO asphyxiations can be categorized by origin as fire, exhaust, or other.

Fire

The type of fire provides valuable information regarding how a case should be worked up. A fire that begins in bedding or clothing in a case with a history of alcohol and/or drug use in a cigarette smoker may suggest an accidental origin. Multiple or unusual points of origin or fires exhibiting features of accelerant use could indicate arson and an attempt to destroy evidence in order to evade detection. The data may also explain how a particular COHb level came to be.

In a typical fire the complete exothermic reaction is

$$C + O_2 \rightarrow CO_2 + heat$$

If the conditions of the fire are altered such that there is an overabundance of fuel (increased carbon) and/or a relative/absolute lack of oxygen, incomplete combustion results:

$$2C + O_2 \rightarrow 2CO + heat$$

The latter is the typical scenario in most fires; therefore, most fire-related deaths are directly attributed to smoke inhalation, primarily from the contained CO therein.

CO itself is a carbonaceous compound. Thus, it too may serve as a fuel. This is most often encountered when a superheated cloud of sooty smoke forms from smoldering fire, following exhaustion of the available oxygen in a relatively confined space. CO may comprise one-sixth to three-quarters of atmospheric volume. As combustion continues, temperature increases to the flashpoint of CO, 1128 °F (608.9 °C). If a source of oxygen is made available, the result is explosive combustion of the smoke cloud, also known as a backdraft or flashover. In order to avoid such a massive advancement of an ongoing conflagration, firefighters are trained to verify manually the temperature of closed doors within a burning building. The same end result can occur during a controlled venting of smoke by allowing fresh air (oxygen) to displace the cloud.

Direct thermal body injuries are most often a secondary effect of fire, dependent on the intensity and duration of the blaze. High-temperature, rapid fires cause extensive skin charring with spared tissues, while cooler but longer ones cause extensive deep-tissue destruction. No direct correlation exists between the extent of damage and CO concentration. The CO level depends on the incomplete combustion of available materials. Most fuel-fed fires have low CO with high CO associated with the plastics and other materials in vehicular fires.

A body severely burned in a fire requires an autopsy to establish identity and determine if the subject was, in fact, alive during the course of the conflagration.

There is no way to correlate the extent of thermal injury with the timing of burns as premortem or postmortem; however, blood associated with other injuries may be significant.

Ideally, a medical examiner is available to examine the fire scene with fire investigators with the body still present. A crude presumptive test for CO toxicity, and thus inhalation of smoke during the fire is possible at the scene, if indicated. The pathologist may incise into muscle in an area of preserved soft tissue and examine for the characteristic monoxide coloration. With an intact barrier, CO does not bind to Hb or Mb to any appreciable degree unless it has been inhaled; thus the presence of pink tissue is a predictor of CO inhalation. However, it is far from definitive. Final assessment is properly deferred to the autopsy.

Incisions into the area of the trachea should be avoided, as this may introduce carbonaceous artifact into the airway and could potentially cloud the issue of smoke inhalation in cases where the CO level is low (e.g., flash fire). Similarly, in cases where the burn is extensive in the area of the neck (**Figure 7**) sooty debris may fall onto the exposed airway surface. In such cases, more distal small airways may be assessed grossly (**Figure 2**) and/or microscopically for the presence or absence of carbon deposits.

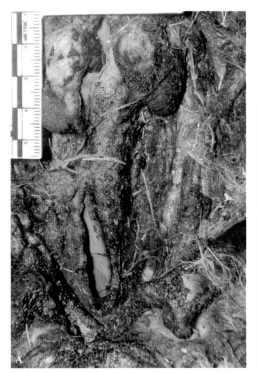 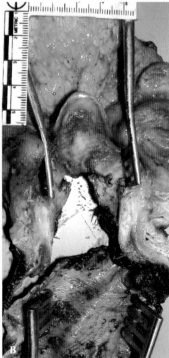

Figure 7 (A) Anterior neck with severe fourth-degree burn, exposing the trachea. In some cases of severe burn, the anterior neck structures are severely charred and may burn through the wall of the trachea. Although examination of the airway for soot is important at the scene, the airway should not be incised in order to prevent artifactual contamination by sooty debris falling into a created defect. (B) Opened trachea with anterior defect showing soot within lumen. This may pose problems as a defect allows sooty material to contaminate the tracheal mucosa.

Exhaust

Most auto exhaust fatalities are more straightforward. Normal incidental automotive exhaust inhalation may result in COHb concentrations between 0.5% and 10%. The typical example of a CO death is an inhalational suicide by means of automotive exhaust via a hose leading from the tail pipe into the cabin (**Figure 8**).

A common nonfire CO death scene involves an automobile in a garage, workshop, or other relatively enclosed space. The deceased succumbs to CO from the engine running and exhaust accumulating. This may be accidental, if the individual had no awareness of the potential danger, as might happen in cold climes when an auto is left running in the garage to "warm up" the heater. The victim(s) may be located elsewhere in the house, as CO is pernicious and easily permeates into the remainder of the dwelling undetected. Suicide is often accomplished in a like manner, with the decedent deliberately sealing the environment (by lowering the garage door or venting the exhaust into the car cabin).

Occasionally, the subject will attempt to conceal a suicide by staging such a scene. A typical scene is a vehicle with the hood up and automotive tools near the decedent's body, giving the appearance that the victim inadvertently succumbed to CO from the exhaust while working on the car. The most compelling argument against such an improbable occurrence is that the non-CO fraction of auto exhaust is highly irritating and would force out an unwilling subject

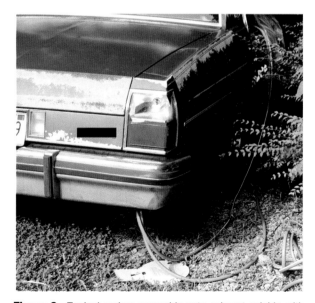

Figure 8 Typical carbon monoxide auto exhaust suicide with hose leading from exhaust pipe to cabin. Most suicides from carbon monoxide result from auto exhaust. These cases often involve running a hose from the vehicle exhaust into the vehicle cabin.

from such an endangering situation within minutes, well in advance of loss of consciousness.

A consideration in any motor vehicle crash is the potential of a mildly elevated CO leaking into the cabin, hindering performance and causing a subsequent vehicular crash. An example of the latter would be the crash of a passenger airliner, wherein the pilots (and passengers) were overcome by the CO produced by a fire in the plane's hold. As a result, the jet crashes shortly after takeoff, killing all aboard.

In a more likely scenario, toxic CO concentrations may accumulate in a driver in traffic. Internal combustion engines operate least efficiently while idling in heavy traffic, especially in an urban environment, and ambient CO levels may reach hazardous concentrations, dependent on the exposure time. Likewise, if a vehicle's exhaust is defective, CO may surreptitiously leak directly into the cabin. If the driver has an elevated COHb, adversely affecting motor skills (as may happen at COHb of 10–30%) with a resultant fatal crash, the CO was a significant factor in the death(s).

Relatively low COHb concentrations may not have any visible pathologic changes, thus the medical examiner can only detect such low-level poisonings with a high index of suspicion. Some advocate routine CO testing in all motor vehicle crash fatalities without clear accident causation, due to the possibility of exhaust leakage into the cabin. Should case circumstances suggest a need, the test may prove of benefit.

Catalytic converters have markedly decreased CO exhaust emissions, as they facilitate the complete oxidation of CO to CO_2. In some cases of auto exhaust asphyxia, the efficiency of the catalytic converter (increased with a warm engine) may be such that the ambient oxygen within the car cabin is consumed and replaced by the exhaust's CO_2. In such instances, CO concentration may be normal or minimally elevated. An ambient cabin air analysis could prove useful in explaining a low or negative COHb (**Figure 9**).

Other

Most other CO exposures are due to inadvertently becoming entrapped in an environment with an elevated CO. The earliest reported CO symptoms date from Aristotle when smoldering coals in a closed room were used for execution. Similar cases still occasionally occur with the use of charcoal grills on porches or in tents.

Electrical generators pose a hazard if used in improperly ventilated sites, such as indoors, in a motor home, or inside a motorboat. Rarely, air-compressor motors can serve as a CO contamination point for compressed air in scuba tanks. If possible, such equipment should be secured and analyzed in a

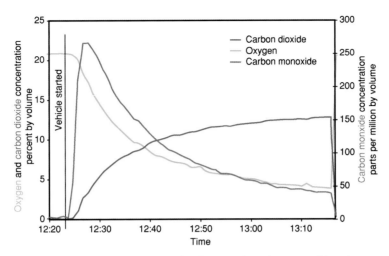

Figure 9 Assay of vehicle cabin with catalytic converter showing decrease in carbon monoxide and oxygen with concurrent increase in carbon dioxide with time. In cases where ambient air composition may be critical, analysis can quantitate the various gases present. In some cases, as in existing disease or with a late-model car, the carbon monoxide may be normal or mildly elevated. With a warm engine, the catalytic converter burns more efficiently and asphyxiation may result from accumulation of carbon dioxide and depletion of oxygen rather than by accumulation of carbon monoxide.

questioned death. The transom of a boat, an unvented deck of a boat, a motorboat ski platform, and the bed of a pickup truck may all be CO hazards, as exhaust may vent to the general passenger area and be retained by a negative-pressure suction phenomenon.

A recent trend of outdoor CO poisonings, specifically associated with boats, has been detected in the last decade. Over 100 such situations have occurred outdoors with almost one-third fatal and another 39% involving loss of consciousness, which potentially could result in drowning. Various identified sources include electric generators on-board, improperly vented engines, stationary position, passenger position at transom/rear, and boat density at or near shore. Over half of the pedestrians on shore have a >5–10% increase in COHb with concurrent symptoms.

Wells and tunnels likewise form contained environments, which can allow lethal collection of CO, especially affecting laborers within such environments. Tragically, these situations often have additional deaths as rescuers, unaware of the hazard, enter the lethal environment – often in an excited state. As with all common asphyxiant gases, detection equipment is available to avoid disasters.

Cause of Death

The general cause of death in most CO exposures is relatively straightforward – asphyxiation due to the inadequate O_2 delivery by Hb; however, fires can be more complicated. In fire fatalities, non-CO noxious gases (most often CN) may be produced. Various

materials, including plastics and padding, can form CN during fires. As CN is another chemical asphyxiant resulting in bright-red livor and tissues, fatal exposure could easily be mistaken for CO poisoning. CO and CN act synergistically as cellular poisons, presumably at the intracellular cytochrome level. In over half of the fires, both CO and CN levels are elevated; thus, the combined action of these toxins (as well as several other potentially nonassayed agents) in concert causes death.

For the sake of accuracy, the medical examiner will often attribute the death to "smoke inhalation" to include such instances. Many pathologists will take this a step further, to include the circumstances of the fire proper and attribute the death to "smoke inhalation and thermal injury." Some contend that "thermal injury" is often euphemistically added to protect the sensibilities regarding how an individual suffered in a fire by basically suffocating to death from the smoke. Such a view ignores the physiology of heat with its impact on human performance and oxygen consumption. In addition, the thought of panic *in extremis* in a conflagration is far from comforting.

Mechanism of Injury

Even relatively low-level CO levels of short duration can be life-threatening. Because CO directly interferes with cellular energy and respiration, high-energy-demand organs such as the heart and brain are most at risk. This is demonstrated by some of the symptoms of acute CO poisoning: headache, seizures, and cardiac dysrhythmias (**Figure 3**).

The heart is especially susceptible to the effects of CO toxicity for myriad reasons. In energy terms, cardiac tissue is high-demand and low-supply, so a continuous ready supply of oxygen is crucial.

Direct CO histotoxicity also occurs at the level of cellular respiration and, if possible, other intracellular processes, as evidenced by the non-COHb level correlative pathology/sequelae: late-phase CO effects after return to a normal COHb, low COHb effects, and extent of CO neurotoxicity in sublethal poisonings. Possible means of delayed neurological effects include direct nerve damage, white-matter demyelination, peroxidation of brain lipids, and/or mitochondrial dysfunction.

Symptomatology

The net result of CO is hypoxic/anoxic anoxemia (the decrease/absence of blood O_2 due to the absence of O_2). In general, symptoms can be estimated based on the percentage of COHb (**Figure 3**). The toxicity and symptoms of CO exposure are highly variable and dependent upon: concentration, duration, O_2 consumption, physical exertion, other toxin(s) present, disease state, and altitude. Of these, the concentration and length exposure are the most critical (**Figure 10**). Although short-term exposure to high CO levels is more likely lethal, chronic or prolonged exposure to lower levels causes far more significant morbidity.

It is possible to predict time to incapacitation experimentally, primarily to compare adverse effects with those of other inhalational toxins. The relationship assumes no existing disease, light activity, and loss of consciousness at 30% COHb. The formula is:

$$FED_{I_{CO}} = (8.2925 \times 10^{-4})(ppm\ CO)(time/30)$$

Adverse effects of CO are not due solely to its direct competition with oxygen binding. A net result of a 50% reduction in O_2 transport results from either a 50% COHb concentration or severe anemia (reducing a normal Hb level from 44% to 22%) and has vastly different potential consequences. In the former case, death is likely without treatment while the latter may have minimal symptoms. In part, this is due to the left shift in the oxygen dissociation curve (**Figure 5**). In addition, there is some direct cytotoxic effect of CO.

CO, as the prototypical suffocating asphyxiant gas, exemplifies the entire essence of forensic pathology. The myriad symptoms and signs lead to a broad differential. Its ubiquity and stealth may conceal its significance in any specific case. The primary target is oxygen (fuel) delivery derangement. This latter is accomplished through the three organs responsible for life in an immediate sense, thus the cause of most forensic pathology casework: the heart (fuel pump), the lungs (fuel source), and the brain (driving force).

The heart in particular is extremely sensitive to CO, with dysrhythmias, angina, and electrocardiographic abnormalities experimentally linked to CO exposure. Existing heart disease may be aggravated with a 5–10% increase of CO. The immediate mechanism of death in CO toxicity is believed to be acute myocardial hypoxia ("heart attack"). Existing disease affecting the oxygen delivery system as a whole, be it blood (e.g., anemia), lungs (e.g., asthma, emphysema, pneumonia), and/or heart (e.g., coronary artery disease) are at increased risk of morbidity and mortality from CO exposure (**Figure 11**). The clinical and pathologic alterations in brain tissue clearly demonstrate CO's toxicity. Any condition (be it increased humidity, temperature extremes, high altitude, or exertion) increasing respiratory rate will also increase CO absorption; cold is a particularly important stressor.

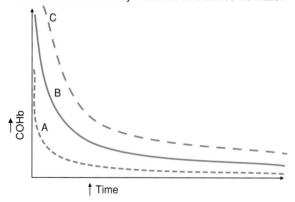

Carbon monoxide toxicity relation to time and concentration

Figure 10 Equilibrium carboxyhemoglobin (COHb) concentrations as a function of ambient carbon monoxide concentration and duration of exposure. The concentration of COHb reaches an equilibrium based on the concentration of carbon monoxide in ambient air and duration of exposure. At lower ambient carbon monoxide concentrations (curve A), the equilibrium is reached more rapidly and the final COHb level is lower. Higher final equilibrium COHb concentrations are reached with higher ambient carbon monoxide concentrations (curves B and C).

Autopsy

Lethal CO Levels

Sudden death from blood loss (due to inability to transport O_2) may occur with a one-fourth decrease in total blood volume (hypovolemic shock). With CO, the functional equivalent holds true. A 25%

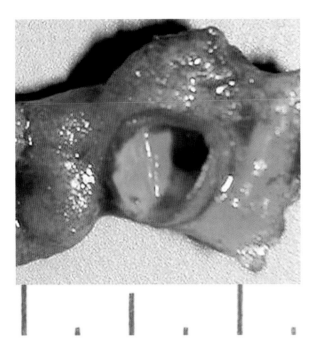

Figure 11 Severe coronary atherosclerosis in carbon monoxide death, 21% carboxyhemoglobin (COHb). In cases where natural disease and/or trauma may be significant prior to carbon monoxide exposure, the subject has an existing difficulty with delivery of oxygenated blood to target organs, most significantly the heart. In this case, the anterior descending coronary artery was 75% stenotic due to existing atherosclerosis. This helps explain why the decedent succumbed to carbon monoxide at 21% COHb.

COHb will most likely be symptomatic and may be fatal (**Figure 3**).

Typical forensic cases involve high CO concentrations. The two major fatal CO sources, fire and internal combustion engine exhaust, have significant differences in COHb levels: COHb in fire averages 59% (range 25–85%) and in exhaust cases 72% (range 48–93%). Other CO exposure sources are significantly less common and may be associated with variable CO levels.

Even low CO levels may be important in death causation. Some have erroneously held that COHb concentrations of less than 10% are not toxicologically significant; however, the recognition of chronic low-level CO toxicity and the phenomenon of "blowing off" (elimination) of CO point to the importance of considering more than just the isolated results of one COHb test. Most authorities believe that many nonlethal CO poisonings go undetected due to the myriad and confusing symptoms. No doubt less obvious death cases are also missed. Data need to be interpreted in light of all the case information and with a degree of suspicion.

An ambient air CO of 1% (1000 ppm) is typically lethal within about 30 min or as quickly as 10 min

with exertion. CO concentrations above 50% are generally considered potentially lethal; however, half of fire fatalities have CO levels of <50%. With significant disease, especially to the heart or lungs, this may be as low as 15–20%. Lower COHb concentrations may be lethal when combined with other central nervous system depressants (e.g., ethanol, sedatives, etc.), toxins, and increased oxygen need (e.g., with exercise/activity).

In fire deaths, the CO may be helpful in assessing potential activity by the decedent during the course of the fire. Higher COHb levels (>50%) suggest survival for a longer period, with exceedingly high levels (>90%) favoring a subject resting, sleeping incapacitated, or otherwise inactive during the blaze. Levels of 20–50% COHb may indicate thermal burns, disease, activity, and/or traumatic factors in the death. A COHb >10% is presumptive evidence of life during the fire and calls for an investigative explanation. Normal CO levels may indicate that the subject was dead prior to the fire. In addition, during a flash fire (such as the explosive combustion of a fireball (e.g., the ignition of an accelerant vapor cloud)), all of the available oxygen in the immediate area is consumed, leaving none to inhale or to react in the fire, forming CO. The only finding at autopsy is a burned body with negligible smoke inhalation discernible (as soot in the airway: **Figure 12**). Extreme caution is urged to consider disease states and other toxins in avoiding conclusions based exclusively on the COHb result.

Both oxyHb and COHb are relatively stable after death. Thus, CO does not bind to blood in the absence of respiration. This can be useful in assessing injuries in a burned body. Areas of premortem trauma, and absent CO inhalation, will be negative for significant COHb. Areas of injury with contusion formed during the course of smoke inhalation will be positive for COHb at varying levels, depending on the temporal relation to ambient CO.

Of special note, CO crosses the placental barrier, where the fetus is more at risk than the mother. Due to delayed maternal COHb dissociation, the gradual build-up in fetal COHb is delayed; however, the final fetal concentration is 10–15% higher. A fetus is much more susceptible to hypoxic damage. Intrauterine fetal death could result in only mild or no maternal symptoms related to CO. Children often succumb at lower percentages of COHb than adults due to increased basal metabolic rate in the former. In infants a 20–25% COHb may prove fatal.

Physical Findings

All the physical findings in CO fatalities are nonspecific. While some features are more common or

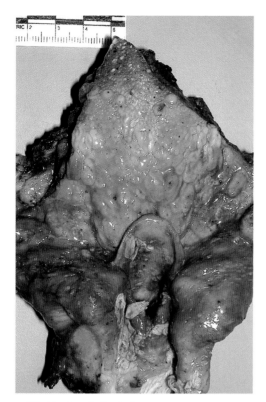

Figure 12 Trachea in flash fire with minimal soot. In a flash fire, all the oxygen in the local area may be consumed in the fireball, leaving no ambient air oxygen for respiration. In such cases, the upper airway may have focal thermal injuries while the remaining airway lacks significant surface soot.

characteristic than others, none is certain or specific. The only definitive observation is an elevated COHb.

Nonspecific Findings

Several features seen in CO-associated deaths are those common to many asphyxial deaths, including: unclotted blood; cerebral edema; acute visceral congestion; and petechial hemorrhages of the skin, serosa, brain, and heart. Also, CO poisoning with concurrent shock or cold temperature delays the onset of rigor mortis.

"Cherry-Red" Livor Mortis and Tissues

The most distinctive and oft-observed finding is neither specific nor uniform. The typical bright-red or "cherry-red" livor mortis (**Figure 1**) may also be seen in numerous other situations. Another electron transport toxin, CN, also produces a similar color but is distinguished by an odor of bitter almonds, detectable by a subset of the population. The red color associated with CN exposure is due to the continued presence of oxyHb after death. In addition, with deaths due to environmental hypoxia and submersion (especially in cold water), the presence of a moist or

damp postmortem environment, early decomposition, and/or fluoroacetate exposure, the livor may appear pink.

With extensive perimortem resuscitative efforts, including extensive artificial respiration, followed very quickly by low-temperature refrigeration, the result may be the same. Focal areas of similar bright-red tissue coloration may be apparent in the vicinity of chest tubes and open chest wounds (from firearms, sharp force, or blunt force), due to a high localized O_2 concentration. Also, contact firearm wounds in any location may have similar tissue coloration due to localized CO resulting from the burning of gunpowder expelling CO gas into the wound.

The typical description of a decedent with CO poisoning is that he/she "looks healthy." That is, the body retains a normal *in vivo* hue due to the continued presence of unutilized oxyHb. As livor may be subtle or unapparent early and/or in darkly pigmented bodies, other easily visualized vascular tissues can be assessed. The typical bright-red color is most readily appreciated in the mucosa of the mouth (**Figure 13**) and the conjunctiva. Fingernails are an excellent site to assess, as the nail beds are usually prominently cyanotic after death. With sufficient COHb, the nail beds appear pink. With a CO of less than 30% and in living patients, the classic "cherry-red" color is absent or barely perceptible, even in lightly pigmented individuals. In clinical cases the bright-red color may be dismissed as mild sunburn or flushing.

Soot in the Airway

An important observation in fire deaths is inhalation of smoke, as confirmed by examination of the upper-airway trachea/bronchi for surface soot (**Figure 14**). If a subject survives in a smoky environment, then soot likely will be present; however, the most reliable indicator of life during a fire is an elevated COHb, not soot deposits within the airway. Soot in the airway is not a reliable predictor of a high or even of an elevated COHb.

Heart

In addition to the brain, petechial hemorrhages can occur in the heart muscle. Microscopic myofiber degeneration may be evident as focal necrosis and/or fatty vacuolation.

Skin Blisters

In some delayed CO-exposure deaths following extended coma, the victim forms distinctive serosanguineous epithelial blisters around the skin of the knees and elbows. This is another nonspecific finding, as

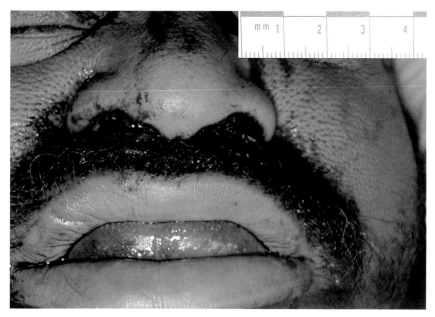

Figure 13 Bright-red tongue in a darkly pigmented individual. In darkly pigmented individuals and in those with low-level carboxy-hemoglobin poisoning, the bright-red livor may not be apparent. In such cases, the mucosae of the mouth and eyes are more easily examined and may allow easier interpretation.

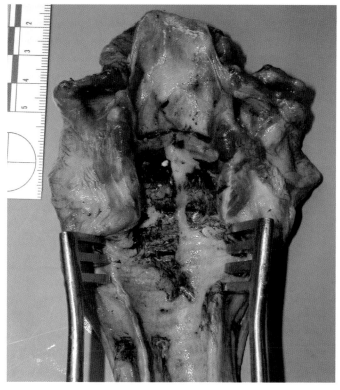

Figure 14 Soot within the trachea. In a typical sooty fire, a film of black smoke lining the tracheal mucosa confirms that the subject was alive during the blaze. In some cases, noncarbon monoxide asphyxiants such as cyanide are produced and kill with low or negative carboxyhemoglobin. In such cases, soot from the fire may be evident in the trachea.

similar damage may be seen following other prolonged comas. In cases where the subject is exposed to heat (e.g., an auto heater), the skin can show similar change.

Neurological

In the brain, CO exhibits pathoclisis, or targeted site-specific pathology. In particular, the extrapyramidal brain and the basal ganglia are most vulnerable to CO. The single most characteristic lesion for significant CO exposure is the delayed development of symmetric necrosis of the bilateral globus pallidus (basal ganglia within brain). The necrotic areas may progress to 1-cm brown cysts.

Lesions of the corpus striatum vasculature and prolonged coma (especially from barbiturate overdose) can cause identical damage. Other brain changes, detectable with specialized radiology techniques, are summarized in **Table 1**. The histologic and gross changes in the brain are nonspecific. The earliest change observed might be gross surface petechial

hemorrhages, which can form within 15 min. At 24 h, pallor is evident. A gradual progression of changes ensues (**Table 2**).

Summary

In CO deaths, the medical examiner serves in a public health role, protecting the decedent's family and the community from similar risks. The critical determinant in detection of hazards is the index of suspicion in the cryptic accidental death. The gross findings may be obvious, as in a significant fire, or unapparent with other CO inhalations. A red blood and tissue color is common with an elevated CO but is neither sensitive nor specific. In investigating the history, a prodrome of afebrile "gastrointestinal disease," especially one affecting multiple persons in the same environment, is a significant clue.

See Also

Asphyxia; **Carbon Monoxide Poisoning:** Clinical Findings, Sequelae In Survivors

Further Reading

Baselt RC (2002) Carbon monoxide. In: *Disposition of Toxic Drugs and Chemicals in Man*, 6th edn., pp. 165–168. Foster City, CA: Biomedical Publications.

Beers MH, Berkow R (1999) Carbon monoxide poisoning, hyperbaric oxygen therapy. In: Beers MH, Berkow R (eds.) *The Merck Manual of Diagnosis and Therapy*, 7th edn., p. 2497. Whitehouse Station, NJ: Merck Research Laboratories.

DiMaio VJM, DiMaio DJ (2001a) Caron monoxide poisoning. In: *Forensic Pathology*, 2nd edn., pp. 389–407. Boca Raton, FL: CRC Press.

DiMaio VJM, DiMaio DJ (2001b) Fire deaths. In: *Forensic Pathology*, 2nd edn., pp. 367–387. Boca Raton, FL: CRC Press.

Fenton JJ (2002) Carbon monoxide, toxic gases. In: *Toxicology, A Case-Oriented Approach*, pp. 257–264. Boca Raton, FL: CRC Press.

Fenton JJ (2003) Carbon monoxide, forensic toxicology. In: James SH, Nordby JJ (eds.) *Forensic Science, An Introduction to Scientific and Investigative Techniques*, pp. 52–53. Boca Raton, FL: CRC Press.

Ferris JAJ (2000) Carbon monoxide, asphyctic deaths. In: Siegel JA, Saukko PJ, Knupfer GC (eds.) *Encyclopedia of Forensic Sciences*, vol. I, pp. 309–310. San Diego, CA: Academic Press.

Finck PA (1977) Exposure to carbon monoxide. In: Tedeschi CG, Eckert WG, Tedeschi LG (eds.) *Forensic Medicine, A Study In Trauma and Environmental Hazards, vol. II. Physical Trauma*, pp. 840–849. Philadelphia, PA: WB Saunders.

Kunsman GW, Levine B (1999) Carbon monoxide/cyanide. In: Levine B (ed.) *Principles of Forensic Toxicology*,

Table 1 Radiology imaging results in carbon monoxide poisoning

Imaging modality	Findings
Computed tomography	Symmetric low-density lesions in cerebral white matter
	Bilateral low-density lesions in globus pallidus
Magnetic resonance imaging	Symmetric hyperintensity in cerebral white matter
	Hypointensity of thalamus
	Bilateral hyperintensity in globus pallidus (T_2-weighted)

Table 2 Progression of microscopic changes in carbon monoxide poisoning with survival interval

Interval to death	Microscopic
34 h	Necrosis in cortex and white matter
	Eosinophilic cytoplasm of the fifth cortical layer and Purkinje cells
2 days	Focal white-matter ring hemorrhages
	Focal hemorrhages without ring
10 days	Globus pallidus axonal swelling
	Subendocardial necrosis papillary muscles
	Lipophages in myofibers
23 days	Transudate
	Neuronal necrosis
	Lipophagocytosis
	Reactive astrocytes
	Glial/capillary proliferation
	Axonal swelling
	Lymphocytic perivascular cuffs
	Decreased/necrotic Purkinje cells
30 days	Ferruginated nerve cells in second cell layer of cortex
40 days	Spongiform foci in globus pallidus
	White-matter lipophagocytosis
$9\frac{1}{2}$ months	Multiple necrotic areas with marked reactive gliosis
	Basal gangliar lipophagocytosis and perivascular lymphocytic cuffs

pp. 330–344. Washington, DC: American Association for Clinical Chemistry Press.

O'Connor JJ (1987) Chemistry and behavior of fire. In: *Practical Fire and Arson Investigation*, pp. 55–79. New York: Elsevier.

Penny DG (2000) *Carbon Monoxide Toxicity*. Boca Raton, FL: CRC Press.

Rutty GN (2003) Carbon monoxide, fire deaths. In: Payne-James J, Busuttil A, Smock W (eds.) *Forensic Medicine, Clinical and Pathological Aspects*, pp. 365–366. London: Greenwich Medical Media.

Rutty GN (2003) Human behavior in fires, fire deaths, Chapter 25. In: Payne-James J, Busuttil A, Smock W (eds.) *Forensic Medicine, Clinical and Pathological Aspects*, pp. 355–356. London: Greenwich Medical Media.

Smith RP (1991) Chemically induced hypoxia, toxic responses of the blood. In: Amdur MO, Doull J, Klaassen CD (eds.) *Casarett and Doul's Toxicology, The Basic Science of Poisons*, 4th edn., pp. 263–268. New York: Pergamon Press.

CHEMICAL CROWD CONTROL AGENTS

K Blaho-Owens, University of Tennessee College of Medicine, Memphis, TN, USA

Introduction

Safe and effective chemical restraint for large numbers of individuals is more challenging than restraining the individual. The goal of restraint of large numbers is to control the crowd by encouraging dispersal into smaller, less threatening numbers. Agents used should have almost immediate effects in low concentrations. The agent should be noxious enough that exposed individuals are quickly aware of their exposure. It should also be noxious enough that those exposed should be motivated to leave the area quickly or follow other commands from law enforcement officers. Injury to the crowd, bystanders, and law enforcement officers from the agent should be minimal. The effects of exposure should be short-lived and readily reversible. The agent should have a short half-life and should be easily degraded, minimizing environmental contamination. There are a few agents that meet these criteria, and their use is discussed in this article.

Chemical restraint methods have been used throughout history. Early forms included drifting clouds of arsenical smoke used by Hunyadi in 1456, arsenical projectiles used in 1672 by the Bishop of Munster's soldiers, and the use of hypnotics by the Danes against King Duncan I in the eleventh century. Even in these early times, weather and wind conditions were appreciated so that the offensive was not to be affected by the agent used. Despite references made to these agents, the best historical account of chemicals used as restraint or for war is from World War I.

Modern chemical crowd control agents were first employed by the French in 1912 when the Paris police used ethylbromoacetate (EBA) against violent offenders. In the early months of World War I, the French launched chlorobenzylidene (CS: tear gas) grenades against the German army. In addition to CS, World War I also introduced chlorine gas and mustard gas, which caused significant morbidity and mortality and resulted in the development of precursors of modern personal protective equipment and riot gear used by law enforcement personnel.

Over the years, chemical restraint agents for control of the individual or crowds have become less lethal and safer than earlier compounds. The three most commonly used agents are chlorobenzylidene (CS), oleum capsicum (OC), and chloracetothenon (CN). Modern incendiary devices and other dispersal methods have made these compounds useful for restraint of the individual violent offender and for mass dispersal for crowd control. There are, however, concerns about the use of these agents by law enforcement officers. These concerns include their possible toxicity to the offender, potential for exposure to the person administering the agent, the potential for any ancillary exposure to healthcare providers or to bystanders, the expansion of their use to nonviolent offenders such as peaceful protesters, and concern about the long-term effects from repeated exposure and from occupational exposure. Some of these issues become more complicated as chemical control agents are increasingly popular with civilians as readily available, often legal, nonlethal, self-defense weapons.

There have been several well-publicized incidents that question the appropriateness of the use of chemical crowd control agents. In one reported incident in the USA, law enforcement officers applied OC liquid via a cotton-tipped applicator directly to the periorbital area of protesters who were illegally trespassing.

The protesters were linked together and refused to disperse. The use of OC against these nonviolent offenders when other methods of control failed generated negative publicity and resulted in legal action against the law enforcement officials. Law enforcement officers opted for this type of application so that exposure to others would be limited rather than to disperse an aerosol in the enclosed space occupied by the protestors.

When used appropriately, crowd control agents have a good safety margin and generally do no permanent harm. In addition to the debate over the agents themselves, there has been some concern over the safety of the delivery vehicles, particularly methylisobutyl ketone (MIBK). While chronic exposure to MIBK has been associated with neurological and respiratory effects, there are no data to support the theory that acute exposure to the low concentrations that occur with CS spray poses these same problems. Flammable compounds used as early vehicles have largely been replaced by water-soluble, less toxic vehicles. Despite all of the controversy surrounding chemical control agents, they offer a less hazardous method of restraint than other potentially lethal alternatives such as firearms. Because some agents can be used from a distance, they provide a method of control for the law enforcement officer without direct contact with a potentially violent individual.

Clinical Features and Treatment

As mentioned above, the three main chemical restraint compounds are OC, CN, and CS. These agents are available in varying concentrations, with several vehicles, in aerosols or foams, and in particulate form with dispersal devices. Some of these are listed in **Table 1**.

Essentially a means of nonlethal chemical warfare, chemical crowd control products are used as defensive agents to incapacitate individuals temporarily, or disperse groups without requiring means that are more forceful. The clinical effects are short-lived once exposure has ended. These agents share common effects, including lacrimation, ocular irritation

and pain, dermal irritation, blepharospasm, conjunctivitis, transient impairment of vision, and mild to moderate respiratory distress. Some corneal defects after exposure have been noted, but whether this is a direct tissue effect of the agent or a result of rubbing the ocular surface is unknown. Contact dermatitis and periocular edema can also result. There have also been reports of allergic reactions to either the compounds themselves or the vehicles used for dispersal. Other more severe effects such as pulmonary edema have been documented when concentrations are several hundredfold above what produces intolerable symptoms or with trauma associated with the explosive device used to deliver the chemical agent.

All of these clinical effects produced by chemical crowd control agents render the recipient temporarily unable to continue violent action or resist arrest. Since they all share a high safety ratio, are effective at low concentrations, and can be used without direct forceful contact by the law enforcement officer, they are ideal agents either for control of the individual offender or for riot control. Because of their relative safety, these agents are generally excluded from international treaty provisions that address chemical weapons. The USA, UK, Ireland, France, China, Korea, Israel, and Russia are just some examples of countries that utilize these compounds as crowd control agents. The legal availability to law enforcement officers and the general public differs between countries; however, most can be easily obtained through international markets or ordered on the internet.

Chemical restraint compounds differ from most agents because some, such as CS, are solid particles with low vapor pressures. They are usually dispersed as fine particles or in a solution. For large crowds, "bombs" have been developed that can be dropped from aerial positions, producing wide dispersal of the compound. They are also formulated in grenades or canisters that can be propelled by either throwing or with a projectile device. The most common method of dispersal is by individual spray cans that deliver a stream, spray, or foam containing the agent. These individual dispersal units were designed to render

Table 1 Examples of chemical restraint products available

Brand name	Ingredients	Delivery system
Cap-Stun	5% oleoresin capsicum	Spray
Alan's Pepper Spray	10% oleo capsicum pepper	Spray
Pepper Foam	10% oleo capsicum	Foam spray
Pepper Gard, Triple Action Spray	10% oleo capsicum plus 10% chlorobenzylidene	Spray
Mark III	5% oleo capsicum plus 5% chlorobenzylidene	Spray

immediate incapacitation to an offender without the use of more forceful methods. Canisters containing a lower concentration of the active ingredient have been marketed to civilians for personal protection. Since there is no formal training for civilians on the use of these devices, there is a significant risk for exposure to the users as well as bystanders.

There are different spray patterns available for practicality of use. A full cone spray pattern is usually a formulation of microscopic droplets that allows a wide dispersion pattern of delivery of the agent. This wide dispersion makes it easy for agent delivery from a distance of 1–3 m (3–8 ft). Full cone sprays are more likely to be affected by wind conditions and generally do not have as many bursts per canister as other delivery systems.

A ballistic stream spray pattern is a concentrated stream that can be used effectively from distances as short as 1 m (3 ft) to as far as 4 m (12 ft). This spray pattern, while having a fairly long range of effectiveness, allows for accuracy in selecting the target while minimizing the risk of contaminating other subjects.

A foam formulation has a greater skin or surface adhesion than other formulations and also reduces cross-contamination. Its effective range is 1–2 m (3–5 ft). A foam product is appropriate for climate-controlled environments and enclosed spaces where contamination of bystanders is likely. An additional benefit of the foam formulation is that it is easy to see the application, especially in low-light conditions.

A fog delivery system uses a full cone spray but is adapted to disperse the chemical agent over a large area, typically an outdoor area. It can contain up to 0.454 kg (1 lb) of agent, and has a range of 2–5 m (6–15 ft). It is not indicated for use in confined spaces or where there are large numbers of bystanders.

Oleum Capsicum

OC or pepper spray (PS) selectively stimulates nociceptors in exposed mucous membranes, releasing substance P, bradykinin, histamine, and prostaglandins. The physiologic effects of these mediators result in vasodilation, increased vascular permeability, pain, and altered neurotrophic chemotaxis. Other common symptoms are listed in **Table 2**. The effects of OC are generally short-lived. The most common effects are a burning sensation and erythema at the site of contact. The effects of exposure can abate without treatment or anecdotally can be shortened by the direct application of baby shampoo followed by irrigation with water. Baby shampoo directly into the ocular area

Table 2 Common clinical findings with exposure to crowd control agents

Finding	Chlorobenzylidene	Chloracetothenon	Oleum capsicum
Ocular			
Lacrimation	✓	✓	✓
Blepharospasm	✓	✓	
Pain and/or burning	✓	✓	✓
Conjunctival injection	✓	✓	✓
Conjunctival edema	✓	✓	
Photophobia	✓	✓	
Corneal abrasion	✓	✓	✓
Impaired vision	✓	✓	✓
Upper airway			
Pain and/or burning	✓	✓	
Shortness of breath	✓	✓	✓
Increased secretion	✓	✓	
Congestion	✓		
Coughing	✓	✓	✓
Throat irritation	✓	✓	✓
Wheezing	✓	✓	✓
Irregular respiration[a]	✓	✓	
Dermal			
Pain	✓	✓	✓
Contact dermatitis		✓	✓
Blistering	✓	✓	✓
Miscellaneous			
Nausea/vomiting	✓		
Bad taste	✓		
Headache	✓		
Increased blood pressure	✓*		

[a]Initial response thought to be associated with pain.

and to other exposed sites is well tolerated. Thorough rinsing with copious amounts of water helps with decontamination. Reapplication of the shampoo product with repetitive rinsing may be needed.

Capsicum in its pure form is a crystalline material. The oleoresin extract of capsicum contains over 100 volatile compounds that act in a similar manner to capsicum. Because of the variability in the individual components of OC, and variation in quality control, products containing this extract have differences in efficacy. Some products describe the capsaicin amount by percentage in the product while others describe the amount of capsaicin in Scoville heat units (SHU). OC described by percentage may differ from preparation to preparation, since different peppers produce different pungencies or a burning sensation. The most consistent method of characterizing OC preparations is by the SHU, described by the American Spice Trade Association analytical methods. Most are formulated in a propylene vehicle to enhance adherence to the skin surface. PS is the most common spray marketed to civilians for nonlethal, noncontact self-defense. For law enforcement it can be purchased in a variety of sprays or foams, in various concentrations or combined with other crowd control agents such as CS (**Figure 1**).

Water-based products are used to reduce the use of more flammable solvents. Water-based agents usually have a lower SHU, and are easier to decontaminate.

Oil-based products are ideal for formulating into fog dispersal units, tend to have a higher SHU, and are more difficult to decontaminate.

The most common complaint after PS exposure is irritation and pain at the site of exposure. The symptoms are transient, and very few require medical treatment. The most significant adverse effects that have occurred in exposure from law enforcement episodes are corneal abrasions, and these can be treated with topical anesthetics and topical antibiotics. There are no clinical data to support the concept that PS exacerbates pulmonary disease or that patients with reactive airway disease are more sensitive to the effects.

The few reports of severe reactions to PS are exceptions rather than the rule. In general, these cases involve exposure in the very young, or in those with other risk factors for poor outcome. Any compound, when used improperly, can cause severe symptoms. Thus far, severe adverse events after PS exposure have been rare.

Of concern were reports of violent prisoners who died after being sprayed with PS or other chemical restraints and then were physically restrained. It was assumed that the police used excessive force and that the prisoners died from "positional asphyxia" from the restraints or that the chemical agent played a role in their deaths. There is no evidence that PS or other agents cause any type of respiratory effects sufficient to cause death. A review of the circumstances

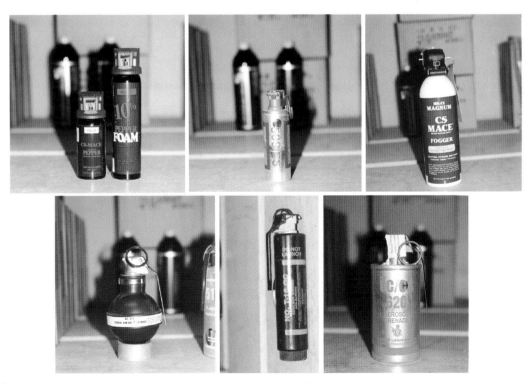

Figure 1 Examples of individual spray containers containing crowd control agents.

surrounding the deaths of the prisoners who died exhibited characteristics consistent with excited delirium from substance abuse. Other contributing factors, such as obesity, hyperthermia, extreme violence, and measurable cocaine on postmortem analysis indicate other causes of death rather than exposure to a chemical restraint. The lesson from these types of in-custody deaths should be that all violent prisoners, whether or not a chemical agent for restraint has been used, might warrant close monitoring and perhaps evaluation by healthcare professionals. A small population of acutely intoxicated individuals is at risk of sudden death, independent of their treatment. Other causes of death or contributing factors should be investigated in cases such as these.

Treatment of exposure to PS is based on severity of symptoms. The first order of treatment should always be the removal of contaminated clothing. Copious irrigation of affected areas will attenuate the burning sensation. However, one must use caution not to contaminate other sites with the irrigant; for example, washing PS from the hair into the eyes or oral pharyngeal mucosa. As mentioned previously, baby shampoo can help to remove PS from skin and eyes and shorten the duration of its effects. A slit-lamp exam of the anterior chamber is warranted to rule out corneal abrasion in patients who remain symptomatic. If present, the abrasion should be treated appropriately with topical antibiotics, cycloplegics, analgesics, and follow-up.

Dermatitis associated with PS can be managed with topical corticosteroids, systemic antihistamines, and analgesics but these cases are relatively rare. An example of rather severe PS dermatitis and ocular swelling is shown in **Figure 2**. This particular patient was sprayed during arrest by police officers and brought to an emergency department for evaluation. He was treated with irrigation, systemic antihistamines, and steroids with resolution of his symptoms within 4 days.

Intense ocular and facial burning prevented opening of the eyes for a short period of time. Decontamination after several minutes of exposure was

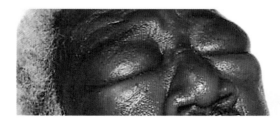

Figure 2 Effects of full-face spray of 10% chlorobenzylidene/10% pepper spray before and after decontamination with baby shampoo.

performed using baby shampoo and rinsing with water. Effects abated about 15 min after using this method of decontamination.

Chlorobenzylidene Malononitrile and Chloracetophenone

CS or tear gas is frequently used by the military and law enforcement officers as a method of controlling both individuals and crowds. The military also uses it during exercises to train personnel in the use of protective equipment. CN, known by its proprietary name Mace, is the oldest of the crowd control agents. CS was developed in the 1950s, and it has largely replaced CN.

CS and CN are both lacrimating agents. CS is usually mixed with a pyrotechnic compound for dispersal in grenades or canisters as a fine particulate that forms the characteristic smoke; CN is usually prepared for aerosol dispersal by individual canisters. Both agents are available in individual containers or large bombs, or they can be dispersed through a handheld aerosolizer. They are formulated with a variety of solvents such as alcohol, ether, carbon sulfide, and methylchloroform or can be dispersed as solid particles. In the USA, a combination of CS (10%) and PS (10%) is used by some law enforcement officers for chemical control.

CS and CN are highly soluble in a variety of agents. When contact with mucous membranes is made, the symptoms described in **Table 2** occur. Even though there is a perception of shortness of breath, pulmonary function tests performed shortly after exposure to either agent have shown minimal alterations. Its mechanism of irritation is not fully understood. The effects of CS are thought to be related to the formation of highly irritating chlorine atoms and hydrochloric acid when it comes in contact with water from mucous membranes. CS and CN have also been described as alkylating agents, targeting sulfhydryl groups. In addition, there is some controversy surrounding the production of cyanide molecules at the tissue level with exposure to high concentrations of CS. Regardless, like OC, the effects of CS and CN are usually manifested without permanent tissue injury. Exposure is most often limited as individuals flee the scene. Exposure can be significant if the affected person is forced into a confined space for extended periods of time.

Most of the dispersal methods achieve concentrations far below what is considered to be lethal. Concentrations achieved in close proximity to grenades or other delivery devices or for those who cannot or will not leave the exposure area may be significantly greater. Based on animal studies it is generally thought that a concentration of $25\,000-150\,000\,\mathrm{mg\,m^{-3}\,min^{-1}}$

or $200\,\mathrm{mg\,kg^{-1}}$ body mass represents the median lethal dose for CS. A grenade can generate a concentration of $2000\text{--}5000\,\mathrm{mg\,m^{-3}}$ at the center, with concentrations becoming significantly less within a few meters from the center of the explosion.

Like OC, the treatment of CS exposure is based largely on the severity of clinical findings. The majority of patients will fully recover within minutes of removal of the agent and will not require medical attention. The most common lasting complaints are facial and ocular irritation. In contrast to other forms of chemical exposure, irrigating the affected area will only intensify and prolong the effects of CS gas or particles. For patients who require medical evaluation, the first order of treatment should always be removal of contaminated clothing with special attention to eliminating secondary exposure by using protective equipment and not placing a contaminated patient in a confined space. Clothing should be removed outside and placed inside a plastic bag, then bagged again. Blowing dry air directly on to the eye assists in vaporizing the dissolved CS gas. Some clinicians have recommended copious ocular irrigation with sterile saline, although this has been thought in some cases to cause an initial acute increase in ocular irritation. A careful slit-lamp exam of the anterior segment of the eye, including evaluation under the lids, should be done for persistent ocular irritation. If particles have become embedded in the cornea or under the lids, they should be removed. If corneal abrasions are present, a few days of topical broad-spectrum antibiotics, cycloplegics, and appropriate analgesics in addition to close follow-up should be prescribed.

Dermal irritation in the form of burning and blistering can be treated with irrigation, preferably with an alkaline solution other than sodium hypochlorite or common household bleach. Erythema can be common in freshly abraded skin, but resolves 45–60 min after exposure. Contact dermatitis can be effectively treated with topical corticosteroids and/or antihistamines.

Typically, dermatitis associated with CS exposure resolves within a few days.

Home remedies such as application of cooking oils are contraindicated and pose an increased risk for irritation and infection. Sodium hypochlorite solutions will exacerbate any dermal irritation and should not be used. Plain soap and water is effective but, in most cases, removal of clothing in a well-ventilated area is all that is needed.

There are conflicting reports about the long-term effects of CS exposure. With an exposure to high concentrations, usually for prolonged periods in a confined space, pulmonary edema, pneumonitis, heart failure, hepatocellular damage, and death have been reported. There are no data to support any claims of teratogenicity. These agents do not appear to exacerbate chronic diseases such as seizure disorders, respiratory disease, or psychiatric illnesses.

The possibility of secondary exposure to healthcare and law enforcement providers exists with the use of chemical crowd control agents. Although published reports are few, effects can be minimized with common-sense practices such as decontamination before the patient is placed in a confined area such as a police car, ambulance, or a confined room in the emergency department. The use of protective personal equipment such as gloves, respiratory and eye protection when appropriate, and careful washing of exposed areas avoids cross-contamination.

The most important considerations in utilizing chemical crowd control agents is that they be used judiciously, in the correct manner, and in place of more forceful means of controlling violent or potentially violent prisoners or crowds. Law enforcement officers should be trained regularly and educated on the appropriate use of agents, their common clinical effects, and the appropriateness of seeking medical care. Medical care should never be withheld from those who request it or those prisoners who have lingering effects. Treatment of exposure is summarized in **Table 3**. To limit injury or potential

Table 3 Options for treatment for exposure to chemical crowd control agents

Treatment	Pepper spray	Chlorobenzylidene	Chloracetothenon
Removal of contaminated clothing	✓	✓	✓
Ocular irrigation	✓		✓
Dermal irrigation	✓	✓	✓
Alkaline-solution irrigation of skin		✓	✓
Soap and water decontamination	✓	✓	✓
Topical steroids for dermatitis	✓	✓	✓
Systemic antihistamines for dermatitis	✓	✓	✓
Systemic steroids for dermatitis	✓	✓	✓
Topical antibiotics for corneal abrasion	✓	✓	✓
Cycloplegics	✓	✓	✓
Analgesics for pain	✓	✓	✓

liability many police forces regulate the use of chemical crowd control agents by establishing policies to guide their use. One example is the "ladder of force." This continuum describes the sequential increase in force and is used to help guide the use of an appropriate method of restraint. Words are used first, followed by more defensive actions such as chemical agents, batons, and finally firearms. It is important to note that some individuals may require more than one exposure to the agent before the optimum effect is achieved or if the agent has been exposed to extreme environmental conditions or has not been replaced in a timely manner. Use of these agents should be monitored and formal reports filed when they are used. Like all equipment, chemical agents should be stored appropriately and replaced according to the manufacturer's guidelines. These agents afford control of violent offenders with much less risk to life and limb than do firearms, explosives, and battering.

See Also

Injuries and Deaths During Police Operations: Shootings During Police Stops and Arrests; **Restraint Techniques, Injuries and Death**

Further Reading

Ballantyne B (1977) Riot control agents: biomedical and health aspects of the use of chemicals in civilian disturbances. *Medical Annual* pp. 7–14.

Karch SB, Stephens BG (1999) Drug abusers who die in custody. *Journal of the Royal Society of Medicine* 92: 110–113.

Stark M (2000) *A Physician's Guide to Clinical Forensic Medicine.* Totowa, NJ: Humana Press.

US Department of Justice (2002) Police Use of Force, Collection of National Data. www.usdoj.gov.GBCPS/pubs/pdexcess.htm

Weaver W, Jett MB (2004) *Oleoresin Capsicum Training and Use.* Quantico, VA: FBI Academy Firearms Training Unit. www.ojp.usdoj.gov/nih/pubs-sum/205293.htm/

CHILDREN

Contents

Stages of Development and Growth

H Hayden-Wade and L K Leslie, Children's Hospital of San Diego, San Diego, CA, USA

Introduction

This section provides a brief overview of children's (defined age 0–18 years) growth and stages of development. In particular, this section will elucidate general patterns of growth (including weight, height, head circumference, brain growth, and puberty) and the acquisition of developmental milestones from childhood through adolescence.

A variety of important forensic issues exist in relation to child growth and development and are discussed in more detail in other selections in this volume, including autopsy.

Growth

Physical Growth

Weight In general, weight increases significantly during the first year and then slows through adolescence. Major weight-related milestones may be tracked from birth through adolescence as follows.

After an initial period of weight loss during the immediate postnatal period, birth weight is regained between the 10th and 14th postnatal day. Between the ages of 2 weeks and 6 months, the average weight gain equals 20 g (0.71 oz) per day and decreases between 6 and 12 months to 15 g (0.53 oz) per day. Across the second year, weight gain slows considerably, with the average monthly weight gain at 25 kg (8.82 oz or 0.55 lb). A quick rule of thumb for the first 2 years of life is that birth weight doubles by 4 months, triples at 12 months, and quadruples at 24 months. After age 2, average weight gain until adolescence is 2.3 kg (5 lb) annually.

Length/height Rough guidelines suggest that birth length is doubled by 4 years of age and tripled by 13 years of age. By the end of the first year, birth length increases by 50%. The average height gain across year 2 is 12 cm (5 in.). From age 2 to the beginning of adolescence, the average child will grow 5 cm (2 in.) per year. Adolescence ushers in a second growth spurt with respect to length/height. In adolescence, a typical (average) maximum growth spurt for a male is 10.16 cm (4 in.), whereas, for female adolescents, their growth spurt averages 7.52 cm (3 in.) during its peak. By the end of the adolescent period, both males and females reach 99% of their adult height.

Head circumference Clinically, head circumference is routinely measured during the first 2 years of life. During this time, the brain is growing immensely and the open sutures between the bones of the skull are closing. Between birth and 2 months, the average head growth in 1 week is 0.50 cm (0.20 in.), and then slows to 0.25 cm (0.10 in.) between 2 and 6 months. The average total head circumference growth from birth to 3 months is equal to 5 cm (1.97 in.), and 4 cm (1.57 in.) average from 3 to 6 months. This trend continues to decelerate across the first year; between 6 and 9 months, head circumference increases 2 cm (0.79 in.) and between 9 and 12 months, head circumference increases only 1 cm (0.39 in.), approximately.

During the second year, a child's head growth slows (i.e., 2.5 cm or 1 in., for the entire year), although attainment of 90% of adult head size occurs by the end of that year.

Brain growth The brain, at birth, is closest to its adult size than any other organ – in fact, it is considered close to 80% of its adult weight. By age 6, a child's brain is closer to 90% of its adult weight. However, while the brain's weight does not change substantially, significant formation of brain neurons

and remodeling of neuronal paths is occurring during childhood and adolescence.

The brain's development is the most rapid during the initial 2 years of life. Prenatally, 250 000 million neurons are formed per minute. Ultimately, between 100 and 200 billion neurons (nerve cells) make up the brain, and are responsible for storing and transmitting information as well as providing neurological interconnection with other neurons. Remodeling is also occurring. Neuronal paths are being remodeled consistently through dendritic branching (i.e., dendrites, or the thread-like extensions of the cytoplasm of a neuron, branch into tree-like processes, composing most of the receptive surface of a neuron) and myelinization (i.e., the process within which a lipid-rich substance coils to form a protective sheath surrounding the axon of nerve fibers to provide efficient transmission of neuronal messages across nerve fibers).

An important developmental aspect of the brain to consider in working with children involves the specific order in which the various areas of the cortex develop. The cerebral cortex, which surrounds the brain and comprises 85% of the brain's overall weight, provides the intellectual capacity that differentiates human beings from our animal counterparts. The order of development of certain areas of control within the cerebral cortex parallels the sequence of acquisition of different developmental milestones and capacities as the child matures. With respect to motoric skills, cortex development dictates a cephalocaudal progression of development, which is marked by truncal coordination at the outset, followed by mastery of the extremities. In the domain of emotional/behavioral/adaptive skills, cortex development continues to mature through adulthood; for example, the last section of the cortex to develop is the frontal lobe (responsible for thought and consciousness).

Changes associated with puberty Adolescents progress through a similar sequence of pubertal changes, although it should be noted that each adolescent varies in the timing and nature of pubertal change.

For adolescent females, the vagina and ovaries become larger, accompanied by cellular and chemical changes, followed by menstruation and ovulation. For males, the testicles enlarge, followed by sperm production. Both females and males develop pubic and underarm hair.

One can judge adolescent physical or reproductive maturity by examining these secondary sex characteristics, which mature in sequential stages, to determine the sex maturity rating (SMR). Clinicians measure

SMR on a five-point scale, with one indicating pre-pubertal stage and five indicating adult status. For adolescent females, the pattern and characteristics of pubic hair, as well as the form and contour of the breasts, help establish the SMR. Around SMR level 4 for breasts and SMR level 3 for pubic hair, adolescent girls experience menarche (first menstrual cycle). In boys, genital changes as well as the quantity and pattern of pubic hair determine SMR. See **Tables 1** and **2** for classification ratings of sexual maturity for males and females, respectively.

Abnormalities of Growth

It is important to keep in mind that a number of medical conditions can impact one or more of these arenas of growth. In addition, several environmental factors can impact growth across population samples. For example, there has been an obesity epidemic among children living in industrialized nations; the weight trajectory information provided by the Centers for Disease Control and Prevention (CDC) only covers average, nonobese weight gain across childhood. At the other end of the spectrum lies the malnourished child, who may exhibit weight gain velocity significantly below that expected for chronological age. In the malnourished child, head circumference and height are relatively spared, especially if the malnourishment is addressed expeditiously.

Measurement of Growth

Because abnormalities of growth may be the first presenting sign of a medical condition or environmental stressor, medical professionals, including forensic scientists, plot an individual child's height, weight, and head circumference on cross-sectional growth charts in order to gather statistical definitions of normality by comparing that child to others of similar age and same sex. In addition, clinicians plot growth velocity in order to determine that a child is growing at an appropriate rate with respect to weight, height, and head circumference.

The CDC growth charts were revised in May 2000 to incorporate more diverse ethnic samples as well as new body mass index (BMI) information for all children 2–20 years of age. These growth charts were originally developed by the US National Center for Health Statistics (NCHS) in 1977. (See **Figure 1** for four of the most recent (2001) standardized growth charts taken from the CDC website (http://www.cdc.gov/growthcharts). Consult the website for additional charts for both boys and girls, including weight-for-stature percentiles, head circumference-for-age, and weight-for-length percentiles for birth to 36 months, and body mass index-for-age percentiles for 2–20 years.)

Development

First quantified by Arnold Gesell in 1925, child development is a dynamic, orderly, and cumulative process by which a child undergoes a series of qualitative changes in skill levels at predictable time intervals called developmental milestones. There are four generally recognized domains of development for a child: (1) motor (both gross and fine); (2) language; (3) cognition; and (4) social/behavioral/adaptive skills. Gross motor skills involve large muscle groups and are essential for skills like running, jumping, rolling, and balancing on one foot, whereas fine motor skills refer to a child's ability to manipulate items with the hands and fingers, such as holding a spoon or turning the pages of a book. Language development reflects a child's ability both to understand and express language. Cognitive skills refer to a child's ability to learn new material and solve problems. Social/emotional skills include abilities such as a child's capacity to relate to and interact with others, to self-soothe, and to self-control.

Table 1 Classification of sex maturity ratings in boys

Rating	Pubic hair	Penis	Testes
1	None	Preadolescent	Preadolescent
2	Scanty, long, slightly pigmented	Slightly enlarged	Enlarged scrotum, pink, less smooth
3	Darker, curls, small amount	Longer	Larger
4	Adult type but less; curly, coarse	Larger, breadth increases	Larger, scrotum is darker
5	Adult pattern; spreads to inner thighs	Adult	Adult

Table 2 Classification of sex maturity ratings in girls

Rating	Pubic hair	Breasts
1	Preadolescent	Preadolescent
2	Scanty, slightly pigmented, straight, on inner part of labia	Breast elevated as small mound
3	Darker, starts to curl, increased amount	Breast and areola enlarged, no separation
4	Coarse, curly, more but less than adult	Areola and future nipple form a secondary mound
5	Adult feminine triangle; spreads to inner surface of thighs	Mature; nipple projects, and areola part of general breast shape

Birth to 36 months: Boys Length-for-age and Weight-for-age percentiles

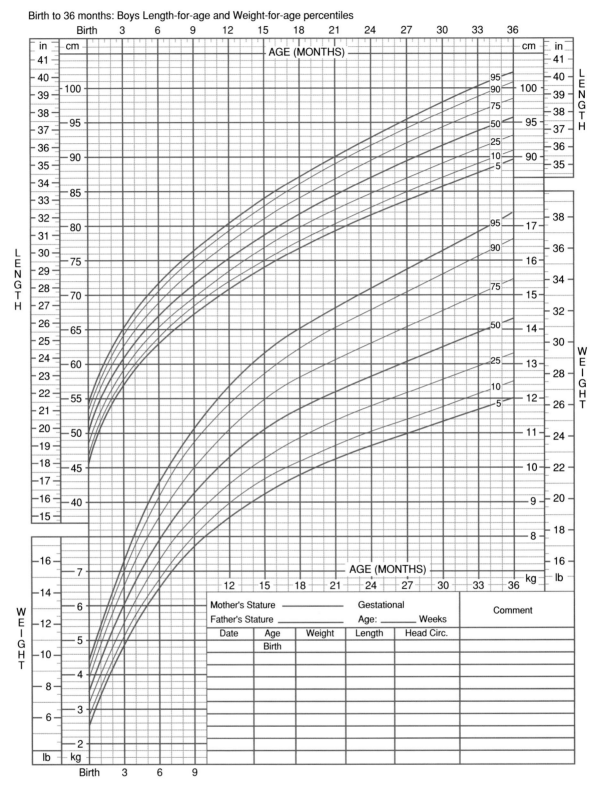

Figure 1A   (continued)

Children who do not reach these developmental milestones at the predicted time intervals may have developmental delay and/or mental health problems.

Motor Development

Motor development encompasses gross motor (involving the large muscle groups) and fine motor (involving the smaller muscle groups) aspects.

Birth to 36 months: Girls Length-for-age and Weight-for-age percentiles

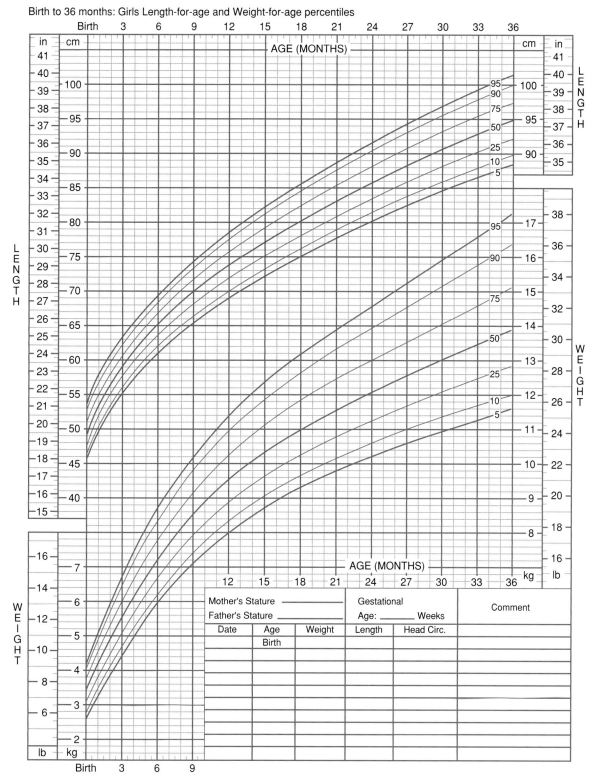

Figure 1B   (continued)

Reflexes   Initially, all infants display a series of primitive reflexes, which are lost as infants develop volitional movement, generalized mass activity, and ultimately specific responses. At birth, there are over 70 reflexes exhibited by infants and tested, most of which are extinguished between 2 and 12 months of age. **Table 3** provides a detailed overview of 11 of these major infant reflexes.

2 to 20 year: Boys Stature-for-age and Weight-for-age percentiles

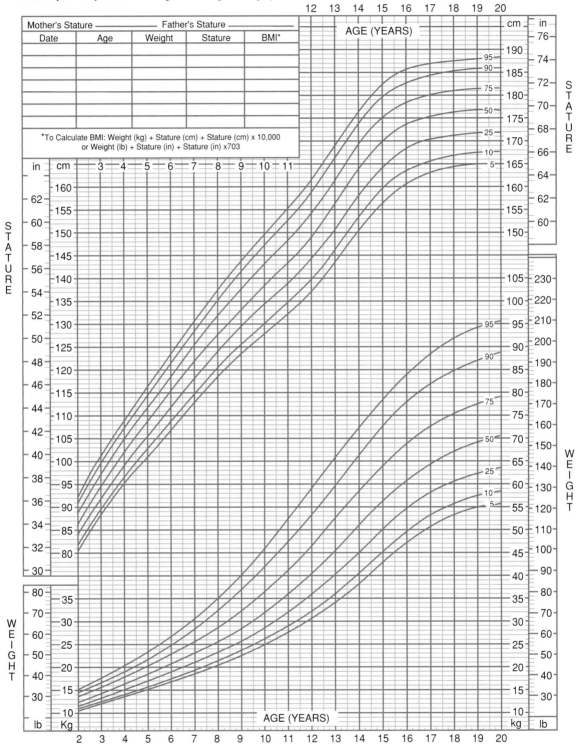

Figure 1C   (continued)

Gross motor development   All children pass through similar sequences of motor development, which progress along with the maturation of the central nervous system in a cephalocaudal (trunk-to-extremity ordered progression of development and control) as well as proximal-to-distal direction. Again, first cephalocaudal progression is marked by truncal coordination, followed by the child's mastery of

2 to 20 year: Girls Stature-for-age and Weight-for-age percentiles

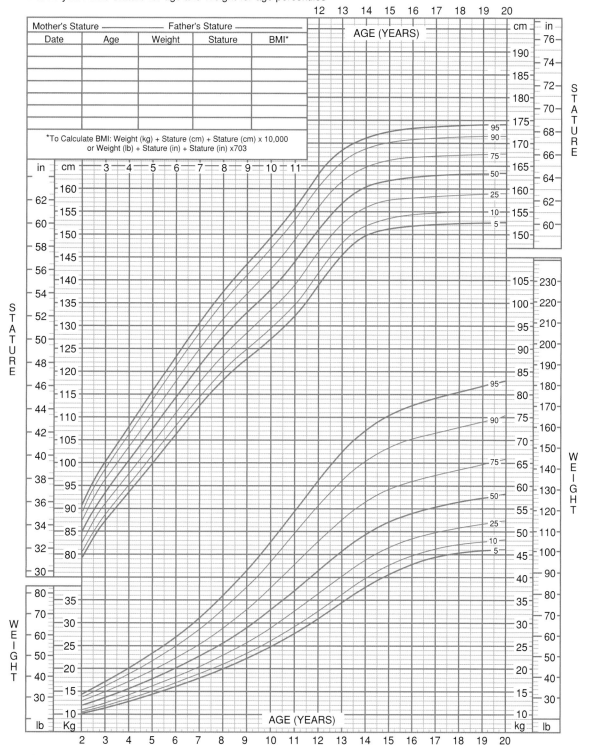

Figure 1D   Source: Center for Disease Control, National Center for Health Statistics.

motor action in the extremities. The proximal-to-distal progression is seen in the coordination of upper extremities first, followed by lower extremities.

In general, the first year of life focuses on cephalo-caudal and proximal–distal development. Growth and refinement of motor skills occur from ages 2 to 4 years. By year 1, the child is able to pull to a stand

Table 3 Newborn reflexes

Reflex	Stimulation	Response	Age of disappearance	Function
Rooting	Stroke cheek near corner of mouth	Head turns toward source of stimulation	3 weeks (becomes voluntary head-turning at this time)	Helps infant find the nipple
Sucking	Place finger in infant's mouth	Infant sucks finger rhythmically	Permanent	Permits feeding
Swimming	Place infant face-down in pool of water	Baby paddles and kicks in swimming motion	4–6 months	Helps infant survive if dropped into body of water
Eye blink	Shine bright light at eyes or clap hand near head	Infant quickly closes eyelids	Permanent	Protects infant from strong stimulation
Withdrawal	Prick sole of foot with pin	Foot withdraws, with flexion of knee and hip	Weakens after 10 days	Protects infant from unpleasant tactile stimulation
Babinski	Stroke sole of foot from toe toward heel	Toes fan out and curl as foot twists in	8–12 months	Unknown
Moro	Hold infant horizontally on back and let head drop slightly, or produce a sudden loud sound against surface supporting infant	Infant makes an "embracing" motion by arching back, extending legs, throwing arms outward, and then bringing them in toward body	6 months	In human evolutionary past, may have helped infant cling to mother
Palmar grasp	Place finger in infant's hand and press against palm	Spontaneous grasp of adult's finger	3–4 months	Prepares infant for voluntary grasping
Tonic neck	While baby lies on back, turn head to one side	Infant assumes a "fencing position"; one arm is extended in front of eyes on side to which head is turned, other arm is flexed	4 months	May prepare infant for voluntary reaching
Body righting	Rotate shoulder or hips	Rest of body turns in same direction	12 months	Supports postural control
Stepping	Hold infant under arms and permit bare feet to touch a flat surface	Infant lifts one foot after another in stepping response	2 months	Prepares infant for voluntary walking

From Berk, Laura E. Child Development, 4/e © 1997. Published by Allyn and Bacon, Boston, MA. Copyright © 1997 by Pearson Education. Reprinted by permission of the publisher.

and begin to take steps. Eventually, the toddler progresses from a wide-based gait to a well-coordinated, sequenced gait that can accomplish more complicated, sequential motor activities such as stair-climbing (by age 2) and skipping (by age 5). School-age children and, later, adolescents, continue to master more complicated sequential motor activities necessary for activities such as sports and driving, for example. **Table 4** lists developmental milestones for the first 6 years of life only, given that this timeframe involves the most rapid change; beyond 6, change occurs across a less rapid trajectory.

Fine motor development   The timing or acquisition of fine motor developmental milestones involves less variability than gross motor development. See **Table 4** for further details.

Speech/Language Development

Table 4 provides an overview of language development from birth to age 6. Although infants do not often have formal word use until age 12 months, the first 12 months are critical to development in terms of understanding that words are concepts for objects. Ultimately, children will comprehend the meanings of various words as they continue to develop. It is not uncommon for a child to display slow mastery or use of new words until 18 months, followed by a burst of language production and comprehension at the end of the second year. Language skills continue to be acquired, including use of prepositions, adverbs, and adjectives (age 3) as well as rules of grammar (age 3–6 years). Language development from age 7 through adolescence focuses primarily upon the social pragmatics of the use of language.

Children display wider variability in speech and language development than any other area due to the variety of individual and environmental factors (e.g., the verbal environment of the child's home or child care facility). For example, children born to large families may exhibit delays in language production given the lowered frequency of attention and opportunities for verbal interaction when compared to single-child families. Bilingual children may also experience temporary (i.e., ameliorates by age 2–3 years) delays in language acquisition, often combining the two languages into a mutant language of their own. Furthermore, poverty can deleteriously affect infants' language development. Although being from a low-income home does not necessarily automatically yield language delay, it is a high-risk factor.

Cognitive Development

Piaget   A plethora of theoretical perspectives regarding childhood development exists; the most famous of which is that of Swiss philosopher Jean Piaget. According to Piaget, children take an active role in working within their environment to incorporate experiences (which he referred to as the act of assimilation) into their personal schema (the way they interpret their world). As children learn and grow, they continually modify their schema when confronted with new events. Piaget labeled the child's modification of schema as accommodation. A child's ability to modify schema depends upon their current particular stage of development.

Piaget's stages include four levels. The first stage is the sensorimotor stage, which occurs between the ages of 0 and 2 years. During this stage, learning is facilitated by sensory means. For example, a baby within this age range prefers to hold and even explore a new object with his/her mouth in order to learn about it fully through sensory stimulation. By the end of the sensorimotor stage, children should master object permanence (i.e., understand that when the mother puts a block out of view behind her back, it is still present, just not visible) and symbolic (representational) thought. The latter may be seen in fantasy play, such as dress-up games.

The preoperational stage (ages 2–6) involves mental processes that are governed by the child's own subjective perceptions. Furthermore, the child does not make a distinction between internal and external reality. By the end of the preoperational stage, a child displays animism (e.g., believing the clouds and flowers smiled at her), egocentrism (i.e., understanding the world from his point of view, with less, if any, empathy for others), idiosyncratic and transductive reasoning (i.e., linking two usually unrelated events such as any woman wearing white and receiving a shot).

Once a child attains the concrete operational stage between ages 6 and 11 (or school age), s/he is able to classify and sort objects using stable concepts such as volume, mass, and number. It is during the concrete operational stage that children learn to conserve, or understand, for example, that a given volume of water remains the same when poured from a short, wide container as when poured from a tall, thin container. This is something that, Piaget proposed, children in the preoperational stage cannot do.

Lastly, there is the stage of formal operations, which covers the full range of adolescence. During this final Piagetian stage, the adolescent can successfully process abstract thought. Piaget suggested that not all human beings reach this level of cognitive functioning. It remains important for any forensic scientist to understand the various cognitive abilities related to each stage of child development. For example, in court questioning, one would not expect a child of 10 to be able to process abstract questions.

Table 4 Selected developmental milestones: birth to 6 years[a]

Age	Gross motor	Fine motor: adaptive	Language	Personal–social: adaptive
Birth	• Moves head laterally		• Vocalizes • Responds to bell	• Regards face
1–3 months	• Improves head control • Able to support head on neck by 3 months • Can bear weight on legs	• Visually follows 90°, 180°, and 360° consecutively • Clenches fists until 3 months • Brings hands together	• Quiets to noise • Coos (e.g., "ooh," "aah") • Laughs • Swipes at objects	• Regards face and hand • Smiles responsively and spontaneously • Chuckles
4–6 months	• Can roll over • Can sit briefly without support • Can lift chest up using arm support	• Can grasp rattle • Grabs and shakes objects • Brings hands to midline	• Demonstrates different needs by producing different sounds • Blows "raspberries" (bubbles) • Turns toward sound (e.g., rattle) or voice • Has raking grasp • Can exchange objects (e.g., cube) from one hand to the other • Brings objects to mouth to feed • Regards objects (e.g., raisin)	• Regards own hand • Works for toy • Imitates speech sounds • Makes single-syllable consonant sounds • Can distinguish between "pleasant" and "angry" voices • Squeals
7–9 months	• Can sit without support • Can crawl on floor • Can stand while holding on to something	• Drinks from cup	• Mimics noises • Responds to spoken name • Understands "no" • Says "mama" or "dada" in nonspecific way • Indicates wants by pointing • Recognizes familiar words (e.g., ball, dog) • Combines syllables	• Can wave "bye-bye" • Puts many objects into mouth • Has object permanence (e.g., will look for lost objects) • Has separation anxiety
10–12 months	• Pulls to stand • Can stand for 2 s • Cruises holding on to furniture • First steps	• Uses pincer (i.e., thumb–finger) grasp • Mimics reading by turning pages • Scribbles	• Says "mama" or "dada" in specific way • Follows gesture command • Can say one specific word (by 12 months)	• Plays repetitive verbal games (e.g., pat-a-cake)
13–15 months	• Can stoop and recover • Climbs stairs using hands and knees • Can sit down from standing • Walks well, with wide-based gait	• Points with fingers • Has more fine motor control (e.g., stacks rings; puts block in cup) • Marks with pencil • Able to use spoon to feed self • Can open boxes	• Can say two specific words • Looks for named object (e.g., "Where's the ball?") • Responds to name • Obeys command: "Give it to me" • Names family members • Verbalizes jargon • Follows one-step commands without gesture • Has knowledge of one or two body parts	• Solves problems via trial-and-error • Has second bout of separation anxiety (first incidence occurs during 7–9-month period) • Can indicate wants (e.g., food preferences) • Can engage in independent play • Imitates household activities

Age	Motor	Fine Motor/Adaptive	Language	Personal–Social
16–18 months	• Can balance on one foot with support • Can walk backwards • Runs	• Enjoys playing with push–pull toys • Can take off/unzip clothing • Can build tower using two cubes	• Can point to simple pictures when asked • Can follow simple two-step commands • Can point to two pictures • Can say 3–5 specific words • Enjoys using the word "no"	• May demand individual attention • Uses inventive solutions to problems • Less mouthing of objects except for food • Helps in house
19–21 months	• Can kick a ball forward • Can jump up • Can walk up steps with support	• Can put lid on box	• Can say 6–10 specific words • Enjoys being read to • Labels actions: "up" = pick me up • Questions: "What's that?" • Combines words • Uses echolalia	• May fear water • Can put on shoes • Washes hands • Imaginary play, e.g., "tea party" • Likes small objects • Uses spoon and fork • Uses pronoun "I"
22–24 months	• Walks up and down steps alone, placing both feet on each step	• Can build tower using four cubes • Can match like objects • Draws horizontal lines • Can dress self	• Enjoys listening to stories • Repeats rhymes • Associates names with familiar objects • Has up to 50 words • Distinguishes "one" from "many" • Communicates feelings using words and gestures • Verbalizes toileting needs • Knows six body parts • Speech is 50% understandable	• Tests limits • "Reads" book to self • Can be easily frustrated • Does not understand concept of sharing • Engages in parallel play with peers
2–2½ years	• Throws ball in overhand fashion	• Has adult grip on crayon • Draws vertical lines • Can build tower using six cubes	• Uses two-word sentences • States name • Sings parts of songs	• Asserts independence • May say "no" often • Brushes teeth with help
2½–3 years	• Runs well • Alternates feet walking up stairs • Balances on each foot for 1 s	• Enjoys 6–12-piece puzzles • Can copy a circle shape • Can build tower using eight cubes	• Learns 50 words per month • Uses three- or five-word sentences • Can state full name • Understands concept of "one" • Can follow three-step directions	• Is able to play cooperatively • Can wash and dry hands • Can name friends
3–3½ years	• Balances on each foot for 2 s • Walks in straight line and backward • Catches and kicks large ball • Controls bowels and bladder during day	• Can copy a cross shape • Capable of stringing beads and other comparable activities • Knows colors and can match objects of similar hue	• Has approximately 900 words • Can repeat back three-digit numbers • Asks "How? Why?" • Understands prepositions • Knows and uses plurals, pronouns, some adjectives and adverbs • Speech is 75–100% understandable • Can talk about remote events	• Has improved attention • Can put on t-shirt
3½–4 years	• Hops	• Cuts with scissors • Puts shoes on correct feet	• Can count to 3 • Can make analogies	• Enjoys board/card games • Has memory for recent events

Continued

Table 4 Continued

Age	Gross motor	Fine motor: adaptive	Language	Personal–social: adaptive
4–5 years	• Somersaults • Learns "heel-to-toe" walking • Balances on each foot for 3–5 s	• Can copy some letters • Can copy a square when demonstrated • Can draw a person in three parts	• Understands and enjoys humor • Makes comparisons between objects • Speech understandable • Has one-to-one correspondence (e.g., counts five blocks) • Understands basic time concepts • Names categories	• May have imaginary friends • Loves to dress up in imaginative play (e.g., superhero, princess) • Aware of gender of self and others
5–6 years	• Capable of gross motor sequenced activity (e.g., skipping, swimming, biking) • Balance on each foot for 6 s • Can catch ball	• Distinguishes directionality (right from left) • Can draw a person in six parts • Can print full name • Can sort various objects by common size	• Speaks primary language fluently • Knows home address and birth date • Sings songs, shares stories • Understands quantity concepts • Understands sequences • Can define seven words • Begins to learn irregular plurals • Uses words to describe inner emotional state • Understands opposites	• Asserts independence • May fear death

Adapted from Batshaw ML (2001) *When Your Child Has A Disability: The Complete Sourcebook of Daily and Medical Care*. Baltimore: Paul H. Brookes; Psychological Corporation (1992) *The Preschool Language Scale III*. Harcourt, Brace, Jovanovich; *Denver Developmental Screening Tool II* (1992) Denver Developmental Materials.
[a]An average age of onset is given; children vary in acquisition of these milestones.

Emotional/Behavioral/Adaptive Development

Freud and psychoanalytic theory Although current developmental theorists view Sigmund Freud's psychoanalytic theory of development as too narrow in focus, most respect and recognize his importance as a pioneer in the field. Freud asserted that all children progressed through a series of five stages. Each stage involves crises to work through, the outcome of which ostensibly affects adult interpersonal and emotional functioning. The earliest phase (0–1$\frac{1}{2}$ years or infancy), or oral phase, revolves around feeding and oral gratification; in order to progress to the next stage, an infant "learns" to separate itself from its mother in learning the centrality of self (which Freud referred to as primary narcissism). The conflict of the second stage (anal; 1$\frac{1}{2}$–3 years) involves rebellion versus compliance with parental demands as well as fear of loss of parental love.

During the middle psychoanalytic stage (phallic; 3–6 years), the child's focus involves genital exploration. Successful transition from the phallic stage of development necessitates identification with like-sex parent after a period of rivalry stemming from sexual attraction to the opposite-sex parent (termed oedipal and Elektra complexes for boys and girls, respectively).

The challenge of defining oneself within the context of same-sex peers comes with the latency stage (ages 6–11 years). Genital exploration subsides and increased control of sexual and aggressive drives emerges. The child immerses him/herself in socially accepted activities during this fourth stage. Lastly, the genital stage of adolescence (beginning with puberty and continuing into adulthood) involves successful separation from parents as well as equally successful extrafamilial relationships (e.g., with peers).

Freud's pychoanalytic theory of development has fueled further theorization and research in the area, inspiring the subsequent theories of Neo-Freudians such as Ann Freud, Mahler, and Erikson. A forensic expert's knowledge of this theoretical perspective on childhood development can certainly assist in the understanding of a colleague or deposed expert who operates from a Freudian or psychoanalytic viewpoint.

Erikson Erik Erikson's theory of emotional development stems from Freudian theory, but with a broader, more advanced point of view. Each of the eight stages involves one central issue, which must be resolved in order for the individual to progress to the subsequent stage. Erikson's first five stages reflect the exact same age ranges as Freud's psychoanalytic stages. Each stage label is fairly self-explanatory in terms of the conflict that the child must overcome: (1) trust versus mistrust of the caregiver; (2) autonomy versus shame and doubt regarding the child's own independent caretaking capabilities; (3) initiative versus guilt in terms of accomplishment of early age-appropriate goals (e.g., toilet training); (4) industry versus inferiority, for example, in the area of early academic achievement; (5) identity versus role confusion for adolescents attempting to establish autonomy and sense of self; (6) intimacy versus isolation for social connection during young adulthood; (7) generativity versus stagnation in adulthood as career paths are established or sought; (8) lastly, old age involves ego integrity versus despair as the elderly individual reflects upon and evaluates his/her life accomplishments.

Abnormalities of Development

Clinicians stress the importance of periodic assessment of developmental milestones in order to chart each child's progress in skills acquisition across the four domains of development. Abnormalities of development are common in about 10% of children and can be global, in which a child shows delayed acquisition of skills across all four domains, or specific to one or more domains. Tjossem's three-category classification system for risk factors for developmental problems in children is commonly cited and includes established, biological, and environmental factors. An infant or child is placed at established risk by a medical disorder, including conditions resulting from genetic and chromosomal abnormalities. An infant or child is at biological risk due to prenatal, perinatal, neonatal, or early developmental insults. Examples include poor maternal nutrition, infectious diseases, or toxins passing through the placenta during pregnancy, and trauma sustained during delivery. An infant or child is placed at environmental risk by life experiences such as onset of a chronic medical condition, poverty, malnutrition, and child abuse and neglect.

Given the fact that each child's individual variability in development is related to a number of factors, any developmental assessment must include a thorough medical history (including birth, infections, hospitalizations, surgeries, medications), family history, physical examination for abnormalities and/or dysmorphic features that might suggest a genetic syndrome, and interviews with primary caretakers regarding the history of that child's acquisition of specific developmental skills (including emotional/behavioral/adaptive skills). In addition, developmental status should be documented.

Measurement of Development

Developmental status can be measured through two types of play-based tests: screening tests and evaluation tests. A developmental screening test is a quick and broad assessment of skills; its purpose is to identify a subpopulation of children who are in need of further, more in-depth evaluation. Screening tests can either rely on a caregiver report of developmental milestones via a questionnaire or involve the standardized administration of items by a professional or paraprofessional. Developmental evaluation instruments are standardized measures that are administered by highly trained professionals such as a psychologist. These tests, more labor-intensive and prolonged (lasting 1–3 h), are used to create a profile of a child's strengths and weaknesses in a variety of developmental domains. The administrator then determines how these strengths and weaknesses will impact a child's interactions within multiple environments (family, school, and larger community). A discussion of specific screening and evaluation tools used to assess developmental progression is beyond the scope of this article; see references below for further reading regarding these types of tools.

See Also

Anthropology: Bone Pathology and Antemortem Trauma; Morphological Age Estimation; Pediatric and Juvenile; **Autopsy:** Pediatric; **Children:** Legal Protection and Rights of Children; Children and Courts; Physical Abuse; Sexual Abuse, Epidemiology; Non-inflicted Causes of Death; **Odontology:** Overview

Further Reading

Aylward GP (1994) *Practitioner's Guide to Developmental and Psychological Testing: Critical Issues in Developmental and Behavioral Pediatrics.* New York: Plenum Press.

Aylward GP (1997) *Infant and Early Childhood Neuropsychology: Clinical Child Psychology Library.* New York: Plenum Press.

Batshaw ML (2001) *When Your Child Has a Disability: The Complete Sourcebook of Daily and Medical Care.* Baltimore, MD: Paul H. Brookes.

Dixon SD, Stein MT (eds.) (1991) *Encounters with Children: Pediatric Behavior and Development.* Chicago: Year Book.

Illingworth RS (1992) *The Development of the Infant and Young Child: Normal and Abnormal,* 9th edn. Singapore: Longman Singapore.

Levine MD, Carey WB, Crocker AC (eds.) (1992) *Developmental-Behavioral Pediatrics,* 2nd edn. Philadelphia, PA: WB Saunders.

Piaget J (1951) *Play, Dreams and Imitation in Childhood.* New York: WW Norton.

Piaget J (1952) *The Origins of Intelligence in Children.* Translated by Cook M. New York: WW Norton.

Rudolph AM, Kamei RK (eds.) (1994) *Rudolph's Fundamentals of Pediatrics.* Norwalk, CT: Appelton & Lange.

Shelov SP (1991) *The American Academy of Pediatrics: Caring For Your Baby and Young Child: Birth to Age 5. The Complete and Authoritative Guide.* New York: Bantam Books.

Tanner JM (1962) *Growth at Adolescence,* 2nd edn. Oxford, UK: Blackwell Scientific Publications.

Trawick-Smith J (2000) *Early Childhood Development: A Multicultural Perspective,* 2nd edn. New Jersey: Prentice Hall.

Legal Protection and Rights of Children

F Orlando and M Seals, Nova Southeastern University, Fort Lauderdale, FL, USA

Introduction

This article will attempt to discuss whether children, by which is meant persons under 18 years of age (as defined by Article 1 of the United Nations Convention on the Rights of the Child (CRC)), are mentally competent to comprehend the complex legal proceedings of an adult criminal court and competent to make decisional choices that will profoundly affect their future life.

We will explore brain development and attempt to connect this science to the law and procedures involving children, especially those charged with horrific crimes. We cannot address the many questions that exist as to these issues in one article but will attempt to give the reader the basis to go further into the subject.

The main questions that we address are:

- Should a "child" (Article 1 CRC) ever be subject to a criminal trial, especially where the sentence can be death or life imprisonment, with no possibility for release, without first being examined by medical, not legal, standards as to competency to understand the process, assist counsel, and have the ability to make decisions as to case outcomes?
- Has the juvenile court in the USA and procedures in other parts of the civilized world been so "criminalized" to have actually eliminated a true separate court and process for children?

We have looked at the original premise of the juvenile court and what today is presumed by many as "a scaled-down second-class criminal court for children" and conclude with questions on how, if possible, the science can be connected to the reality of present-day law.

There is no doubt that today children are involved in many violent and horrific crimes. This question remains: how does a civilized and humane society deal with these issues?

Discussion

Legal protection and rights of children are concerned with the theory that children are incapable of functioning mentally on an adult level because of immaturity. Current scientific research shows that the child's brain is vastly different from that of an adult. Research indicates that during childhood the brain continues to develop, contrary to what researchers believed in the past. While a child may physically appear to have developed into an adult, his/her brain has not fully developed into an adult brain. Because of this lack of development, the child may be mentally unable to make decisions on an adult level. This inability becomes particularly troublesome when the child enters the court system charged with committing a crime.

Throughout the USA and the world there is great concern about children committing horrific crimes at younger and younger ages, as exemplified by the recent cases involving Lionel Tate and Lee Boyd Malvo. In March 2001, the Florida court sentenced 14-year-old Lionel Tate to life in prison without parole for killing a six-year-old child. Tate's defense counsel argued that the child's death occurred as a result of Tate "demonstrating wrestling techniques" on her, but did not request a mental competency proceeding. Tate was 12 years old at the time. Lee Boyd Malvo, 18, confessed to the sniper shootings that occurred in Washington, DC, Virginia, and Maryland in 2002. He is currently being tried as an adult in Virginia. The state is seeking a death sentence. Malvo was 17 when the shootings occurred, in which 10 people died and three were wounded. Malvo is raising the insanity defense, in which he claims that his actions were the result of "indoctrination" and "transference" by John Muhammad, the 40-year-old adult involved in the shootings together with Mr. Malvo. Malvo confessed to the police officer after a lengthy interrogation. Psychiatrists have testified that because of the influence Muhammad had over Malvo, Malvo was unable to distinguish between right and wrong and committed the shootings to please Muhammad. This influence began when the child was much younger.

To deal with situations such as these, many jurisdictions in the USA have chosen to subject these children to adult court and adult sentences, including the death penalty. However, since many children may be unable to function mentally on an adult level, there are serious questions of whether the juvenile will be able to aid his/her attorney competently in the defense or even understand the court proceedings. There is no question as to the level of violence involved in the cases referred to and the public's right to expect accountability. The question is: what is accountability and are children, even those who commit horrific crimes, redeemable? Recent developments in child brain research may help to answer this concern.

In December 2003, Lee Boyd Malvo was convicted of the murder of Federal Bureau of Investigation analyst Linda Franklin. By convicting Malvo of capital murder, the jury rejected medical opinions and scientific findings on child brain development as to Malvo's competency to formulate intent and the idea that he was "programmed" by an adult. Psychiatrists had testified that because of Malvo's impressionability, youth, and unstable home environment, John Muhammad had been able to "brainwash" and "indoctrinate" Malvo into committing the sniper shootings. The fact that the jury was unable to accept these evaluations is evidence of the difficulty in transmitting to a fact finder the impressionability and mental development of children. However, his youth and immaturity played a major role in the penalty phase of Malvo's trial. On December 23, 2003, the jury sentenced Malvo to life in prison. This sentence does show some consideration for Malvo's immaturity because he was spared the death penalty. The jury used the medical evidence to mitigate but not excuse his actions with a "not guilty by reason of insanity" verdict.

Such actions taken by the jury raise the question of how do the medical and legal systems come to accept each other? In March 2004, the judge formally sentenced Malvo to life in prison without the possibility of parole. Sentencing a child to life without the possibility of parole violates Article 37 of the United Nations CRC, which prohibits the death penalty and any sentence that does not have a reasonable time for completion and release of the child. Article 1 of CRC defines a "child" as anyone under the age of 18. However, the sentence of life in prison did not appease the victims' groups connected with Malvo's case. In the USA, victims' rights groups have gained significant influence in criminal cases and often seek vengeance and not justice. Vengeance is an unconstitutional punishment. Malvo's sentence of life in prison without possibility of parole illustrates how vengeance may have influenced the judge and jury, regardless of the fact that he was a child.

Brain Development in the Child

The human brain weighs approximately 1.35 kg (3 lb) and is composed of different parts, called lobes.

The parietal and temporal lobes control the ability to learn languages and understand spatial relations. The frontal lobe makes up the largest portion of the brain. The prefrontal cortex, a small part of the frontal lobe located behind the forehead, controls abstract thinking, prioritization of thoughts, planning, the ability to anticipate possible consequences of actions, and the ability to control impulses. Up until now, scientists had believed that the human brain was fully developed in early childhood. However, Dr. Elizabeth Sowell, working in brain research at the University of California – Los Angeles (UCLA), discovered that the frontal lobe is the final part of the brain to develop completely and that it is the lobe that changes the most during childhood. Dr. Sowell and other UCLA researchers are working together with researchers at Harvard Medical School and the National Institute of Mental Health to map the development of the child's brain.

The researchers used magnetic resonance imaging (MRI) to scan the brains of children every two years from early childhood through adolescence and into the early 20s. Dr. Judith Rapoport of the National Institute of Mental Health conducted the first study in 1999. She and her colleagues studied brain development of 145 children and found that the brain undergoes a thickening process in a second overproduction of gray matter, the "thinking" part of the brain, just before the onset of puberty. This overproduction is mostly concentrated in the frontal lobe. Until that study, scientists only knew that the brain overproduced gray matter for a short time period from before birth through the first $1\frac{1}{2}$ years of life. Research shows that the brain's gray matter increases and decreases in different brain areas at different times of development. However, the overproduction of gray matter peaks at age 11 in females and age 12 in boys. Afterwards, gray matter is shed and discarded at the rate of 1–2% a year. However, the brain's white matter (wire-like nerve fibers connecting different parts of the brain) thickens progressively from birth and an insulating layer of myelin envelops the fibers. This insulation helps the brain focus and work more efficiently.

Researchers have discovered that a growth spurt of white matter starts at the front of the brain in early childhood, moves to the back of the brain, and stops after puberty. There are also growth spurts from age 6 to age 13 in the temporal and parietal lobes. However, researchers have found that production of gray matter occurs in the opposite direction from the back to the front of the brain, meaning that the frontal lobe does not fully develop until the early 20s. Researchers at UCLA have studied MRI scans of adults between the ages of 23 and 30 and of children ages 12–14. The study showed that the parietal and temporal lobes of the brain were fully developed in the child's brain. However, they found that adults have much more myelination in the frontal lobe than children. The research suggests that production of gray matter in the frontal lobe relates to the maturation of cognitive processing but the sensory, auditory, and language centers of the brain are fully developed in the child's brain.

In a correlating study led by Dr. Deborah Yurgelun-Todd of Harvard Medical School, researchers studied functional MRI scans of children viewing various pictures of faces showing different expressions. The study revealed that children in their early teen years used the amygdala center of the brain that mediates fear and "gut" reactions. Males tended to use the amygdala center more than females because the male frontal lobe develops slower in males. As the children age, they begin to use the frontal lobe in identifying the expressions. This suggests that as the children age they use reason more than "gut" instinct.

Dr. Ruben C. Gur has argued that current research strongly suggests that the human brain does not fully mature until the early 20s. The last areas to mature are the regions of the brain that control impulsivity, judgment, planning, and foresight of consequences. Dr. Gur suggests that the age of 21 or 22 is closer to the "biological" age of maturity.

Legal Consequences of the Research

If the brain does not mature until the age of 21 or 22, there may be significant legal consequences involved in the processing of juvenile offenders. The above research suggests that children are not emotionally or cognitively mature enough to understand the ramifications of their actions or the legal process. The juvenile justice system is based on the common-law presumption that children are mentally mature by the age of 14 and thus have all the reasoning abilities of an adult to formulate intent. The American court system currently operates under this idea and allows states to impose the death penalty for offenders who commit capital crimes as young as 16 years of age. However, it must be noted that, because of the lengthy appeals process in the USA, it is not uncommon for offenders to spend between 10 and 20 years or more on death row awaiting execution. At the time of execution, the offender is no longer a child. But the new research findings suggesting the brain does not fully develop until the early 20s brings to light issues of whether the teenage offender is mentally culpable for actions taken during childhood. The issue is not when the person is executed, but when the sentence was imposed.

The US practice of executing offenders who commit capital crimes during childhood has drawn criticism from the European Union, the United Nations, and the Inter-American Commission on Human Rights (IACHR), a branch of the Organization of American States. In October 2002, the IACHR ruled that the USA violated the norm of *jus cogens* (internationally recognized standards of decency) when it allowed the imposition of the death sentence for Michael Domingues. Domingues, a Mexican national, broke into a woman's home in Nevada at the age of 16 and murdered her and her four-year-old son. He was sentenced to death at the age of 17 for the two murders and currently awaits execution. Even though he was ruled competent to formulate the necessary intent to commit the crimes, there are questions of whether he was competent to comprehend the judicial process that led to his death sentence.

On October 31, 2003, the IACHR issued a report to the US government regarding the case of Napoleon Beazley. The state of Texas executed Beazley on May 28, 2002 for the April, 19, 1994 murder of John Luttig while burglarizing Luttig's vehicle in the driveway of his home. Beazley was 17 years old at the time of the murder. The IACHR found that the USA violated the international norm of *jus cogens* and also violated Beazley's right to life under Article I of the Commission's Declaration of the Rights and Duties of Man. The IACHR recommends that the USA review its laws that allow execution of individuals who were under 18 years of age at the time of their capital offense. It is cases such as these that call into question the developmental immaturity of juvenile offenders and the concept of legal competency.

Legal Competency of the Child

While there is no precise legal definition of competency, the issue of competency has mostly been used in the legal processing of adult offenders who are mentally ill or retarded. However, as scientific research shows, juveniles are developmentally immature and thus, seemingly, are less competent to make decisions effectively on an adult level. These observations are reinforced by the results of the MacArthur Foundation Juvenile Competency Study.

The MacArthur study tested individuals between the ages of 11 and 24 to compare the capacities of children and adults as trial defendants. The test analyzed their responses to a series of questions about hypothetical situations and the decisions available in each. The reasons for the responses were evaluated to determine psychosocial maturity, including the "ability to evaluate risk, to think about future consequences, and to resist peer pressure." Extrapolating

the test results to the US population as a whole suggested that approximately one-third of 11–13-year-olds and one-fifth of 14–15-year-olds are probably not competent to stand trial. Many of the children in the study did not understand the judicial process, including the role of the jury and judge. Also, they were less likely to understand their legal rights even with an explanation of what the rights contain. These findings were consistent even for the children who had prior contact with the legal system. Other studies indicate that when juveniles are questioned by authority figures they are more likely to answer in a manner they believe the questioner wants. It is arguable that this may have been what happened in the Lee Boyd Malvo murder case. When questioned by the authorities, Malvo admitted the shootings and even that he enjoyed committing them. Because of Malvo's impressionability and immaturity, he may have been trying to please the adult authority figures in order to be released, as many children do with parents, school officials, or when involved in the justice system. These findings are significant in that even though juvenile offenders have the right to remain silent and to have an attorney, most states allow the juvenile to decide whether or not to waive these rights without a prior finding of competency.

The practice of allowing juveniles to waive these important rights assumes that juveniles are competent to make these decisions knowingly and intelligently. This assumption is contrary to the research findings outlined above. While the juvenile offender may waive these rights, a judge, but most often the prosecutor in the USA, will make the decision of whether the juvenile offender will be tried in juvenile court or waived over to adult court. In *Kent* v. *United States*, 383 US 541 (1966), the US Supreme Court outlined a list of factors judges must consider in making this decision. Among these are:

- the seriousness of the alleged offense
- whether community protection requires the waiver
- whether the offense was committed in an aggressive, violent, premeditated or willful manner
- the sophistication and maturity of the juvenile as determined by his/her home environment, emotional attitude, and pattern of living.

However, this analysis may be moot when the state gives the prosecutor the right to transfer the juvenile offender to adult court, on the basis of the offense charged as opposed to the maturity and competency of the child, or the state lowers the age of automatic transfer to age 16 or, in Florida and New York, even 14, and for murder cases presumably any age. This fact raises the question of whether or not prosecutors should have to follow the same standards as judges, outlined in Kent. It seems that it would be a mistake not to make the decision to transfer a juvenile offender to adult court based on competency and the Kent standards.

Juvenile courts were developed on the basis that children do not have the same decision-making capabilities of adults and are therefore less culpable for their actions. As the Court pointed out in Kent, "the juvenile court is engaged in determining the needs of the child and of society rather than adjudicating criminal conduct. The objectives are to provide measures of guidance and rehabilitation for the child and protection for society, not to fix criminal responsibility, guilt, and punishment." This finding may be questionable under present laws and procedures. Special safeguards were built into the juvenile justice system but should contain no less due process than for adults, especially as to competency and assistance of competent legal counsel. If the juvenile courts do not recognize this as a legitimate role for a separate court for children, then the question of whether there is still a need for a separate judicial venue for children arises. The eminent legal scholar Professor Barry Feld argues that there may no longer be a need for a separate juvenile court because in adult courts the defendant would receive full due process protections, including competency exams. Feld concludes that the juvenile court of today has been "criminalized" without including the full due process of an adult court.

The two elements of legal competence are: (1) competence to assist counsel; and (2) decisional competence.

The US Supreme Court stated a two-part test of whether a juvenile offender can competently assist counsel in *Dusky* v. *United States*, 362 US 402 (1960). The test is whether the youth has "sufficient present ability to consult with his lawyer with a reasonable degree of rational understanding" and "whether he has a rational and factual understanding of the proceedings against him." Dr. Thomas Grisso and other justice researchers have recognized that a juvenile may be able to assist counsel but be incompetent to make decisions about his/her defense. The Lionel Tate case is illustrative of this point.

In Tate's case, the state of Florida offered Tate a three-year sentence in a juvenile facility as opposed to the sentence he ultimately received, which was life without any chance for parole in prison, i.e., until death! Tate rejected this offer. It is questionable whether such a decision can be conceived of as understanding the legal process. Decisional competence involves understanding, appreciation, reasoning, and choice. These abilities are governed by the frontal lobe, which research now shows does not fully

develop until the early 20s. The holding of the Florida Fourth District Court of Appeal of Florida overturning Tate's sentence reinforces these findings. The court concluded that Tate's due process rights were violated when the lower court did not *sua sponte* order a competency evaluation of Tate to see if he was mentally capable of aiding in his own defense. The court stated that, because of Tate's extremely young age and lack of prior exposure to the judicial system, a "competency evaluation was constitutionally mandated to determine whether he had sufficient ability to consult with his lawyer with a reasonable degree of rational understanding and whether he had a rational, as well as factual, understanding of the proceedings against him."

The court recognized that Tate is entitled to a new trial because a competency hearing done three years after he was sentenced "to determine the present competency of a maturing child cannot adequately retroactively protect his rights."

However, it must be emphasized that the court did not solve the problem of whether any juvenile is really competent to aid in his/her own defense. The court limited its holding to the Tate case and stated that "competency hearings are not mandated simply because a child is tried as an adult." Furthermore, the court recognized that the trial court should have inquired whether Tate may be "competent" and not whether he is "incompetent." But the Tate court also emphasized that in Florida children do not have an absolute right to be treated in a "special system for juvenile offenders." Florida and other state legislatures have chosen to use a statutory system that specifies at what age a child may be tried as an adult instead of utilizing the common-law "infancy" defense. Because these statutory systems leave the decision whether to try the child as an adult to the state prosecutor, perhaps those prosecutors should be under the same standards applicable to judges under Kent.

Since current research indicates that the human brain is not fully developed until the early 20s, juvenile offenders may not have the mental capacity to waive any of their rights. This issue raises the question of whether the child and society would be better served if these rights could not be waived. To safeguard these rights, it would seem the law should require a Kent-like proceeding to determine competency in the juvenile court with counsel present at every stage of the proceedings. Such safeguards should be especially required in cases where the child is being tried as an adult and the death penalty or life without parole is a possible sentence. With the new indications about brain development in adolescents, justice researchers could argue that it is neither legally right nor morally right to try juvenile offenders as adults, especially when the sentence could be death or life imprisonment. International standards of juvenile justice might better protect the legal rights of children under those circumstances. It should be noted that Article 37 of the CRC prohibits the incarceration of any child for life without possibility of release and also prohibits a death sentence for a child.

Conclusion

The issues surrounding the legal protection of children are greatly determined on how children are treated once they enter the legal process. Juvenile courts were established to rehabilitate juvenile offenders based on the theory that children differ mentally from adults. Recent scientific research lends credit to this theory by showing that the human brain is a "work in process" until the early 20s. Since the frontal lobe is the last part of the brain to develop and given that it controls reasoning ability, childhood immaturity is arguably a component of incompetency to stand trial. It is questionable whether an alleged juvenile offender really has the mental capacity to understand the charges against him/her and the possible outcomes to be able to assist a lawyer in the child's defense. Because the USA allows imposition of the death penalty for crimes committed as a juvenile, the American justice system attempts to turn juvenile offenders into adults because of the crimes they commit. The juvenile court was created to prevent this happening. Perhaps it is time to consider returning to the common-law presumptions as to a child's ability to formulate intent and as a last resort, accept the findings and recommendations of Professor Feld and totally abolish the separate judicial process for children. We must also ask, when will the legal system connect the reality of process to the science of childhood brain development?

See Also

Children: Stages of Development and Growth; Children and Courts

Further Reading

Beyer M (2000) Immaturity, culpability, and competency in juveniles: A study of 17 cases. *Criminal Justice Magazine* 15: 26.
Convention on the Rights of the Child. UN General Assembly, November 20, 1989.
Feld B (1997) Abolish the juvenile court: Youthfulness, criminal responsibility, and sentencing policy. *The Journal of Criminal Law and Criminology* 88: 68–136.
Feld B (1999) *Bad Kids: Race and the Transformation of the Juvenile Court.* Oxford University Press, Inc.
Grisso T (1980) Juveniles' capacities to waive Miranda rights: An empirical analysis. *California Law Review* 68: 134.
Grisso T, *et al.* (2003) Juvenile competency to stand trial. In: Flynn-Robinson C (ed.) *National Association of Counsel for Children, Children's Law Manual Series,* Ch. 4. pp. 35–59.
Howell A Examining juvenile culpability and adjudicative competence with new research. *The Southern Juvenile Defender Center.* Available online at: www.childwelfarenet/SJDC/Juvenileculpability.pdf.
McCord J, *et al.* (2001) *Juvenile Crime, Juvenile Justice: Panel on Juvenile Crime, Prevention, Treatment, and Control,* p. 166. National Academy Press.
National Institutes of Mental Health. *The Teenage Brain: A Work in Progress.* NIH Publication No. 01-4929. Available online at: www.nimh.nih.gov/publicat/teenbrain.cfm.
Ortiz A (2003) *Adolescent Brain Development and Legal Culpability.* American Bar Association, Criminal Justice Section. Available online at: www.abanet.org/crimjust/juvjus/juvdp.html.
Ortiz A (2003) Juvenile death penalty: Is it "cruel and unusual" in light of contemporary standards? *Criminal Justice Magazine* 17(4).
Sheperd R (1998) Juvenile's waiver of the right to counsel. *Criminal Justice Magazine* 12(1): 38.
Steinberg L (2003) Juveniles on trial: MacArthur Foundation Study calls competency into question. *Criminal Justice Magazine* 18(3).

Children and Courts

R N Parrish, Office of the Guardian ad Litem, Utah, UT, USA

Introduction and Scope

During the last half of the twentieth century, court cases involving children as victims of various types of crime became a common fixture of courtrooms in the USA, the UK, and many other parts of the world. In addition, judges in many countries have concentrated more attention on protecting children from various forms of abuse, neglect, and abandonment caused by their primary caretakers. The phrase "child abuse" or "child maltreatment" was rarely used in the USA until the seminal works of Dr. John Caffey and Dr. C. Henry Kempe made the phenomenon emerge and remain in the public conscience (**Figure 1**).

The huge increase in numbers of reported cases of child maltreatment has resulted in a new courtroom focus on the forensic abilities of various experts from

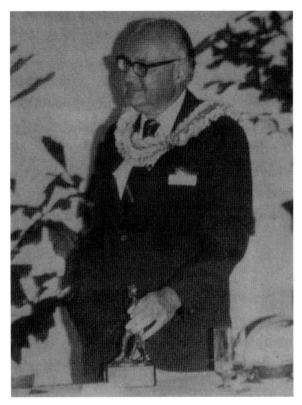

Figure 1 Dr C Henry Kempe. Reproduced with permission of J Lauridson, © 2004.

a variety of fields. Expert medical witnesses have become a vital and indispensable part of courtroom proof in cases involving children and this has resulted in an unprecedented interaction between medical professionals and lawyers. Those whose task is to prove, or disprove, allegations of child physical abuse, child neglect, or homicide have turned to medical science to answer a number of perplexing questions. Medical forensic experts are regularly asked to assist in identifying the cause and possible mechanism of a child's injuries, determine the likely time when such injuries were caused, and sort between accidentally caused and intentionally inflicted lesions. In all countries where child maltreatment has become a regular fixture in the legal process, those who attempt to prove that caretakers purposely inflict injuries on children in their care have faced the difficult task of overcoming general disbelief among the populace. The vast majority of the public does not mistreat the children in their charge. The concept itself is so foreign that when such people sit in judgment of others charged with such an offense, they often struggle with finding another guilty of such conduct. When this is coupled with the facts that most child victims are either too young or too injured to assist in identifying the cause and mechanism of their injuries, and that proof in the courtroom is often made up exclusively of circumstantial

evidence, judges and juries often look to forensic medical experts to provide the ultimate answers.

An equally important revolution has occurred in the field of child sexual abuse, where the forensic challenges may be even more difficult. Medical experts are asked to make fine distinctions between genital injuries that could have been self-inflicted by the child or accidentally caused and those that are consistent only with sexual conduct by some other person. This article will focus primarily on physical injuries and homicide of children related to abuse or neglect.

This article will also focus on the role of the medical forensic expert as a vital contributor to the modern child maltreatment courtroom process. A subsidiary focus will be on the expert's ability to perform the dual role in educating the trier of fact as to sometimes complex medical concepts and then expressing opinions based on the state of forensic knowledge as to the key issues in a child maltreatment trial. Examples will be offered showing how forensic experts can use visual illustrations, computer-generated diagrams and animations, and other media to simplify and enhance this vital role.

Identification of Cause, Manner, and Timing of Physical Injuries to Children

Identifying the Cause

Since there are rarely any eyewitnesses to acts of abuse causing injury to children, unless those eyewitnesses are too young to testify or are in league with the abuser, courtroom proof of the cause of injuries depends upon the expertise of forensic pathologists and/or clinicians. In most cases, whether the child died from the abuse or not, both types of expertise may be helpful, since clinicians regularly see and diagnose the cause of a wide variety of usually nonfatal injuries, while the pathologist must regularly interpret the cause and manner of fatal injuries to children. The range of injuries found in victims of child abuse run the gamut from subtle marks that are quite difficult to interpret to severe closed-head injuries caused by violent forces to marks that were clearly caused by impact with some object where the only issue is what object and who wielded it? Forensically trained experts use the collective knowledge gained by those in their respective fields to answer such questions. Most such questions are ultimately resolved, though, by common sense.

Given the general public disbelief concerning child abuse, getting a judge or jury to accept that someone intentionally or knowingly harmed a child is often very difficult. Experts must give the trier of fact a basic education about the medical issues in the case, and attorneys must then trust that the persons sitting in judgment are capable of applying that education to the facts of the case. As with most types of learning in the twenty-first century, those issues reinforced with graphic support make the most impact. The modern forensic expert must master not only his/her science, but the art of persuasion and teaching, as well.

One of the first tasks in identifying the cause and manner of an injury or set of injuries is to examine the history provided by the person providing care for the child when the injury likely occurred. Although defalcation about the cause of injury is likely in cases of inflicted trauma, the perpetrators rarely lie about the onset of symptoms. The most important information for a forensic expert asked to express an opinion as to when an injury occurred is often examination of the behavior of the child over the last several days before the significant injury or death. Indeed, some experts have said that the cardinal sign of child abuse or inflicted injury is discrepant or evolving history to explain an injury. Where the story just doesn't fit the severity and nature of the injuries to the child, or where the caretaker should know what happened, but claims that nothing occurred, inflicted trauma should be suspected.

Modern technology has greatly simplified the sometimes painstaking process of matching injuries to their cause. A simple example of this is offered in **Figures 2–4**.

Forensic experts are often asked to match an injury of unclear etiology with its cause. In this case, a search

of the crime scene yielded the object responsible for the injury. Often, a well-trained forensic pathologist or physician can deduce that several different injuries are in fact related in cause. In the case illustrated in **Figures 5–7**, the child victim was identified at autopsy to have a small amount of blood at the tail of the pancreas, but no other apparent abdominal bleeding; a small amount of subdural blood in the spinal cord; and unusual marks and bruises apparently overlying this area on her back near the spine. Although it was possible the injuries were unrelated to each other in mechanism and even timing, the possibility was raised during investigation that they were in fact related. Through this series of still graphics, the expert pathologist illustrated a cause that would explain all three injuries having been caused by a severe blow to the back of the child (**Figure 7**). This same child had several paired sets of punctate marks in various locations on her body. The pathologist conducting the autopsy requested the police investigators to search the victim's environment for an object that might account for these marks. The police discovered a corncob skewer in the child's toy box, which, when matched to the scale of the injuries through overlays, perfectly matched the puncture marks on her body. Given the fact that some of these marks were in the middle of her back, the expert pathologist was later

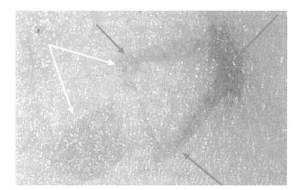

Figure 3 Scaled pattern of object suspected to have caused injury. Reproduced with permission of J Downs, © 2004.

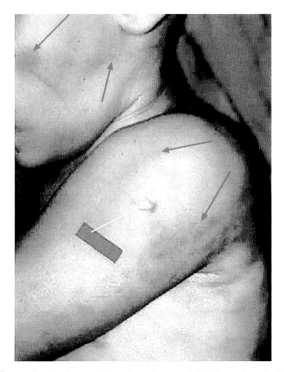

Figure 2 Unclear patterned-mark on a child. Reproduced with permission of J Downs, © 2004.

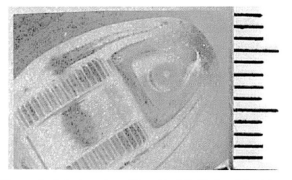

Figure 4 Actual overlay of the object (lighter) and the injury. Reproduced with permission of J Downs, © 2004.

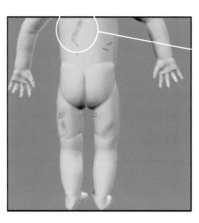
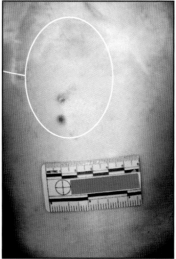

Figure 5 External bruises/marks on back. Reproduced with permission of J Lauridson, © 2004.

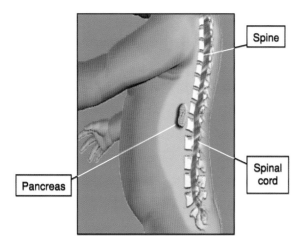

Figure 6 Blood at tail of pancreas and in spinal cord. Reproduced with permission of J Lauridson, © 2004.

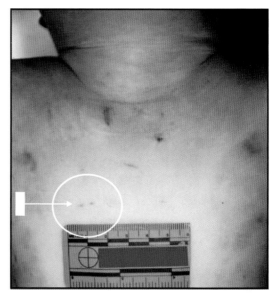

Figure 8 Punctate marks on the child's chest. Reproduced with permission of J Lauridson, © 2004.

able also to opine that these were inflicted by some other person, not self-inflicted (**Figures 8–11**).

One of the most difficult aspects of forensic medical work in child abuse cases is determining which injuries might have been caused by accident and contrasting those which are consistent only with inflicted trauma. The task is made somewhat simpler when all the injuries of similar age are considered together as a pattern, since when some injuries were quite obviously inflicted, it makes it more likely that all were part of the same assault on the child. Thus, although certain bruises might, if they happened in isolation, have been caused by accident, when they

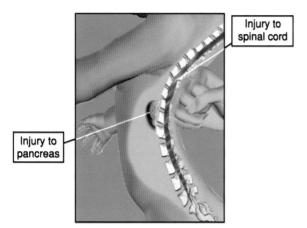

Figure 7 Mechanism accounting for all three injuries being contemporaneous. Reproduced with permission of J Lauridson, © 2004.

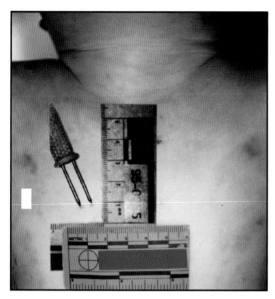

Figure 9 Matching overlay showing corncob skewer. Reproduced with permission of J Lauridson, © 2004.

are considered together with other inflicted injuries the cause becomes clear.

In the case illustrated in **Figures 12–16**, a 9-month-old infant was allegedly found on her back having supposedly smothered under a stack of blankets. The lividity pattern shown in **Figure 12** allowed the expert pathologist to opine that the baby had been in a face-down position for at least a significant period of time after her death, which had likely occurred hours before she was discovered, contradicting the caretakers' version of events. The remaining figures illustrate other injuries documented at the time of autopsy, which included a blunt-force tear of the ear (**Figure 13**); multiple facial bruises in various stages of healing (**Figure 14**); a grab mark on the child's forearm (**Figure 15**); and healing damage to the gums at the position of the frenulum (**Figure 16**). Although the caretakers offered accidental explanations for each of these injuries, their stories were inconsistent with the mechanism, timing, and severity of the injuries. For instance, the child's

Left wrist

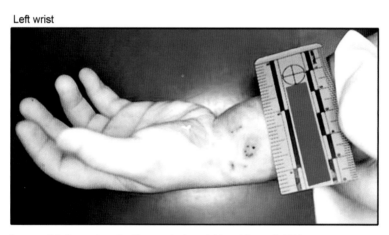

Figure 10 Punctate marks on wrist. Reproduced with permission of J Lauridson, © 2004.

Left wrist

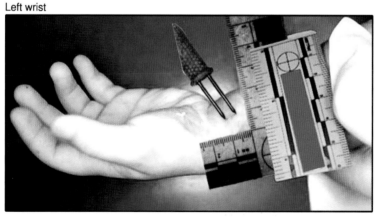

Figure 11 Overlay showing corncob skewer match. Reproduced with permission of J Lauridson, © 2004.

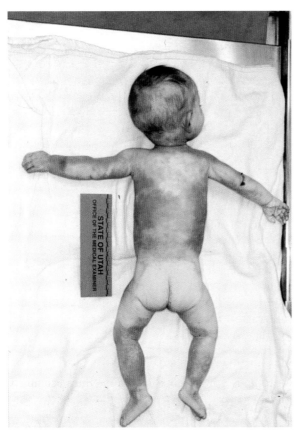

Figure 12 Lividity. Reproduced with permission of J Lauridson, © 2004.

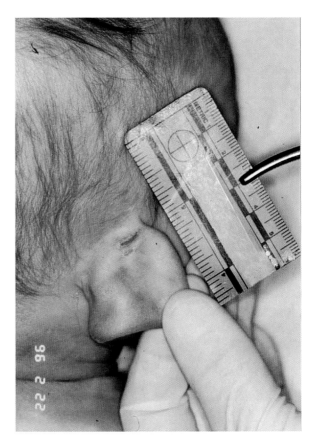

Figure 13 Tear behind ear. Reproduced with permission of J Lauridson, © 2004.

mother claimed that the gum injuries were caused by the paramedics who performed life-saving measures on the child. The forensic expert pathologist was able to refute this claim by pointing out that when the paramedics arrived the child had been dead for at least a couple of hours and since the gum injuries show evidence of inflammation and inflammation cannot occur postmortem, the paramedics could not have caused the injuries. In addition, the medical experts refuted the mother's claims that the child's facial bruises, leg and arm fractures, and other injuries were caused when the baby was trapped in the crib. Ultimately, a jury rejected all of the mother's and her boyfriend's accidental explanations for the injuries and convicted the mother of murder and the boyfriend of child physical abuse.

Verbal descriptions by forensic medical expert witnesses of such things as internal abdominal injuries are simply insufficient to convey the force that would be necessary to cause such an injury. In **Figures 17–19**, a simple computer animation was used to illustrate the position of the injured internal organs, the nature of the force that would have been required to cause the injury, and the resulting leakage of intestinal contents into the abdominal cavity, ultimately causing peritonitis and the child's death. Similarly, the pattern of a burn injury alone can allow an experienced forensic expert witness

to explain and illustrate in court the difference between an inflicted burn and one caused by accident. In most cases of inflicted burn injuries to children, the caretaker attempts to account for the injury by claiming the child turned the water on him/herself, or climbed into a bathtub which already had extremely hot water in it. The expert can explain that, in either scenario, the child's burns would have appeared to be irregular, splash-type patterns, since the child would have struggled to get out of the burning water. By contrast, when the burns are distinguished by clear and even lines of demarcation between burned and spared skin, and especially when certain parts of the skin are spared from burning, it becomes clear that someone must have held the child in the burning water to create the pattern of injury (**Figures 20–23**).

In many jurisdictions, there are limitations placed by courts upon what types of demonstrative evidence may be introduced, and most restrictions apply in jury trials. Photographs of the victim's injuries taken during the autopsy process are often considered gruesome and unfairly prejudicial to the accused. Some courts make a distinction between preevisceration and postevisceration autopsy photographs, holding that the latter are always presumed to be too gruesome to be admissible as evidence unless there is a particularized and unique need to introduce such photographs. Attorneys whose task is to illustrate and prove the cause of internal injuries face the further problem that internal autopsy photographs are very difficult for the untrained to interpret, and may be so distasteful that jury members cannot look at them and thus risk missing the point. Computer diagrams and animations can greatly enhance the expert's ability to explain and illustrate in a manner understandable to everyone the nature, location, and cause of internal injuries to a child. Such diagrams and animations, if based upon the original findings at the autopsy, may be the preferable method for illustrating forensic expert testimony.

Possibly the most difficult medical and anatomical concepts to teach to those who have no prior training, such as judges and juries, are those associated with closed-head injuries in children. Concepts such as axonal injury, subdural hematoma, retinal hemorrhages, and retinoschisis are virtually impossible to convey successfully by words alone. Modern computer technology has allowed easier methods not only to teach basic anatomy of each of these concepts, but also to illustrate the mechanism that results in various forms of trauma to the brain and eyes during severe rotational trauma inflicted upon the child's head. Figures 24–30 represent still images which are part of computer animations illustrating the mechanism of injury of such conditions as subdural hematoma and retinal hemorrhages.

Identifying the Timing of Injury

For virtually any injury or set of injuries inflicted upon a child, there are fairly well-recognized symptoms that would appear a particular amount of time following infliction of the injury, assuming the child is otherwise neurologically normal. With severe head injuries, there is a consensus among qualified experts that the

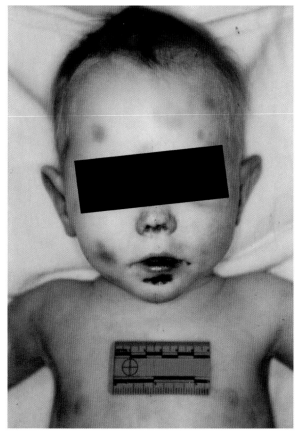

Figure 14 Facial bruises and lacerations. Reproduced with permission of J Lauridson, © 2004.

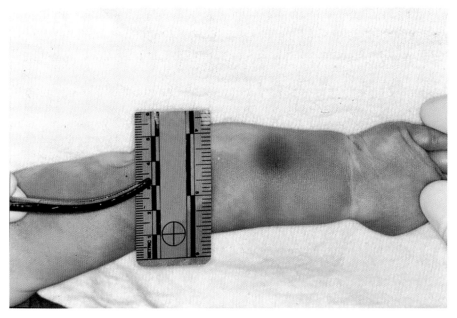

Figure 15 Grab mark on forearm, overlying radius fracture. Reproduced with permission of J Lauridson, © 2004.

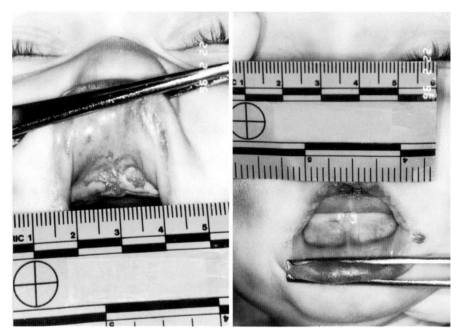

Figure 16 Healing damage to gums, not caused by postmortem. Reproduced with permission of J Lauridson, © 2004.

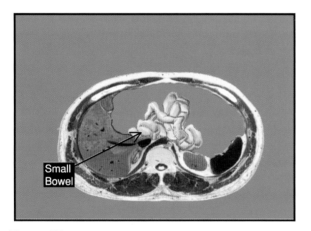

Figure 17 Anatomy of abdominal cavity. Reproduced with permission of J Lauridson, © 2004.

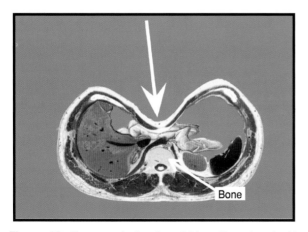

Figure 18 Nature and direction of blow. Reproduced with permission of J Lauridson, © 2004.

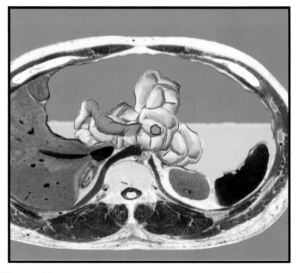

Figure 19 Peritonitis resulting from tear of the lower bowel. Reproduced with permission of J Lauridson, © 2004.

onset of symptoms would be immediate and even laypersons observing the child would recognize that the child is not "normal," but has suffered a serious injury. With bruises, internal injuries, and other forms of injury the symptoms may take some time to appear, but should be noticeable. For instance, when a child suffers a blow or compressive trauma sufficient to cause a bruise, it causes pain which should be obvious if a person is present. Fractures of the bone are painful not only when first caused, but remain persistently painful when the part of the body is manipulated in certain ways, often for several days.

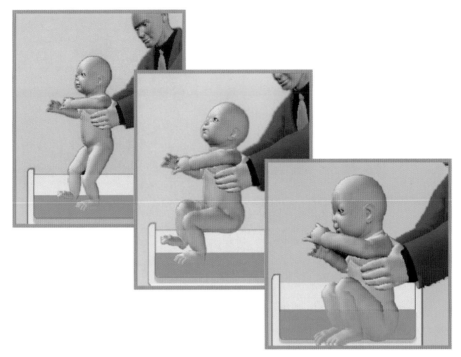

Figure 20 Diagram showing mechanism of immersion burn to infant. Reproduced with permission of J Lauridson, © 2004.

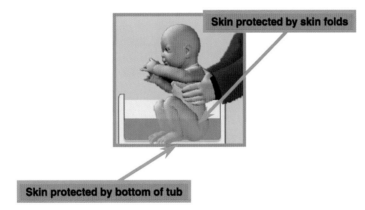

Figure 21 Diagram showing burned and spared areas of skin. Reproduced with permission of J Lauridson, © 2004.

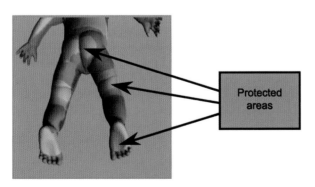

Figure 22 Actual injuries suffered by child. Reproduced with permission of J Lauridson, © 2004.

The medical forensic expert, if limited to only medical information gleaned from the nature of the injuries, can only express qualified opinions about when an injury was caused. Such an expert must be provided with information concerning what others have said about the child's behavior surrounding the apparent time when the child was injured. It is the application of known medical science to the facts in each case concerning when the child changed from apparently well to injured or symptomatic which allows the qualified expert to express a helpful opinion concerning timing of injuries in court. Developing

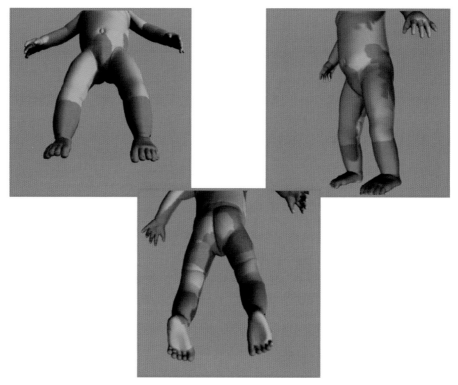

Figure 23 Several views of the burns. Reproduced with permission of J Lauridson, © 2004.

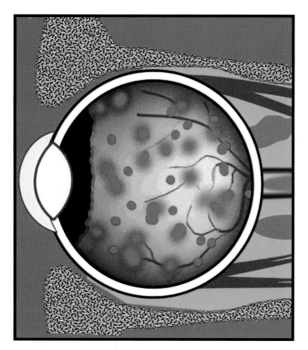

Figure 24 Pattern of retinal hemorrhages associated with severe angular/rotational trauma. Reproduced with permission of J Lauridson, © 2004.

a reliable opinion about timing in a closed-head injury case is particularly challenging, since there is a continuum of symptoms based on the severity of the head injury. In the most severe cases, where children suffer death or permanent brain impairment from the assault, forensic experts can be quite clear in stating that the child would have shown symptoms immediately and those symptoms would progress in a fairly predictable fashion over a short period of time. Even where the caretakers for the child are unwilling to describe what they saw, if they call for assistance from police or paramedics, the rapid deterioration of the child's condition is well documented from the first contact of trained professionals with the child through the hospital emergency room and through to the final outcome for the victim.

Identifying the Perpetrator

Identifying the person who caused injuries to a child is a complicated matter, which usually requires more than the forensic skill of the clinicians and pathologists involved in a case. However, the medical experts provide the most important assistance in the courtroom on the issue of identification. First, the forensic expert identifies the likely age of the injury by comparing the expected onset of symptoms with what was described by witnesses. Next, the expert narrows the "window" during which the injuries could have occurred by applying what is known about the onset of symptoms to the witnesses' descriptions of the victim's behavior. Finally, the expert may express the opinion that someone who was in the role of a caretaker for the child during that "window" of time was likely the cause of the victim's inflicted injury. The proponent of the evidence must

Hemorrhages in Orbit

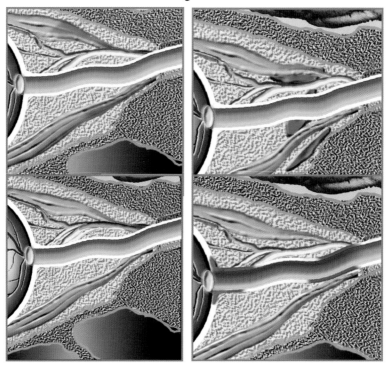

Figure 25 Images showing mechanism which causes optic nerve sheath hemorrhages anterior to the apex. Reproduced with permission of J Lauridson, © 2004.

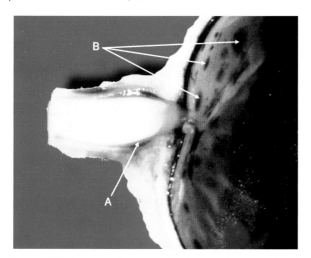

Figure 26 Autopsy photo showing both optic nerve sheath hemorrhages and retinal hemorrhages. Reproduced with permission of J Lauridson, © 2004.

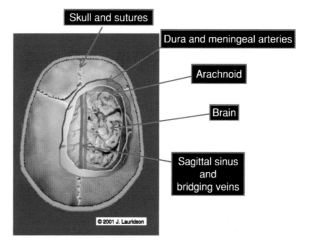

Figure 27 Computer diagram showing basic anatomy of the head from above. Reproduced with permission of J Lauridson, © 2004.

then invite the trier of fact to consider a number of factors to narrow the proof of exactly who the perpetrator was. The remainder of that proof comes from other witnesses who describe what happened to the child both before and after the child's health became compromised.

Figure 31 illustrates a simple timeline prepared by hand during the investigation when the injury occurred, based on descriptions of the child's

behavior from several witnesses, then illustrates that the fatal head injury must have been inflicted while the child was alone with only one person. **Figure 32** is a simple courtroom timeline suitable for use in a closing argument to illustrate what happened to the child victim, when it occurred, and who was with the child when the fatal injuries were inflicted.

Cases in which the perpetrator of abuse was a complete stranger to the child victim are quite rare.

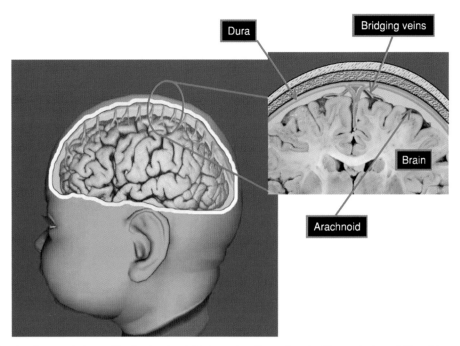

Figure 28 Lateral and coronal views of brain showing bridging veins. Reproduced with permission of J Lauridson, © 2004.

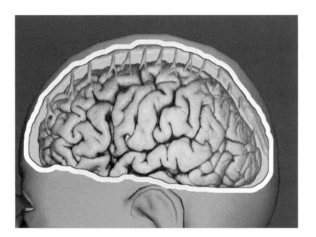

Figure 29 Mechanism of shearing of bridging veins during violent trauma. Reproduced with permission of J Lauridson, © 2004.

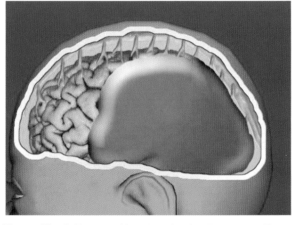

Figure 30 Collection of blood under the dura mater. Reproduced with permission of J Lauridson, © 2004.

In such cases, and assuming that the report to law enforcement authorities is made within a short time after the assault, processing the victim's body for traces of body fluids, hair, or clothing associated with the suspect may be helpful. The same is true for cases involving sexual abuse of children, although stranger abductions of children are even rarer than physical abuse or homicide committed by a complete stranger.

The Forensic Expert in Sexual Abuse Cases

Contrary to the intuitive beliefs of most members of the general public, most forms of sexual assault upon young children do not leave clear medically identified injuries which allow the forensic expert to say with certainty that the injury was inflicted by some other person. Even intercourse with young children does not always leave injuries. In addition, the younger the child, the more rapidly injuries to the anogenital area heal and since most reports are not made contemporaneously with the assault, it is often the case that no medical signs remain because of the rapid healing process. Those tasked with proving sexual abuse cases in the courtroom must use a forensic expert to explain why the absence of medically identifiable signs of injury does not rule out the possibility of the assault disclosed by the child.

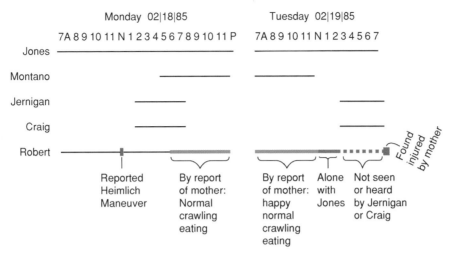

Figure 31 Investigative timeline created as each new witness is interviewed. Reproduced with permission of J Lauridson, © 2004.

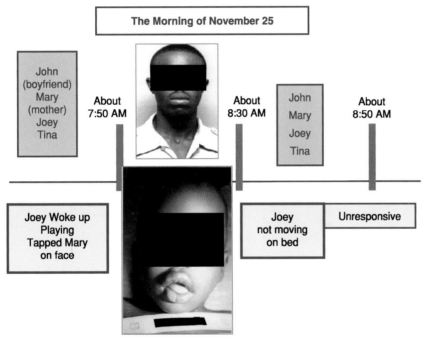

Figure 32 Courtroom timeline for closing argument. Reproduced with permission of J Lauridson, © 2004.

In general, obvious medical signs identifying sexual abuse as even a potential cause will be present in only one-third of valid cases. Those cases where the forensic expert is able to identify assault by another person as the only possible cause are fairly rare, and usually involve signs of repeated, penetrating trauma. As with physical injuries, courtroom persuasion depends upon illustration of the anatomy, especially focusing on the three-dimensional aspects of the anogenital structures. Quite often in cases involving penetrating injury to the hymen of a young girl, for instance, the claim made by the person accused of assaulting the child is that the child suffered some sort of accidental straddle injury. The well-trained expert can explain

that, unless the object which the child straddled could have penetrated the outer genital structures without leaving any sign of trauma, the inner damage to the hymen with no other injuries is inconsistent with the described straddle injury. Of course, whether the child was wearing clothing and/or a diaper is also critical in considering whether penetrating injury to the internal hymen could have occurred from the straddle injury. Illustrations used to make this point must show the difference between contact with external genital structures and penetrating trauma. **Figures 33–38** are simple computer-generated diagrams useful for illustrating various forms of sexual abuse of a young female child.

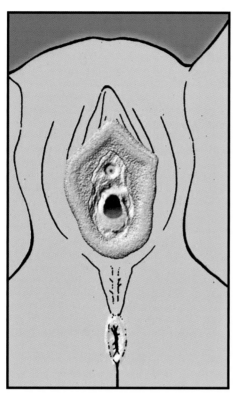

Figure 33 Basic genital anatomy, showing three-dimensional nature of structures. Reproduced with permission of J Lauridson, © 2004.

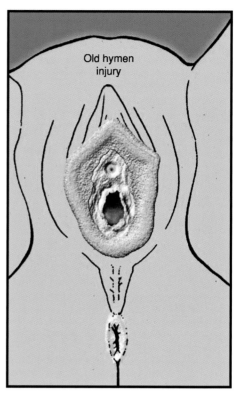

Figure 35 Diagram showing an old, healing injury to the hymen. Reproduced with permission of J Lauridson, © 2004.

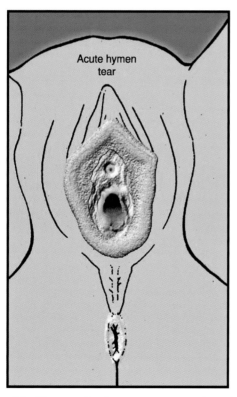

Figure 34 Diagram showing an acute tear of the hymen. Reproduced with permission of J Lauridson, © 2004.

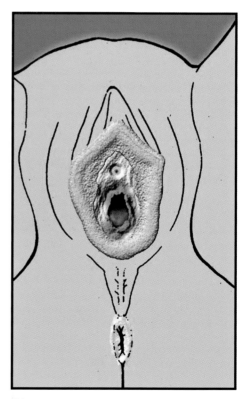

Figure 36 Redness or irritation of the hymen. Reproduced with permission of J Lauridson, © 2004.

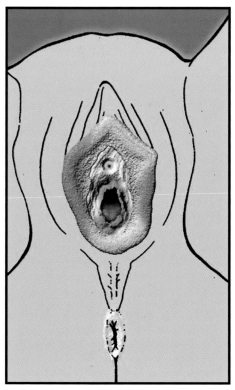

Figure 37 Redness or irritation of both labia and hymen. Reproduced with permission of J Lauridson, © 2004.

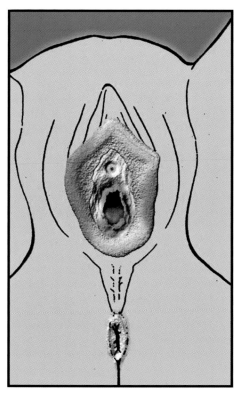

Figure 38 Hymenal injury along with anal redness and edema. Reproduced with permission of J Lauridson, © 2004.

Conclusion

Forensic medical experts have ushered in a novel era for attorneys tasked with proving all forms of child abuse in the courtroom. The collective expertise of expert pathologists in homicide cases, and of clinicians in all forms of abuse cases, is a powerful scientific basis for courtroom opinions explaining how the child was injured, when the child was injured, and in most cases the identity of the person who caused those injuries to the child. Persuasion in the courtroom now requires not only a sound scientific basis for opinions expressed, but also expert competence in educating the trier of fact concerning complex medical concepts through creative use of demonstrative materials. The combination of continued enhancement of the ability to identify the cause of injuries to children as well as to illustrate those concepts in courtrooms should result in providing justice for the youngest victims of crime.

See Also

Children: Legal Protection and Rights of Children; Sexual Abuse, Overview; Sexual Abuse, Epidemiology; **Imaging:** Radiology, Pediatric, Scintigraphy and Child Abuse

Further Reading

American Prosecutors Research Institute/National Center for Prosecution of Child Abuse (2004) *Investigation and Prosecution of Child Abuse*, 3rd edn. USA: Sage Publications.

Caffey J (1972) On the theory and practice of shaking infants. *American Journal of Diseases in Children* 124: 161–169.

Case ME, Graham MA, Corey Handy T, *et al.* (2001) Position paper on fatal abusive head injuries in infants and young children. *American Journal of Forensic Medicine and Pathology* 22: 112–122.

Kempe CH, Silverman FN, Steele BF, Droegemueller W, Silver HK (1962) The battered child syndrome. *Journal of the American Medical Association* 181: 17.

Lauridson J, Parrish R (2001) *Computer Graphics in Child Abuse and Neglect.* 13 APSAC Advisor 2, Spring 2001, pp. 14–16.

Lauridson J, Levin A, Parrish R (2001) *The Shaken Baby Syndrome: A Visual Overview.* version 2.0, CD-ROM. Ogden, UT: National Center on Shaken Baby Syndrome.

Levin AV (2000) Retinal haemorrhages: a review. In: David TJ (ed.) *Recent Advances in Paediatrics*, pp. 151–219. London: UK: Churchill-Livingstone.

Reece R and Ludwig S (eds.) (2001) *Child Abuse: Medical Diagnosis and Management*, 2nd edn. Philadelphia, PA: Lippincott, Williams & Wilkins.

Policy statement (2001) *Shaken Baby Syndrome: Rotational Cranial Injuries.* Technical report (T0039): policy statement. *Pediatrics* 108: 206–210.

Emotional Abuse

T Donald, Women's and Children's Hospital, North Adelaide, SA, Australia

Introduction

The psychological harm that occurs in all forms of serious child abuse, as well as that which exists as an entity in its own right, has only been systematically studied since the mid-1980s.

It is now accepted that its occurrence is central to the harm that serious abuse of any type produces in children as well as being the basis of the long-term effects of abuse.

The concepts, classification, identification, recognition, and intervention are still being researched and developed.

The material to be covered in this article includes:

- an overview of psychological/emotional maltreatment and its central role in the harm manifest by abused children
- epidemiological aspects of psychological/emotional maltreatment
- psychological/emotional maltreatment, child protection legislation and the legal system
- clinical aspects of psychological/emotional maltreatment, including its recognition and categorization.

General Concepts Related to Psychological/Emotional Abuse

The Central Position of Psychological Maltreatment in Any Type of Serious Child Abuse

Child abuse and neglect are phenomena that adversely affect children's development, and sometimes their physical well-being and survival.

Overall, most children who suffer child abuse are harmed by their primary carers, who are usually their parents. Children who experience sexual abuse invariably know the person who harmed them, but it is frequently an individual who does not have primary responsibility for their care.

When considering child abuse and neglect in general, the basic premise is that parents (the commonest primary carers of children) are responsible for ensuring that their interactions with their children are nurturing and neither abusive nor neglectful. In other words, that their care facilitates (at least) adequate growth and development of their child.

Parents may be stressed or disturbed and may find it difficult to achieve an adequate parenting role. The child for whom they are responsible may be temperamentally difficult or have a physical or psychological condition, which makes parenting arduous. The general societal expectation is that if parents are unable to manage their parenting role adequately it is their responsibility to seek assistance. If they do not, or they are unable to do so, others have the duty to intervene for the sake of the child as well as the parent.

Even though four categories of abuse are described (physical, sexual, psychological or emotional, and neglect), the harm resulting from abuse is of either a physical or psychological nature. For instance, most children who experience sexual abuse are not harmed physically. They do, however, manifest psychological harm, which is the critical issue and has significant and often serious effects over time.

Similarly, most children who are physically harmed through physical assault have no residual effects from the injuries. However, these children also suffer short- and long-term psychological effects.

Therefore, the harmful effects of abuse, manifest as the child grows and develops, emanate from the psychological damage inherent in the abusive acts and interactions.

In fact, the level of psychological maltreatment that occurs, irrespective of the abuse category present, is the best predictor of long-term adverse effects of any form of abuse.

When psychological harm occurs in association with other forms of abuse, the harmful incidents are either few in number but seriously traumatic (for example, because they threaten the child's survival) or alternatively the abuse occurs over a longer period of time, with the child being repeatedly exposed to the harmful behaviors of the perpetrator.

When children have been sexually abused the factors that will lead to psychological harm include the extent of trust betrayal experienced by the child and the level and seriousness of the threats used to ensure the compliance of the child with the abusive sexual acts.

The Emergence of Psychological Maltreatment as an Entity

With the development of a better understanding of the dynamics of physically abusive families, it became clear that physically abused children were often harmed in nonphysical ways. The harm seen in these children resulted from the damaging way in which they were parented and in the failure of their parents to meet their emotional needs.

Similarly, in children who had suffered sexual abuse, there were frequent signs of psychological or emotional damage that resulted indirectly from the harmful behavior of the abuser.

The concurrence of psychological abuse with physical or sexual abuse is now recognized during the evaluation of physically or sexually abused children. Its presence should always be sought to ensure optimal management of the child.

Psychological harm is now well accepted as an entity in its own right and the harmful patterns of interaction between caregivers and children, which cause emotional and psychological damage, have been identified.

As with all types of child maltreatment, parenting dysfunction is central to the problem of psychological abuse, but in this form it is at its most severe. Harm to the child's emotional/psychological health results from various combinations of damaging parental behaviors and lack of parental availability or responsiveness.

Children are vulnerable to any form of abuse, including psychological, by virtue of their position of differential power compared with their adult caregiver.

Emotional–Psychological Maltreatment and Child Abuse Statistics

In child abuse data collections, the lowest rate for reporting psychological maltreatment is in the 0–2-year age group and the highest in those children 12 years or older.

Also, psychological maltreatment is up to five times more commonly reported in lower-income groups. In part this is related to the higher reporting rates of all forms of abuse in these groups. Generally psychological maltreatment is likely to be underreported unless it is linked to other forms of abuse (for example, physical or sexual abuse). It is generally considered that, in higher socioeconomic groups, verbal and other "psychological" methods are used by choice to control others. Consequently, it seems likely that psychological maltreatment would be more common in this social group. It is not established as such because of the overall lower rate of notification of suspected abuse in this social group.

Some comparison of national statistics is possible using data from the USA, Canada, England, and Australia.

Statistical collection in England is centralized, and the statistical material can be gathered in a consistent manner, with each area of the country using the same definitions and interpreting information in the same way. However, a different system of "confirmation" of abuse is used and, because there is no mandatory reporting, many children who in other countries would enter the child protection system are managed in alternative ways.

The USA, Canada, and Australia are federal systems with individual states collecting their child protection data as they see fit. This may contribute to interstate variation in data but the overall outcome can generally be regarded as representative of the respective country as a whole.

English Data

In England children are designated as "in need" and may then be entered on the child protection register after a multidisciplinary case conference. Inclusion on the child protection register is the closest equivalent to the category "abuse substantiated," that is used in other countries. Overall, the rate of children to age 16 years on the child protection register is 4/10 000.

Since 1998 the proportion of children on the register under the category "emotional abuse" has been fairly stable at between 16% and 18%. Emotional abuse is most prevalent in the 5–15 year age group (21% of those on the child protection register are in this age range). In each age group neglect remains the most common reason for children to be on the register.

US Data

Child abuse statistics in the USA are compiled from individual states. The published figures from 2001 show that 3 million children were subject to a child protection investigation and 30% of these were considered to be victims (i.e., the abuse was considered substantiated). Children who were victims of psychological/emotional abuse comprised 6.8% of victims, compared with 59.2% who were considered victims of neglect. In 2001 the rate of psychological maltreatment was 0.9/1000 (a constant rate since 1997).

Canadian Data

The Canadian *Incidence Study of Reported Child Abuse and Neglect* relates to data collected from the Canadian provinces in 1998, when a total of 135 573 children were subject to a child protection investigation. Child maltreatment was substantiated in 45% of the investigations. Emotional maltreatment was one of the four primary categories (i.e., physical abuse, sexual abuse, neglect, and emotional maltreatment) and comprised 19% of the investigations.

Fifty-four percent of the investigations into suspected emotional maltreatment were substantiated (compared with a substantiation level of 34% for suspected physical abuse, 38% for sexual abuse, and 43% for neglect).

Australian Data

The Australian child protection statistics for the financial year 2002–2003 (July 1, 2002–June 30, 2003) show that over this year 198 355 notifications of suspected child abuse were made and 66 456 investigations finalized (these were the notifications considered necessary to investigate). The substantiation rate overall was 33.5% but was 60.4% for those notifications that were considered necessary to investigate.

Overall, emotional abuse comprised 34% of the substantiated cases, compared with 27.8% for neglect and physical abuse and 10.2% for sexual abuse.

Psychological Maltreatment and the Legal System

Following the first modern description of physical abuse, which occurred in the late 1960s, it became clear that specific child protection legislative provisions needed to be introduced to enable the state to intervene to protect children who had been abused or who were considered to be at high risk of abuse.

Child protection legislation also led to the establishing of state statutory agencies whose primary responsibility was and remains the assessment of children suspected of having been abused and their subsequent protection from further abuse, if needs be through court action.

Child Protection Legislation and Psychological/Emotional Maltreatment

The primary purposes of child protection legislation are to provide a legal basis for receiving notifications of suspected abuse; to authorize the assessment of children in whom abuse is suspected; to guarantee the ongoing safety of children, either through placement outside their family of origin or successful intervention within their family of origin, to ensure that further abuse does not occur; to ensure that, when necessary, legal intervention is appropriate and optimal; to organize the provision of appropriate therapeutic services directed at helping the child resolve the effects of abuse.

The central focus in the development of child abuse definitions is whether the primary emphasis should be on the maltreating behavior of the carers, or the consequences of the behavior on the child. For instance, sexual abuse is usually defined in terms of the maltreating behavior (the child being subjected to inappropriate sexual contact), whereas physical abuse is defined by the outcome for the child, namely physical injury.

Child Protection Legislation and the Categorization of Child Abuse

In most jurisdictions child protection legislation defines physical abuse, sexual abuse, emotional or psychological abuse, and neglect. Such categorization is not meant to imply that abuse of different forms does not occur in the same child; in fact more than one category of abuse can be identified in most abused children. Legal intervention in cases of child abuse in part depends on how closely the situation of suspected harm matches the abuse definitions incorporated in child protection legislation. Therefore, reports of child abuse tend to be assessed categorically, reflecting the requirements of legal definitions.

Categorization of abuse is also important in those jurisdictions where the legislation incorporates the concept of "mandatory reporting." Mandatory reporting refers to the legal requirements placed on certain individuals, usually professionals, to report to a specifically identified agency any child in whom the mandated notifier has reasonable grounds to believe abuse has occurred. Sometimes, the legislative requirement is broader, and includes those children in whom abuse is considered highly likely to occur. The categories and definitions of abuse present in child protection legislation give guidance to mandated notifiers in the identification and then the reporting of suspected abuse.

Whether or not child abuse (of any category) has occurred is not predicated on the intent by the abuser to harm the child. Therefore, legislative definitions of abuse do not include any intentional requirements. This does not mean that intentional acts of child abuse do not occur but intent is not required either for abuse to be suspected or confirmed. Generally speaking, the level of intent associated with abusive acts is an indication of the seriousness of the abuse.

Usually child protection legislation incorporates the concept that behaviors are abusive when they are outside the norm for the accepted community standards of parent–child interaction. This concept is particularly relevant when considering emotional or psychological maltreatment. The parental behavior involved may not be considered abusive when it occurs as an isolated event but is harmful when it is repetitive and occurs consistently.

The legislative emphasis in the definitions that form the basis for assessment and intervention in suspected cases of psychological maltreatment varies between:

- the evidence of harmful behaviors by parents
- the evidence of harm to the child
- a combination of both.

In most jurisdictions the legislation will require that to substantiate that psychological maltreatment has occurred, it is necessary to show both ill-treatment by the parents and evidence of harm in the child. This may limit the provision of intervention services to families where parental behaviors have the potential to harm but the effects on the child are not yet obvious.

Clinical Aspects of Psychological Maltreatment

The Development of a Suspicion That Psychological Maltreatment Is Present

The recognition of physical abuse depends on the presence of suspicious injury; sexual abuse is most often recognized after an allegation has been made by the child. Because psychological maltreatment has no external physical signs and children who experience it are not usually aware of the abusive nature of their parents' interactions with them, the suspicion that psychological abuse is occurring in its own right is based primarily on observations of, or reports of, harmful patterns of repetitive parent–child interaction.

Psychological maltreatment refers to the harm caused to a child's mental or emotional state by abusive caregiver behaviors. Generally, psychological maltreatment in its extreme forms is referring to harmful patterns of behavior that are repetitive and convey to children that they are worthless, and neither wanted nor loved. This produces a belief in children that their only value is in meeting their parent's needs.

A child is also indirectly psychologically harmed by serious threats imposed by another on the person with whom the child has established a primary relationship (usually the mother) and other loved ones. Such harm most commonly occurs in situations of family violence.

Those who work with children and families have been aware for many years that certain forms of parent–child interaction cause obvious distress and potential harm to children. The commonest and most obviously damaging parental behavior of this type recognized is verbal abuse, which ridicules and belittles a child.

When a child has been psychologically abused, the "evidence" of harm is not always apparent. Signs of harm include a deterioration in, or lower than expected, cognitive function, and an immaturity, and therefore vulnerability, in the child's capacity to manage social or emotional challenges competently. Children who have been psychologically harmed are not usually aware themselves of the harm to which they have been subject. Compared with the obvious injury of a physically abused child and the allegations made by sexually abused children that bring to light the harm they have suffered, the recognition of psychological maltreatment depends on observations of potentially harmful parental behavior linked with the manifestations of harm seen in the child.

The Terminology That Describes Inflicted Psychological Harm

In general terms, "emotion" refers to a mental feeling or affection, whereas "psychology" refers to the cognitive or volitional states of consciousness that affect the attitude or outlook of an individual. It has been suggested that emotional and psychological abuse should be distinguished from each other. However, there is a close interdependence between cognition and emotion and this distinction is no longer considered useful.

The most acceptable and appropriate term is considered to be psychological maltreatment or abuse.

A Framework for the Recognition and Definition of Psychological Maltreatment

When considering psychological maltreatment the following issues need to be addressed.

First, the parental behaviors that cause psychological or emotional harm in children do so when they are sustained and repetitive. They do not necessarily produce any significantly adverse effects when occurring intermittently in the context of an otherwise satisfactory parent–child relationship. Therefore, definitions of psychological maltreatment should incorporate the concept of threshold of harmful parenting behavior, above which intervention on the child's behalf should be considered and below which intervention should be directed at improving the parent–child relationship.

Second, some of the behavioral and developmental consequences of psychological maltreatment are seen in children in whom psychological maltreatment cannot be established. Therefore, such behaviors and developmental disturbances should only be attributed to psychological maltreatment when the harmful parental behaviors are apparent.

Psychological maltreatment indicates the presence of a harmful relationship between the parent and child. The American Professional Society on the Abuse of Children states that: "Psychological maltreatment means a repeated pattern of caregiver behavior or extreme incidents that convey to the caregiver's children that they are worthless, flawed, unloved, unwanted, endangered, or of value only in meeting another's needs."

This definition is linked by the American Professional Society on the Abuse of Children to six forms of psychological maltreatment:

1. spurning (verbal and nonverbal hostile rejection or degradation)
2. terrorizing (behavior that threatens or is likely to harm physically the child or place the child or the child's loved objects in danger)

3. exploiting/corrupting (encouraging the child to develop inappropriate behaviors)
4. denying emotional responsiveness (ignoring the child's need to interact, failing to express positive affect to the child, showing no emotions in interactions with the child)
5. isolating (denying the child opportunities for interacting/communicating with peers or adults)
6. mental, health, medical, or educational neglect (ignoring or failing to ensure provision of the child's needs).

These six categories of psychological maltreatment describe patterns of parental behavior which, when repetitive and severe, will significantly harm a child. Even though each of these categories of psychological maltreatment contains a continuum of seriousness of behavior, from minor to serious, they tend to be used to describe the most serious occurrences of psychological abuse, those in which legal intervention is usually considered necessary.

For lesser degrees of psychological maltreatment, when a mental health approach rather than legal intervention is indicated, an alternative system of categorization of psychological maltreatment may be found useful. This approach is particularly helpful in planning interventions. As previously mentioned, the carer behaviors that have been identified as emotionally/psychologically harmful to children have their most detrimental effect when they are repetitive and inflicted with intent to harm.

The severity of psychological maltreatment is then established by a combination of the intent to psychological abuse and the level of resulting harm in the child.

The least severe form of psychological abuse is not associated with intent and is not likely to lead to harm. For example, the isolation imposed on a child through parents resorting to time-out or grounding is not intended to cause harm and will not unless it becomes repetitive and intended to harm.

Moderately severe psychological abuse is associated with a significant level of malicious intent and is therefore associated with a high probability of harming the child.

Severe psychological maltreatment occurs when the repetitive, harmful acts are malicious and continue to occur with the abuser knowing that they are harmful. Inherent in the following alternative categories of psychological maltreatment is the lack of intent by the carers in the harmful acts they inflict upon their children. The lack of intent indicates that a mental health rather than legal intervention approach is more appropriate. If, in the process of intervention it is discovered that intent to harm is present in the maltreating behaviors then legal intervention must be considered.

The following five categories overlap with the six APSAC categories. They are given as follows.

1. Lack of emotional availability and responsiveness. Primary carers in this category often have significant mental health problems or are substance abusers. Therefore, they are not able to respond to their child's emotional needs adequately. It is important to note that sometimes, although one primary carer is unavailable, another is able to meet the child's needs. In such a situation there is no evidence of significant harm manifest by the child. Intervention should focus on the psychosocial circumstances of the potentially abusive carer.
2. Lack of positive attribution to or acknowledgment of the child. There is a significant level of denigration and rejection focused on the child. However in this context, it is not consistently present and is not associated with intent. When the child is perceived by the carer to be deserving of such treatment and it is persistent and pervasive, then legal intervention must be considered necessary.
3. Interactions with the child, which are developmentally inappropriate or inconsistent. These carer behaviors are typified by either the expectation that a child should be involved in matters that are more the responsibility of adults or by failing to acknowledge the need for a developing child to have appropriate freedom to participate in independent activities and explorations. Examples include carers who burden young children with their own emotional or psychosocial difficulties and carers who oversee their child to the extent that little developmentally appropriate exploration or self-learning is possible.
   When the developmentally inappropriate behaviors involve the exposure of the child to traumatic events (for example, repeated episodes of domestic violence), then the harm which invariably occurs indicates that the psychological abuse is serious and that legal intervention must be considered.
4. Lack of regard for the child's individuality and own psychological boundaries. In its most severe form this category of maltreatment includes illness induction or symptom fabrication, so-called Munchausen syndrome by proxy. The harm associated with this degree of psychological maltreatment invariably indicates that legal intervention is necessary. However, when physical or psychological symptoms are exaggerated or carers become preoccupied with their child's health and well-being, to the detriment of the child's emotional and psychological state, then a mental health

approach is appropriate. The transition point between these two extremes occurs when the carer does not respond to planned intervention, persistently and vigorously exposes the child to repeated medical assessments, and insists on lines of medical management not indicated by the child's clinical condition.

5. Disregard for the child's need for social adaptation. When a carer fails to supervise a child adequately so that the child is adversely affected by corrupting and other missocializing experiences, nonlegal intervention may be appropriate if the carer accepts the inappropriateness of his/her acts of omission. However, active corruption of children (for example, by having them involved in overtly criminal behavior) requires legal intervention.

Stepwise Approach for Managing Suspected Psychological/Emotional Maltreatment

1. Establish the presence of harmful/potentially harmful carer behaviors:
   a. reported
   b. directly observed.
2. Define the nature of the carer–child interaction and the adequacy of the level of physical and psychological care in the context of the harmful/potentially harmful carer behaviors.
3. Consider the presence/absence of intent to harm in the harmful/potentially harmful care behaviors:
   a. intent to harm present – notification to statutory authority
   b. intent to harm absent – mental health-based management.
4. Mental health management:
   a. establish the level of carers' acceptance of their harmful/potentially harmful behaviors towards their child
   b. review the child's need for protection and the psychological adequacy of the child's care environment
   c. formulate a program of intervention.

See Also

Children: Legal Protection and Rights of Children; Physical Abuse; Sexual Abuse, Overview; Sexual Abuse, Epidemiology

Further Reading

APSAC (1995) *Psychosocial Evaluation of Suspected Psychological Maltreatment in Children and Adolescents. Practice Guidelines.* Chicago, IL: American Professional Society on the Abuse of Children.

Binggeli N, Hart S, Brassard M (2001) *Psychological Maltreatment of Children; the APSAC Study Guides 4.* Thousand Oaks, CA: Sage.

Brassard M, Hardy D (1997) Psychological maltreatment. In: Helfer M, Kempe R, Krugman R (eds.) *The Battered Child,* pp. 392–412. Chicago, IL: University of Chicago Press.

Brassard M, Germain B, Hart S (eds.) *Psychological Maltreatment of Children and Youth.* Elmsford, NY: Pergamon Press.

Cicchetti D, Nurcombe B (eds.) (1991) *Development and Psychopathology* 3: 1–124.

Garbarino J, Guttman E, Seeley JW (1986) *The Psychologically Battered Child.* San Francisco, CA: Jossey Bass.

Glaser D (1993) Emotional abuse. In: Hobbs C, Wynne J (eds.) *Child Abuse,* pp. 251–267. London: Baillière Tindall.

Hart S, Brassard M, Karlson H (1996) Psychological maltreatment. In: Berliner L, Briere J, Bulkley J, Jenny C, Reid T (eds.) *The APSAC Handbook on Child Abuse and Neglect,* pp. 72–89. London: Sage.

Iwaniec D (1995) *The Emotionally Abused and Neglected Child: Identification, Assessment, and Intervention.* Chichester, UK: Wiley.

O'Hagan KP (1993) *Emotional and Psychological Abuse of Children.* Buckingham, UK: Open University Press.

Physical Abuse

C Jenny, Brown Medical School, Providence, RI, USA

Introduction

Physical abuse of children is a common problem worldwide. The definition of physical abuse may vary from one culture or community to another. For example, physical punishment of children is outlawed in some countries, while other countries have few barriers to families administering draconian punishments to their children. In countries with organized child protection laws and systems, the medical examination and documentation of inflicted injuries to children are important for the children's protection. The recognition and documentation of abusive injuries are needed in cases involving living children as well as in child homicide cases. In addition to forensic pathologists, many other types of physicians and nurses require expertise in caring for abused children.

The World Health Organization (WHO) defines the physical abuse of a child as "that which results in actual or potential physical harm from an interaction

Table 1 Risk factors identified in studies of physical child abuse

Victim characteristics
Male sex
Premature birth
Age under 4 years
Minority race
Physical or mental handicap
Family characteristics
Poverty
Unmarried parents
Unrelated male living in household
Maternal depression
Intimate partner violence between adults in household
Young maternal age
Offender characteristics
Male sex
Unemployment
Substance abuse
History of abuse in childhood

or lack of interaction, which is reasonable within the control of a parent or person in a position of responsibility, power, or trust." WHO considers children to be human beings below the age of 18 years. They estimate that worldwide 57 000 children under 15 years of age die yearly as a result of child abuse. The homicide rate for children under 5 years of age is twice that of children 1–14 years of age. Nonfatal abuse occurs much more frequently. Abuse can lead to disabling physical and mental illness. The cost to society of caring for victims of childhood physical abuse has never been estimated.

While no "profile" of child abusers can be assumed, several risk factors for victimization have been identified. **Table 1** includes generally accepted epidemiologic factors that have been identified to be associated with increased risk of physical abuse.

This article will address the general principles in the diagnosis of physical abuse, including taking a history, performing physical examinations, recommended radiologic examination, photodocumentation, and medical chart documentation. Following this, abusive injuries will be discussed by organ system. Finally, the role of medical personnel in the multidisciplinary evaluation of child abuse will be discussed, and the need for cooperation and communication between disciplines will be emphasized.

Medical and Forensic Evaluation of Cases of Suspected Physical Abuse

The Medical History

General principles It is important to obtain a careful medical history in any case of suspected physical abuse. Generally, caretakers are interviewed separately. For medical professionals, a caring, nonjudgmental approach should be used. Since many medical conditions can mimic child physical abuse, the history must be comprehensive. The components of the complete history are as follows. At the end of the interview, caretakers should be given the opportunity to ask questions and to express their opinions about what they think is wrong with the child.

History of the presenting symptoms or injuries The history of the current event should begin before the child became symptomatic. The time previous to the onset of symptoms is documented, including the child's activities, level of alertness, sleep patterns, meals, bowel movements, vomiting, and mood. Was some precipitating event noted, such as a fall, a tantrum, or a sudden change in affect or activity level? When was the child last noted to be completely normal? What was the first change noted? How have symptoms changed over time?

When documenting the period after the child became symptomatic, the interviewer should review each change in status and document the surrounding events. Where was the child when changes in status occurred? Who was with the child? What was the child doing? How was the child functioning? This minute-by-minute history of every aspect of the child's life during this time can lead to important information about what actually happened to the child.

Past medical history The entire medical history should be reviewed, starting with the mother's pregnancy. Was the pregnancy planned? Was the pregnancy welcomed? Did the mother consider terminating the pregnancy? A history of the mother's symptoms and illnesses during pregnancy as well as any complications should be documented, as well as her use of medications, drugs, and alcohol, or other toxic exposures. Record mother's weight gain during pregnancy and when and if prenatal care was sought.

The labor and delivery history is next obtained, including complications, procedures, Apgar scores, need for resuscitation at delivery, problems in the newborn nursery, length of hospitalization, and birth weight.

The child's entire medical history should be reviewed, including illnesses, growth, immunizations, medications, and allergies.

Emotional, behavioral, and developmental history The course of the child's development, including school performance and achievement, can influence the evaluation of presenting signs and symptoms.

Delayed development may be a sign of underlying illness, previous injury, or environmental deprivation. The appropriateness of the child's emotional attachment and bonding should be explored. Behavioral problems or disorders can increase the risk of abuse, or may be the result of ongoing abuse.

Nutritional history   Take a history of regular intake, type of feeding (if infant), diet characteristics, and food intolerance.

Family history   It is important to record a family history of unusual illness. Include a history of genetic or inherited disorders, premature deaths and sudden infant deaths, fetal wastage, consanguinity, unusual bleeding problems, brittle bones or tendency to fracture easily, poor wound healing, early teeth or hearing loss, and mental retardation.

Social history   The level of family functioning should be assessed, including employment, economic stress, substance abuse, marital dysfunction, criminal history, and domestic violence. Potential family stressors should be identified, and sources of family support documented, including financial resources, extended family support, housing, and community support.

Environmental history   While the medical practitioner would rarely conduct a home visit, others can provide information about the child's environment, including temperature, unsafe conditions, exposure to toxins such as lead or carbon monoxide, overcrowding, the safety and quality of housing, the general level of cleanliness and order, and adequacy of the home's condition.

Physical Examination

A careful head-to-toe examination is critical, including vital signs, measurement of height, weight, head circumference, height-to-weight ratio, and body mass index. Description of the child's affect and state of consciousness is noted. As part of a good physical exam, a careful genital and anal exam is necessary. In suspected head trauma cases, an indirect ophthalmoscope examination done by an ophthalmologist is indicated. Any suspicious skin lesions are carefully documented and photographed. When bruising is noted, serial examinations over time are required to document progression of the lesions. A rape kit is performed if sexual assault is suspected.

It is important not to miss physical findings that might not be obvious, including scalp trauma, pulled hair, bruising behind the ears or of the pinna, blood or effusions behind the tympanic membrane, scleral lesions, trauma to the pharynx, mouth, teeth or frenula, crepitus over ribs or long bones, or signs of abdominal or chest trauma.

Review previous growth parameters if the child's growth is abnormal to aid in diagnosing chronic neglect or failure to thrive.

Radiologic Studies

A radiographic skeletal survey should be done in all cases of suspected physical abuse in children under 2 years of age. In children between 2 and 5 years of age, it is less useful, although may be used when occult fractures are suspected. It is not likely to be useful in children over 5 years of age. Table 2 lists the parameters of an adequate skeletal survey. Repeat skeletal surveys done 2 weeks after the initial survey may increase the yield of occult fractures diagnosed, because some very new fractures are sometimes difficult to visualize radiographically.

Radionuclide bone scans may be a useful adjunct to skeletal survey, but should not replace the skeletal survey. Any positive findings should be confirmed with radiography.

Computed tomography (CT) is the modality of choice for the initial evaluation of suspected abusive head trauma. Magnetic resonance imaging (MRI) should be done at 5–7 days postinjury because it is more sensitive and specific for diagnosing subacute and chronic head injuries. Techniques useful in diagnosing abusive head trauma include T_1 and T_2 weighting with proton-density or inversion-recovery sequences, gradient echo sequences, and diffusion weighted images.

Table 2   Parameters of the skeletal survey

Required images	
Views of appendicular skeleton	*Views of axial skeleton*
Humeri (AP)	Thorax (AP and lateral)
Forearms (AP)	Pelvis (AP; including mid and lower
Hands (oblique PA)	lumbar spine)
Femurs (AP)	Lumbar spine (lateral)
Lower legs (AP)	Cervical spine (lateral)
Feet (AP)	Skull (frontal and lateral)

Technique
   Use high-resolution film (spatial resolution of at least 10 line pairs per millimeter)
   Screen/film speed not to exceed 200
   Low kVp (bone technique)
   Single emulsion or special film-screen combination

Reproduced with permission from American Academy of Pediatrics Section on Radiology (2000) Diagnostic imaging of child abuse. *Pediatrics* 105: 1346.
AP, anteroposterior; PA, posteroanterior.

Table 3 Laboratory evaluation of suspected physical abuse

Test	Purpose
Blood count	Screens for anemia and unsuspected disease, helps determine cardiovascular status
Urinalysis	Screens for occult renal trauma
Liver function studies	Screen for occult liver trauma
Amylase	Screens for occult pancreatic trauma
Calcium, phosphorus, vitamin D	Screen for metabolic bone disease
Coagulation studies	Determines coagulation status. May include partial thrombin time, prothrombin time, platelet count, bleeding time, tests for activated coagulation
Urine organic acids	Screens for metabolic disease in cases of suspected head injury
Electrolytes and pH	Determine fluid status

Trauma to the thorax and abdomen is best imaged by CT. Upper gastrointestinal studies and abdominal ultrasound may be useful in specific situations.

Laboratory Evaluation

When physical abuse is suspected, certain laboratory tests will be helpful in confirming the diagnosis, detecting occult injury, and ruling out medical conditions that might mimic abuse. **Table 3** lists these tests and describes the role of each test. The list is not exhaustive. Individual cases may require other diagnostic tests, depending on the clinical presentation.

Photodocumentation of Physical Abuse

When physical abuse is suspected, liberal use of photographs of visible lesions is an important part of the medical and forensic work-up. Digital cameras, film cameras, and video cameras have all been shown to be useful. It is important that the photographer has adequate equipment and training before taking the responsibility of documenting abusive injuries.

All photographs should be carefully identified and labeled, including the time and date of the image. Using multiple exposures and magnification levels can increase the yield of useful photographs. Size and color standards should be included in the field. Images should be labeled with the name of the subject, as well as with other identifying data. On anatomic images, a referential body part should be included to orient the viewer.

Generating the Medical Record

Generating a complete record is an important part of the forensic work-up in cases of suspected child abuse. Histories should be carefully documented. The source of the information recorded should be noted. Direct quotes from the victim can be archived in the record. Drawings of physical findings should supplement physical descriptions. A carefully constructed and preserved record can be helpful in substantiating abuse cases.

Physical Injuries Resulting from Abuse

Any injury can be the result of an accident, and any injury can be the result of physical abuse. However, certain types of injury have been noted to be more frequently caused by child abuse. In evaluating the cause of any injury, the history, the forces involved, and the circumstances of the injury should be carefully evaluated. The following injuries will be discussed by body region.

Abusive Head Trauma

Trauma to the head and central nervous system is the most fatal type of child abuse, especially in infants and small children. Several types of trauma may involve the head and central nervous system.

Traumatic alopecia and subgaleal hemorrhage
Traumatic alopecia results from traction or pulling on the hair (**Figure 1**). The child is left with bald

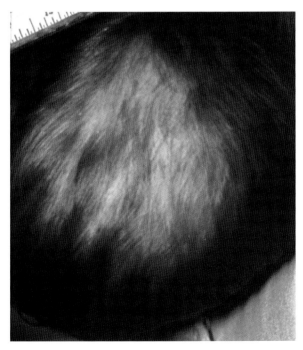

Figure 1 Traumatic alopecia resulting from traction or pulling on the hair.

patches on the scalp where the hair grows back readily. Small petechiae may be seen at the site of the avulsion of hair roots. Traction on the scalp can also cause bleeding under the scalp (subgaleal hemorrhage) and separation of the aponeurosis through accumulation of blood. In children, large amounts of blood can be lost into the subgaleal space, leading to significant anemia.

Epidural hematoma Epidural hematomas in children are more likely caused by accidental trauma. About 5% of epidurals are the result of child abuse. An epidural can occur even in the absence of skull fracture because of the malleability of the developing skull. Blunt trauma can cause significant in-bending of the skull, damaging the vessels below the skull. The onset of symptoms following an epidural hematoma may be delayed hours to days. Epidural hematomas are commonly the cause of "lucent intervals" after head injury, followed by delayed development of serious symptoms.

Subdural hematoma Subdural hematomas can be caused by blunt trauma and/or rotational acceleration and deceleration of the head (**Figure 2**).

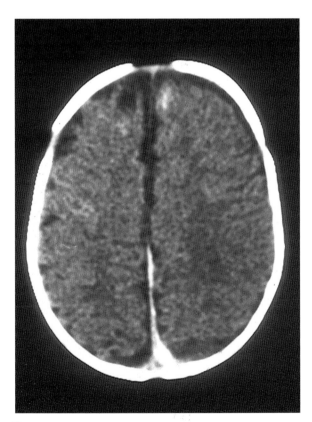

Figure 2 Subdural hematomas from abusive head trauma seen on magnetic resonance imaging of the head.

In infants and small children, subdural hematomas are commonly the result of inflicted injuries. The bleeding occurs between the dura mater and the arachnoid layer of the meninges. Rotation of the head causes rupture of delicate vessels between the two layers. Acute hematomas can be quickly resorbed, or can lead to the formation of hygromas in the subdural space, which can lead to the formation of chronic subdural effusions of high-density, protein-rich fluid. In infants, chronic subdurals can expand because of the plasticity of the skull, leading to rapid growth of the head (**Figure 3**).

Subdural hematomas caused by abusive head trauma are more likely to extend into the midline falx cerebri. Posterior fossa subdurals are also more common in inflicted injuries.

Preexisting subdural hematomas are known to be susceptible to rebleeding with fairly minor trauma. These rebleeds rarely lead to a change in the child's neurologic status unless a large amount of fluid accumulates, leading to increased intracranial pressure.

Dating subdural hematomas by imaging studies is problematic. Often very acute subdurals can appear on CT and MRI scans as fluids of two different densities because of the separation of formed and liquid components of blood.

Abusive brain injuries Brain injury can result from abusive head trauma. Diffuse brain injuries range from concussion (a change in physiologic and neurologic function without obvious changes on imaging studies) to diffuse axonal injury (disruption of axons in the subcortical white matter). Diffuse axonal injury can be detected postmortem using specific stains for beta-amyloid protein precursors.

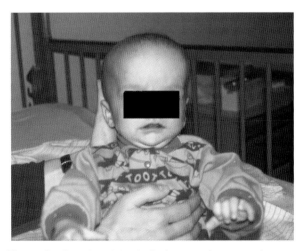

Figure 3 Chronic subdural effusions causing unusual expansion of the infant skull.

Cerebral edema causes secondary injury to the brain as intracranial pressure increases, decreasing cortical blood flow. After brain injury, a cascade of neurotoxic chemicals is released from the injured tissue, leading to further brain injury.

In addition to diffuse injuries, focal contusions and hemorrhage can occur in the brain tissue. A common finding in abusive head trauma is "gliding contusions" or "gray–white-matter shearing tears" (**Figure 4**). These lesions occur at the gray–white-matter junction, often in the cortical frontal lobes. The lesions are thought to be caused by the different tissue densities moving at different rates during rotational acceleration.

Recent research has focused on the changes in the cervical cord seen after violent shaking of infants. Subtle signs of axonal injury can sometimes be found in the cord at the cervicomedullary junction, where the brainstem becomes the spinal cord (**Figure 5**). These injuries are hypothesized to cause apnea that leads to severe, diffuse cerebral edema and extensive brain damage in infants who have been violently shaken. To diagnose these injuries, the brain and upper spinal cord must be removed *en bloc* at autopsy, and section must be taken through the junction for microscopic examination.

Shaken-baby syndrome   Shaking as a mechanism for causing brain injury has been reported in the literature on many occasions. In spite of a wealth of clinical data that exists, there is some doubt whether shaking alone can cause brain injury, or whether impact is also required. Newer anatomic testing devices and computer models have reaffirmed the dangers of shaking. Certainly, shaking and impact are both likely to be dangerous in infants and young children. By using the term "abusive head trauma," the mechanism of injury is not presumed. The concept of shaken-baby syndrome remains useful, especially in the context of child abuse prevention.

Shaking is thought to be the mechanism of formation of the extensive retinal hemorrhages often found in infant victims of abusive head injury (**Figure 6**). The hemorrhages characteristically involve multiple layers of the retina and extend throughout the retinal surface out to the ora serrata. These hemorrhages are

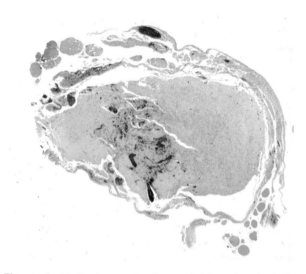

Figure 5 Photomicrograph of axonal injury found at the cervicomedullary junction in an infant who was violently shaken.

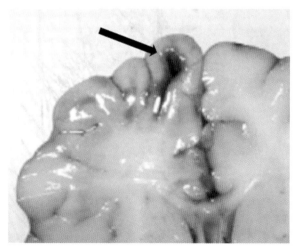

Figure 4 Gliding contusions (gray–white-matter shearing tears) of the brain tissue found at autopsy in an abused infant (arrow).

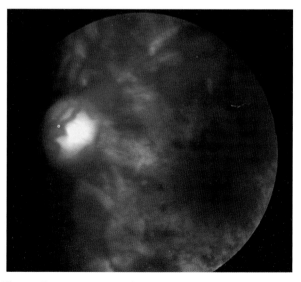

Figure 6 Extensive retinal hemorrhages characteristic of the findings in shaken-baby syndrome.

not isolated to the posterior pole of the retina alone. Detachment or folding of the retina can also occur, leading to retinoschisis.

Abusive Skin Injuries

Bruises Injuries to the skin and soft tissues are common manifestations of abuse. Accidental bruises are more likely to be located on the lower arms and legs of children. Bruising is rarely found on nonabused infants who are not yet pulling to standing. The appearance of bruises is influenced by many factors, including the depth of the bruise, the amount of blood pooling to form the bruise, the thickness of the skin in the bruised area of the body, and the status of circulation to the body part. Yellow coloration is not likely to be seen in a bruise before it is 18 h old.

Pattern marks Abusive skin injuries will sometimes resemble the object used to inflict the injury (**Figure 7**). Hand prints can appear as the outline of the hand on the child's face or body. Careful measurement and examination of pattern marks can lead to the discovery of the offending object in the child's environment.

Burns Burns are often associated with child abuse or neglect. Immersion burns are the most common type. Typically the child will show clear lines of demarcation with few splash marks (**Figure 8**). A careful investigation, including measuring the water temperature and flow rate of the water at the scene of the event, is needed to analyze the purported mechanism of the burn. Often abusive scald burns appear in a "stocking or glove" pattern on the affected extremity.

Hot objects, such as lighters, cigarettes, or kitchen implements, can be used to inflict burns on children, leaving a pattern of the hot object on the skin (**Figure 9**).

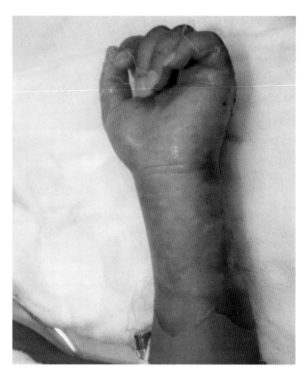

Figure 8 Abusive immersion burns. Note the clear demarcation between burned and normal skin, and the absence of splash marks.

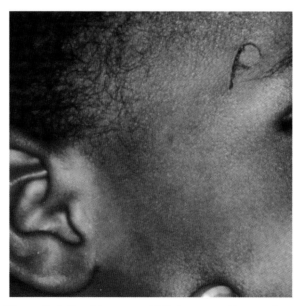

Figure 9 Inflicted burn on a child's face caused by applying a hot cigarette lighter.

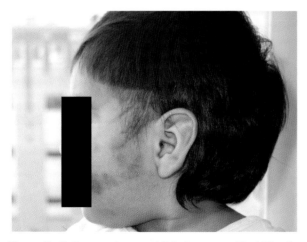

Figure 7 Pattern marks on a child's face caused by hitting the child with a hand.

Abdominal and Chest Injuries

Hitting, kicking, or throwing a child can cause injuries to the thorax and abdomen. The mortality rate from abusive injuries to these body regions is generally higher than it is in accidental injuries. Liver lacerations or contusions, splenic lacerations, pancreatic injury, and stomach and bowel lacerations and hematomas have all been described as resulting from abuse. Kidney and adrenal injuries are less commonly seen. All these injuries can be "silent" and not obvious on initial evaluation. A careful trauma work-up is important in cases of suspected abuse.

Lung contusions and lacerations, pericardial hemorrhage, ruptured aorta or vena cava, disruption of the thoracic duct, and cardiac contusion can all be caused by abuse. Commotio cordis, the onset of serious cardiac arrhythmia caused by a blunt impact to the chest, can be a cause of sudden death following abuse.

Abusive Fractures

Any type of fracture can be a result of abuse or accidental injury. Multiple fractures and fractures of different ages would suggest the possibility of abuse in children with normal bones and no history of major trauma.

Some types of fracture are more specific for abuse than others. "High-risk" fractures include the following.

Subperiosteal new bone formation The periosteum of the long bones of infants is somewhat loosely attached to the bone. Traction on the long bone can cause "stripping" and elevation of the periosteum leads to calcification of the tissue below the periosteum (**Figure 10**). Periosteal elevation can also occur in any area of increased bone metabolism. In the first 6 months of life, diffuse periosteal elevation can be seen in the absence of trauma.

Classic metaphyseal lesions The most vulnerable part of the developing skeleton in young children is the zone of provisional calcification in the metaphyses of the long bones. This is an area of active growth, where calcified tissue is being laid down in the primary spongiosa. Pulling, twisting, shaking, and mishandling of infants and toddlers cause typical "bucket-handle" or "corner" fractures at the metaphysis (**Figures 10** and **11**). These fractures actually represent planar fractures through this growing tissue.

Rib fractures Accidental rib fractures are rare in infants and young children. When abuse occurs, rib

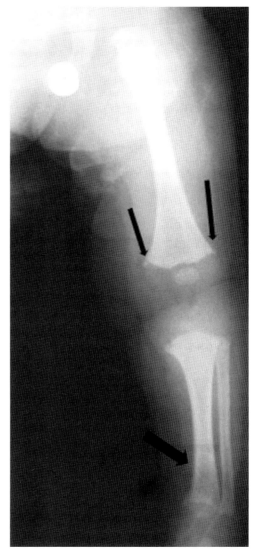

Figure 10 Subperiosteal new bone formation of the tibia resulting from abuse (thicker arrow); classic metaphyseal lesions presenting as "corner fractures" (thin arrows).

fractures are commonly found laterally and posteriorly on the ribcage. Abusive rib fractures usually result from squeezing of the chest. Anterior–posterior compression of the chest often causes the ribs to break where the rib heads articulate with the vertebrae and where the lateral curvature of the ribs occurs.

Acute rib fractures are difficult to visualize by radiographs. Alternatively, healing and the development of callus reveal infant rib fractures more easily (**Figure 12**). Skeletal surveys repeated 2 weeks after the initial evaluation for abuse will often yield healing fractures that were missed on the initial radiographs.

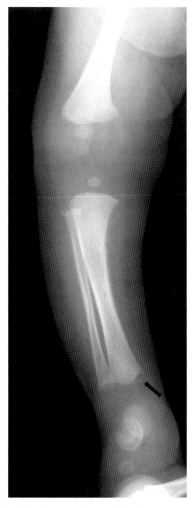

Figure 11 Classic metaphyseal lesion presenting as a "bucket-handle fracture".

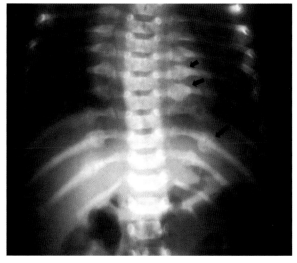

Figure 12 Multiple healing rib fractures seen on a skeletal survey (some of the many fractures are indicated by arrows).

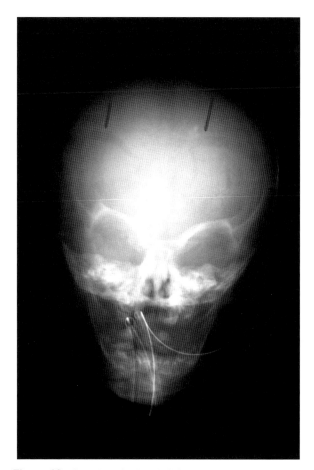

Figure 13 Complex abusive skull fractures.

Sternal and scapular fractures Again, fractures of the sternum and scapula are rare in infants and young children, but both types of fracture can be seen associated with other types of abusive fracture to the upper arm and shoulder girdle. The acromion process of the sternum is particularly vulnerable to fracture.

Vertebral body fractures These fractures are more likely seen in children who have suffered abusive head trauma. The mechanism of injury is thought to be from hyperextension and hyperflexion of the spine during vigorous shaking, or from slamming the child down in a sitting position on to a hard surface.

Complex skull fractures Simple, linear parietal and occipital skull fractures are commonly the result of minor household trauma in infants and toddlers. The infant skull is quite plastic and in-bends readily. Complex, multiple, diastatic, or depressed fractures are less likely to occur after a simple fall and are more suggestive of abuse (**Figure 13**).

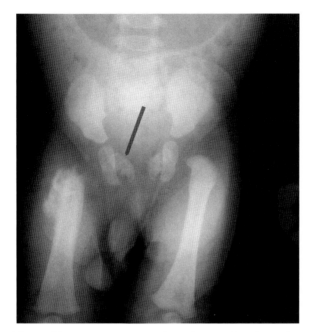

Figure 14   Pubic rami fracture (arrow) caused by abuse of an infant. Note the displaced femur fracture also present on the left.

Pelvic fracture   Pelvic fractures are rare in infants and toddlers in the absence of major trauma. In abuse, fractures of the pubic rami can be seen as a result of excessive pressure on the pelvis during diapering (**Figure 14**).

The Multidisciplinary Evaluation of Child Abuse

Diagnosing abuse is a complex and difficult task. Cooperation between professionals in different disciplines is of great value. Physicians are often the first to suspect that a child has been abused. The physician has the unique opportunity to perform a careful study of history and physical examination. Physicians should be aware of medical conditions which are likely to mimic abuse and to be misdiagnosed as abuse. However, the physician's role is limited to the medical setting. Law enforcement officers and child protection workers are charged with the investigation of families and homes to ensure a child's safety and to determine whether or not a crime has been committed. The physician must communicate his or her findings and medical opinions to other professionals to facilitate the investigation.

Many communities have recognized the value of the multidisciplinary child protection team meeting to enhance communication between professionals. By having an opportunity to discuss complex cases, all views are aired and potential strengths and weaknesses of an investigation can be determined. It is important that physicians cooperate with other agencies to assure the safety of children.

See Also

Children: Emotional Abuse; Sexual Abuse, Overview; Sexual Abuse, Epidemiology; Non-inflicted Causes of Death; **Injury, Fatal and Nonfatal:** Documentation; Burns and Scalds

Further Reading

Beaty JH (1997) Orthopedic aspects of child abuse. *Current Opinion in Pediatrics* 9: 100–103.
Chapman S, Hall CM (1997) Non-accidental injury or brittle bones. *Pediatric Radiology* 27: 106–110.
Duhaime AC, Christian CW, Rorke LB, Zimmerman RA (1998) Nonaccidental head injury in infants – the "shaken-baby syndrome." *New England Journal of Medicine* 338: 1822–1829.
Kini N, Lazoritz S (1998) Evaluation for possible physical or sexual abuse. *Pediatric Clinics of North America* 45: 205–219.
Kleinman PK (1998) *Diagnostic Imaging of Child Abuse,* 2nd edn. St. Louis, MI: Mosby.
Kocher MS, Kasser JR (2000) Orthopaedic aspects of child abuse. *Journal of the American Academy of Orthopaedic Surgeons* 8: 10–20.
Lonergan GJ, Baker AM, Morey MK, Boos SC (2003) From the archives of the AFIP. Child abuse: radiologic-pathologic correlation. *Radiographics* 23: 811–845.
Nimkin K, Kleinman PK (2001) Imaging of child abuse. *Radiologic Clinics of North America* 39: 843–864.
Peck MD, Priolo-Kapel D (2002) Child abuse by burning: a review of the literature and an algorithm for medical investigations. *Journal of Trauma-Injury Infection and Critical Care* 53: 1013–1022.
Reece RM, Ludwig S (2001) *Child Abuse. Medical Diagnosis and Management,* 2nd edn. Philadelphia, PA: Lippincott/Williams and Wilkins.
Schwartz AJ, Ricci LR (1996) How accurately can bruises be aged in abused children? Literature review and synthesis. *Pediatrics* 97: 254–257.
Stephenson T (1997) Ageing of bruising in children. *Journal of the Royal Society of Medicine* 90: 312–314.
The Ophthalmology Child Abuse Working Party (1999) Child abuse and the eye. *Eye* 13: 3–10.
Wardinsky TD, Vizcarrondo FE, Cruz BK (1995) The mistaken diagnosis of child abuse: a three-year USAF Medical Center analysis and literature review. *Military Medicine* 160: 15–20.
Wissow LS (1995) Child abuse and neglect. *New England Journal of Medicine* 332: 1425–1431.

Sexual Abuse, Overview

B Marc and M Nathanson, Compiegne Hospital, Compiegne, France

Introduction

Very few areas of pediatrics have expanded so rapidly in clinical importance in recent years as that of sexual abuse of children. A risk assessment conducted for the 2002 *World Report on Violence and Health* has shown that 8% of male and 25% of female children up to age 18 experience sexual abuse of some kind. Other studies have suggested that approximately 1% of children experience some form of sexual abuse each year, resulting in the sexual victimization of 12–25% of girls and 8–10% of boys by age 18. Children may be sexually abused by family members or nonfamily members and are more frequently abused by males. Boys may be victimized nearly as often as girls, but may not be as likely to disclose the abuse. Adolescents are perpetrators in at least 20% of reported cases; only a small minority of sexual abuse allegations involve women. Emergency physicians, clinical forensic physicians, and pediatricians may encounter sexually abused children in their practices. Child abuse and neglect, sometimes also referred to as child maltreatment, are defined in the *World Report on Violence and Health*, published by the World Health Organization, as: "All forms of physical and/ or emotional ill-treatment, sexual abuse, neglect or negligent treatment or commercial or other exploitation resulting in actual or potential harm to the child's health, survival, development, or dignity in the context of a relationship of responsibility, trust, or power."

Child sexual abuse is defined as the involvement of a child in sexual activity that he/she does not fully comprehend, is unable to give informed consent to, or for which the child is not developmentally prepared and cannot give consent, or that violate the laws of society.

Sexual activities encountered may include all forms of oral–genital, genital, or anal contact by or to the child, or abuse without physical contact, such as exhibitionism. Sexual activities may include the inducement or coercion of a child to engage in any unlawful sexual activity; the exploitative use of a child in prostitution or other unlawful sexual practices; and the exploitative use of children in pornographic performances and materials.

The evaluation of alleged sexual assault of a child presents the most difficult challenge to the medical professional. The role of the medical professional in assessing child sexual violation is further complicated by the frequent delay in disclosure and the very nature of child sexual abuse. Most children who report that their genitalia have been subjected to sexual contact, from touching by hand even up to full penetrative sexual intercourse, show no evidence of old or fresh injuries to the genital area. There are several reasons for this paucity of diagnostic findings. On the one hand, children are naturally reticent about reporting such conduct, so that the opportunity to see and record acute changes is lost; on the other hand, children are seldom subjected to great violence because a pedophile intent on maintaining access to a child is careful to avoid attracting attention. On those rare occasions when a child has been violently assaulted, the injuries are obvious and may require surgical repair. The history given by the child remains the bedrock of any evaluation. Knowledge of how child sexual abuse takes place and the acts involved helps doctors take better histories from carers and children and promotes understanding of the significance of genital findings.

Child sexual abuse is directly linked to further risks for the victimized child. Sexual abuse may result in other sequelae including depression, panic disorder, and attempted suicide. For all these reasons, child sexual abuse must not be neglected by any physician who may encounter such cases in his/her professional experience.

Medical examination of sexually abused children or adolescents must be undertaken in specialized centers by trained physicians. The medical examination has three aims: (1) to identify clinical evidence of genital or extragenital lesions; (2) to diagnose sexually transmitted infections or pregnancy; and (3) to evaluate the needs for medical care, psychological support, and social investigation. Laboratory investigations differ according to the delay between the abuse and the examination. Testing for human immunodeficiency virus (HIV) and hepatitis B and C virus antibodies and detection of pregnancy is realized in all cases, especially if a long delay between sexual assault and child examination is encountered. Good knowledge of child genitalia, use of magnifying lenses, training, and experience of the physician are important points of the medical intervention. Careful and precise examination allows the writing of a descriptive medical certificate, which is also a very important part of the medical intervention.

Various Circumstances of Examination of Child Victims of Sexual Abuse

Sexually abused children are seen by pediatricians and forensic physicians in a variety of circumstances:

1. children seen for a routine physical examination or for care of a medical illness, behavioral condition, or physical finding that would include child sexual abuse as part of the differential diagnosis
2. children thought to have been sexually abused and who are brought by a parent to the pediatrician for evaluation
3. children brought to the pediatrician by social service or law enforcement professionals for a medical evaluation for possible sexual abuse as part of an investigation
4. children brought to an emergency department after a suspected episode of sexual abuse for evaluation, evidence collection, and crisis management.

The presenting symptoms of sexual abuse may be so general (e.g., sleep disturbances, abdominal pain, enuresis, encopresis, or phobias) that caution must be exercised when the examiner considers sexual abuse. Nonacute genital findings indicative of sexual abuse are better examined by a physician with training in child abuse. Forensic physicians and pediatricians evaluating children who have these signs and symptoms should at least consider the possibility of abuse and, therefore, should make a report if no other diagnosis is apparent to explain the findings. For example, the French penal law, which is very strict about medical confidentiality, permits reporting of sexual abuse of children under 15 to judicial, sanitary, or social authorities. Since January 2004 reporting of sexual abuse of minors under 18 to judicial, sanitary, or social authorities has been allowed even if minors do not consent.

A complete history, including behavioral symptoms and associated signs of sexual abuse, should be sought. The primary responsibility of the physician is the protection of the child, sometimes requiring a delay in informing the parent(s) while a report is made and an expedited investigation by law enforcement and/or child protective services can be conducted.

Interviewing and Preparing the Child before a Medical Examination

In many countries, the suspicion of child sexual abuse as a possible diagnosis requires a report to both the appropriate law enforcement and child protective services agencies. All physicians need to know their state law requirements and where and when to file a written report.

The diagnosis of sexual abuse has protective and criminal consequences. The courts have allowed physicians to testify regarding specific details of the child's statements obtained in the course of taking a medical history to provide a diagnosis and treatment. Occasionally, children spontaneously describe their abuse and indicate who abused them. When asking young children about abuse, line drawings, dolls, or other aids can be used by professionals trained in interviewing young children such as in rape crisis centers and in clinical forensic units. Children may also describe their abuse during the course of the physical examination. It is desirable during the interview to use open questions and to avoid showing strong emotions such as shock or disbelief; moreover, if possible, the child should be interviewed alone.

The conversation should begin with topics which interest the child and which are nonthreatening. The evaluator should use the child's language and be reassuring. Children referred for medical examination may have been exposed to an abusive environment, or have medical or behavioral indicators of possible abuse. Children should be asked if they know why they have been brought to the doctor and to relate what has happened; what they say should be recorded in their own words. Whenever possible, the nature of the sexual contact, including pain, penetration, and ejaculation, should be ascertained, using this opportunity to give reassurance and explain the nature of the medical examination.

When children are brought for evaluation little or no history may be available other than that provided by the child. The pediatrician or clinical forensic physician should try to obtain an appropriate history in all cases before performing a medical examination. The child may spontaneously give additional information during the physical examination, particularly as the mouth, genitalia, and anus are examined.

History from the child remains a most important diagnostic feature in coming to the conclusion that a child has been sexually abused. History-taking should focus on whether the symptoms are explained by sexual abuse, physical abuse to the genital or anal area, or not. Written notes in the medical record or audiotape or videotape should be used to document the questions asked and the child's responses. Most expert interviewers consider that it is very difficult or impossible to interview children younger than 3 years.

Behavioral Indicators of Children Sexual Abuse

A behavioral history may reveal events or behaviors relevant to sexual abuse, even in the absence of a clear history of abuse in the child. The relationship of the abuser impacts on the severity of the abuse. Newly manifested behavioral changes in young child victims of sexual abuse include: clinging behavior and irritability; loss of bowel and bladder control; thumb-sucking; withdrawal; night terrors; bedwetting; and inability to sleep alone. In school-age children, manifestations include: feeding difficulties; anorexia nervosa; overeating; change in school performance; loss of concentration; anger; and altered levels of activity with either shortened attention and hyperactivity or depression and inactivity. In preadolescents and young adolescents, behavioral changes include poor peer relationships, restricted social life, inappropriately sexualized behavior, poor self-esteem, depression, guilt, suicidal gestures, acting in a sexually inappropriate way for age, e.g. delinquency, absconding, substance abuse, and even prostitution.

Physical Examination and Medical Evaluation

The medical professional who evaluates the child who is potentially a victim of sexual abuse becomes part of an investigative team gathering information and evidence of an alleged crime. In the case of a child, the medical examiner can provide essential information about the circumstances of disclosure, behavior patterns, environmental history (where the child has been), medical history, and any past infections, interventions, or procedures that might influence the interpretation of the medical findings.

The examination should be carefully explained to the child before it is performed, in order to obtain his/her full cooperation and not to result in additional emotional trauma. It is useful to have someone present, such as a supportive adult not suspected of involvement in the abuse. Children may be anxious about giving a history, being examined, or having procedures performed. Time must be allotted to relieve the child's anxiety.

The examiner must also know that only a small proportion of all children referred for medical evaluation of sexual abuse have abnormal examinations at the time of evaluation. This may be because of the delay between facts and examination or when abuse is not so severe as vaginal or anal penetration, as occurs frequently in child sexual abuse.

If great care is taken to prepare the child it will be possible to perform an appropriate examination without sedation or anesthesia. What is to happen during the examination must be explained simply and gently to the child. Children feel better when they are allowed to choose, for example who they would like to keep with them during the examination. The experienced examiner needs to anticipate their fears and answer all questions.

The child should have a complete pediatric examination, including brief assessments of developmental, behavioral, mental, and emotional status. Special attention should be paid to the growth parameters and sexual development of the child. In the rare instance when the child is unable to cooperate and the examination must be performed because of the likelihood of trauma, infection, and/or the need to collect forensic samples, consideration should be given to using sedation with careful monitoring. Instruments that magnify and illuminate the genital and rectal areas should be used: colposcopic examination is very useful. Signs of trauma should be carefully documented by detailed diagrams, illustrating the findings, or photography. The consent for, storage of and release of such images must be strictly controlled. Specific attention should be given to the areas involved in sexual activity – the mouth, breasts, genitals, perineal region, buttocks, and anus.

Genital Examination

Appropriate positioning of the child can facilitate the examination for both child and doctor, especially to visualize the posterior portion of vaginal introitus in a young girl. In female children, the genital examination should include inspection of the medial aspects of the thighs, labia majora and minora, clitoris, urethra, periurethral tissue, hymen, hymenal opening, fossa navicularis, and posterior fourchette.

Various methods for visualizing the hymenal opening in prepubertal children have been described. Many factors will influence the size of the orifice and the exposure of the hymen and its internal structures. These include the degree of relaxation of the child, the amount of traction (gentle, moderate) on the labia majora, and the position of the child (supine, lateral, or knee-to-chest). The technique used is less important than maximizing the view and recording the method and results. Of course, speculum or digital examinations should not be performed on the prepubertal child.

Gentle labial separation and traction help to visualize the hymen within the vaginal introitus. Sterile cotton-tipped applicators can be used to delineate the hymen.

The use of colposcopy and photodocumentation has improved the detection rate for findings associated with sexual assault; they have been the basis for research into normal genital anatomy and post-traumatic changes associated with child sexual abuse in many published papers (**Figures 1** and **2**).

In the prepubertal child, vaginal penetration (past the level of the hymen) usually results in the hymen tearing between 3 and 9 o'clock. Lacerations may be associated with bruising or abrasions ventrally as well

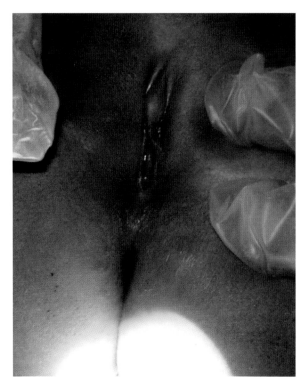

Figure 1 Hymenal lesions.

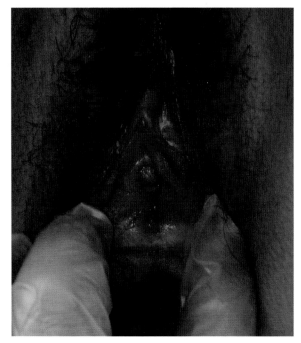

Figure 2 Hymenal lesions.

as to the posterior fourchette and lateral introital tissues.

Anal Examination

Anal examinations can be performed in either the supine or the left lateral position; most children are

less comfortable in the knee-to-chest or prone position. Anal penetration often results in lacerations, abrasions, and bruising, but examinations of any other than freshly assaulted victims may be negative (normal) in 90% of cases.

In both sexes, the anus can be examined in the supine, lateral, or knee-to-chest position. It is important to note the presence of bruises around the anus, scars, anal tears (especially those that extend into the surrounding perianal skin), and anal dilation. Anal penetration results in trauma when there has been significant force, resistance by the child, or lack of lubrication (**Figures 3** and **4**). However, careful penetration (finger in the young children, penis after careful lubrication in older ones) will not show any trauma, except anal dilatation in the very first times. Injuries such as bruising, abrasions, or lacerations of the anal verge will heal in a few days. Rarely,

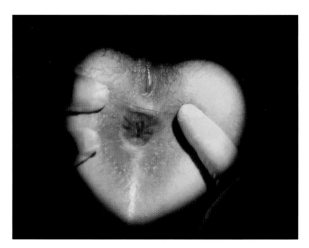

Figure 3 Anal lesions in a preadolescent girl.

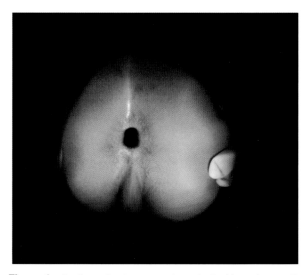

Figure 4 Anal opening in a young boy who had been frequently sexually abused.

extensive damage such as deep fissures or rupture of the sphincter will need surgical repair. Very traumatic lesions are mostly observed in sexual abuse of children associated with murder. Laxity of the sphincter, if present, should be noted. If the child reveals any events that may have occurred to the areas of the body being examined, these details should be noted.

Poor and Delayed Examination

If the alleged sexual assault has occurred within 72 h, or there is bleeding or acute injury, the examination should be performed immediately. In this situation, protocols for child sexual assault victims should be followed to secure biological trace evidence such as epithelial cells, semen, and blood, as well as to maintain a chain of evidence. When more than 72 h has passed and no acute injuries are present, an emergency examination may not be necessary, although each case must be considered on its own merits. An evaluation therefore should be scheduled at the earliest convenient time for the child, physician, and investigative team.

In children, several factors tend to lessen the chances of finding injuries diagnostic of sexual assault. Most reports of child sexual abuse note positive findings in only 43–76% of examinations. On the one hand, most children delay reporting the assault, so that many or all of the injuries disappear by healing; on the other hand, assaults upon children may be limited to fondling, simulated intercourse such as intercrural connection (penile friction between the inner thighs and external genitalia), when no injuries will ever be present.

Examination of a Male Child Victim of Sexual Abuse

In male children, the thighs, penis, and scrotum should be examined for bruises, scars, ecchymosis, and bite marks.

Photographic Documentation of the Lesions

In most major referral centers, photodocumentation has become standard practice in evaluating allegations of sexual assault. In specialized centers, examiners have mainly relied upon the use of the colposcope. This instrument has been long and widely used in sampling and screening for cancer of the cervix. In the hands of most examiners it has also been used to diagnose lesions of the external genitalia and hymen. The main value of photodocumentation of the sexual assault victim is to record the findings permanently and so avoid the need for delayed reexamination.

Forensic Sampling in Child Sexual Abuse

It is appropriate to take forensic samples if sampling is performed when the examination occurs within 72 h of acute sexual assault or sexual abuse. Some form of forensic evidence can be identified in one of four children examined within 48 h of their assault. Over 90% of children present positive forensic evidence findings when seen within 24 h of their assault. The decision to collect evidence is best made by the timing of the examination. Swabbing the child's body for evidence is unnecessary after 24 h (mouth, anus) or 48 h (skin, genitalia).

Clothing and linen yield most evidence and should be pursued vigorously for analysis. The clothing should be kept in glazed brown paper; the kind used for wrapping parcels is ideal because it is robust. The underwear should especially be kept as possible evidence. It should be checked that all areas of the clothing that are wet with secretions have dried before sealing each item in a separate evidence bag bearing an appropriately signed label.

Skin Examination

It is essential to sample, document, and process all foreign matter found on the child's body. Dried blood or secretions can be collected with saline-moistened swabs, although some laboratories prefer dry swabbing. The examination may be facilitated by appropriate ultraviolet irradiation; fluorescent material often consists of ejaculate, and the procedure helps to locate areas to be swabbed.

Oral Examination

Any trauma should be documented, if seen in a short delay. If any oral penetration has occurred, the buccal mucosa will need to be swabbed, including the areas under the tongue and around the pillars of the fauces. Swabs should be saved for microscopical examination.

Vaginal Examination

If the female child is examined shortly after the sexual abuse, the first action is to document trauma to the external genitalia and vaginal introitus. For this purpose, all secretions should be swabbed or sampled as appropriate, with great care in a nonpubertal girl. When possible, in the postpubertal victim, examination with a transparent speculum should follow to determine the degree of internal injuries. Vaginal wall and cervical injuries are common. The vaginal pool should be swabbed, once again retaining one swab for microscopic examination.

Anal Examination

In an early examination, any injuries should be documented and the perianal area swabbed, followed by the anal canal and rectum, for the presence of ejaculate and lubricants, if any; again one swab should be retained for microscopical examination. If there is any evidence of serious anorectal injury, proctoscopy may be necessary under general anesthesia.

Searching for Sexually Transmitted Diseases in Children

The predominant sexually transmitted diseases (STD) observed among children with histories or signs of abuse are syphilis, vulvovaginal candidiasis, condyloma acuminata, herpes progenitalis, and hepatitis B; very rare cases are HIV-positive.

To avoid pediatric STDs after sexual abuse, it is necessary, when not delayed, to treat promptly and adequately, in order to avoid diseases that could result in significant sequelae in children.

Gonorrhoea, syphilis, *Chlamydia*, herpes simplex and human papillomavirus, and HIV can be diagnosed by means of serology. The diagnosis of STD is important not only to the care of the victim but also in determining the fact of sexual contact. As laboratories become more sophisticated, these infections may become important forensic markers as organisms become traceable between assailant and victim. This evidence may be direct, e.g., gonorrhea, trichomoniasis, syphilis, or HIV, or confirmatory, such as *Chlamydia*. It is even possible in some cases to type individual strains of microorganisms that can also be typed on the suspected perpetrator.

Searching for STDs in abused children also means that medical professionals should provide appropriate disease prophylaxis for sexual assault victims, as well as pregnancy prophylaxis in postpubertal girls. This will vary depending on the susceptibility of organisms in different countries or local legal constraints on the use of drugs. Recent data indicate that appropriate early treatment of HIV exposure may influence the course of the infection.

All laboratory specimens must be treated carefully to protect them from contamination and degradation. The chain of evidence must be maintained using signed labels and evidence books according to local requirements. Specimens must be maintained in reliable environments before reaching the reference laboratories.

Assessing the Diagnosis of Sexual Abuse of Children

Diagnosis of child sexual abuse can often be suspected from a child's history. Its assessment is not simple. Physical findings are often absent, since many types of abuse leave no physical evidence, and mucosal injuries often heal rapidly. Occasionally, a child presents with clear evidence of anogenital trauma without an adequate history. Moreover, abused children may deny abuse. Findings that are concerning, but in isolation are not diagnostic of sexual abuse, include: (1) abrasions or bruising of the inner thighs and genitalia; (2) scarring or tears of the labia minora; and (3) enlargement of the hymenal opening. Findings that are more concerning include: (1) scarring, tears, or distortion of the hymen; (2) a decreased amount of or absent hymenal tissue; (3) scarring of the fossa navicularis; (4) injury to or scarring of the posterior fourchette; and (5) anal lacerations.

Comparison of mean hymenal diameters demonstrates that children with a history of penetration had a significantly larger transverse opening than nonabused children. Children with previous penetration are more likely than nonabused children to have a horizontal opening measuring >6.5 mm in the knee-to-chest position, and less than 1.0 mm of hymenal tissue is detected at 6 o'clock only in those with a history of penetration.

Abrasions, hematomas, and lacerations of the external genitalia heal without definitive evidence of sexual assault in a prepubertal girl. However, in cases where evidence of penetration beyond the hymen has been documented, with a resulting acute tear, the hymen will heal with clear evidence of forensic considerations. This will present as focal disruption of the hymen with loss of hymenal tissue. At puberty, all estrogen-sensitive tissue will respond, but the focal absence of hymenal tissue will persist.

Just as in the preadolescent, trauma to the external genitalia after puberty tends to heal quickly and completely. Minor lacerations and hematomas of the hymen may result in some minimal changes to the hymenal edge, which may appear similar to a redundant hymen. Major tears extending to the base of the hymen will persist and can be visualized more easily with the use of cotton-tipped swabs.

Unless the victim of anal penetration is seen within days of the assault, there will be little, if any, evidence of injury. The presence of decreased tone and fissures may be corroborative of penetration. Anal lacerations, by contrast, have rarely been found in circumstances other than those of blunt-force penetrating trauma.

In postpubertal females, the interpretation of healed trauma consistent with penetration must be made with caution. An adolescent girl who is sexually active will show hymenal injury due to consensual sexual intercourse. In cases of postpubertal vaginal assault, signs include: abrasions or hematomas; partial or complete hymenal tears; posterior fourchette injuries; lacerations; abrasions; and hematomas. Anal fissures, lacerations, and changes in anal tone may be associated with traumatic anal penetration.

The differential diagnosis of genital trauma also includes accidental injury and physical abuse. This differentiation may be difficult and may require a careful history and multidisciplinary approach. Because many malformations and infections or other causes of anal–genital abnormalities may be confused with abuse, familiarity with these other causes is important.

Physicians should be aware that child sexual abuse often occurs in the context of other family problems, including physical abuse, emotional maltreatment, substance abuse, and family violence. If these problems are suspected, referral to a child abuse specialist or assessment center for a more comprehensive evaluation is imperative.

Other Treatments Needed

It is appropriate to consider in all children who have been sexually abused that they be reviewed by a child psychiatrist to assess many factors including the need for treatment. The need for treatment varies depending on the type of sexual assault (whether the perpetrator is a family member or nonfamily member), the duration of the assault, and the age and symptoms of the child. Poor prognostic signs include more intrusive forms of abuse, more violent assaults, longer periods of sexual molestation, and closer relationship of the perpetrator to the victim.

Conclusion: Sexual Abuse and Judicial Proceedings

The evaluation of sexually abused children is increasingly a part of clinical forensic and general pediatric practice. Medical examiners are part of a multidisciplinary approach to prevent, investigate, and treat the problem and need to be competent in history-taking, physical examination, selection of laboratory tests, and differential diagnosis.

In many countries, an expanding clinical consultation network is available to assist the primary care physician with the assessment of difficult cases.

Because the likelihood of criminal court action is high, detailed records, drawings, and/or photographs should be kept. The submission of written reports to justice departments is encouraged by many penal laws. Physicians required to testify in court are better prepared and may feel more comfortable in making assessments when their records are complete and accurate. In general, the ability to protect a child may often depend on the quality of the physician's records, especially in criminal court.

See Also

Children: Legal Protection and Rights of Children; Emotional Abuse; Physical Abuse; Sexual Abuse, Epidemiology

Further Reading

Adams JA, Harper K, Knudson S, Revilla J (1994) Examination findings in legally confirmed child sexual abuse: it's normal to be normal. *Pediatrics* 94: 310–317.

American Academy of Child and Adolescent Psychiatry (1997) American Academy of Child and Adolescent Psychiatry practice parameters for the forensic evaluation of children and adolescents who may have been physically or sexually abused. *Journal of the American Academy of Child and Adolescent Psychiatry* 36: 423–442.

American Academy of Pediatrics (1999) Guidelines for the evaluation of sexual abuse of children: subject review. *Pediatrics* 103: 186–191.

Berenson AB, Chacko MR, Wiemann CM, et al. (2000) A case-control study of anatomic changes resulting from sexual abuse. *American Journal of Obstetrics and Gynecology* 182: 820–834.

Berenson AB, Chacko MR, Wiemann CM, et al. (2002) Use of hymenal measurements in the diagnosis of previous penetration. *Pediatrics* 109: 228–235.

Christian CW, Lavelle JM, De Jong AR, et al. (2000) Forensic evidence findings in prepubertal victims of sexual assault. *Pediatrics* 106: 100–104.

Heger A, Ticson L, Velasquez O, Bernier R (2002) Children referred for possible sexual abuse: medical findings in 2384 children. *Child Abuse and Neglect* 26: 645–659.

Hymel KP, Jenny C (1996) Child sexual abuse. *Pediatric Review* 17: 236–249; quiz 249–250.

Jones JG, Lawson L, Rickert CP (1990) Use of optical glass binocular magnifiers in the examination of sexually abused children. *Adolescent and Pediatric Gynecology* 3: 146–148.

Makoroff KL, Brauley JL, Brandner AM, Myers PA, Shapiro RA (2002) Genital examinations for alleged sexual abuse of prepubertal girls: findings by pediatric emergency medicine physicians compared with child abuse trained physicians. *Child Abuse and Neglect* 26: 1235–1242.

Pandhi D, Kumar S, Reddy BS (2003) Sexually transmitted diseases in children. *Journal of Dermatology* 30: 314–320.

Sexual Abuse, Epidemiology

E Baccino and **L Martrille**, Centre Hospitalier
Universitaire de Montpellier, Montpellier, France

Introduction

Epidemiological surveys of child sexual abuse (CSA) have several objectives:

- to assess the extent of the phenomenon, through incidence, defined as the number of new cases occurring each year within a group of individuals, and prevalence, which represents the proportion of individual victims of CSA within the population
- to improve the knowledge of the various aspects of CSA, such as: risk factors, subclinical symptoms, evolution, and severity of the outcome in order to help professionals to make the earliest diagnosis and to provide the most appropriate care; it is also of interest for the judicial system to know the true impact of a crime on the victims to pronounce the most relevant sentence
- to make people aware of this public health concern.

Unfortunately, and due to the sensitive nature of this topic, the above-mentioned goals are far from being achieved.

In the first part of this article, the main and demonstrated data are presented, the second part focuses on the remaining problems that generate debate and/or may be the subject of future research.

Essential Data

There are only three methodologically sound studies about CSA epidemiology: one was conducted in the UK in 1985, and the two others were carried out in Canada and France in 1989.

These studies concern children under 16 years of age, representative of the general (nonclinical) population, and who were the victims of precisely defined sexual abuse, ranging from fondling of breasts and genital areas to more severe sexual assaults such as fellatio, masturbation, sexual intercourse, and sodomy.

Prevalence of CSA

- in both genders: 3–5%
- in females: 4–8%
- in males: 2–4%.

The age of maximum risk is 10 years, and CSA is repetitive in one-third (33%) of cases.

CSAs occur within the family in almost 20% of cases, and the perpetrator is the so-called 'functional father' (i.e., father, stepfather, or mother's partner) in 10% of cases.

The CSA is reported to judicial or health services in only 10% of cases.

In a country like France (60 million people), roughly 2 million people are victims of CSA before the age of 15 (prevalence), and the incidence is 50 000 cases each year.

A 1988 US study suggested that the incidence of CSA was around 1%, and that teenagers were the perpetrators in at least 20% of cases.

A comparison of prevalence in two French studies, one in 1989 and the other one in 2000, showed similar results for females (4.1% in 1989 versus 3.4% in 2000).

In France the legal definition of rape is restricted to sexual penetration (fellatio, vaginal intercourse, sodomy); the prevalence of this crime among females under 15 years is 300 000 in a population of 60 million, of which 50% is female.

CSA is not only a frequent and difficult judicial problem but also a major public health challenge for civilized societies; unfortunately, it is far from being controlled, as the first step of a satisfactory solution (prevention and early diagnosis) is rarely taken. This results, at least partly, from flaws found in most published epidemiological studies.

Epidemiological Studies: Flaws and Suggestions

An extensive international literature review carried out in 1994 showed large variations in prevalence and incidence ratios not linked to national specificities but rather to methodological problems such as the following.

Selection of Population

Studies based on student population, medicolegal group activities (clinical populations), or police data are not representative of the general population considering the large underreporting rate (10%).

Age Limit of Victims and Perpetrators

For legal and cultural reasons, the term "child" does not mean the same thing all over the world. With regard to the age limit of childhood, the range extends through literature from 12 to 18 years.

In the published literature, there is disagreement on the age of the perpetrator: most authors do not mention this criterion; for others, in order for the offense to be considered as an assault, the perpetrator must be an adult or at least 5 years older than his/her victim (this would exclude consensual sexual activities between peers).

Definition of Sexual Abuse

The definition is quite broad; it includes exhibitionism, exposure to pornographic materials such as publications and movies, pinching and even the use of obscene words. As a result, in one report, although the population was well defined, the prevalence rate reached an unrealistic 51%; unfortunately, this percentage was mentioned too often in further reports. This broader definition carries the risk that these publications will not be taken seriously and may strengthen the case of those who do not want to admit the reality and the importance of CSA.

Data Collection

Fourteen of 17 publications reviewed for this article were excluded because the nonresponse rate was considered to be too high (above 50% with prevalence 5%).

The studies that had the best response rates were those in which the questions about CSA were not the primary aim of the questionnaire.

Incest

In the literature, there is no agreement on the definition of the perpetrator: for some, only the biological father could be involved; for others, all biologically linked family members could be involved, and for some, the perpetrator is the functional father, one who plays the role of the father from the victim's point of view (whether biological father, stepfather, or adoptive father). As a consequence, prevalence rates vary from 1% to 15%.

Long-Term Effects of CSA

Severity (of a crime or a disease) is a concept accepted by both the judicial and the health systems; accordingly, harshness on the part of law enforcement depends at least in part on the negative clinical effects of CSA on the victims. Therefore, in most countries sentences are more or less in proportion to the clinical type and supposed gravity of CSA, e.g., rape is more severely punished than fondling, and incest between a father and his daughter is more severely punished than the same sexual assault committed by an unknown assailant.

This rationale is backed by many physicians who consider that a history of CSA will increase the risks of mental disorders such as depression and suicide, and of becoming an abusive parent. However, these hypotheses have not yet been scientifically demonstrated; they are based on retrospective studies evaluating the number of CSA cases in clinical groups (prostitutes or psychiatric patients generally), but not on prospective studies. Only the previously mentioned UK study provided limited information of this kind, showing that responders and nonresponders, CSA victims and nonvictims, did not differ with respect to either social professional groups or geographic location at the time of the study.

Of course, there is no question that some types of CSA will have short-term, mid-term, and long-term severe adverse effects (clinical, social, and judicial), but basing judicial policies on highly hypothetical medical beliefs might also be regarded as an abuse.

Historical Evolution of CSA

Due to the dramatic increase in cases reported to police, especially in the early 1990s in countries where information campaigns were undertaken, one might think that there is a real increase in CSA cases. However, the only study designed to answer this question did not show any difference in prevalence rates among victims aged between 15 and 65 years (the low rate found in victims aged over 65 at the time of the study might be due to the victims' memory problems).

Thus, it seems that the increase in cases is due to an improvement in reporting rates. There are great prospects for further improvement, considering that CSA is still the tip of an iceberg, with 90% of its mass underwater.

Physicians' Role

Unfortunately, physicians play a minor role. Various studies in France and the USA have shown that they played an active role in fewer than 10% of CSA cases reported to authorities. Another French study showed that they were not intentionally underreporting (for reasons of confidentiality, for instance): they are just unable to detect CSA in patients who consult for other reasons.

In Finistère (Brittany, France), a survey showed that all physicians in this area (general practitioners and specialists) diagnosed only 15% of the CSA which occurred during the year 1993.

Conclusion

The epidemiological studies about CSA provide us with some clear facts:

- the victims are twice as likely to be female as male
- the age at which children are most at risk is 10 years
- the aggressor is often known by the victim and there is a high rate of relapse if nothing is done to stop the abuse
- unfortunately, the low rate of reporting to authorities (10%) shows that all too often, nothing is done.

These studies also provide a long list of features, among which ignorance of early symptoms (medical, psychological, or social) should be stressed, which lead to poor diagnostic conclusions and the unknown severity of the effects of each type of CSA. This results in a lack of evaluation of the appropriate care that should be provided for this large public health problem.

Indeed, further studies are needed. However, it is important to mention that they are difficult to realize, expensive, and often limited by ethical considerations.

CSA is one of the least tolerable crimes in public opinion. Building a CSA-free world should make it a priority to undertake an international effort to fight this outrage – this should begin with properly designed longitudinal and collaborative epidemiological studies based on consensual definitions of all the variables to be evaluated.

See Also

Children: Sexual Abuse, Overview; **Imaging:** Radiology, Pediatric, Scintigraphy and Child Abuse

Further Reading

Baccino E (1994) Données épidémiologiques des abus sexuels chez les mineurs en France. *Med Mal Infect* 425–439.
Finkelhorn D (1994) The international epidemiology of child sexual abuse. *Child Abuse and Neglect* 409–417.
Merrick J, Browne KD (1999) Child abuse and neglect: a public health concern. *Public Health Review* 279–293.

Sudden Natural Infant and Childhood Death

R W Byard, Forensic Science Centre, Adelaide, SA, Australia
H F Krous, Children's Hospital and Health Center, San Diego, CA, USA

Introduction

Sudden death in infancy and childhood has many natural, inflicted, and noninflicted causes. This article concentrates on the wide range of natural diseases that may result in sudden and unexpected deaths of previously well, or medically stable, infants and children. Deaths due to inflicted and noninflicted injuries are dealt with elsewhere, and, due to its unique position, characteristic and postulated mechanisms for sudden infant death syndrome (SIDS) are dealt with in detail separately.

Accuracy of diagnosis is of prime importance in cases of unexpected infant and childhood death in order to understand underlying mechanisms, optimize outcomes for grieving families, enable future pregnancy counseling, and ensure that data and information supplied for vital statistics are correct.

Determining the incidence of sudden childhood death is not necessarily an easy task as rates vary among populations and within communities over time. Death certificate and autopsy diagnoses may not always be correct, as there is often regional bias in preferred diagnoses, and investigations may not always be comprehensive or follow standard protocols. Rates for sudden natural death have varied between 1.1 and 13.8 cases per 100 000 of the pediatric population, accounting for 2–5% of deaths in the age range of 1–20 years. The most common causes of sudden natural death also vary according to age. For example, lethal infections tend to occur at a younger age than cardiac abnormalities. Infections are more often lethal in nonwestern countries. Causes of sudden natural childhood death are summarized in **Table 1**. Only selected conditions have been discussed in the following article. Further details of these and other conditions are available in standard texts.

Sudden Infant Death Syndrome

SIDS, or crib death or cot death, is defined as "the sudden death of an infant less than one year of age which remains unexplained after a thorough case investigation, including performance of a complete autopsy, examination of the death scene, and review of the clinical history." Despite dramatic falls in rates following "reduce the risk" campaigns characterized by changes in infant care practices, SIDS remains the most common cause of postneonatal death in western countries.

The term SIDS can only be applied after other causes of unexpected infant death such as accidents, inflicted injury, and natural diseases have been excluded. If investigations and autopsies are not meticulously performed there is, therefore, a danger that other causes of death may be incorrectly termed SIDS. This possibility led the late John Emery to warn against using SIDS as a "diagnostic dustbin." The following article details a range of conditions that may be confused with SIDS. An important concept that cannot be overemphasized is that "not every infant who dies in a crib dies of crib death."

The characteristic features and possible causes of SIDS deaths are summarized elsewhere.

Table 1 Differential diagnosis of unexpected infant and childhood death due to natural diseases

Idiopathic
Sudden infant death syndrome

Cardiac
Congenital cardiac defects (before and after surgery)
Cardiomyopathies
Tumors
Conduction defects
Infections
Miscellaneous: endocardial fibroelastosis

Vascular
Aortic abnormalities: supravalvular stenosis, coarctation,
  William syndrome, DiGeorge syndrome
Coronary artery abnormalities: anomalous coronary arteries,
  aplasia/hypoplasia, idiopathic arterial calcinosis, coronary
  arteritis (Kawasaki disease)
Venous abnormalities: total anomalous pulmonary venous
  drainage
Vascular malformations
Pulmonary hypertension
Miscellaneous: fibromuscular dysplasia, thromboembolism

Infectious
Cardiovascular: myocarditis
Respiratory: acute bronchopneumonia
Central nervous system: meningitis, encephalitis
Gastrointestinal: gastroenteritis, botulism
Genitourinary: pyelonephritis
Generalized: septicemia, endotoxemia

Respiratory
Asthma
Upper-airway obstruction
Bronchopulmonary dysplasia
Infections
Miscellaneous: massive pulmonary hemorrhage, tension
  pneumothorax

Central nervous system
Hemorrhage: bleeding diathesis, vascular malformations
Tumors
Epilepsy
Metabolic disorders
Infections
Miscellaneous: tuberous sclerosis

Hematological
Hemoglobinopathies: sickle-cell disease
Malignancies: lymphoma, leukemia
Bleeding diathesis
Anemia
Miscellaneous: infections, polycythemia, splenic disorders

Gastrointestinal
Intestinal obstruction: intussusception, volvulus
Intestinal perforation
Late-presenting congenital diaphragmatic hernia
Gastroesophageal reflux/aspiration
Infections: gastroenteritis
Miscellaneous: cystic fibrosis, malnutrition

Genitourinary
Wilms tumour
Hemolytic–uremic syndrome
Complications of pregnancy
Primary renal disease: pyelonephritis, glomerulonephritis
Urinary tract obstruction

Metabolic
Fatty acid oxidation defects: acyl-coenzyme dehydrogenase
  deficiencies (medium-chain, long-chain)
Reye's syndrome
Carbohydrate disorders: glycogen storage diseases
Organic acid disorders

Endocrine
Insulin-dependent diabetes mellitus
Congenital adrenal hypo/hyperplasia

Miscellaneous
Connective tissue disorders: Marfan syndrome, Ehlers–Danlos
  syndrome type IV
Skeletal disorders: achondroplasia
Chromosomal disorders: trisomy 21

Adapted from Byard RW (2004) *Sudden Death in Infancy Childhood and Adolescence*, 2nd edn. Cambridge: Cambridge University Press.

Cardiac Conditions

A multitude of structural, infectious, cardiomyopathic, and neoplastic cardiovascular disorders may cause sudden infant and childhood death.

Congenital Defects

Congenital defects include cyanotic, acyanotic, and obstructive conditions, the two most common being tetralogy of Fallot and transposition of the great vessels. Complications resulting in sudden death include rhythm disturbances and cerebral or myocardial infarction associated with polycythemia. Even after successful surgical repair, there remains a significant risk of sudden death due to heart block and arrhythmias.

Ventricular septal defects are the most common congenital heart defect, but rarely cause sudden death. In clinically significant cases affected infants and children usually manifest signs of cardiac failure, with failure to thrive, feeding difficulties, and sweating. Uncomplicated atrial septal defects are not a cause of sudden death in infancy or early childhood.

Cardiomyopathies

Cardiomyopathies represent a heterogeneous group with variable inheritance patterns. A number of familial metabolic disturbances are also characterized by secondary cardiomyopathies. Hypertrophic cardiomyopathy is characterized by a marked increase in the size and weight of the heart. Inheritance may be autosomal dominant or recessive, involving gene defects in at least eight chromosomes with disruption in coding for contractile proteins actin and myosin. Typical pathological features include marked reduction in the size of the left ventricular cavity with typical myofiber disarray on light microscopy.

Other cardiomyopathies associated with unexpected death are dilated and restrictive, and both have heterogeneous etiologies. Arrhythmogenic right ventricular cardiomyopathy (**Figure 1**) refers to a specific familial condition that primarily affects the right ventricle with fibrolipomatous replacement of muscle tissue. Rarer entities that may cause unexpected infant death include histiocytoid cardiomyopathy (**Figure 2**) and noncompaction of the left ventricle.

Endocardial fibroelastosis associated with structural abnormalities or metabolic conditions may also be associated with sudden death (**Figure 3**).

Outflow Obstruction

Any lesion that causes obstruction to the outflow of blood from the left ventricle may result in cardiac hypertrophy with its attendant risk of lethal arrhythmia. Examples include coarctation or disruption of

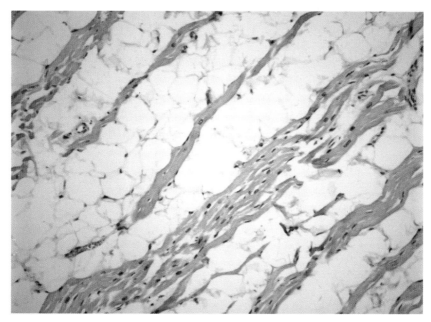

Figure 1   A case of sudden death of a young child caused by arrhythmogenic right ventricular cardiomyopathy with fat replacing right ventricular myocardium. Hematoxylin & eosin, 200×.

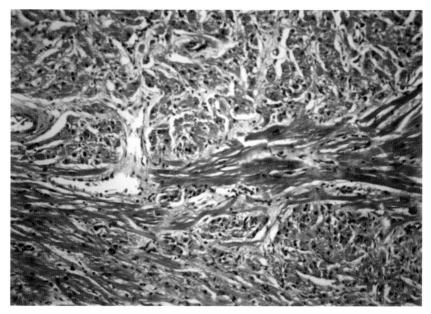

Figure 2   Islands of altered myocytes with eosinophilic granular cytoplasm (upper and lower fields) replace normal myocardium (center) of the heart of an infant with histiocytoid cardiomyopathy who died suddenly and unexpectedly. Hematoxylin & eosin, 200×.

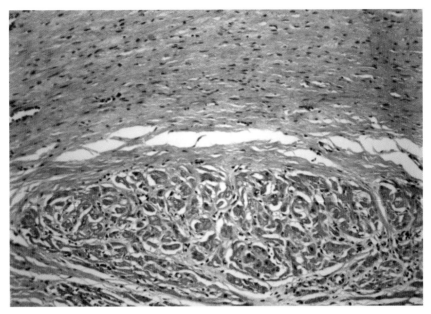

Figure 3 Endocardial fibroelastosis of left ventricle showing marked thickening with fibrous and elastic tissue. Masson trichrome, 200×.

the aortic arch and stenosis of the aortic valve, which may be unicuspid or bicuspid. Subaortic stenosis caused by either a fibromuscular membrane or diffuse narrowing of the outflow tract is another cause of sudden death in infancy or childhood.

Tumors

Tumors such as rhabdomyomas, fibromas, or myxomas may occur within the heart in infants and young children and cause significant problems from outflow tract obstruction, embolization, or conduction tract disruption. Rhabdomyomas may be a "forme fruste" of tuberous sclerosis, a condition characterized by mental retardation, epilepsy, and an increased risk of sudden death.

Conduction Tract Disorders

Conduction tract problems may also arise with a variety of other conditions and include entities such as the prolonged QT interval syndromes. Disturbances in genes controlling cardiac sodium and potassium channels result in prolongation of the QT interval and have significant association with sudden death. Swimming may be a trigger to a lethal arrhythmia in children with long QT syndrome (LQTS) and in infancy there has been confusion with SIDS. More than 35 LQTS gene mutations have now been identified in LQTS. The diagnosis can be established by epinephrine (adrenaline) challenge of a decedent's mother, or by analysis of the decedent's blood or paraffin-embedded cardiac tissue using exon-specific amplification by polymerase chain reaction and direct DNA sequencing to identify the various gene mutations.

Vascular Conditions

Again there are a wide range of disorders that may cause sudden childhood death.

Aortic Abnormalities

Outflow obstruction, as with cardiac conditions described above, may cause significant cardiac hypertrophy with an increased risk of lethal arrhythmia. Supravalvular stenosis, due to an autosomal dominantly inherited disorder of elastin, has several forms, including membranous, tubular, and hourglass narrowing of the aorta distal to the aortic valve. Coarctation due to a discrete narrowing near the ligamentum arteriosum has a similar effect.

Williams syndrome is due to a mutation or deletion on chromosome 7q11.23 and is characterized by infantile hypercalcemia, abnormal facies, peripheral pulmonary artery stenosis, supravalvular aortic stenosis, and growth and developmental retardation. Sudden death results from the effects of coronary artery stenosis or ventricular outflow tract obstruction.

DiGeorge syndrome results from a microdeletion of chromosome 22q11.2 causing abnormalities of tissues derived from the third and fourth pharyngeal pouches. Affected children have characteristic dysmorphic facies and suffer from thymic and parathyroid aplasia or hypoplasia, with aortic arch anomalies, truncus arteriosus, or tetralogy of Fallot.

Coronary Artery Anomalies

The coronary arteries must be evaluated for the positions of their ostia, as well as variations in the angles of their take-off from the aorta, and initial and subsequent courses. Ostial ridges or membranes may also result in significant compromise of blood flow. Coronary artery anomalies may be part of complex congenital malformations of the heart or an isolated defect, and are a well-recognized but rare cause of sudden death in infancy and childhood.

Anomalous coronary arteries may arise from the opposite sinus of Valsalva, the aortic arch, the opposite coronary artery, or the pulmonary trunk. Sudden death has occurred with all variants when there is sufficient angulation or luminal narrowing to compromise blood flow.

Idiopathic arterial calcinosis is a rare disorder characterized by calcification of arterial walls. Lethal consequences result from coronary artery narrowing.

Kawasaki disease, or mucocutaneous lymph node syndrome, is now the major cause of acquired heart disease in children in western countries. The etiology is uncertain; however, it is characterized by transmural coronary arteritis with medial degeneration, thrombosis, and aneurysmal dilatation.

Venous Abnormalities

Total anomalous pulmonary venous connection (TAPVC) occurs when there is drainage of pulmonary veins into the systemic venous system rather than into the left atrium. Drainage may be above or below the diaphragm. Significant obstruction of the common draining vein may be associated with the development of pulmonary hypertension.

Other vascular disorders associated with sudden infant and childhood death include vascular malformations, other causes of pulmonary hypertension, and arterial fibromuscular dysplasia. Fatal pulmonary thromboembolism may also rarely occur in infancy and childhood associated with similar predisposing conditions to adults such as immobilization, recent surgery, venous stasis, sepsis, and malignancy.

Infectious Disorders

Fulminant infections of the heart, lungs, and/or central nervous system can cause rapid deterioration and sudden death, even in infants and children who have not appeared particularly unwell prior to collapse.

Myocarditis

Inflammation of the heart may be caused by a variety of infectious and noninfectious agents. Viral infection is most likely due to coxsackie B viruses but may also occur with coxsackie A, echo, polio, cytomegalo, human immunodeficiency, parvo, influenza, and adeno viruses. Although infants and children may present with a febrile illness and/or cardiac failure a significant percentage may have minimal or no symptoms prior to their terminal collapse. At autopsy, variable degrees of inflammation, edema, and fibrosis with myocyte necrosis (**Figure 4**) will be found. A giant-cell variant also occurs. Sudden death is caused by lethal arrhythmias.

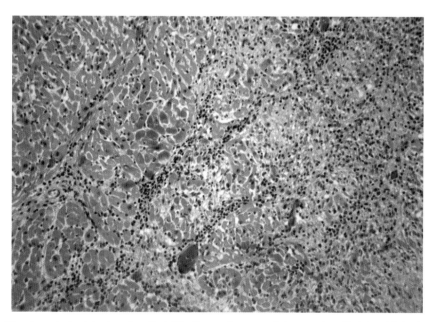

Figure 4 Myocarditis characterized by lymphocytic infiltration and myocardial necrosis with interstitial edema and fibrosis that caused the sudden death of an infant. Hematoxylin & eosin, 200×.

Rheumatic Fever

The incidence of rheumatic fever has declined markedly in western communities. It follows a group A streptococcal infection and causes, amongst other lesions, inflammatory foci within the heart and valves, with vegetation formation. Sudden death results from myocarditis with arrhythmias, or from embolization of friable valvular vegetations into the coronary arteries.

Upper Respiratory Infections

Acute inflammation from infection around the upper aerodigestive passages may result in sudden death if there is compromise of airway patency. The classic example is acute epiglottitis where infection with *Haemophilus influenzae* type B causes swelling of the epiglottis with obstruction of the inlet to the larynx. Cases are rare now that immunization for *Haemophilus* has been undertaken.

Acute bacterial infection of the tonsils, posterior portion of the tongue, or retropharyngeal spaces may also cause lethal airway occlusion, as may infections of the trachea. Pseudomembranes in diphtheria, and less often in bacterial tracheitis, may dislodge and obstruct upper airways.

Lower Respiratory Infections

Acute bacterial pneumonia (**Figure 5**) may be fulminant, especially with organisms such as *Streptococcus pneumoniae*, *H. influenzae*, and *Staphylococcus aureus*. In established cases there will be filling of alveoli and distal airways with neutrophils with early organization. Lung and blood cultures are required in the autopsy assessment.

Meningitis

Bacterial infection of the cerebrospinal fluid and the meninges may cause a rapidly progressive clinical disorder resulting in death. This is particularly so with meningitis due to *Neisseria meningitidis*. Other pathogens that cause meningitis in infants and children include *H. influenzae* and *Streptococcus pneumoniae*. These latter organisms are now uncommon given the widespread administration of immunizations during infancy and early childhood.

The clinical presentation may be nonspecific in infants, compared to older children, who may complain of photophobia and nausea. Autopsy findings may not necessarily include characteristic acute inflammation of the meninges, as death may result from endotoxemia before overt acute inflammation becomes established. Brain swelling with vessel thrombosis and/or infarction may occur and bilateral intraadrenal hemorrhage, Waterhouse–Friderichsen syndrome, may be present.

Gastroenteritis

Globally, gastroenteritis is one of the major causes of infant and early childhood death. Dehydration and electrolyte imbalances may result in fatal outcomes. At autopsy typical features of dehydration include sunken eyes, sunken fontanelle, wrinkling of

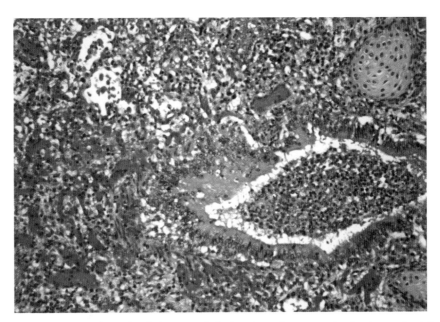

Figure 5 A section of lung from an infant who died unexpectedly from bronchopneumonia showing neutrophils infiltrating a distal bronchus (right) and adjacent alveoli. Vascular congestion and intraalveolar hemorrhage are also present. Hematoxylin & eosin, 200×.

the liver capsule, and drying of mucosal and serosal surfaces. Vitreous humor analyses will show sodium levels of greater than $155 \, \text{mmol} \, l^{-1}$. Hyperkalemic cardiac arrhythmias may cause sudden death, as may central nervous system venous thromboses. Neglect or deliberate withholding of water must be considered.

Respiratory Conditions

Acute upper-airway obstruction by foreign material such as food (**Figure 6**) or a toy part is not uncommon in infants and young children. Other respiratory causes of sudden death in children are less frequent.

Asthma

Although acute asthma may cause sudden death in the pediatric age range it usually involves older children who have either a history or autopsy findings of significant disease. Death may be due to asphyxia, cardiac arrhythmia, or electrolyte disturbance. Anti-asthma drugs have been implicated in some cases and full toxicological screening is required. At autopsy there is usually hyperinflation of the lungs with mucus plugging of airways. There may be a pneumothorax or changes of alveolar overdistension.

Upper-Airway Obstruction

Apart from airway blockage from foreign materials, there are a range of natural disorders that may encroach upon the upper aerodigestive tract producing critical narrowing. These include choanal atresia, lingual thyroglossal duct cysts, nasopharyngeal tumors, heterotopic tissues, vascular malformations, and upper-airway infections. Micrognathia in conditions such as Pierre–Robin syndrome may cause a retro-positioned tongue to occlude the airway, as may macroglossia. Structural defects such as laryngo- and tracheomalacia may also narrow the airway, as may upper-airway infections.

Bronchopulmonary Dysplasia

This chronic lung disease develops in infants after a period of prolonged assisted ventilation. It is characterized by scarring of lung parenchyma with obliteration of alveolar spaces. Pulmonary hypertension, ventilation–perfusion mismatch, bronchial hyper-reactivity, and reduced lung compliance may all be associated with an increased risk of sudden death.

Neurological Conditions

Conditions that interfere with neural control of respiration and cardiac function may cause sudden death. Due to the unique characteristics of the skull, space-occupying lesions in the form of tumors or hemorrhage may not only compromise cerebral function by destroying tissue, but may also cause elevation of intracranial pressure. This compresses vital centers and interferes with blood flow and oxygenation.

Hematological Disorders

Any conditions that predispose to spontaneous hemorrhage, such as hemophilia or thrombocytopenia,

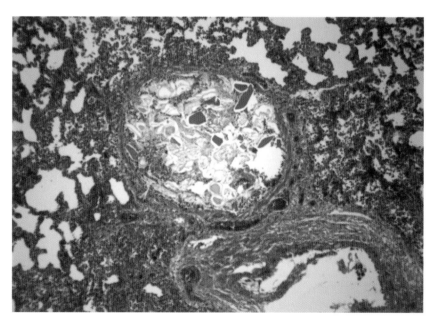

Figure 6 A case of fatal aspiration in a young child with occlusion of a bronchiole by gastric contents including meat fibers. Hematoxylin & eosin, 200×.

may be associated with lethal intracranial hemorrhage. Similarly, hematological conditions with a tendency to spontaneous thrombosis such as deficiencies in plasminogen, antithrombin III, and proteins S and C, may cause ischemic stroke in children. This may also occur with the hemoglobinopathies.

Vascular Disorders

Vascular malformations or aneurysms may cause death due to spontaneous hemorrhage from weakened vessel walls. Both vascular malformations and aneurysms may be solitary or associated with more generalized conditions, including Osler–Weber–Rendu syndrome (hereditary hemorrhagic telangiectasia), cystic renal and liver disease, and connective tissue disorders.

Tumors

Tumors located at critical sites in the brain may cause death due to compression of brainstem autonomic control centers or to acute hydrocephalus from obstruction to cerebrospinal fluid drainage. Presenting symptoms may be entirely nonspecific and treatment for a presumed viral gastroenteritis may have been mistakenly initiated in the preceding days. Even quite slow-growing tumors within the cranial cavity may precipitate clinical deterioration if there is hemorrhage into the tumor or into adjacent cerebral tissue.

Epilepsy

While it is recognized that there is an increased risk of sudden death in epileptic children, underlying mechanisms are far from clear. Certainly there is a risk of traumatic death such as drowning in children with epilepsy, or to death from an underlying syndrome such as tuberous sclerosis. However, other children may be found dead with minimal findings. Suffocation, respiratory arrest, and/or cardiac arrhythmias are likely mechanisms in fatal cases. Autopsy examinations should include neuropathological evaluation of the brain, looking for underlying abnormalities that may have been responsible for the epileptic discharges, or for evidence of chronic hypoxic–ischemic damage due to previous fitting.

Metabolic Disorders

Familial or acquired metabolic disorders may be associated with thromboembolism and ischemic stroke (e.g., homocystinuria), or hemorrhage (e.g., scurvy).

Structural Abnormalities

Children with Arnold–Chiari malformation, in which there is downward displacement of the medulla and cerebellum into the cervical spinal canal, are at risk of sudden death due to a variety of problems. Brainstem compression may cause respiratory arrest and recurrent laryngeal nerve paralysis may result in laryngeal obstruction. Shunts inserted for hydrocephalus may block, or cause lethal thromboembolism, pulmonary hypertension, or ascending infection.

Miscellaneous Disorders

Unexpected death has also occurred in children with a wide range of disorders that affect the central nervous system including Friedreich's ataxia, tuberous sclerosis, von Recklinghausen disease, septo-optic dysplasia, Guillain-Barré syndrome, and Déjérine–Sottas disease.

Hematological Conditions

Hemoglobinopathies

The most significant hemoglobinopathy is sickle-cell disease due to replacement of glutamic acid by valine in the sixth position on the β-chain of the hemoglobin molecule. Reduced plasticity of red blood cells results in a sickled shape with blood vessel obstruction. Sequestration crisis occurs when sickled red cells become trapped within the spleen, causing circulatory collapse. Homozygous children are also at risk of sudden death due to overwhelming sepsis.

Hematological Malignancies

Acute leukemias may present as sudden death due to intracerebral hemorrhage from primary or secondary thrombocytopenia. Mediastinal lymphomas have been associated with external compression of the upper airway with lethal obstruction.

Disorders of Coagulation

Inherited or acquired defects in coagulation pathways may result in life-threatening hemorrhage, particularly if bleeding occurs inside the skull. Accidental and inflicted injuries must be considered in cases of intracranial hemorrhage given they are far more common than disorders of coagulation.

Gastrointestinal Conditions

Intestinal Obstruction

Intussusception and volvulus are causes of potentially lethal intestinal obstruction in children. Although the usual presentation involves abdominal pain and vomiting, occasional cases are clinically silent, resulting in serious electrolyte disturbances and dehydration with established sepsis occurring before a diagnosis is made. These cases may, therefore, not be identified until autopsy. Predisposing lesions such as hyperplastic Peyer patches or Meckel diverticulum in cases of intussusception and cystic fibrosis in cases of volvulus should be looked for.

Gastric Dilatation and Perforation

Marked gastric dilatation with fatal perforation may occur in children with cerebral palsy due to air swallowing and autonomic neuropathy, in children with eating disorders, and in children with Prader–Willi syndrome. In the latter instance excessive appetite with decreased vomiting and a high pain threshold predispose to gastric rupture.

Late-Presenting Diaphragmatic Hernias

Small defects in the diaphragm may not be associated with intrauterine herniation of abdominal organs into the pleural cavity. As a result, defects may be plugged by the spleen or liver until much later in life. When herniation occurs there may be sudden death from mediastinal shift with compression of the heart and lungs. Occasional cases survive for some time with nonspecific symptoms until gastric or intestinal perforation occurs into the pleural space. Cases have presented in a similar manner to SIDS.

Genitourinary Conditions

Although diseases of the renal system are not usually associated with sudden death, certain conditions may have catastrophic outcomes.

Wilms Tumor

Wilms tumor, or nephroblastoma (**Figure 7**), is a primary malignancy of the kidneys that occurs mainly in childhood and is now associated with a good prognosis. Occasional cases may, however, present with sudden death, for example, if there has been extensive hemorrhage into tumor parenchyma, or if a portion of this angioinvasive tumor extends into or embolizes to the lungs.

Hemolytic–Uremic Syndrome

This systemic thrombotic microangiopathy is characterized by thrombocytopenia, hemolytic anemia, and renal insufficiency. It often follows infection with vero-toxin producing *Escherichia coli* and may cause sudden death from intracerebral hemorrhage.

Complications of Pregnancy

Pregnancy should be excluded as a possible cause of sudden death in any sexually mature female adolescent. Conditions such as amniotic fluid embolism, ruptured ectopic pregnancy, placental hemorrhage, peripartum cardiomyopathy, or vascular rupture should be checked for at autopsy.

Metabolic Conditions

More than 30 metabolic disorders that may cause illness and death in infancy and childhood can now be detected by tandem mass spectrometry, which is indicated in essentially all cases of unexplained infant and childhood death. Even though they are rare, their

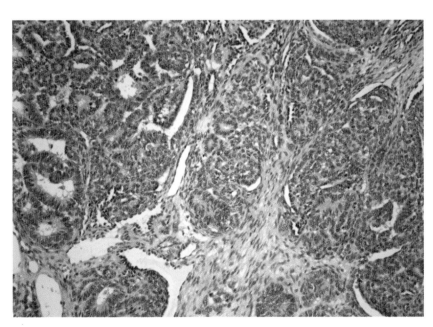

Figure 7 Wilms tumor characterized by epithelial, blastemal, and ill-defined mesenchymal differentiation. Hematoxylin & eosin, 200×.

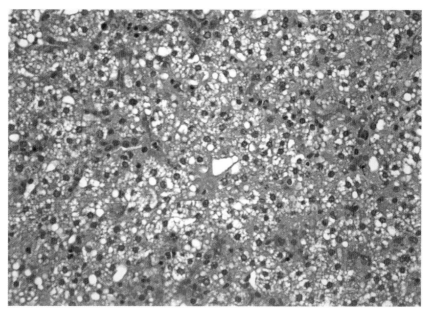

Figure 8 A section of liver from a neonate who died suddenly at 3 days of age with very-long-chain acyl-coenzyme A dehydrogenase deficiency revealing diffuse microvesicular fatty change. Hematoxylin & eosin, 200×.

diagnosis is critical in not only explaining death, but also in future pregnancy planning. Although amino acid and organic acid disorders are usually characterized by obvious illness and deterioration, fatty acid disorders such as medium-chain acyl-coenzyme A dehydrogenase deficiency (MCAD), long-chain acyl-coenzyme A dehydrogenase deficiency (LCAD), and very-long-chain acyl-coenzyme A dehydrogenase deficiency (VCLAD) (**Figure 8**), long-chain L-3-hydroxy acyl-coenzyme A dehydrogenase deficiency (LCHAD), and carnitine palmitoyltransferase deficiency type II (CPT II) may have subtle courses before sudden death occurs.

Endocrine Conditions

Insulin-Dependent Diabetes Mellitus

Sudden death may occur in affected children from ketoacidosis, or from excessive insulin administration. There is also a group of young diabetics who have been found dead in bed for no obvious reason. Nocturnal hypoglycemia may be the cause of death in these cases.

Adrenal Hypo- and Hyperplasia

Congenital hypoplasia of the adrenal gland may be associated with an Addisonian crisis and death. Conversely, hyperplasia of the adrenal glands, due to enzymatic defects in the cortisol synthetic pathway, may lead to excessive sodium loss and collapse.

Miscellaneous Conditions

A variety of other rare and unusual conditions may be found at autopsy in cases of sudden and unexpected infant and childhood death. These include connective tissue disorders such as Ehlers–Danlos and Marfan syndromes; skeletal disorders such as achondroplasia; dermatological disorders such as hypohidrotic ectodermal dysplasia; muscular disorders such as malignant hyperthermia; chromosomal disorders such as trisomy 21 and fragile X syndrome; and immunological conditions such as anaphylaxis and myasthenia gravis.

Conclusions

While SIDS remains the most common cause of postneonatal sudden unexpected infant death, a wide range of other conditions may cause sudden and unexpected death in infancy and early childhood. Accurate delineation of the cause and manner of death is dependent upon meticulous review of the medical history, careful examination of the death scene, and thorough postmortem examination. Scene reconstruction may be especially illuminating in understanding potential mechanisms of death in cases of noninflicted injury. Ancillary studies, including tandem mass spectroscopy screening for metabolic disorders and measurement of vitreous electrolytes, are also critically important in the evaluation of cases in which the cause of death is not immediately apparent. Unfortunately, unless autopsy examinations are scrupulously undertaken, many of the cases of subtle natural disease described above will remain undiagnosed or misdiagnosed.

See Also

Children: Physical Abuse; Non-inflicted Causes of Death; **Sudden Infant Death Syndrome, Etiology and Epidemiology**

Further Reading

Adams EJ, Chavez GF, Steen D, *et al.* (1998) Changes in the epidemiologic profile of sudden infant death syndrome as rates decline among California infants: 1990–1995. *Pediatrics* 102: 1445–1451.

Berger S, Dhala A, Friedberg DZ (1999) Sudden cardiac death in infants, children, and adolescents. *Pediatric Clinics of North America* 46: 221–234.

Byard RW (1996) Vascular causes of sudden death in infancy, childhood and adolescence. *Cardiovascular Pathology* 5: 243–257.

Byard RW (2003) Unexpected infant and childhood death. In: Payne-James J, Busuttil A, Smock W (eds.) *Forensic Medicine: Clinical and Pathological Aspects*, pp. 231–245. London: Greenwich Medical Media.

Byard RW (2004) *Sudden Death in Infancy, Childhood and Adolescence,* 2nd edn. Cambridge, UK: Cambridge University Press.

Byard RW, Krous HF (2001) The differential diagnosis of sudden infant death. In: Byard RW, Krous HF (eds.) *Sudden Infant Death Syndrome – Problems, Progress and Possibilities*, pp. 209–227. London: Arnold.

Byard RW, Krous HF (2003) Sudden infant death syndrome: overview and update. *Pediatric and Developmental Pathology* 6: 112–127.

Corey H, Andy T, Buchino JJ (1998) Sudden natural death in infants and young children. *Clinics in Laboratory Medicine* 18: 323–338.

Denfield SW, Garson A (1990) Sudden death in children and young adults. *Pediatric Clinics of North America* 37: 215–231.

Gillette PC, Garson A (1992) Sudden cardiac death in the pediatric population. *Circulation* 85: I-64–I-69.

Goodwin JF (1997) Sudden cardiac death in the young. A family history of sudden death needs investigation. *British Medical Journal* 314: 843.

Klitzner TS (1990) Sudden cardiac death in children. *Circulation* 82: 629–632.

Krous HF (1995) The differential diagnosis of sudden, unexpected infant death. In: Rognum TO (ed.) *Sudden Infant Death Syndrome: New Trends in the Nineties,* Vol. 16, pp. 74–80. Oslo: Scandinavian University Press.

Morentin B, Aguilera B, Garamendi PM, Suarez-Mier MP (2000) Sudden unexpected non-violent death between 1 and 19 years in north Spain. *Archives of Disease in Childhood* 82: 456–461.

Non-inflicted Causes of Death

R W Byard, Forensic Science Centre, Adelaide, SA, Australia
T S Corey, University of Louisville School of Medicine and Office of the Chief Medical Examiner, Louisville, KY, USA

Introduction

Nomenclature has been changing in recent years, and proposals have been advanced that the term "accident" should be abandoned, as most noninflicted injuries are predictable and preventable. While the authors can see certain merit in this concept it is not completely correct, as some injuries are not preventable. In addition, "accident" is a standard classification that is used for manner of death and it is a word with which most readers would be quite familiar. For these reasons the term has continued to be used in this article when referring to traumatic episodes arising from noninflicted injury.

Causes of accidental death in childhood vary considerably depending on the age group and community studied, but overall are due in large part to motor vehicle-associated events. Other common scenarios involve drowning, thermal injuries, falls, poisoning, and choking. Mechanical suffocation is the second most important cause of accidental death in infants after motor vehicle crashes, compared to adolescents where drowning occupies the second position, well behind motor vehicle accidents. Firearm deaths occupy third position in 15–19-year-olds in the USA but are quite rare in this age group in other communities such as Australia.

Rates of accidental death are also quite different in different countries with rates as high as 30.5 per 100 000 of the population reported in the age range 1–19 years in the USA in the 1980s, compared to 10.8 per 10 000 for children under 4 years, 5.3 in 5–9-year-olds, 6.4 in 10–14-year-olds, and 29.2 in 15–24-year-olds in Australia in the 1990s. Reported rates from other countries are summarized in **Table 1**.

Motor Vehicle Deaths

Children may suffer lethal injuries in motor vehicle crashes as passengers, pedestrians, cyclists, or drivers (at older ages). The extent of injuries to passengers and drivers is determined by the circumstances of the crash, the speed of impact, and whether restraining harnesses or seatbelts were used. Unusual behavior by a parent prior to a single vehicle crash when all of

Table 1 Rates of accidental death per 100 000 of the population in the age range 1–19 years in various countries

USA	30.5
Canada	26.1
Norway	22.3
France	21.5
England and Wales	15.6
The Netherlands	13.1

the children in a family are in a vehicle raises the possibility of murder suicide.

Injuries in high-speed impacts are often multiple, involving head, chest, and abdominal trauma. Head injuries are often lethal in isolation with closed head injuries, atlantooccipital fracture–dislocations, and brainstem lacerations. Severe skull and facial skeletal fractures are often associated with lacerations and disruption of the brain. Other lethal injuries that are not uncommonly encountered are aortic transection, cardiac lacerations, flail chest, and extensive parenchymal disruption of the liver and spleen. Chest injuries may occur without significant rib fractures due to the elasticity of the juvenile ribcage.

While seatbelts and restraining harnesses have undoubtedly reduced morbidity and mortality from vehicle crashes, they must be correctly worn; additionally, caregivers must ensure that the child is tall enough for proper fit of standard, factory-installed restraint devices. Loosely fitting belts have been associated with carotid artery and aortic transection, in addition to other intraabdominal organ injuries when children have "submarined" under webbing. Shoulder harnesses that contact the neck in children who should be in booster seats may cause carotid artery injury. Booster seats that are used to elevate a small child in an adult car seat may predispose to slipping under belts if they are not firmly and correctly tethered. Unfortunately, assessment as to whether a seatbelt was used at the time of a fatal crash is often difficult, as markings on the skin may be absent or may be masked by the interposition of clothing.

Pedestrians tend to be older than passengers, reflecting increased independent mobility with age. Fatal injuries again involve the head and neck followed by the abdomen and chest. Childhood pedestrian fatalities occur in a bimodal distribution. In one group, a common scenario may involve a child running across a road into traffic without being aware of the dangers involved. A somewhat younger group involves events occurring in domestic driveways when a parent backs a vehicle over a toddler. Assessment of patterned injuries or the direction of brush abrasions may assist in determining a likely sequence of events.

Cyclists tend to be an older group: injuries occur in children or adolescents who are considered old enough to ride bicycles in, or near, traffic. Injuries may result from direct impact with a vehicle, or from secondary impact against the ground or another vehicle. Alternatively, falling on to bicycle handlebars has also been responsible for a percentage of injuries to abdominal organs.

Drowning

Children are at increased risk of drowning at two age ranges: under 4 years and 15–19 years. These particular ages reflect young children's inability to understand and/or deal with potentially dangerous environments, and risk-taking behavior by adolescents. The diagnosis of drowning may not be straightforward and depends on circumstantial evidence and the exclusion at autopsy of underlying natural diseases or inflicted trauma. As infants and very young children can be held under water with minimal effort by an adult, the possibility of homicide may be difficult to exclude in the absence of independent verification of the history.

Infants and young children are at particular risk of drowning in swimming pools and baths if left unattended. Curious children playing in water may overbalance into pools and be unable to extricate themselves. Baths also have slippery bases and sides and it may not be possible for an infant with immature physical coordination and strength to remove him- or herself from water once immersed. Parents and child carers may have been lulled into a false sense of security if an infant is in a bath with an older sibling, or in an infant bath seat (**Figure 1**). However, no infant should be left in water unattended

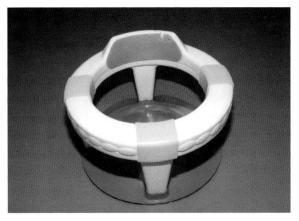

Figure 1 A 7-month-old boy was found drowned in a bath after slipping through the sides of a plastic baby bath seat and becoming entrapped. His 2½-year-old brother was in the bath with him at the time. They were left alone by their mother.

by an adult carer, either alone or with a sibling. In fact, it has even been suggested that an infant may be at increased risk of drowning if left in a bath with a stronger, more active sibling. Bath seats may also tip over and entrap infants, and infants may slip down in such seats and get trapped under water.

Toddlers are also at risk of drowning in industrial buckets that are partially filled with water. Curiosity, combined with infants' high center of gravity, predispose children to slip headfirst into buckets and remain trapped. Similar deaths have occurred in infants slipping into toilet bowls.

The average time that infants who have drowned have been left unattended has been cited as less than 5 min, with only small amounts of water necessary to cause death. For example, children have drowned in as little as 5 cm of water in bathtubs.

At autopsy there may be changes such as skin wrinkling associated with prolonged immersion and marked pulmonary edema. However, if laryngospasm has occurred there may be minimal fluid present in the lungs. Diatom examinations and assessment of differential chloride levels between the right and left sides of the heart have not been proved as useful tests for drowning. Layer dissections of the neck and back may reveal occult bruising if a young child has struggled while being intentionally held under water.

An important part of an autopsy examination is exclusion of natural disease that may either have caused death while a child was in water, or incapacitated the child, facilitating drowning. A classic example of the latter situation is epilepsy. The effects of other natural diseases may be exacerbated by exercise from swimming such as myocarditis, aortic stenosis, hypertrophic cardiomyopathy, or prolonged QT interval resulting in a lethal outcome.

Thermal Deaths

There are a variety of types of lethal and nonlethal thermal injury, including flame burns which char skin and singe hair, scalding from hot fluids, and contact burns from touching hot objects. Scalds are the most frequent type of nonlethal accidental thermal injury in children, followed by contact and flame burns. In fatal cases, however, deaths from residential fires are more common than lethal scalds. Scalds may be due to spills, splashes, or immersion. Spills usually occur when a young child pulls over a container of hot liquid. Resultant injuries are characterized by irregular margins and a nonuniform depth of injury with an "arrowhead" pattern as liquids flow downward, cooling with distance, resulting in progressively shallower and narrower lesions. Accidental scalds usually involve the head, face, arms, and upper torso. Splash

scalds occur when a child immersed in hot water moves and attempts to get out of the tub.

Children who die in house fires may be incinerated, making autopsy assessment difficult due to charring of remains, heat-induced fractures, and loss of body parts. In cases in which the circumstances are considered suspicious, radiographs may be helpful in identifying bullets or other foreign bodies prior to postmortem examination. More intact bodies may show cherry-pink discoloration typical of carbon monoxide toxicity. The presence of soot in the airways indicates that the deceased had been alive for some time during the fire. Absence of these features suggests that death occurred prior to a fire that may have been set in an attempt to disguise a homicide.

Occasionally, blood carboxyhemoglobin levels may be quite low. This will occur if there has been survival for some time after a fire with attempted resuscitation, resulting in blood carbon monoxide levels falling. It is also possible that cyanide poisoning derived from burning plastic materials contributed to death. Measurement of blood cyanide concentration may be helpful in cases where there is some doubt about the toxicity of the level of carbon monoxide. All bodies should be carefully assessed for signs of injury. Levels of carboxyhemoglobin may also not be high in cases where there has been a rapid flash fire involving solvents, as minimal carbon monoxide may be generated in such cases. Children may also have lower levels of carboxyhemoglobin than adults in fatal cases, as they may be more vulnerable to the effects of fire due to their higher respiratory rates and smaller airways that are more susceptible to mucus obstruction. Additionally, very young babies may succumb to carbon monoxide at lower environmental concentrations due to the higher affinity of fetal hemoglobin for the carbon monoxide molecule.

Cases are not uncommonly encountered where more than one child in a family has died in a house fire. This generally occurs because children tend to practice avoidance behavior rather than escape. For example, if a fire starts in a bedroom where a child has been playing with matches or a cigarette lighter, children may gather in the part of the room that is furthest from the flames rather than trying to exit by a door or window. Another scenario involves a young mother with multiple children who tries to gather the family to escape. In such a scenario, the bodies of the family members may be found commingled near an exit. In such commingling of remains, it is recommended that the remains be transported as a "unit" and separated in the autopsy suite. This allows the pathologist an opportunity to observe the spatial relationships that may alter thermal patterns on the bodies, and prevents loss of potentially important evidence such as teeth or small bones.

Fire deaths have also occurred in cars when, for example, bored children have been playing with matches or electric car lighters. The interiors of modern vehicles are highly flammable and there may be papers, rubbish, and other combustible material present that will add to the conflagration. Again, children who were left in the front of cars may be found in the back seat due to avoidance rather than escape behavior. Locked car doors may be another impediment to escape. Deaths from thermal injuries may be immediate or protracted, resulting from sepsis with contributions from metabolic disturbances and dehydration.

Asphyxia

Asphyxial fatalities occur when there has been sufficient deprivation of oxygen to cause death. Accidental suffocation may occur in a variety of ways, including:

- smothering if the external airways are covered
- choking if there is obstruction of the internal airways
- external pressure on the chest in mechanical asphyxia
- oxygen deprivation in entrapment or where there has been replacement of oxygen by inert gases.

Sleeping Accidents

Infants and young children are at risk of asphyxial deaths in cribs from a number of causes. Smothering may occur if an infant becomes wrapped in, or pressed against, plastic that has been used to cover a mattress, crib, or pillow to prevent soiling (**Figure 2**).

Particularly dangerous are thin plastic dry-cleaning or garbage disposal bags. Infants may also asphyxiate if they are left sleeping face-down on polystyrene-filled cushions or pillows. No specific autopsy features will be present in such cases, which will not be able to be differentiated from sudden infant death syndrome based purely on pathological findings. Such deaths demonstrate the importance of scene investigation, and integration of this information into the case facts considered when determining the cause and manner of death.

Strangulation occurs when external pressure on the neck obstructs blood vessels and air passages. The vessels become occluded at much lower external pressures than the actual airway, so the vast majority of strangulations are due to compromise of blood flow to the head rather than actual airway compression. Infants and young children are again at risk in their cribs and beds if clothing becomes caught on bolts or projections inside a crib. Once balance is lost, an infant may become suspended. If the child is not discovered immediately, hanging usually results in a clearly defined parchmented ligature mark around the neck. If the venous return is occluded prior to arterial flow into the head, an infant who has hanged may also have petechiae of the face and conjunctivae. Hanging may also occur if an infant slips down through the floor or side of a broken crib and becomes suspended by the neck, or hangs over the side of a crib or seat (**Figure 3**).

Wedging deaths may occur in cribs when a thick mattress does not completely fit the crib, leaving a space at the side into which an infant may roll or slip, or in gaps between pieces of sectional furniture or between "adult furniture" and an interior wall. Death results from a combination of mechanical asphyxia due to pressure on the chest and smothering

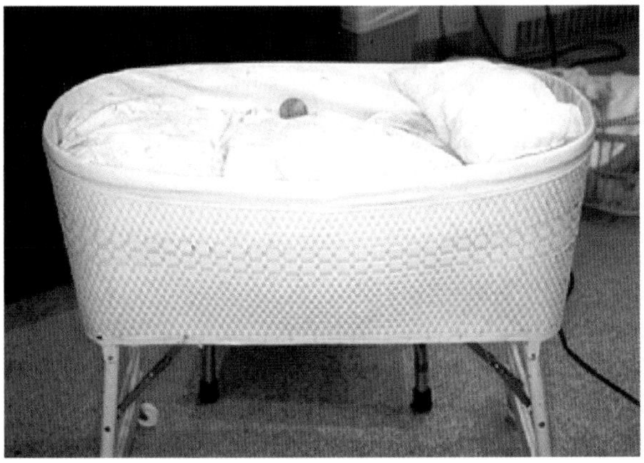

Figure 2 A young infant was found wedged between pillows and the plastic-lined side of the old borrowed bassinet. Fluffy pillows had been added by the parents. Suffocation had resulted when the infant's face had pressed against the plastic liner.

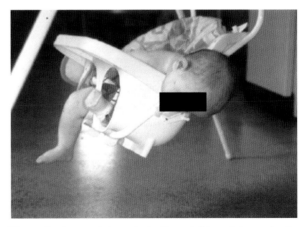

Figure 3 A young infant who had been left in an infant swing for several hours was found dead with his head hanging over the edge. Death was due to neck compression.

from the mattress covering the nose and mouth. Portable mesh-sided cribs are a particular problem if a thicker mattress has been added to the crib, as the distensible sides easily allow an infant to slip between the mesh and mattress and suffocate. Similar deaths have occurred when infants or toddlers have slipped between adult mattresses and walls or headboards. While facial and conjunctival petechiae are uncommon in such circumstances, lividity patterns and impressions from mattresses and bed clothing may help to corroborate histories.

Toddlers may also wind window cords or electric flexes around their necks and hang if their cribs have been left within reach of curtains or electrical appliances such as fans. Hanging may also occur if infants have been left unattended in seats with restraining harness such as infant bouncer or car seats.

Choking

Infants and young children are at risk of choking from inhaled foreign bodies; the peak age is between 2 and 3 years with most cases occurring under 5 years. Young children develop their incisor teeth well before their molars and so are able to bite off pieces of firm food before being able to masticate them adequately. Rounded and/or hard foods such as hot dogs, candy, carrots, nuts, and grapes present particular problems, as do parts of toys, balloons, metal screws, and plastic pen components.

While most children present with a history of wheezy breathing, gagging, or coughing, in some cases foreign bodies may remain asymptomatic until fatal airway obstruction occurs. Objects may also lodge in the esophagus rather than the airways. Deaths from inhaled foreign bodies may also be due to vessel perforation or sepsis.

Autopsy assessment of these cases may be difficult if the obstructing object has been removed during resuscitation attempts. Reliance on the history will be vital in formulating a likely cause and manner of death.

Mechanical Asphyxia

Fatal accidental compression asphyxia in childhood is a rare event. Younger children tend to be trapped under furniture or by industrial equipment while playing, whereas older children become trapped in excavated ditches or under motor vehicles in similar circumstances to adult traumatic asphyxial deaths.

Overlaying

Suffocation of an infant who has been sleeping in the same bed as an adult may be difficult to prove, given that there are usually no specific autopsy findings. Evaluation of these cases requires a clear description of the positions that the infant was placed to sleep in, and then found. Softness of the mattress, amount of bedding and parental fatigue, sedation, or intoxication should all be documented. Examination of parental clothing may reveal staining by serosanguineous infant oral secretions, demonstrating close contact between the parent and child at some time during the night. Although in some cases no decision may be able to be made, the diagnosis is sustainable when there is a clear history of an infant being found beneath the body, limb, or breast of a sedated adult.

Other Asphyxial Deaths

Accidental hanging may occur in adolescent males engaging in sexual asphyxia where hypoxia is used to augment solitary sexual activities. The presence of fetish items and pornography, and the secluded nature of the scene, usually mean that the diagnosis presents no difficulties.

Falls from Heights

While there is no doubt that infants and children may be severely injured or die from falls, there is considerable debate regarding the amount of force that is required to cause lethal injuries. Unfortunately, much of the early literature relied upon the unchallenged histories of cases, which were subsequently shown to be potentially unreliable. For example, if the presenting history in several series is believed, then short falls around the house are far more lethal than witnessed falls from considerable heights. The reality is that inflicted injuries sustained in the company of only one adult are often blamed upon accidents.

Characteristic features of inflicted craniocerebral trauma blamed on short falls are described elsewhere. The investigation of such cases requires a full autopsy with clear documentation of injuries, including radiographs, with independent verification of the history if possible and examination of the scene or scene photographs. Significant bruising and soft-tissue swelling may occur if a young child or toddler falls on to a hard sharp object such as a plastic toy or the edge of furniture (**Figure 4**).

Poisoning and Drug Toxicity

Deaths from poisoning tend to occur in two age groups: toddlers and adolescents. Young children are at risk of ingesting a variety of mainly household toxins while exploring. These commonly include plants, medicines prescribed for adult caregivers but left within reach of children, and household products such as cleaning agents, insecticides, and petroleum derivatives. Toxicological screening may be hampered

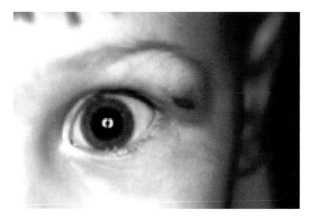

Figure 4 Thirty minutes after a healthy toddler was witnessed falling on to a table edge, significant periorbital edema and redness, with an overlying superficial abrasion, can be seen around the left eye. The injury resolved without sequelae.

by the range of possible substances ingested in a suspected case, and so a full inventory of household medications and materials should be obtained. Organic toxins may be even more difficult to detect.

Adolescents are at risk of unintentional death from illicit drug or alcohol ingestion, or suicide from intentionally ingested prescription medications. The nature of drug deaths varies depending on the community involved and toxicological screening should be based on local drug-taking practices.

Adolescent drowning and motor vehicle accident deaths are often characterized by alcohol consumption. Alcohol also causes death from respiratory depression, positional asphyxia, or inhalation of gastric contents. Rural communities have reported deaths from gasoline inhalation, whereas other types of volatile agent tend to be used in urban areas. Deaths from drugs such as cocaine and opiates tend to involve older individuals, although designer amphetamines have caused a number of deaths of adolescents in so-called "rave" dance clubs.

Electrocution

Electrocution deaths are uncommon in children and occur either when a child is playing with or near a faulty electrical device at home, or when an older child climbs a tree or building near high-voltage power lines.

Farm Deaths

Farms are quite dangerous places for children and adolescents: there are high rates of unintentional injury and death compared to cities. Deaths occur in young children from vehicle run-overs, falls, drowning, or from animal kicks. Older children may

fall from horses or be fatally injured while using machinery unsupervised. Injuries tend to be extensive, with amputations, crush injuries, and evisceration.

Deaths Related to Animal Activity

In addition to falls from horses or kicks from farm animals, a range of potentially lethal injuries may arise from animals, including envenomation from spiders and snakes, anaphylaxis from insects, and mauling from domestic dogs. Dog attacks are characterized by lacerations and puncture wounds around the head and limbs: deaths may occur from cranial trauma, neck injuries, or exsanguination from deep lacerations involving vessels. Young children are particularly vulnerable to dog attacks as they are small, defenseless, and may provoke animals. Fatal dog attacks may involve more than one dog, with "pack behavior" precipitating the fatal event, despite otherwise placid behavior by all dogs but the "alpha" member of the pack (**Figure 5**).

Sports Deaths

Children playing sport may collapse due to the effects of occult or known underlying organic diseases, such

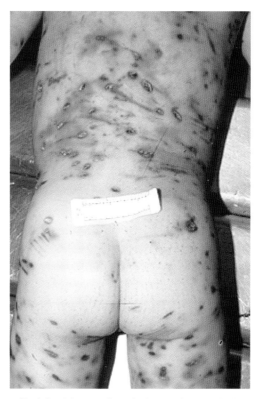

Figure 5 A fatal dog mauling of a 3-year-old boy who had been attacked by a number of mixed-breed dogs in a fenced backyard. Multiple sets of puncture wounds from canine incisors are present with patterned abrasions from dragging of incisors over the skin surface.

as asthma, hypertrophic cardiomyopathy, congenital heart disease (with or without surgery), and myocarditis, exacerbated by activity. Alternatively, trauma may play a role in death, with head and neck injuries accounting for a number of cases. A specific entity that may occur in children or adolescents who have been hit in the chest by a hardball or hockey puck is commotio cordis. Impact is followed by collapse with intractable cardiac arrest/arrhythmias.

Environmental Temperature-Related Deaths

As at all ages, deaths may be caused by exposure to high or low environmental temperatures. Infants are particularly predisposed to hyperthermia as they have high metabolic rates and are generally not able to extricate themselves from hot environments. Infants heavily swaddled in warm rooms and children left in cars on hot days are at increased risk of lethal hyperthermia. If exposure occurs over several hours, there may be evidence at autopsy of dehydration with skin slippage and elevated vitreous humor sodium levels. If, however, the child is extricated more quickly, autopsy findings may be minimal, and the diagnosis will be dependent on historical information such as first responder reports, and body temperature on arrival at the emergency department. Children may die from lethal cardiac arrhythmias if exposed to low environmental temperatures.

Hospital Deaths

Unintentional deaths of children in hospital may result from failure to monitor adequately or from misadventure due to surgery, anesthesia, drug therapy, or diagnostic procedures. The investigation of such cases requires careful review of the hospital record, including surgical and anesthetic notes and medication history. Equipment that may be implicated in a death should be seized and independently examined, and toxicological analyses should be conducted for a full range of medications, not only those prescribed to the victim.

Conclusion

Full investigation of childhood deaths caused by unintentional trauma requires a clear description of the lethal event with corroboration of the history by independent observers if possible. In fact, many of these deaths in infancy may be misdiagnosed as sudden infant death syndrome if an adequate scene investigation with integration of information into the case history has not occurred. Complete investigation of such deaths is important not only to determine the correct cause and manner of death in an individual case, but also for public health reasons to identify potentially hazardous situations or products. The likelihood of an injury from a described incident must be determined from the autopsy findings and a reconstruction of events. The developmental level of a child must also be taken into account, particularly in very young children, before an event can be accepted as a plausible cause of death or not.

See Also

Children: Physical Abuse; Sudden Natural Infant and Childhood Death; **Falls from Height, Physical Findings:** In Children; **Sudden Natural Death:** Cardiovascular

Further Reading

Buchino JJ, Corey TS, Montgomery V (2002) Sudden unexpected death in hospitalized children. *Journal of Pediatrics* 140: 461–465.

Byard RW (1996) Hazardous infant and early childhood sleeping environments and death scene examination. *Journal of Clinical Forensic Medicine* 3: 115–122.

Byard RW (1996) Mechanisms of unexpected death in infants and young children following foreign body ingestion. *Journal of Forensic Science* 41: 438–441.

Byard RW (2000) Accidental childhood death and the role of the pathologist. *Pediatric and Developmental Pathology* 3: 405–418.

Byard RW, Cohle SD (2004) *Accidents* (Chapter 2). *Sudden Death in Infancy, Childhood and Adolescence*, 2nd edn. Cambridge, UK: Cambridge University Press.

Byard RW, Lipsett J (1999) Drowning deaths in toddlers and pre-ambulatory children in South Australia. *American Journal of Forensic Medicine and Pathology* 20: 328–332.

Byard RW, Gilbert J, James R, Lipsett J (1999) Pathological features of farm and tractor-related fatalities in children. *American Journal of Forensic Medicine and Pathology* 20: 73–77.

Byard RW, Lipsett J, Gilbert J (2000a) Fire deaths in children in South Australia from 1989 to 1998. *Journal of Paediatric and Child Health* 36: 176–178.

Byard RW, Green H, James RA, Gilbert JD (2000b) Pathological features of childhood pedestrian fatalities. *American Journal of Forensic Medicine and Pathology* 21: 101–106.

Byard RW, James RA, Gilbert JD (2002) School sports deaths. *American Journal of Forensic Medicine and Pathology* 23: 364–367.

Byard RW, Hanson K, James RA (2003a) Fatal unintentional traumatic asphyxia in childhood. *Journal of Paediatric and Child Health* 39: 31–32.

Byard RW, Hanson K, Gilbert JD, James RA (2003b) Death due to electrocution in childhood and early adolescence. *Journal of Paediatric and Child Health* 39: 46–48.

Corey TS, McCloud LC, Nichols GR, Buchino JJ (1992) Infant deaths due to unintentional injury. An 11 year autopsy review. *American Journal of Diseases of Children* 146: 968–971.

Division of Injury Control, Centers for Disease Control (1990) Childhood injuries in the United States. *American Journal of Diseases of Children* 144: 627–646.

Nixon JW, Kemp AM, Levene S, Sibert JR (1995) Suffocation, choking, and strangulation in childhood in England and Wales: epidemiology and prevention. *Archives of Disease in Childhood* 72: 6–10.

Peclet MH, Newman KD, Eichelberger MR, *et al.* (1990) Patterns of injury in children. *Journal of Pediatric Surgery* 25: 85–91.

CLINICAL TRIALS

Contents

Good Clinical Practice and Ethical Aspects

C M Saunders, QEII Medical Centre, Perth, WA, Australia
M J Millward, University of Western Australia, Perth, WA, Australia
A Provis, Mount Hospital, Perth, WA, Australia

Introduction

Evidence for the usefulness of medical treatments is gained in a variety of ways, the "gold standard" of which is a clinical trial. Clinical trials are the tool used to test the safety and efficacy of most new diagnostic and therapeutic measures in patient populations. Although some medical developments (such as surgical techniques) become accepted as standard practice based on careful clinical observations without a comparative clinical trial, most new therapeutic treatments follow from laboratory experiments performed in tissue culture or in animals. It would be unreliable to translate any of these ideas into medical practice without careful controlled clinical trials. These are phase I–IV clinical trials. The first phase (phase I) is to study, for example, drug delivery and toxicity in healthy volunteers or patients with advanced or incurable diseases. Then in phase II to study drug efficacy and activity in a larger group of patients. Following successful phase I and II studies, a new treatment must be tested against the best existing conventional therapy by means of the phase III study, or randomized controlled trial (RCT). If the new treatment proves superior, it will be submitted to government regulatory authorities for approval, which allows the producers to market the drug and doctors to use it in the treatment of patients. After approval, further trials may be done and ongoing surveillance of treatments is carried out either by individual doctors and institutions auditing results or by reporting of adverse events (phase IV). This article will concentrate on the RCT and, in particular, how this applies to new drug treatments, although it should be borne in mind that these observations apply to any therapeutic intervention.

The Randomized Controlled Clinical Trial

The first clinical trial was ascribed to the British naval surgeon James Lind who wrote in 1753:

> On the 20th of May, 1747, I took twelve patients in the scurvy aboard the Salisbury at sea. Their cases were similar...Two of these were ordered a quart of Cyder a day. Two others took twenty five drops of elixir vitriol...Two others took two spoonfuls of vinegar...Two were put under a course of Seawater. Two others had each 2 oranges and one lemon. Two remaining the bigness of a nutmeg...The consequence was the most sudden and visible good were perceived from the use of the oranges and lemons.

In the modern context, the RCT was first developed by RA Fisher in the 1920s for agricultural research, and was introduced some 20 years later into medicine in a trial evaluating antibiotic treatment for tuberculosis. An RCT is a study in which a cohort of subjects with a defined disease is randomly allocated to one or other treatment (which may be an established versus either a new treatment, or using a placebo drug as the control) and their outcomes recorded. The advantages of an RCT are that randomization avoids the types of bias inherent in observational studies, such as confounding, which may result in apparent differences between treatment groups which do not in fact exist, and that by recruiting large numbers of subjects to a trial the chance that the outcomes between the two arms will differ because of unequal distribution to risk factors becomes small. It is possible to calculate this probability – the P-value. If a trial is designed to encompass any patients with a given condition the results can be generalized to the prevention or treatment of the disease as a whole.

The disadvantages of RCT include the randomization process and the difficulties this causes both subjects and researchers, in particular with regard to consent and the effects on the doctor–patient relationship, the concept of equipoise, and the use of a placebo arm in trials. These will be explored in this article.

Design, Conduct, and Review of RCT

An RCT is a carefully designed test to see if one treatment (usually a new one) is superior to an existing treatment. Performing an RCT is a substantial undertaking, requiring cooperation between doctors, scientists, statisticians, and usually a pharmaceutical or biotechnology company (the "sponsor") that has discovered the product to be tested. The first step is to decide how the efficacy of the treatment will be decided (e.g., survival rate of patients with cancer, level of neurological function in patients with multiple sclerosis) and what level of improvement over current treatment the new treatment is expected to produce. For example, if a certain type of cancer has a survival rate of 75% of patients being alive at five years with current treatment, a promising new treatment might be expected to increase this percentage to 85%. The statistician will be able to calculate how many patients will need to be included in the trial to detect this difference reliably if it exists, and how long the patients will need to be followed up. To detect reliably relatively small differences in outcomes, RCTs may involve many hundreds or even thousands of patients.

All RCTs (and indeed all clinical trials of any phase) are set down in detailed written protocols. The protocol is basically an "instruction manual" for undertaking the trial. As well as the prespecified statistics, the protocol will include a list of precisely which patients will be able to enter the trial (called "eligibility criteria"), what treatments they will receive, what tests will be done and when, and what modifications will be made to the treatment if it produces side-effects.

Before the trial can commence, the protocol will be subjected to extensive review by doctors and other experts in the field of medicine relevant to that trial. As well as this, all hospitals and clinics where patients in the trial will be treated must have the trial approved by their ethics committee.

In all clinical trials, patients can only be entered on to the trial after they have provided informed consent. Nearly always, this consent is written and patients are given an information sheet that explains to them the reasons they are being invited to join the trial, what the trial treatments are, and what the potential side-effects and risks are. This written information sheet is also reviewed by the ethics committee to ensure it is sufficiently clear and contains the relevant information. As well as written information, patients will be given a verbal explanation of the trial by the principal investigator, or a member of his/her research staff.

To undertake a study which is not likely to answer the scientific question posed is not only bad science, but also unethical: the patient is being subjected to tests or treatments of which the efficacy cannot be proven in the study. To overcome this, major funding agencies and many ethical committees insist that any proposed research is carefully scrutinized by peer-review processes. When an RCT commences, the sponsor will often set up a committee to review the progress of the trial and assess any problems that may arise. This committee will contain independent medical experts and statisticians who are not involved in the conduct of the trial, and reports regularly to the sponsor. Their recommendations may range from minor matters, such as small changes to the trial treatment and tests done, to recommending the trial be stopped if they think there are new data that may indicate a serious risk to patients.

An example of this "early stopping" happened in May 2002 when an arm of the Women's Health Initiative Study was stopped four years early. In this study, otherwise healthy older women were randomized to receive hormone replacement therapy (HRT) or placebo, the hypothesis being that HRT would prevent a number of diseases, including heart disease. In fact, a little over halfway through follow-up it was found that there was an excess of heart disease (as well as excess breast cancer and stroke, a more expected outcome) and that this very small increase had exceeded the stopping rules. Ethically the trial monitors had to stop the study – it appeared that women in the study had more heart disease, not less, as a result of taking HRT, although there were no excess deaths recorded. However, many clinicians and scientists in the field were disappointed, as stopping the trial early meant that we will never know if taking HRT makes women more or less likely to die from heart disease, and it is unlikely we will ever again be able to repeat this kind of study.

International Guidelines

The ethics of human experimentation were first widely debated following the disclosure of Nazi practices during World War II. In 1946, at the trial of 23 German doctors charged with "war crimes" and "crimes against humanity" for their experimentation on prisoners of war and civilians, the Nuremberg Code was established. This code aimed to protect the interests of human participants in research. Building upon this, the World Medical Assembly in 1964 adopted the Declaration of Helsinki containing "recommendations guiding physicians in biomedical research involving human subjects." This was most recently adopted at the 52nd World Medical Association General Assembly in 2000.

These guidelines recommend that a patient should firstly be assured of the best proven diagnostic or therapeutic method, and that any new treatment being tested will be at least as advantageous as any other, with a reasonably low chance of side-effects. The patient must be informed of the benefits and hazards of all possible treatments, and must be free to refuse to participate in a trial or withdraw at any time. The physician must also be free to change to another treatment if he/she feels this will benefit the patient. The patient may also anticipate that the doctor/investigator will keep any excess investigations in the trial to a minimum.

A number of other international agencies are involved in research guidelines. The European Directive on Good Clinical Practice in Clinical Trials, published in May 2001 (adopted in the UK in May 2004, administered by the Medicines and Healthcare Regulatory Agency (MHRA)) is one of the most far-reaching of these research guidelines. It stipulates tight control and reporting guidelines for clinical research which may well prove costly and unwieldy in practice – in fact, the UK Medical Research Council (MRC) and main UK cancer charity, Cancer Research UK, have assessed the impact of this on UK research and estimated the added bureaucracy and cost could lead to a fall in research output of 90%.

In the USA, the National Committee for Quality Assurance and the Joint Commission on Accreditation of Healthcare Organizations have collaborated to form the Partnership for Human Research Participation, which accredits institutions, and has a national set of standards and a voluntary oversight process that complements current regulatory efforts. Driven by a number of disasters in research, the American Society of Clinical Oncology has developed policies for conduct of clinical research that aim to enhance

public trust in clinical trials by ensuring safety and informed consent, ensuring the integrity of research, encouraging training of researchers, providing accountability and support for the oversight process, and enhancing efficiency and cost-effectiveness of this process. They recommend centralized ethics approvals, education in both science and ethics for researchers, a focus on the process rather than document of consent, federal oversight of research, improved local infrastructures, and avoidance of conflicts of interest.

In the UK, a number of individual medical bodies have also developed guidelines. These include the MRC, the Royal College of Physicians, the King's Fund, the British Medical Association, the Medical Sterile Products Association, and the Association of the British Pharmaceutical Industry (ABPI). There is no statutory legislation on human experimentation (except the Human Fertilization and Embryology Act 1990); however, pharmaceuticals are regulated via the MHRA.

A Patient's Journey through a Clinical Trial

The clinical trial process is described in **Figure 1**.

Ethical Dilemmas in Clinical Trials

RCTs provoke ethical controversy for several reasons. One of the main reasons is that, in an RCT, the treatment a patient receives will be determined by random allocation rather than directly by the doctor and patient themselves. This is contrary to the usual model of medical care where treatment decisions are made by the doctor advising the patient of his/her recommendation and what alternatives there are. In an RCT, both the doctor and the patient must be comfortable with the process of randomization.

An RCT is aiming to test whether a new treatment is better than the "best" current treatment. The concept of "equipoise" has been used to describe the situation where the doctor believes that the patient's best interests would be equally served regardless of which treatment he/she was randomized to. In that circumstance, deciding treatment by random allocation is ethical. However, if the doctor honestly believes that, for an individual patient, one of the treatments in the trial is likely to be less effective or more risky than another treatment, then the doctor is not in equipoise and should not recommend that patient enter the trial.

Equipoise has also been extended beyond the individual doctor to encompass the body of expert

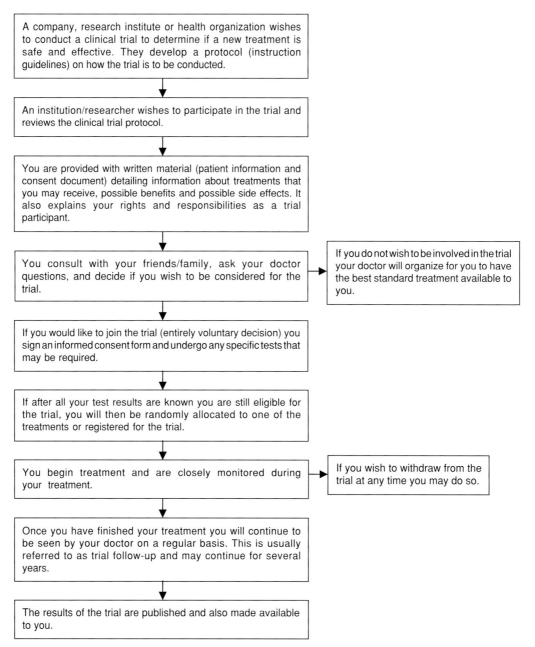

Figure 1   The clinical trial process.

medical opinion about the best treatment for a disease. Suppose there are two ways of treating that condition and among the medical community some doctors always use method A, some always use method B, and others use either A or B depending on individual circumstances. In this scenario, there is "professional equipoise," even though some individual doctors honestly believe A or B is the best treatment. It is ethical to perform an RCT that determines exactly which is the best treatment and all doctors could ethically participate, although many of the "committed" ones may not wish to do so.

Another ethical dilemma in RCTs involves the use of placebos. A placebo is an inactive inert substance with no therapeutic effect, made to look like the treatment being tested (e.g., a pill of the same color). In an RCT involving a placebo, the patient and often the doctor will not be told if the pill the patient is taking is the active treatment or the placebo. Some patients who are treated with placebo report that their symptoms do improve (placebo effect), probably as a result of the positive psychological effect associated with receiving "treatment." However, placebos cannot be ethically used if there is a proven effective treatment for that condition. The only time it is ethical for patients to receive the placebo treatment is where there is genuinely no other treatment or (rarely) where the disease is so mild that no treatment is required at that time.

The placebo issue has recently come into focus again because some placebo trials have been carried out in developing countries for conditions such as human immunodeficiency virus (HIV) where there is proven effective treatment in the developed world. Some researchers have argued that such trials are ethical because the effective treatment is not available to these patients because of their cost and thus there is really "no effective treatment" for them. Thus they could not be worse off by receiving a placebo. However, others have argued that performing such trials only exploits already suffering populations deprived of healthcare by using them to gain knowledge that is primarily intended to benefit developed world patients.

Consent in Clinical Trials

To allow a patient to make an autonomous decision to enter a trial, he/she must be fully informed about his/her disease and its treatment. This will include details of the clinical trial the patient is being requested to join, along with the risks and benefits of all possible treatments (of course, a patient outside a trial should also be informed of all possible treatments and not simply the one he/she is offered). If the patient then consents to the treatment or trial then there is informed consent.

But we may be faced with another dilemma: although it is ethically imperative to obtain a patient's fully informed consent before initiating any treatment within a clinical trial, there may be situations in which full disclosure is harmful to the doctor–patient relationship, in particular if the doctor is no longer viewed as offering the patient the "best" individualized treatment, but instead acting as researcher with treatment allocated "randomly". This predicament has been shown to be a major factor in poor accrual rates into clinical trials as the clinical researcher needs to spend considerable effort to explain the trials process to a patient.

The Incompetent Patient

Clinical trials generally require patients to be competent to make informed decisions on whether to enter the trial or not. However in some areas of medicine patients may not be competent to make such decisions. New treatments for childhood diseases must be performed in children below the age of legal consent.

Their parent or guardian is able to consent on their behalf, although for older children the doctor will normally give some explanation to the child, and aim to get an understanding if the child at least assents to the trial treatment. Adolescents just below the legal age of consent (18 years in most countries) may formally sign a consent form with their parent/guardian.

Other situations where issues of competency arise are in trials for patients with head injuries, for patients in intensive care units, and for patients with Alzheimer or similar diseases. International guidelines provide some direction on when it is permissible to enroll such patients in trials, and what safeguards need to be in place.

Some writers have suggested that all patients with serious illnesses are incapable of giving fully informed consent to enter trials, as their judgment is clouded by the possibility of death or serious disability. However, serious illness *per se* is not considered sufficient to make a patient incompetent to make other important decisions such as making a will, appointing a power-of-attorney, or deciding to refuse treatment, so it is unlikely that a patient would become incompetent to decide on participation in a trial.

Industry-Sponsored Trials

Development of any new medical product, in particular a new drug, takes at least a decade and many millions of dollars. The final pathway in such drug development is the RCT, thus many are sponsored and run by pharmaceutical companies anxious to prove the worth of their investment. To run such trials requires close cooperation with clinicans who have access to the appropriate patient population and are willing to participate. By necessity there is a cost to this and the pharmaceutical company must recompense the clinical research team. This is often over and above the actual cost of running the trial, with the excess going to fund other research of the team. However, the clinical researcher must walk a fine ethical line in order not to be coerced by financial gain into participation in a trial which does not meet the ethical requirements outlined above. Equally the researcher has to outline any financial gain for him/herself or the department to the potential trial participant.

Ethics Committees

Ethics committees (or institutional review boards in the USA) are tasked with reviewing applications for research projects on human subjects, and can look at a wide range of aspects, from the science of the project, to its ethical viability, to practical aspects such as whether the institution and researchers have the facilities and expertise to undertake the treatment proposed. A detailed description of the work of these committees can be found on the Central Office for Research Ethics Committees website (www.corec.org.uk).

Conclusions

The RCT is the most useful tool of the clinical researcher, providing the most secure method for evaluating medical treatments. In the 60 years since it has been in use in medicine it has evolved into a scientific discipline in its own right, with complex multidisciplinary methodology and biostatistical tenets, and with accompanying ethical predicaments both for the clinical researcher and for a patient offered participation in an RCT. These issues include trial monitoring, randomization, the use of placebos, and informed consent. These issues need careful consideration in the design and conduct of any RCT, and must meet both international guidelines and the scrutiny of a local institutional ethics committee.

See Also

Clinical Trials: Legal Aspects and Consent

Further Reading

Anonymous (1948) Streptomycin treatment of pulmonary tuberculosis: a Medical Research Council investigation. *British Medical Journal* ii: 769–782.
European Directive on Good Clinical Practice in Clinical Trials: http://www.mca.gov.uk/ourwork//licensingmeds/types/clintrialsbriefnote.pdf.
National Committee for Quality Assurance and the Joint Commission on Accreditation of Healthcare Organisations: www.jcaho.org/.
Roddis L (1950) *James Lind*. New York: Henry Schuman.
Saunders CM, Baum M, Haughton J (1994) Consent, research and the doctor–patient relationship. In: Gillon R (ed.) *Principles of Health Care Ethics*. Chicester, UK: Wiley.
Taylor KM, Margolese RG, Soskoline CL (1984) Physicians' reasons for not entering eligible patients in a randomised clinical trial of surgery for breast cancer. *New England Journal of Medicine* 310: 1363–1367.
US Government (1949) *Trials of War Criminals Before the Nuremberg Military Tribunal under Control Council Law*, vol. 2, pp. 181–182. Washington, DC: US Government Printing Office.
World Medical Assembly (1964) *Declaration of Helsinki*. Recommendations guiding medical doctors in biomedical research involving human subjects. Adopted by the 18th World Medical Assembly, Helsinki, Finland 1964. *British Medical Journal* 313: 1448–1449.
World Medical Assembly (2000) *Declaration of Helsinki*. Amended by the 52nd World Medical Assembly, Edinburgh, Scotland, 2000. *British Medical Journal* 313: 1448–1449.
Writing Group for the Women's Health Initiative Investigators (2002) Risks and benefits of estrogen plus progestin in healthy postmenopausal women: principal results from the Women's Health Initiative Randomized Controlled Trial. *Journal of the American Medical Association* 288: 321–333.
www.asco.org: the official website of the American Association of Clinical Oncology.

Legal Aspects and Consent

K L Cerminara, Nova Southeastern University, Fort Lauderdale, FL, USA

Introduction

Legal and ethical concerns overlap closely in the area of clinical trials. Both legal and ethical experts focus on informed consent as the touchstone for the validity of human experimentation in the form of clinical trials. Additional concerns addressed by the law relate to the confidentiality of subjects' information, the type of controls used in clinical trials, and the potential for conflicts of interest that exist in clinical trials. In addition to the availability of possible litigation-based remedies, the law has established independent review bodies to protect research subjects in these areas.

Informed Consent

The doctrine of informed consent applies to both medical treatment and medical research. The United Nations' International Covenant on Civil and Political Rights provides that "no one shall be subjected without his free consent to medical or scientific experimentation." Just as treating physicians must obtain the voluntary, informed consent of their patients who have capacity to consent (or of the legally authorized representatives of their patients without capacity to consent), researchers similarly must obtain voluntary, informed consent from subjects or their legal authorized representatives to experiment on those human subjects.

In the clinical trials context, informed consent has been explicitly addressed in the USA as a matter of federal regulation. Other US laws and various sources of international law and policy similarly address informed consent, in accordance, for the most part, with US regulatory informed consent requirements. Universally, informed consent is seen as the optimal result of a process of communication between researchers and subjects to ensure that subjects with legal capacity to make decisions understand the nature of the research and its risks and benefits, and voluntarily agree to participate in the research. Formally, an informed consent document, signed by both researcher and subject, must specify the information provided during that process, to memorialize both that the communication occurred and that the subject voluntarily agreed to participate.

The required contents of such informed consent documents may be clearly delineated by law, as they are under US regulations and as suggested by international medical and medical ethical organizations such as the Council for International Organizations of Medical Sciences (CIOMS). Under the US regulations, for example, all clinical trial informed consent documents must include: (1) a statement that the activity in which the subject is participating constitutes research; (2) further details about that research, its purposes, and its procedures; (3) a description of foreseeable risks and benefits to subjects; (4) discussion of treatments or procedures from which the subject (if ill) might benefit rather than participating in the trial; (5) information about the manner in which and the extent to which the researcher will maintain confidentiality of subject records; (6) for certain research, information about whether and to what extent compensation or treatment will be available if the subject is injured during the research; (7) identification of a contact person in case of questions or concerns; and (8) assurance that the subject is agreeing voluntarily and the researcher is not engaging in certain activity that would tend to coerce the subject. The informed consent document may also include additional information.

While required, and while constituting strong evidence, the informed consent document is not definitive evidence of whether the human subject gave informed consent to participation in a clinical trial. Rather, the document should serve as a memorialization of the conversation that is at the heart of the informed consent process. Various members of the team of researchers on any clinical trial, not simply the researcher whose name appears on the informed consent document, may be involved in the conversations during which subjects are told about the clinical trial and are given an opportunity to ask questions about it.

Special Populations

Certain categories of research subject have been deemed worthy of special protection in clinical trials, both generally and particularly with regard to the

clinical trials' informed consent process. Children, pregnant women, fetuses, neonates, the mentally ill or compromised, and prisoners are often singled out as deserving of special consideration. More broadly, any potential subject considered to be "vulnerable" might require special care to ensure that the consent provided by that "vulnerable" subject or his/her legally authorized representative is truly informed and voluntary. CIOMS defines "vulnerable persons" as "those who are relatively (or absolutely) incapable of protecting their own interests," meaning people who "have insufficient power, intelligence, education, resources, strength, or other needed attributes to protect their own interests." Among the vulnerable, then, can be the elderly, the economically or socially disadvantaged, subordinate members of hierarchical groups such as medical or nursing students, and the seriously ill.

Persons who are ill and are contemplating participation in a clinical trial merit special consideration in the informed consent process for two reasons. First, a seriously ill person, especially one with a terminal diagnosis, is often less likely than a healthy person to listen to and comprehend information at the level that might be required to ensure informed consent to participate in a clinical trial. Such a person may also not be acting voluntarily in agreeing to participate in a clinical trial, even if there is no apparent source of coercion. This is because persons in such a position are often compliant and needy; they rely on others to be decision-makers rather than making decisions for themselves.

Second, any ill person considering participation in a clinical trial is vulnerable to the so-called "therapeutic misconception." Persons who are ill who consider participating in clinical trials to test the efficacy of proposed treatments for their illnesses usually enter into such trials seeking cures. Although a clinical trial is, by definition, experimental, and although they may be randomly assigned to control groups in which they will not receive the new treatment (and may not receive any treatment), such persons suffer from the misconception that they are being treated through the trial. Clinical trials are not the same as treatment, yet persons who are ill who sign on to be subjects in them often treat them as if they are. To the extent a subject agrees to participate in a clinical trial while operating under this "therapeutic misconception," then that subject's consent may not be informed and voluntary.

The Mentally Incapacitated

Those who are mentally incapable of giving informed consent to participation in clinical trials represent a distinct special population worthy of mention. While researchers must obtain informed consent directly from subjects who are mentally capable of giving such consent, some researchers may desire to engage in research on subjects who do not have the ability to hear or to understand information about the clinical trials proposed. In such situations, to the extent it is appropriate to proceed at all, researchers must obtain informed consent to participation in those clinical trials by competent persons who are authorized under the law to speak for the incapacitated subjects.

The question of whether it is appropriate to proceed at all requires consideration of the level of risk to which this category of research subject may be subjected. US regulations and CIOMS guidelines, for example, emphasize that research on such subjects must involve no more than slight or minor increases above the amount of risk involved in routine examination. In some instances, as under US regulations, the amount of risk that might be tolerated may vary with the amount of benefit the research may offer either to the subjects or to the population to which the subjects belong.

Additionally, whether it is appropriate to proceed at all may depend on the type of research the researcher intends to perform and whether that research is appropriately performed on the type of mentally incapacitated subject the researcher wishes to utilize in his/her experimentation. Some subjects' inability to understand information may stem from their age; children, for example, are generally presumed by the law to be incapable of appreciating information regarding clinical trials sufficiently to consent to their own participation in them. Yet it may be important to conduct certain research on children because, again for example, children are likely to react differently from adults to certain medications; children may require different procedures than do adults; and some diseases or conditions only appear in children or are best studied when those suffering them are still children rather than adults. In such situations, it would likely be appropriate to proceed with research on children, after complying with particularized safeguards that might apply (for example, under US regulations) when obtaining the informed consent of competent persons who are authorized by the law to speak for the child-subjects. With children above 4 or 5 years of age, some form of child assent to the research is appropriate, in addition to consent from a person legally capable of giving it.

It might be less appropriate to proceed with research on subjects in certain other categories of mental capacity. The mentally ill or retarded, for example, arguably should not be used as research subjects unless the research in question relates in some way to their mental state. Research that could be conducted on the mentally capable should not be conducted on those who are mentally incapacitated. Examples of research on the mentally ill or retarded that could be appropriate, however, could include research into the neurological processes of a person with a certain level of mental retardation, or a study of the types of brain wave activity observable in a schizophrenic patient. In such situations, the research necessarily would require the participation of subjects falling into such categories of mental incapacity. Again, with special safeguards in place, then, it could be appropriate for such research to continue with the informed consent of competent persons who are authorized by law to speak for the subjects.

Yet another category of mentally incapacitated research subjects could include those who once possessed decision-making capacity but who currently are not conscious. Some researchers may desire to engage in clinical trials involving subjects in persistent vegetative states or comas. Once again, this research should not proceed if the research could be performed on subjects with mental capacity. If, however, the proposed research investigated issues related distinctly to the person in a persistent vegetative state or coma, then it might be possible for the research to proceed, as long as the researcher took special care to design the study appropriately to minimize risk and to inform and obtain consent from a competent person authorized by law to speak for the subject.

In all these situations, a variety of persons could be legally empowered to consent to research on behalf of mentally incapacitated subjects, as long as the research at issue was of the type that required participation of mentally incapacitated subjects rather than mentally capable subjects. An incapacitated research subject who once had decision-making capacity may have designated, through a legal instrument such as a durable power of attorney, a person to make decisions on his/her behalf in such situations; such a designation would accord the designee presumptive ability to consent on the subject's behalf. If the incapacitated research subject previously had not designated such a decision-maker – either through inactivity or through legal inability to do so, as with children or those who have always lacked mental capacity – the law generally will provide a list of persons (proxy decision-makers) who can, in the absence of contrary designation, make decisions on behalf of incapacitated persons.

The courts offer resources that should be accessed if there exist any questions. Questions could range from whether proposed research involving the incapacitated should proceed at all, whether a designee or proxy decision-maker can consent to research rather than or in addition to medical treatment, or whether a particular designee or proxy decision-maker is an appropriate person to consent on a particular subject's behalf. Guardianship proceedings may be instituted to ensure that the person consenting to a research subject's participation is acting in the subject's best interests, or the court may be asked otherwise to decide whether the subject him/herself – assuming he/she was once mentally capable of consenting to participation in clinical trials research – would have consented to the research in question.

Use of Placebos

Another concern arises from the potential for subject misunderstanding when placebos are used as controls in clinical trials. Placebos are inert or ineffective substances or procedures. Examples include sugar pills and sham surgery. In a clinical trial, placebos may be administered to or used with a control group because the researchers conducting the trial wish to test how well subjects receiving a new drug or treatment do in comparison with subjects receiving no drug or treatment. To ensure blindness or double-blindness, all subjects in such a trial must receive something that looks like a drug or treatment. Otherwise, the subjects or the researchers (or both) would know exactly which subjects were receiving the drug or treatment being tested (those getting something) and who were not (those getting nothing).

Some argue that clinical trials should never incorporate placebos if a standard drug or treatment exists for the condition in question. In such cases, the argument goes, the new drug or treatment should only be tested against the current standard drug or treatment. Others respond that even if a current drug or treatment exists, it is valuable to know how effective the new one is as compared with both the current standard and the result occurring when people take or do nothing to treat the condition in question. The law does not prohibit use of placebos in clinical trials, but it does require (1) that use of placebos be appropriate under a risk/benefit analysis of the design of each clinical trial and (2) that those subjects participating in placebo-controlled clinical trials truly give informed consent to such participation.

In some cases of placebo use, true informed consent may not be possible. Misunderstandings can easily arise, and can rise to the level of legal problems, when a subject participates in a clinical trial involving the administration of placebos to a control group without understanding that to be the case. Such misunderstandings are particularly probable in two settings. First, they may be particularly probable when the subject is ill and is participating in a clinical trial testing a drug or treatment for his/her illness. Second, they may be particularly probable when physicians from the developed world are conducting clinical trials in developing countries. In either case, the vulnerable nature of the population being studied in the trial suggests a need to be particularly careful in the informed consent process. The subject who is ill may be likely not to focus on the information provided about placebos because of his/her desire to participate in the trial as a chance for a cure. The subject from a developing country may be likely not to understand information provided about placebos because of communication difficulties, cultural differences, or other variables.

Other Legal Concerns

In addition to informed consent, two additional subjects raise particularly important potential legal issues, although they do not constitute an exhaustive list of legal concerns that could arise in the course of a clinical trial. These additional issues are confidentiality and conflicts of interest.

Confidentiality

Medical information always receives a special level of protection under the law. The confidentiality of medical records must be maintained except in particularly delineated situations, and so it is with information about a subject in a clinical trial. While information about the subjects' reactions to and success or lack of success with the treatment or drug being studied is important to the clinical trial, the identities of subjects are never to be reported and in most cases are not to be revealed to anyone except researchers. Similarly, other information about the subject learned during the course of the trial may not be revealed except in certain narrow circumstances. One example might be information learned during the taking of the subject's medical history.

Exceptions do exist. In some cases, the law requires disclosure despite the general rule of confidentiality. For example, if something learned during a medical exam in the course of a clinical trial indicates currently ongoing elder, child, or spousal abuse, most jurisdictions will require that the information be reported to the appropriate authorities. Similarly, if something learned indicates that a crime has been committed, the law may require reporting to the appropriate authorities. So too must researchers report medical information tending to suggest the existence of a public health problem, such as a sexually transmitted disease or a communicable disease considered a threat to public health.

Conflicts of Interest

Two types of conflicts of interest may exist between researcher and subject in a clinical trial. The first, which is inherent in any setting involving medical research, does not necessarily lead to a legal problem. Specifically, the interests of researchers are always at odds in some senses with the interests of the human subjects of their clinical trials. Researchers and subjects often have different goals, and subjects often expect researchers to have mindsets corresponding to the subjects' goals rather than to the researchers' actual goals. Especially if they are operating under the "therapeutic misconception" described above, subjects often expect researchers to be looking out for their (the subjects') well-being or best interests. Such expectations are enhanced when the subjects participating in a trial are both ill and patients of the physician conducting that clinical trial. Physicians seek to benefit their patients, but researchers engage in clinical trials to obtain generalizable data tending to prove or disprove a hypothesis rather than to benefit any particular subject. Researchers thus have different focuses than subjects, and their goals likely differ from the goals of the subjects. Such an inherent conflict of interest does not necessarily create a legal concern, for if it did, all clinical trials would be legally suspect. Rather, legal implications may arise from this inherent conflict of interest if, among other scenarios, a subject were found to lack sufficient knowledge or understanding of the parties' roles and goals to have given valid informed consent.

Conflicts of interest may also arise in the clinical trials context in a more explicit way. A researcher may have a monetary or prestige-based stake in a clinical trial's outcome. If significant enough, that stake may give the researcher an incentive to falsify data, to ignore data, or otherwise to manipulate data so that the trial produces the outcome that most benefits the researcher. Thus, conflicts of interest may give rise to legal issues of fraud or other research misconduct.

For example, it is often the case that a number of researchers are conducting clinical trials on the same or very similar drugs or treatments. The researcher who first reaches a scientifically supportable conclusion and publishes his/her findings has the prestige of having made the discovery in question, even if

others follow closely. A researcher conducting a trial that is substantially the same as or similar to trials others are conducting thus has an incentive to ignore inconsistent data or signs of problems in an effort to publish his or her findings first. Similarly, if a researcher owns a significant amount of stock in the pharmaceutical company that manufactures a drug the researcher is testing in a clinical trial, the researcher has an incentive to manipulate data so that the drug is shown to be safe and effective. If the drug is shown to be safe and effective, it can be marketed, earning money for the pharmaceutical company and indirectly producing a monetary gain for the researcher because his/her stock in that company will rise in value due to increased earnings from the drug.

Both these situations, should they materialize and cause injury to a subject, would present legal issues of fraud or other research misconduct. The law sometimes attempts to deal proactively with the latter situation. In such instances, in which there exists tangible evidence tending to suggest in advance special cause for concern about a potential conflict of interest, the law (at least under US regulations) will require up-front disclosure by the researcher. Such disclosures must be made to bodies overseeing the clinical trials, although some argue that such disclosures should be made to the human subjects themselves.

Reviewing Committees or Boards

Independent bodies have been established to review the protocols, or descriptions, of clinical trials before such trials begin. Review by such independent entities ensures that the legal and ethical concerns described above, as well as others, have been considered by someone other than the researcher or another interested party. Such reviewing bodies are called institutional review boards, or IRBs, in the USA and names such as ethical review committees, research ethics committees, or ethics review committees in other countries. Although based at the institutions through which the clinical trials are conducted, they are required by law to have what is hoped to be sufficient diversity of membership and a sufficient number of unaffiliated members to ensure independence. They exist to protect the human subjects of clinical trials by considering, among other things, whether it appears the subjects will be given every opportunity to give informed consent, the extent to which the subjects' confidentiality will be maintained, and whether the risks and benefits of each proposed trial seem to be reasonable, both absolutely and in comparison to each other. Not only must a clinical trial protocol be submitted to such an independent body for review and approval before a trial may be conducted, but the reviewing body will also continue to monitor the trial until the trial has concluded.

These bodies are expected to take special care in reviewing clinical trials being performed on vulnerable populations. International research raises special concerns when the researchers hail from a developed country and the subjects of their clinical trials reside in poor, developing countries. Some of the main concerns that have arisen include whether the subjects in those developing countries are truly giving voluntary, informed consent and whether the risks those subjects are being asked to take are reasonable in relation to the benefits that may accrue to them or to citizens of their country. With regard to the latter concern, some have suggested that the law should provide that clinical trials cannot take place in developing countries unless the drugs or treatments resulting from the trials will be made available in those countries after the conclusion of the trials.

See Also

Clinical Trials: Good Clinical Practice and Ethical Aspects; **Consent:** Treatment Without Consent; Confidentiality and Disclosure; **Medical Records, Access to**

Further Reading

Annas GJ, Grodin MA (1992) *The Nazi Doctors and the Nuremberg Code: Human Rights in Human Experimentation*. New York: Oxford University Press.

Bankowski Z, Levine RJ (1993) *Ethics and Research on Human Subjects: International Guidelines*. Geneva, Switzerland: Council for International Organizations of Medical Sciences.

Beecher HK (1966) Ethics and clinical research. *New England Journal of Medicine* 274: 1354–1360.

Beh HG (2002) The role of institutional review boards in protecting human subjects: are we really ready to fix a broken system? *Law and Psychology Review* 26: 1–46.

Capron AM (1989) Human experimentation. In: Veatch RM (ed.) *Medical Ethics*, 2nd edn., pp. 135–184. London: Jones and Bartlett.

Council for International Organizations of Medical Sciences (2002) *International Ethical Guidelines for Biomedical Research Involving Human Subjects*. Geneva, Switzerland: CIOMS.

Department of Health, Education and Welfare (1978) *The Belmont Report: Ethical Principles and Guidelines for*

the Protection of Human Subjects of Research, Report of the National Commission for the Protection of Human Subjects Research. DHEW Publication [OS] 78-0012. Washington, DC: US Government Printing Office.

Goldner J (1993) An overview of legal controls on human experimentation and the regulatory implications of taking professor Katz seriously. *St. Louis University Law Journal* 38: 63–134.

Hoffman S (2001) The use of placebos in clinical trials: responsible research or unethical practice? *Connecticut Law Review* 33: 449–501.

Hoffman S (2003) Regulating clinical research: informed consent, privacy, and IRBs. *Capital University Law Review* 31: 71–90.

Jones JH (1993) *Bad Blood: Tuskegee Syphilis Experiment*. New York: Free Press.

Katz J (1972) *Experimentation With Human Beings: The Authority of the Investigator, Subject, Professions, and State in the Human Experimentation Process*. New York: Russell Sage Foundation.

Katz J (1993) Human experimentation and human rights. *St. Louis University Law Journal* 38: 7–54.

Kuszler PC (2001) Conflicts of interest in clinical research: legal and ethical issues: curing conflicts of interest in clinical research: impossible dreams and harsh realities. *Widener Law Symposium* 8: 115–152.

Levine RJ (1988) Uncertainty in clinical research. *Law, Medicine and Health Care* 16: 174–182.

Levine RJ (1988) *Ethics and Regulation of Clinical Research*, 2nd edn. New Haven, CT: Yale University Press.

Meier BM (2002) International protection of persons undergoing medical experimentation: protecting the right of informed consent. *Berkeley Journal of International Law* 20: 513–554.

Orentlicher D (2002) Universality and its limits: when research ethics can reflect local circumstances. *Journal of Law, Medicine and Ethics* 30: 403–410.

Permissible Medical Experiments ("The Nuremberg Code") (1949) II *Trials of War Criminals Before the Nuremberg Military Tribunals Under Control Council Law* no. 10, pp. 181–182. Washington, DC: US Government Printing Office.

Shimm DS, Spece RG (1991) Conflict of interest and informed consent in industry-sponsored clinical trials. *Journal of Legal Medicine* 12: 477–513.

Spece RG, Shim DS, Buchanan AE (eds.) (1996) *Conflicts of Interest in Clinical Practice and Research*. New York: Oxford University Press.

US Department of Health and Human Services (2002) Protection of human subjects. *Code of Federal Regulations*. Title 45, Part 46. Washington, DC: US Government Printing Office.

US Food and Drug Administration (2002) Protection of human subjects; standards for institutional review boards for clinical investigations. *Code of Federal Regulations*. Title 21, Parts 50, 54, 56. Washington, DC: US Government Printing Office.

COLD CASE REVIEW – UK EXPERIENCE

J Fraser, University of Strathclyde, Glasgow, UK

Introduction

In the UK, cold-case reinvestigations involve a fresh start based on original witness statements and other primary documentation, such as the pathologist's report. The expectation of progress is mainly based on physical evidence and increasingly on the reassessment of the crime in the light of behavioral and other information. Offenses are typically close-contact, sexually motivated homicide, rather than the fleeting or absent contact of gun crimes, where opportunities for physical evidence transfer are much less. Although reinterviewing witnesses is essential for investigative purposes, it is primarily used to confirm or deny hypotheses as to the sequence of events, rather than providing new eye-witness evidence. An advantage in the UK is the relatively small number of jurisdictions and police forces. There are 43 police forces for a population in excess of 50 million. There are also a very small number of forensic suppliers. These factors taken together enable the introduction of unified processes and procedures across the UK. They also facilitate the availability of national crime analysis systems and specialist support for cold cases via the UK National Crime and Operations Faculty (NCOF), a support service funded by the police service.

What is Forensic Science?

A clear understanding of the nature, potential, and usage of forensic science in case reviews is essential for effective outcome. Forensic science is the interpretation of scientific tests and observations in the context of an individual case. Literally, it is any science in the service of the courts and in cold cases there are no limitations to the usual services provided by a typical forensic laboratory; this includes pathology, fingerprints, and any scientific discipline that can assist.

There are some basic principles of forensic science that are particularly important in cold cases. One of these is Locard's principle: "every contact leaves a trace." What is sought in cold cases is to identify contact points between offender, scene(s), and the victim. This is often by reworking the original sequence of events in light of new behavioral, pathological, or forensic observations.

Science in Context

Forensic science is the interpretation of results in the context of the case circumstances, not the tests themselves. Forensic science is completely context-dependent, and failure to interpret findings in this manner is an abdication of the responsibility of the scientist. However, the probative value of the evidence is a matter for the court and it follows that if either the test result or the context changes, a new interpretation is required. In cold cases, both the results and the context may have to be revised as further work is undertaken. This cannot be done unless the scientist is close to the inquiry and there are good lines of communication.

Understanding and Using Physical Intelligence

The most important aspect of the work of forensic scientists is the provision of physical intelligence during the investigative phase, often before a suspect is identified. However, forensic scientists often consider their primary purpose to be the provision of evidence in court. Perhaps 90% of their observations can contribute to the investigative phase of an inquiry, a fact that is sadly lost on most scientists and many senior investigative officers (SIOs). Even their actual evidence is more likely to be used to eliminate suspects or negate hypotheses than be of use in a court case against a named individual. Forensic science can be used during an investigation to:

- clarify the sequence of events
- identify critical facts (particularly important in cold cases)
- provide elimination factors
- direct lines of inquiry, such as targeting house-to-house interviews
- assist in interview or crime-scene examination strategies.

It is vital then that the importance of integrating physical intelligence into the investigation is recognized and implemented in cold cases. Physical intelligence has the unique benefit that, after the offender has been identified, generally physical intelligence could be transformed to the physical evidence that is essential for a prosecution in cold cases. Intelligence detects cases but evidence is required for prosecution.

The National Crime and Operations Faculty

The NCOF is the body that supports cold-case investigations across the UK, although some UK forces have their own specialist units. NCOF supports cold cases with behavioral profilers, crime analysts, and senior detectives but primarily through forensic science advisors who take an investigative overview. The NCOF has developed a template for reviews of physical evidence in case reviews, which is the major part of a case. This template is shown in **Table 1**. This work requires an extensive and detailed analysis of any materials that can be recovered and a reassessment of their potential. This may include extracts or samples retained in the laboratory, which could be analyzed by current techniques. In some cases possessions of the victim are returned to relatives and retained. This is an important source to investigate. It is common for exhibits to be recorded as destroyed when this is not the case; therefore, persistence and imagination can yield considerable benefits in this element of the review.

Universal Principles for Cold-Case Reviews

Make a fresh start This means a new team of officers who approach the crime completely fresh and are prepared to question every assumption. This avoids being contaminated by mindsets associated with the old inquiry, which may have been based on a single or incorrect hypothesis. Typically, the original

Table 1 National Crime and Operations Faculty template of physical evidence in cold-case reviews

Stage	Typically includes
1. Initial assessment	• Establishing previous and new lines of inquiry • Identification of investigative problems which require solutions
2. Physical evidence review	• Production of a detailed plan before commencing work • Fingerprint and exhibit review and retrieval • Identifying items originally examined, items not examined, and new items encountered • Establishing tentative sequence of events on the basis of available information and any new information (e.g., behavioral analysis) • Review and reinterpretation of all physical evidence, including pathology, scene, photographs, and videos
3. Identify what is known	• Draft a formal report based on physical evidence and its interpretation • Draft a formal forensic strategy identifying potential for case
4. Develop policies and tactics	• Prearrest policy for crime-scene investigation • Forensic search strategy • Interview strategy • Review of evidence postinterview

documentation may indicate that events have been defined, actions taken, or suspects eliminated when this is not the case. To begin with, a reinvestigation from the finishing point of the old one is to build on sand. A fresh start also avoids the constraints arising from justifiable rejection of physical items in the original inquiry but which now could (and would) be analyzed successfully. DNA on items originally tested for blood grouping is the classic, but by no means only, example of this. Lack of understanding of the potential of physical evidence by police officers and poor knowledge of the investigative process and case context by scientists are barriers that only a fresh start to the case can overcome. The approach required is that of mature and self-critical teamwork in order to identify previously overlooked or new opportunities.

Crime assessment The work of the Federal Bureau of Investigation behavioral science unit at Quantico, USA, has led to improved understanding of areas such as victimology, attack and deposition methods in homicides, and the behavior of sexual offenders. A new inquiry will be in a much better position to undertake crime assessments taking behavioral aspects into account with the totality of forensic results, rather than crime-scene assessment, which is often limited to day 1 or 2 of the inquiry, and the immediate findings. Often the availability of a relatively trivial forensic test such as the presence or absence of alcohol will radically change the direction of an inquiry when set in context.

Use systematic processes Given the scope of any one inquiry and the potential for it to be revisited, it is essential that clear processes are followed and good discipline in recording progress, findings, and decisions is followed. The NCOF recommends a five-step process for cold-case reviews, which is outlined in **Table 2**.

Selection of Cases for Review

Many police forces will have a number of cold cases that could be reinvestigated and therefore cases will need to be selected and prioritized. Transparent selection criteria are required to inform relatives in those cases that are not selected for reinvestigation to explain why this is so. One method of achieving this is to use declared and published criteria agreed by a panel in advance of case selection. The panel might include one or more experienced senior investigating officers (SIOs), a crime-scene manager or crime-scene coordinator, a fingerprint expert, and a specialist advisor. A specialist advisor in this sense is a highly experienced forensic scientist who can take a forensic overview and is fully aware of the latest scientific developments. Selection criteria typically include:

Table 2 Stages in the cold-case review process recommended by the National Crime and Operations Faculty

Stage	Typically requires
1. Formal case assessment	• An independent assessment group covering a range of disciplines • May need an independent advisory group in high-profile or sensitive cases
2. Retrieval of items	• Documentation and exhibits in police forces • Documentation and exhibits in forensic laboratories • Bringing all documentation up to current standards • Materials recovered in laboratory analyses • Scene and postmortem examination photographs
3. Assess present potential	• Constant focus on case context and investigative problems • Information and intelligence (not just evidence) • Clarification of key events, timings, etc.
4. Obtain new information	• Use of lateral thinking • Assessment of items originally overlooked • Following previous processes to exhaustion • Reassessment of scene, motivation, and actions • Use of new techniques and technologies
5. Reevaluate	• A generalist rather than specialist scientist • Integration of all specialist evidence and intelligence • Focus on the needs of the investigation • Production of reports for interview and arrest strategies

- the nature of the crime (i.e., close contact)
- age of the crime
- present age of the probable offender
- availability of physical items and therefore potential
- potential impact of new technology, e.g., DNA
- miscarriages of justice or high-profile cases
- likelihood of successful prosecution.

It is important to realize that a large amount of reinterviewing witnesses and checking will still have to be done and therefore any review will require significant resources.

New Science and Technology

One of the major factors influencing cold-case reviews is development of new science and technology. This is not confined to forensic science but includes any relevant useful science technique or technology. Some examples include:

- the National Injuries Database
- new methods for fingerprint enhancement
- the national fingerprint identification system (NAFIS)
- new technology for comparing palm prints
- new and more sensitive DNA methods
- national DNA databases
- low copy number DNA analysis
- mitochondrial DNA sequencing
- familial DNA analysis
- behavioral and geographical profiling.

It must be stressed that it is rarely the science in isolation that leads to new breakthroughs. Most frequently, it is the appraisal of test results that leads to clarifying circumstances, directing resources, setting elimination criteria, pointing to a suspect, or assisting in interview strategies. However, most lost opportunities result from lack of thought, not lack of technology. The investigation of such a case is described below.

Case History of Lynette White: A Cold-Case Review and Miscarriage of Justice

Lynette White was a strikingly pretty teenage prostitute stabbed to death in the early hours of Valentine's Day 1988. She was murdered in a dingy apartment above a betting office in the seedy Butetown area of Cardiff, where she took punters. The apartment contained only a bed and had no electricity. A blanket covered the window, with the only source of light being a street lamp. Consequently, the apartment was dark and cold with a narrow exit route out and down the stairs to the street. Lynette was stabbed around 50 times in a frenzied attack with something like a large kitchen knife. Most of the wounds were concentrated on the breasts and throat. She had bled out in the confined space between the bed and the window, and after the attack her body had been dragged away from the wall by the ankles. Attempts were made to obtain the then nascent DNA evidence from her body, but this was unsuccessful, and blood-grouping evidence obtained from the scene turned out to be a red herring.

Initial inquiries focused on her lifestyle, in particular her pimp and his associates, with whom she had allegedly been in dispute. Eventually, five black males were charged with the murder and three were convicted in 1990, primarily on the evidence of police interviews and despite some alibi evidence. Two years later the Cardiff Three were released, with the court of appeal particularly criticizing the nature of the interview and confession evidence.

In early 1999 South Wales police decided to undertake a full review of the case. The Head of Physical

Evidence at NCOF, Dave Barclay, was appointed to undertake a full forensic review with the assistance of other NCOF services such as behavioral advice and crime analysis. An independent advisory panel was appointed to monitor the work on behalf of the community. This enabled religious, educational, and ethnic-minority groups to be represented and fully exposed to the process, including complete access to the police files.

In mid-1999 an experienced SIO, Bill Hacking, from a different police force was appointed to lead the investigative element of the review.

By then the physical evidence review had identified three general areas:

1. Existing opportunities. Attempts had been made throughout the 1990s as new DNA techniques were developed to obtain a profile from intimate swabs and from known contact areas, such as the socks and bottom of her jeans. Lynette's body was known to have been dragged away from the wall area. This attempt was unsuccessful because of swamping with her blood and pigment from jeans.
2. Disregarded items. The examples of disregarded items are a speck of blood on a cellophane wrapper from a condom packet and blood on the key ring to the apartment – both too small for analysis in 1988 and subsequently overlooked. The importance of the cellophane wrapper had not been fully appreciated; it had been removed from a full, closed packet of condoms, which was lying on the bed. Any fingermarks or blood from the offender would place him in the room at the time of the crime.
3. New opportunities. These opportunities arise from a complete reassessment of the case, including actions at the scene.

From the above it can be seen that any cold-case review should not just be a laboratory-based reassessment of items already submitted, and certainly not simply a "DNA review," as this will uncover only one category of opportunities.

A complete case assessment by a behavioral scientist and the forensic scientist working together, and a reenactment in the apartment at the same hour the crime was committed in the 1990s, provided new information. The police version, which involved more than five Afro-Caribbean males, the victim, and a female witness all being present and active during the crime, could not be true. There was an absence of physical evidence, including footwear marks in blood, which defied all logic. On the scene assessment alone, the original scenario and suspects could be discounted. DNA later confirmed this elimination of the "Cardiff Three."

The behavioral advice pointed toward a different motivation and suspect group – a young single male of white or Asian origin, following a dispute in the course of Lynette's work. A reenactment by the scientist undertaking known actions at the scene and then running from the house in conditions of complete darkness identified a number of possible contact points between offender and scene. These areas contacted by the scientist on the way out were marked and cross-referenced to the scene observations in the 1990s. Actual opportunities emerged following mapping of this sequence of events on to the original scene photographs, photographs of finger marks, and retained materials such as some sections of wallpaper.

As a result of this work, it became apparent that the offender might well have cut himself at the scene (not unusual with 50 stab wounds with an unguarded blade) and that one particular drop of blood which had run down the wall under the window did not fit the general pattern of blood staining. Although there was very considerable arterial and cast-off blood from Lynette at the scene, this particular drop had impacted the wall from a different angle. It appeared to be cast-off and was 1 m from the majority of the pattern. However, the area had not been sampled nor was the wallpaper retained. The scientist suggested removing the skirting board and a small amount of blood was found, protected, and painted over, in the crack between the skirting board and the wall.

Areas of contact on the exit route that were re-examined showed some evidence of edge detail in blood; the amount of blood, though minimal, did not diminish as would be expected if it were simply secondary transfer from Lynette. A small area of blood smear inside the apartment door had been overlooked, but mapping the areas contacted by the scientist by close examination of the scene photographs revealed it. The door had been painted over with gloss paint before returning the apartment to the owner in 1988, and also repainted subsequently. The paint was removed in the target area and a swab from the area removed for DNA analysis.

These three new opportunities, together with the fleck of blood on the cellophane which had been disregarded, and the socks and jeans were the subject of considerable and innovative DNA work at Forensic Alliance, a major UK supplier. All eventually gave either full or almost complete DNA profiles from the same unknown male.

While the work on the jeans and socks had already been planned, all the other opportunities were identified and reprioritized by the combination of behavioral information and physical-case assessment.

The DNA profile, which was obtained from the UK national DNA database system of 20 alleles giving a match probability of around 1 billion, did not match any of the previous suspects and thus absolutely eliminated the Cardiff Three, as well as their colleagues and all other original suspects. However, there was no match on the national database and the source of the DNA remained unknown.

In an innovative attempt to identify the offender, the allele pattern of the DNA from the scene was compared to other nonmatching profiles on the basis that alleles are statistically similar between relatives, and that criminality runs in families. In late 2002, a voluntary intelligence sample was requested from Jeffrey Gafoor, a local security guard whose relative was on the database and had a similar familial pattern. He attempted suicide after providing the confirmatory buccal sample and in July 2003 pleaded guilty in court to the murder – 15 years after the crime.

Lynette White is an excellent example of the need to set physical evidence in context with the inquiry as a whole and to integrate the assessment process. Without that close integration and communication, valuable opportunities will be overlooked. It also provides a regrettable, but hopefully historic, illustration of the "making things fit your sole hypothesis" trap for investigators.

Managing Exhibits and Results

Exhibit tracking is an essential element of case reviews. This must use a common source of information, which describes the life history of all relevant items. The system should clearly show what has gone for analysis, when it went, why it went, when results were obtained, and where the item is stored. This is not only an aid to the review process but an essential part of the criminal justice process, should the review result in a trial. A schematic approach is useful to show items which still await analysis or results or which have been overlooked, as can be identified at a glance instead of plowing through page after page of laboratory documentation. The tracking system must be constantly refreshed and act as a definitive source of accurate information to the review team.

The Concept of Scenelines

Another concept, which is used to prevent anomalies in the logical thinking behind a hypothesis or sequence of events, is the sceneline. This was first developed at NCOF and involves plotting all the actual known significant facts and scientific inferences in relation to the crime against the proposed hypothesis developed by the investigators. This is analogous to a timeline, which is constructed (usually by commercial software such as I2) to test witness statements and express spatial relationships. The investigative hypothesis becomes a sceneline – a physical sequence of events on which every one of the actual events must lie, or be connected to by a provable logical inference. It follows that if factual events lie off the sceneline, then that hypothesis is wrong. This technique has proved particularly powerful in cold cases where there may be a considerable feeling that investigators "know" what happened, based on previous media coverage or work by the force. Often relatively small observations by the pathologist or overlooked laboratory results can completely disprove the initial hypothesis if it is tested in this way.

Conclusion

Effective cold-case reviews are based on:

- a structured approach which uncovers overlooked-opportunities and identifies new ones such as identification of contact points
- integration of science with the investigative process
- reevaluation of previous findings such as sequences of events in a more rigorous and constructively critical manner
- informed planning for key events such as interviews and searches
- use of management tools such as sceneline and exhibit-tracking software.

Crucially, it is not just about science but science in context, focused clearly on investigative problems and the needs of the criminal justice system.

See Also

Crime-scene Investigation and Examination: Collection and Chain of Evidence; Death-scene Investigation, United States of America; Major Incident Scene Management; Suspicious Deaths

Further Reading

Association of Chief Police Officers (2000) *Murder Investigation Manual.*
Association of Chief Police Officers (2000) *The Manual of Standard Operating Procedures for Scientific Support Personnel at Major Incident Scenes.*

COMA, DEFINITIONS AND DIFFERENTIAL DIAGNOSES

Contents
Pediatric
Adult

Pediatric

S Keeley, Women's and Children's Hospital, North Adelaide, SA, Australia

Introduction

Coma is a medical emergency and as such, no discussion, even one essentially confined to definition and etiology, can occur without appreciating the complexity of the task facing the clinician. Whilst attending to the support of vital functions, the clinician will endeavor to answer the following questions:

1. What is the level of functional impairment (the extent of the lesion's effect)?
2. What is the rate of progression?
3. What is the likely pathological process?
4. Is there an immediately treatable cause?

Coma in children, particularly the infant, has added complexity introduced by the developmental stage of the child. Alterations in consciousness leading to coma are only noticeable when the behavioral responses vary from those a carer has come to expect. Where the repertoire of behaviors is limited to the simple reflex responses of the very young, which can remain almost unchanged until coma supervenes, the early recognition of alterations in conscious state requires both experience and frequent observation. It is not surprising, therefore, that conditions that in an adult may be recognized early, appear in the child to present late and often in an immediately life-threatening manner. Early recognition, prompt management, and intervention are infinitely preferable to resuscitating the moribund.

Regardless of age, coma can be produced only by processes that either depress cortical function bilaterally or directly impinge on the brainstem reticular activating formation. Broadly categorized, coma is caused either by a metabolic insult of sufficient severity to create diffuse, bilateral cortical dysfunction or by structural lesions directly affecting the reticular activating system. It is expected that the reader will be familiar with the definition of coma. Aspects of particular relevance in this article are those that help appreciate the nuances required to see the pediatric perspective.

Definition

Coma is a term used to describe the point in a process of evolving unconsciousness at which the sufferer is no longer capable of a purposeful response to the most vigorous of stimuli. It is, therefore, a behavioral description rather than a single clinical state and represents a state anywhere between the unimpaired to the completely unresponsive.

A variety of descriptions of the intermediate states of responsiveness are possible. "Lethargy" is often used to describe the state of diminished arousal that is responsive to a light stimulus such as voice. "Obtundation" is typically used to describe the poorly sustained but purposeful arousal elicited by mild stimulus (e.g., touch), whereas "stupor" requires vigorous (e.g., painful) stimuli for the elicitation of a purposeful response. Coma supervenes when it is no longer possible to elicit a purposeful response. This, of course, does not mean that no response is elicitable. A comatose patient may exhibit a range of reflex nonpurposeful responses of diminishing complexity culminating in a total absence of response to even the most intense of painful stimuli.

This complexity of stimulus/response is captured in the Glasgow Coma Scale (GCS). Though initially developed as a means to objectify the altered states of consciousness caused by head trauma, it can serve as a useful tool in nontraumatic coma. It also allows one to rephrase the definition of coma more specifically – coma requires the GCS to be <9. The obvious limitations of this scale for children have led to many attempts at modification, particularly of the verbal component (see **Table 1**).

It can be readily seen that for the purposes of defining coma (GCS <9), both the adult and pediatric versions are equivalent.

This, of course, does not mean that the scales are equally useful to detect the presence of coma.

Table 1 Glasgow Coma Scale (modified for pediatrics)

		All ages (best function)[a]		Score
Eye opening		Spontaneous		4
		To speech		3
		To pain		2
		None		1
	<1 year		>1 year	
Motor response	Spontaneous movement		Obeys commands	6
	Localizes pain		Localizes pain	5
	Flexion to pain		Withdraws to pain	4
	Abnormal flexion		Abnormal flexion	3
	Extension to pain		Abnormal extension	2
	Flaccid		Flaccid	1
	0–2 years	2–5 years	>5 years	
Verbal response	Smiles/coos	Appropriate words	Oriented and converses	5
	Consolable cry	Inappropriate words	Confused	4
	Inconsolable cry	Cries/screams	Incomprehensible sounds	3
	Grunts	Grunts	Grunts	2
	No response	No response	No response	1

[a]Whilst coma is defined as a GCS <9 condition, the changes in consciousness that precede it can also be defined by the GCS. Children <9 months do not localize pain.

Considerable debate has centered on the individual components of the GCS and their precision as predictors of severity/outcome as compared to the composite score. A nonlocalizing flexor response to a painful stimulus is sufficient to determine the presence of coma in children over the age on 1, the total score adding little. Reliance on the motor scale as the sole determinant of coma in those below the age of 1, and in particular those less than 9 months old (who at their best do not consistently localize pain) is clearly inappropriate. In such patients, the composite score is a better representation of their capacity.

Some investigators have commented that an inexperienced observer tends to score the same patient lower than a more experienced counterpart. This is even more likely to be the case in children. Finally, a number of common situations can make the scale inapplicable – endotracheal intubation precludes assessment of the verbal component, whereas facial swelling can prevent eye opening. There is no common agreement as to how to score such patients.

Despite the obvious utility of the GCS in describing coma, additional observations of signs such as pupillary response, brainstem reflexes, and respiratory pattern will be necessary for the assessment of likely cause.

Developmental Considerations

Coma is easy to define but hard to detect. This seemingly incongruous statement deserves explanation. The appearance of the comatose child can resemble the sleeping child. Newborns and infants up to 2 months of age can spend more than 90% of their day asleep. Whilst sleep, for the most part, can be readily differentiated from coma by the application of a stimulus and subsequent arousal, both the intensity of the stimulus needed to provoke arousal and the duration of that arousal can vary. A normal newborn, recently fed, may require a painful stimulus to wake and, when eventually woken, may fall asleep as soon as the stimulus ceases.

The limited reflex behaviors exhibited by the newborn are primarily those consequent to arousal, or the capacity for wakefulness. With maturation, the infant increasingly exhibits signs of awareness – visible actions consequent to sensations, emotions, or thoughts triggered by environmental stimuli. The observer must therefore have sufficient experience of the range of child behaviors across the developmental spectrum such that their expectations match the capacity of the child. Consistent purposeful responses to pain are readily observable to most (including lay) observers by 1 year of age. Whilst the experienced observer will be able to readily discern alterations of conscious state at all ages, it should be remembered that it is the parents who initiate most healthcare visits. A variable ability to detect subtle and early changes is to be expected.

Indeed, the readily observable consequence of this difficulty is on the perceived rate of onset of some of the common causes. In general, coma of acute onset suggests causes such as trauma, ingestion, seizure, or cerebrovascular event. Onset over hours to days suggests infection, metabolic disorder, or mass lesions. The frequency of emergency presentations of conditions in the latter category points to the difficulty in the recognition of early alterations in conscious state.

Pediatric Vulnerability

The development of the central nervous system commences in the 3rd week of gestation and continues rapidly for at least the first 2 years of life. Progressive increase in cell number, myelinization, dendritic interconnections, and axonal growth leads to a rapid increase in brain weight. At birth, the brain is already 25% of its adult weight, whilst the child's total weight represents only 5% of adult weight. Not surprisingly, cerebral blood flow and oxygen consumption are proportionately greater in the infant than the adult. This equates to an increased vulnerability to the so-called metabolic causes of coma that interfere with substrate availability – hypoglycemia, hypoxia, shock, etc. The frequency of hypoxic–ischemic injury at postmortem in patients succumbing to coma is a clear reflection of this vulnerability. The capacity for wakefulness (arousal) is dependent on a region of interconnected neurons located ventral to the ventricular system and extending from the mid-brain to the lower pons. Known as the reticular activating system (RAS), it receives information from multiple sources and disseminates widely into the cortex. This region of the child's brain is susceptible to trauma consequent to the imbalance between the relative size of the head versus torso and the strength of the supporting musculature. Extremes of rotation or flexion/extension of the head and neck are readily generated, creating rotational/shear forces sufficient to disrupt the function of the RAS leading to abrupt onset of coma. It is believed the relatively fixed brainstem acts as a fulcrum around which the more mobile cortex can move during which it is subject to rotational/distraction injury. Magnetic resonance imaging (MRI) has confirmed that, in up to 60% of pediatric traumatic coma victims, brainstem injury is not only present but that its extent determines prognosis.

The pediatric brain, with its incomplete myelination, seems more susceptible to injury consequent to textural differences, variable rates of deformation in adjacent tissue creating shear stress, and the lack of protection offered by the thin calvarium. The corpus callosum appears particularly vulnerable. Somewhat paradoxically, the capacity for tolerating expanding lesions is enhanced by the incomplete fusion of sutures.

Apnea is a frequent accompaniment to pediatric brain injury, adding the risk of secondary injury from hypoxia/hypercarbia.

Finally, and perhaps most telling of all, is the physiological vulnerability to hypoxia of the young in any circumstance where airway patency and ventilatory adequacy are challenged. Airway obstruction and hypoventilation with the accompanying hypoxia and hypercarbia are all believed to potentiate the central nervous system (CNS) injury and are thought to be key triggers for acute brain swelling seen in some cases of trauma.

The prognosis for children suffering coma is commonly underestimated. Indeed it was once believed that for an equivalent injury children, with the plasticity of function believed to exist, had an improved outcome compared to that experienced by adults. It is now clear that the opposite is the case – indeed, the earlier the injury the more occult its consequence and the more delayed and extensive the effect.

Etiology

The differential diagnosis of coma is broad. The nonspecific nature of coma, with causes as diverse as septicemia and inborn errors of metabolism, requires a planned approach to diagnosis. Knowledge of the common categories of cause and their typical presentation as well as the age-specific frequency of individual diagnoses can help structure examination and investigation as well as ensure the rapid recognition of the treatable.

Typically, one of four pathophysiologic categories is suggested by the history and examination: (1) supratentorial expanding lesion; (2) infratentorial expanding lesion; (3) brainstem lesion; and (4) metabolic disorders. Whilst the overall incidence of pediatric coma is unknown, and is likely to be location and health system specific, some broad generalizations are possible.

In most of the published literature, children under the age of 1 year are not only the group most likely to suffer coma from any cause but also are those most likely to suffer from nontraumatic coma. The age group at greatest risk from traumatic coma is the 15–18-year-old group. That the likely cause varies with age is not surprising. Congenital causes are more likely in the first few months, infections more common in the young child, and trauma/intoxications in the older age groups.

Where only nontraumatic causes of coma are considered, infectious causes make up the clear majority of cases. This is in contrast to most adult series and requires the clinician to be particularly vigilant in

Table 2 Etiology of coma by age

<1 year		1–12 years		13–18 years	
Cause[a]	Frequency (%)[b]	Cause[a]	Frequency (%)[b]	Cause[a]	Frequency (%)[b]
Infection[c]	50	Infection[c]	30	Trauma	40
Congenital	15	Seizures	20	Intoxication	25
Seizures	10	Trauma	20	Infection[c]	20
Metabolic	5	Metabolic/ingestion	10	Accidental[d]	5
Trauma	5	Accidental (nontrauma)[d]	10		

Source: Data from multiple sources, reflects the case for developed countries and is approximate only.
[a]Infrequent causes are omitted.
[b]Frequency in descending order by age; in up to 10% of cases the cause may remain unknown.
[c]Infection includes CNS-specific and systemic infections.
[d]Accidental: category includes causes such as asphyxiation, carbon monoxide poisoning, etc.

exploring the possibility of occult infection (**Table 2**). As indicated, the cause may remain undetermined. In many of these instances, the explanation is likely multifactorial. Hyperthermia, electrolyte abnormalities, hypovolemia, and acidosis coexist in many of the common infectious diseases of childhood, and whilst individually insufficient to explain the coma, in combination they can cause profound CNS depression.

The initial presentation of the child reflects not only this diverse etiology but also the difficulties inherent in the assessment of the under-1-year age group. Presentations in this age group are as likely to be nonspecific (e.g., vomiting, poor feeding, pallor) as they are to be CNS-specific (e.g., seizures, altered conscious state).

It is not uncommon for children to arrive at emergency medical services already intubated, having been given sedatives/relaxants. In these patients, examination can be limited to purely evaluation of the pupillary response. In such instances, management should reflect the broad possibilities. It should be particularly emphasized that it is important not to ignore any incongruities in the history or examination – what may have appeared to emergency personnel as a tonic seizure may be the early indication of central herniation. Mortality overall is in the range of 40–60%; it is cause-specific and time-weighted. The longer the duration of coma, regardless of cause, the worse the outcome. Coma consequent to complications of congenital abnormalities has a much higher mortality than intoxications for example. The low mortality from accidental ingestions, intoxications, and some metabolic causes supports the focus on supporting vital functions and treating the immediately treatable.

A number of "coma-like" conditions have been known to cause some initial confusion in diagnosis. The locked-in syndrome caused by a bilateral anterior pontine lesion is rare in pediatrics. Coma can,

however, be mimicked by conditions causing severe neuromuscular weakness. Infantile botulism is one such condition where widespread weakness, often with early bulbar weakness, ophthalmoplegia, and ptosis, can cause the child to appear comatose. Psychogenic coma is unlikely.

The minimally conscious child is used to describe the chronic state where a child may exhibit arousal (clear sleep/wake cycles) but absent to nonpurposeful responses to stimuli.

Finally, in a brief discussion focused on definition and etiology, the clinical imperatives of this life-threatening complication have been given only passing mention. It is fitting to conclude that the challenge of the resuscitation, examination, investigation, and diagnosis and treatment of the comatose child is one that even the most experienced practitioner will find daunting.

See Also

Coma, Definitions and Differential Diagnoses: Adult

Further Reading

Giancino JT, Ashwal S, Childs N, *et al.* (2002) The minimally conscious state: definition and diagnostic criteria. *Neurology* 58: 349–353.

Plum F, Posner JB (1995) *The Diagnosis of Stupor and Coma*, 4th edn. Philadelphia, PA: F.A. Davis.

Rennick G, Shann F, de Campo J (1993) Cerebral herniation during bacterial meningitis in children. *British Medical Journal* 306: 953–955.

Robinson S (1992) The Glasgow Coma Scale: a critical look. *Axon* 4(1): 21–23.

Tasker RC (1999) Coma. In: Macnab A, Macrae D, Henning R (eds.) *Care of the Critically Ill Child*, pp. 68–75. London: Churchill Livingstone.

Wong CP, Forsyth RJ, Kelly TP, Eyre JA (2001) Incidence, etiology and outcome of childhood non-traumatic coma: a prospective, population based study. *Archives of Disease in Childhood* 84: 193–199.

Adult

P Marks, The General Infirmary at Leeds, Leeds, UK

Definition of Coma

Coma can be defined as a state of unresponsiveness in which an individual is unaware of him/herself and the environment and cannot be aroused into a state of awareness or respond to the environment.

The Anatomical Substrate of Consciousness

Consciousness depends upon the interaction between the reticular formation within the brainstem and the cerebral hemispheres. The reticular formation is a complex polysynaptic pathway consisting of a network of small and large neurons that are present within the brainstem and extend to the diencephalon. All major sensory pathways have projections to the reticular formation where interaction takes place before there is projection to the cerebral cortex. The reticular activating system in particular is chiefly concerned with arousal and the maintenance of a wakeful state.

In principle, coma may be caused by dysfunction of the reticular activating system within the brainstem or diencephalon, notably the thalamus, or by bilateral problems affecting the cerebral hemispheres.

Pathophysiology

Lesions in the supratentorial compartment may cause a depression in the level of consciousness by displacing the brain laterally or caudally, with resultant dysfunction of the reticular formation. Infratentorial mass lesions initially compress adjacent structures, then with further expansion, downward herniation of the cerebellar tonsils and medulla through the foramen magnum occurs, as does upward herniation of the brainstem through the tentorial hiatus (**Figure 1**).

Within the supratentorial compartment, two types of brain herniation are recognized: first, subfalcine herniation, where the cingulate gyrus passes beneath the falx cerebri and, second, transtentorial herniation, where the parahippocampal gyrus and uncus pass through the tentorial hiatus.

An expanding lesion in one cerebral hemisphere will cause the cingulate gyrus on the medial surface of the hemisphere to herniate under the falx cerebri (**Figure 2**). This can cause displacement of the internal cerebral vein and the anterior cerebral artery and its

branches. Although often clinically silent, such herniation can result in infarction in the territory of the anterior cerebral artery.

Transtentorial herniation takes place when an expanding lesion results in downward herniation of the parahippocampal gyrus and uncus through the tentorial incisura (**Figure 3**). Three structures of importance are compromised as a result:

1. the ipsilateral oculomotor nerve, resulting in pupillary dilatation due to the now unopposed sympathetic innervation of the pupil

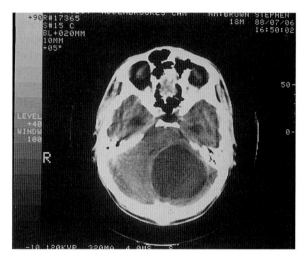

Figure 1 This computed tomography head scan shows a large cystic lesion in the right cerebellar hemisphere. It is producing a mass effect and is displacing the brainstem and cerebral aqueduct. The patient presented in a coma and at operation was found to have a hemangioblastoma, which was resected with good result.

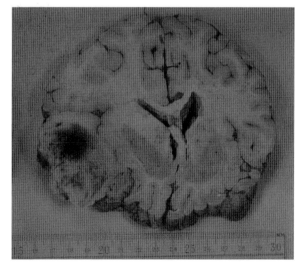

Figure 2 This coronal brain slice shows a glioblastoma multiforme in the left temporal lobe. Note the shift of midline structures and the herniation of the cingulated gyrus.

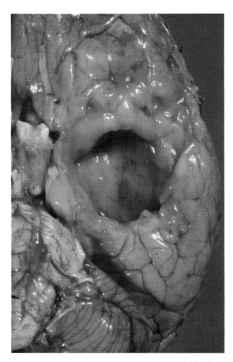

Figure 3 This patient had a cystic astrocytoma of the left temporal lobe and died. This autopsy photograph of the base of the brain shows the lesion and how the medial temporal structures have been displaced by transtentorial herniation.

2. the brainstem, resulting in a depression of the level of consciousness due to dysfunction of the reticular activating system. Long tract signs may also occur

3. the posterior cerebral vessels, leading in agonal cases to infarction of the medial aspect of the occipital lobe (calcarine infarction) (**Figure 4**).

It should be clearly appreciated that it is not just mass lesions such as tumors, abscesses, or hematomas that may result in coma, but other diffuse disturbances of the brain may also produce coma. These are classified into metabolic disturbances; toxic problems such as drug overdose and alcohol ingestion; inflammatory problems such as meningoencephalitis; epilepsy; and other causes such as subarachnoid hemorrhage or primary psychiatric illness. With metabolic disturbances, a general rule is that "all the failures" may produce coma, for example, renal failure, hepatic failure, cardiac failure, and so forth. **Table 1** outlines the primary intracranial causes of coma while **Table 2** looks at conditions of other etiologies that may result in coma.

Causes of Coma

It is important to have a systematic approach to managing patients in coma and a useful way to analyze the etiology of coma is described in **Table 3**.

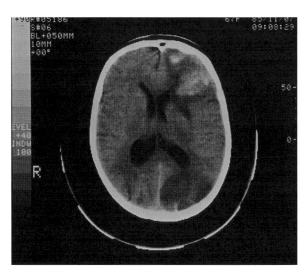

Figure 4 An area of low density is seen in the right occipital region. This represents infarction of the occipital lobe consequent upon transtentorial herniation. The confluent frontal contusion has resulted not only in transtentorial herniation but also in subfalcine herniation in this patient who fell downstairs.

Table 1 Primary intracranial causes of coma

- Head injury
- Intracranial tumor
- Meningitis
- Encephalitis
- Intracranial suppuration, e.g., abscess, subdural empyema
- Thrombosis of the venous sinuses of the dura mater
- Cerebral infarction

Table 2 Other conditions resulting in coma

- Toxic states, e.g., drugs, alcohol
- Generalized seizures
- Hypoxia
- Hyponatremia
- Hyperglycemia
- Hypoglycemia
- Hepatic failure
- Renal failure
- Disorders of calcium metabolism
- Thyroid problems, e.g., hypothyroidism
- Hypothermia
- Thiamine deficiency

Glasgow Coma Scale

This is the most universally accepted measure of the level of consciousness (**Table 4**). It is measured by assigning a patient a score relating to three parameters: first, the stimulus necessary to cause the patient to open his/her eyes; second, the best motor response in the limbs; and third, the best verbal response obtained from the patient. The maximum

Table 3 Etiology of coma

Coma with focal neurological signs or evidence of head injury
Supratentorial or infratentorial space-occupying lesion, e.g.,
   tumor, hematoma, abscess
Hypoglycemic encephalopathy
Hepatic coma
Coma with meningism with no focal or lateralizing neurological signs
Meningoencephalitis
Subarachnoid hemorrhage
Coma without focal or lateralizing neurological signs or meningism
Hypoxic encephalopathy
Hyponatremia
Hypoglycemic encephalopathy and hyperglycemia
Liver failure
Renal failure
Hypocalcemia
Hypothermia
Hypothyroidism
Thiamine deficiency
Drug overdose
Generalized epilepsy, including postictal states
Nonneurological causes
Malingering
Hysteria
Catatonic schizophrenia

Table 4 Glasgow Coma Scale

	Score
Eye-opening	
Nil	1
To pain	2
To verbal stimuli	3
Spontaneously	4
Best verbal response	
No response	1
Incomprehensible sounds	2
Inappropriate words	3
Disoriented and converses	4
Oriented and converses	5
Best motor response	
No response	1
Extension	2
Abnormal flexion	3
Flexion	4
Localizes to pain	5
Obeys commands	6

score that can be obtained is 15 for a patient who is fully oriented with eyes open and obeying commands. The minimum score is 3 – it is impossible to score less than 3. It is important to record the score a patient obtains in each area of the Glasgow Coma Scale so that deterioration or improvement can be monitored.

Investigations

In patients in coma with evidence of head injury or who have focal neurological signs, a computed

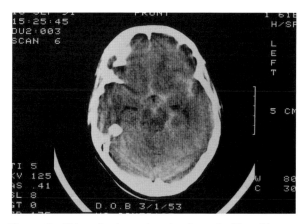

Figure 5 This patient was found collapsed with a Glasgow Coma Scale of 5. The computed tomography head scan shows widespread blood within the subarachnoid spaces. At autopsy, a saccular aneurysm of the anterior communicating artery was found to be the source of the hemorrhage.

tomography (CT) or magnetic resonance imaging (MRI) scan of the brain will detect the presence of mass lesions in the supratentorial or infratentorial compartments. Blood glucose should be estimated and liver function tests performed. Lumbar puncture should not be performed in the presence of space-occupying lesions as this may precipitate coning.

In patients who are in coma and have evidence of meningism but in whom no focal or lateralizing neurological signs are present, a CT head scan should be performed. This will detect the presence of blood within the basal cisterns and subarachnoid spaces as well as other focal collections of blood or pus (**Figure 5**). Lumbar puncture is indicated in the investigation of these patients if there is no contraindication on CT scanning and in these circumstances, it is important to examine the cerebrospinal fluid for the presence of blood, microorganisms, protein, and inflammatory cells.

In patients who are in coma but who do not exhibit focal or lateralizing neurological signs or evidence of meningeal irritation, the following investigations should be performed:

- full blood count and erythrocyte sedimentation rate
- urea electrolytes and blood glucose
- liver function tests
- red blood cell transketolase
- plasma and urine osmolality
- serum calcium
- thyroid function tests
- arterial blood gases
- thiamine
- toxicology screen of urine and blood

- an electroencephalogram should be carried out, as this may show characteristic patterns in the hepatic and renal failure and may also detect nonconvulsive status epilepticus.

In patients without focal and lateralizing signs it may still be necessary to perform a CT or MRI scan and again, a lumbar puncture may be indicated if the other diagnostic tests fail to disclose the etiology of coma.

Management

A detailed management plan for all the various causes of coma is beyond the scope of this article and readers are referred to the Further reading section at the end of this article. However, certain principles of management should be clearly understood and these are outlined below:

- Resuscitation – ensure that the airway is clear, breathing is occurring, and that an adequate circulation is being maintained.
- Intravenous access should be adequate and may necessitate the insertion of central lines.
- At the same time as intravenous access is secured, blood should be withdrawn for various biochemical and hematological tests.
- As resuscitation is proceeding, clinical, laboratory, and radiological evaluation of the patient should be taking place and this is obviously aimed at detecting why the patient is in a coma.
- Certain etiological factors that result in coma may be treated specifically. For example, hypoglycemia can be managed by intravenous glucose infusion, opiate intoxication can be treated with naloxone and Wernicke's encephalopathy caused by thiamine deficiency may be treated with intravenous thiamine.
- The continuing care of patients in coma includes attention to pressure areas, monitoring of fluid and electrolyte balance, cardiac function and the maintenance of breathing, and control of epileptic seizures within or without the intensive care setting.

Prognosis

This is determined by a number of factors:

1. the etiology of the coma
2. the depth and duration of coma
3. clinical signs relating to brainstem reflexes.

Differential Diagnosis

A number of important conditions need to be distinguished clearly from conditions producing coma.

Brain Death

This refers to irreversible loss of function of the brain and brainstem irrespective of whether the heart is beating or not.

Etiology

1. head trauma
2. drug toxicity
3. central nervous system infections, including encephalitis and meningitis
4. cerebrovascular disease, including hemorrhagic and ischemic stroke
5. hypoxic–ischemic insults, including cardiac arrest, carbon monoxide poisoning, and status asthmaticus.

Diagnosis

This is clinical and assessment should be carried out by two doctors experienced in the performance of these tests on two separate occasions 12–24 h apart.

The essential diagnostic criteria are that:

- The patient is unconscious.
- The patient is apneic.
- The patient has absent brainstem function with the following features: (1) absent pupillary responses; (2) absent corneal reflexes; (3) absent oculovestibular reflexes, that is, doll's eyes, and caloric-induced eye movements are absent; (4) absent cough and gag reflexes; and (5) absent ventilatory reflexes, that is, there is no spontaneous respiration when the patient's respirator is disconnected and sufficient time elapses to allow arterial carbon dioxide tension to rise above the threshold required for the stimulation of respiration ($PaCO_2 > 8$ kPa).
- Stimulation of any region within the cranial nerves should not elicit a motor response.
- Patients should not be hypothermic or hypotensive. The patient should exhibit a flaccid tone and absent spontaneous or induced movement.

Although the diagnosis of brain death is essentially clinical, it is important to ensure that a remediable or reversible condition has been eliminated by appropriate imaging and other investigations, including blood tests and toxicology screens.

It is well recognized that in the presence of brain death the electroencephalogram shows electrical silence and that cerebral angiography shows no blood flow through the brain.

Persistent Vegetative State (PVS)

At one stage this condition was known as coma vigil. It is defined as a condition of wakefulness

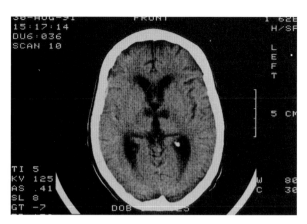

Figure 6 This computed tomography scan shows bilateral thalamic damage from carbon monoxide poisoning. The victim was found in a room that was heated by a defective gas fire. He remains in a persistent vegetative state.

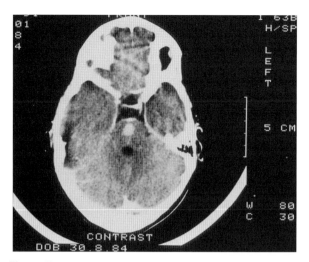

Figure 7 This computed tomography scan through the posterior cranial fossa shows a high-density area within the pons. This was due to a hypertensive hemorrhage and the patient was locked in.

Table 5 Principal causes of persistent vegetative state

- Head injury
- Cerebrovascular disease
- Hypoxia–ischemia, e.g., carbon monoxide poisoning, cardiac arrest
- Intracranial infection, e.g., meningitis, encephalitis
- Terminal stages of degenerative central nervous system disorders

without awareness. In the vegetative state the patient displays unawareness of him/herself and the environment and has a stable circulation, breathes spontaneously, and exhibits cycles of eye opening and eye closure with periods of sleep and wakefulness. For a vegetative state to be classified as persistent, it must continue for more than 4 weeks and it is therefore unlikely that it represents a phase in the recovery from coma.

When a vegetative state continues for more than 12 months after head injury or 6 months after other etiological causes of this condition, it is referred to as a permanent vegetative state.

In broad terms of neuropathology, PVS is attributable to severe and diffuse damage to the cerebral hemispheres in the presence of an intact brainstem. It should however be noted that damage to the rostral part of the brainstem in conjunction with damage to the cerebral hemispheres can also be consistent with the development of PVS. Diffuse axonal injury is a frequent cause of PVS, as is extensive laminar necrosis of the cerebral cortex consequent upon global cerebral ischemia or hypoxia. Thalamic necrosis of whatever etiology, for example, carbon monoxide poisoning, may also result in PVS (**Figure 6**). The principal causes of PVS are listed in **Table 5**.

Locked-In Syndrome

This is a particularly unpleasant and unfortunate condition in which patients are aware of themselves and their environment but are unable to respond due to loss of motor and speech function. The condition may be caused by supranuclear lesions affecting the corticospinal tracts, usually in the region of the ventral pons below the level of the oculomotor nerve nuclei (**Figure 7**). Alternatively the condition may be attributable to nuclear or infranuclear disease of motor nerves. Causes within the brainstem include head injury, tumor, demyelination, central pontine myelinolysis, and hemorrhage or infarction usually of hypertensive origin. Nuclear or infranuclear causes include Guillain–Barré syndrome or polyneuropathy.

Other Differential Diagnoses of Coma

These include narcolepsy, a condition characterized by excessive sleepiness, with abnormally regulated rapid eye movement sleep. The other important differential diagnosis of coma is syncope. This is essentially due to a variety of causes, all of which result in loss of postural tone and consciousness from an acute reduction in the blood flow to the brain. Disorders of cardiac rhythm, reduction in stroke volume, and reduced peripheral resistance of whatever etiology can result in syncope.

See Also

Carbon Monoxide Poisoning: Clinical Findings, Sequelae In Survivors; **Coma, Definitions and Differential Diagnoses:** Pediatric; **Head Trauma:** Pediatric and Adult, Clinical Aspects; Neuropathology

Further Reading

Andrews K (1999) The vegetative state – clinical diagnosis. *Postgraduate Medical Journal* 75: 321–324.

Plum F, Posner JB (1980) *The Diagnosis of Stupor and Coma,* 3rd edn. Philadelphia, PA: FA Davis.

Teasdale G, Jennett B (1974) Assessment of coma and impaired consciousness: a practical scale. *Lancet* 2: 81–84.

Widjicks EF (1995) Determining brain death in adults. *Neurology* 45: 1003–1011.

COMPLAINTS AGAINST DOCTORS, HEALTHCARE WORKERS AND INSTITUTIONS

C G M Fernie, University of Glasgow, Glasgow, UK

Introduction

The well-known maxim reminds us that common things occur commonly and this is not simply in respect to clinical conditions. Whilst there are now a considerable variety of routes of accountability that members of the healthcare professions might face, the most common of these in the UK almost certainly continues to be the National Health Service (NHS) complaints procedure given that the majority of consultations with healthcare workers in the UK will take place in this context.

This article will consider the different ways in which healthcare professionals may have to justify their actions by reference to the systems in place in the UK. Attempts have been made in recent years to reduce the burgeoning use of litigation to call these workers to account as this adversarial approach may not only not have the desired effect, but also result in potential economic disadvantages to society generally in that costs frequently exceed any settlement to the claimant.

The NHS Complaints Procedure

A frequent error amongst these groups continues to be the difference between a complaint and a claim. The generally accepted definition of a complaint within the NHS complaints procedure is "an expression of dissatisfaction that requires a response." Commonly, professionals believe that because there is no "formal" complaint they do not have to furnish a reply. However, if a patient is unhappy with the care he/she has received and wishes to have an explanation, surely by definition the preceding criteria are fulfilled? In contrast, a claim is undertaken through the branch of private law that in England and Wales is known as tort but in Scotland as delict. Here the objective is to obtain financial recompense for harm suffered by a patient. There are three fundamental parts to a medical negligence claim: (1) a duty of care; (2) a breach of that duty; and (3) harm suffered as a consequence (the causative link). Although in England and Wales there has been some moderation of the inherent adversity in the system with the introduction of the new civil procedure rules subsequent to Lord Woolf's reforms, there continues to be a distinctly different approach and the emphasis in the NHS complaints procedure is very much on achieving local resolution.

Of course, it may not simply be double jeopardy that the healthcare worker faces. An adverse event may initially be dealt with through the NHS complaints procedure, then be referred to the Health Service Commissioner (ombudsman) by route of appeal. Thereafter it may be reported to the General Medical Council (GMC) and can even end up in the criminal courts. Ultimately the case may turn to the civil courts in an attempt to obtain restitution. The use of the complaints procedure as a dry run for civil litigation is not unknown despite guidance to the contrary and there appears implicit acceptance of the futility of this in the proposed NHS General Medical Services regulations (the statute governing the provision of general practitioner services in the UK) where there is an acceptance that the two processes can go ahead simultaneously. Even at the present time, there is nothing to stop a solicitor being instructed by a complainant to act for him/her in taking the preliminary steps within the procedure.

Civil actions may ultimately (leaving aside the unifying influence of European law) reach the definitive court of appeal in the House of Lords and, while academics may try and argue on the distinguishing features of cases such as *Hunter* v. *Hanley* ((1955) SC 200, 1955 SLT 213) or *Bolam* v. *Friern HMC* ((1957) 2 All ER 118, [1957] 1 WLR 582, 101 Sol Jo 357, 1 BMLR 1), subsequent case law modifying these principles as found in *Bolitho* v. *City and Hackney Health*

Authority ((1997) 4 All ER 771 HL) has almost certainly affected the way we deal with negligence claims throughout the UK, albeit the new "civil procedure rules" emanating from the Woolf reforms only apply in England and Wales. These new rules came into force in 1999 and represented the greatest change in the civil justice system for over a century. Woolf had concluded that public access to civil justice could only be improved by making litigation simpler, quicker, and cheaper.

After the formal consultation by the Wilson Committee, resulting in the publication *Being Heard*, the new NHS complaints procedure came into effect on April 1, 1996, and thereafter most medical defense organizations found an increase of at least 50% in cases both within the general practitioner sector, which makes up about two-thirds of their workload, and against hospital doctors.

Within the new procedure there were a number of key objectives, including ease of access and simplification, plus common features for complaints about services provided within the NHS. The intention here was that all healthcare workers would be accountable through the same process. Importantly, there was a separation of complaints from disciplinary procedures and the hope was to avoid apportionment of blame, making it easier to differentiate lessons on management and service delivery from complaints in order to achieve improvement. It is easy to see where the concept of clinical governance emanated from within this process. The hope was that there would be fairness to staff and complainants alike, with more rapid, open procedures and a degree of honesty and thoroughness where the prime intention was not only to resolve the problem, but also to satisfy the concerns raised by the complainant.

Rather than a confrontational, adversarial approach the process envisaged was much more of an investigative one. The overall concept was of the type found within alternative dispute resolution that has attracted considerable interest within the legal profession who had become increasingly aware of the disadvantages of formal litigation.

Accountability for healthcare workers may arise through a number of routes:

- NHS hospital complaint
- NHS family health services complaint
- ombudsman
- civil litigation
- GMC
- General Dental Council
- National Council for Nursing and Midwifery
- criminal prosecution
- fatal accident inquiry/coroner's inquest.

Of course, not only may that professional be required to submit to one of these processes but, if unlucky, the practitioner can end up going through all of these, either simultaneously or sequentially.

Medical defense organizations will look after the professional interests of doctors and dentists, whereas the British Medical Association (BMA) will assist with issues of personal conduct, although it is quite possible that there is overlap. It is not unknown for a doctor's medical defense organization to exercise its discretionary function by helping in this area in cases where a doctor is not, perhaps, a member of the BMA. Likewise, the Royal College of Nursing will cater for a nurse's professional interests and in primary care may also have responsibility for indemnity.

With the separation of complaints from discipline since the inception of the NHS complaints procedure, the number of disciplinary hearings has fallen dramatically, certainly compared to the previous terms of service hearings where general practitioners were often involved in an acrimonious exchange with complainants who were present at the same time in a quasilegal setting. Fewer than 1% of NHS complaints are dealt with through the disciplinary process, although this is still available for certain allegations.

Where a complaint is made on behalf of a patient who has not specifically authorized another individual to act for him/her, care should be taken not to disclose personal data to the complainant. The advice given by medical defense organizations is that one should not be deemed obstructive, although it may be valid to "flag up" this particular issue.

The healthcare worker should avoid disclosing any incidental information and in the case of a medical practitioner should ensure that there is compliance with the GMC guidance contained within its booklet *Confidentiality: Protecting and Providing Information*. Similar obligations apply to the other professions, although the doctors' national regulatory body has increasingly refined its advice in recent years.

Increasing use has been made of private healthcare, especially in England and Wales, and although the complaints procedure will cover any complaint made about a trust staff or facilities relating to that trust's private pay beds, this does not extend to the private medical care provided by the consultant outwith his/her NHS contract.

At the time of writing, there is a time limit on initiating complaints and a complaint should normally be made within six months of the incident resulting in the dissatisfaction, or within six months of the date of becoming aware of that problem, provided that is within 12 months of the problem. However, there is discretion that, more often than not, can be invoked to extend this time limit and there are proposals within the new family health services regulations to extend the primary limitation period to one year. *Prima facie,* this may appear unfair on the doctor but one has to contrast this with the GMC's ability to look into complaints within a five-year period, although this may be extended if the gravity of the offense merits it.

There is a recognized philosophy that, if a personal response is in order, then a simple explanation may often resolve that patient's concern, but if the preliminary response does not address the complaint to the complainant's satisfaction, there is a route of appeal. To that end, trusts are required to appoint at least one person to act in the role of the convenor to whom such requests are made.

Conciliation

Conciliation is considered to be a voluntary process where both parties agree to participate with the intention and hope of resolving the complaint at a local level.

Lay conciliators are required to be made available by trusts in order to optimize the conditions to achieve resolution. The purpose of this process is to permit the complainant and respondent to address the relevant outstanding issues in a nonconfrontational manner so that an acceptable agreement may be reached but not to impose a solution upon the parties concerned.

An integral part of the process is confidentiality so that the conciliator might encourage both parties to consider the reasons for the complaint in an open way. Whilst neither the conciliator nor the participants should provide information from the process to any other person, it is in order for the conciliator to inform the trust when conciliation has ceased and give an indication of whether or not resolution has been achieved.

Although not strictly forbidden, it is not normal to have a representative from a professional body present or for a solicitor to accompany a complainant, although it would be usual for the complainant to have another person there for support.

The Independent Review Panel (IRP)

There is a route of appeal in that complainants who are dissatisfied with the preliminary response. They may make a request for an IRP to the convenor either orally or in writing within a period of 28 calendar days from completion of the local resolution process.

In deciding whether to convene a panel, the convenor has to consider, in consultation with an independent lay chair from the regional list, whether the

trust can take any further action short of establishing a panel to satisfy the complainant and also if establishing a panel would add any further value to the process.

Whilst there was a tendency to grant a request for such a hearing, this is by no means automatically granted and has now decreased, so that only 22% of requests in 2000–2001 resulted in a panel going ahead.

Where clinical issues are involved there is an obligation for the convenor to take appropriate clinical advice in deciding whether to convene such a panel.

As well as informing the complainant in writing of the decision on whether or not a panel should be appointed, the convenor must set out clearly the terms of reference if there is to be a hearing or the reasons for any decision resulting in refusal.

Should the convenor refuse to hold an IRP; there is a further right of appeal to the ombudsman.

It is a decision for the panel how to conduct its proceedings having regard to guidance issued by the NHS within the following rules:

- The panel's proceedings must be held in private.
- The panel must give both parties a reasonable opportunity to express their views.
- Should any of the panel members disagree how the panel should go about its business, the chairperson's decision will be final.
- When being interviewed by the panel, the complainant and any other person interviewed may be accompanied by a person of their choosing who, provided the chairperson agrees, may speak to the panel, except that no one may be accompanied by a legally qualified person acting as an advocate.

Whilst the approach is discretionary, there is normally not an impediment to a professional adviser with a law degree actually assisting a doctor provided the adviser is not acting as a solicitor or advocate/barrister.

Subsequent to receipt of the panel's report, the Chief Executive of the trust must write to the complainant informing him/her of any action the Trust propose to take as a result of the panel's deliberations and of the right of the complainant to take the grievance to the ombudsman if he/she remains dissatisfied.

There are, of course, various time limits set out within the guidance, and it is safe to say there is often difficulty in achieving these targets (only 9% of IRPs were concluded within target in 2000–2001), although with greater familiarity, progress is being made to reach them.

An evaluation of how the new NHS complaints procedure was performing was undertaken, and the result was a consultation document published in 1993, *NHS Complaints Reform – Making Things Right*. Of the 140 000 people who made a formal complaint the preceding year, only 3500 felt the need to request an independent review. However, the overwhelming consensus was that this stage caused the most dissatisfaction with users of the procedure.

It "is not perceived by complainants to be impartial. Improving this aspect of the current procedure is the single most commonly cited suggestion for reform." The proposal is for Commission for Healthcare Audit and Inspection (CHAI) in England and Wales or an extension of the ombudsman's role in Scotland to permit a more independent and robust review to take place than currently exists.

The Ombudsman

The NHS ombudsman looks into complaints made by or on behalf of people who have suffered because of unsatisfactory treatment or service by the NHS. He/she is completely independent of the NHS and the government. The ombudsman's services are free.

Anybody wishing to complain to the ombudsman must first have put their complaint to the NHS organization or practitioner concerned, such as the hospital trust, health authority, the general practitioner, or the dentist, who should give the complainant full details of the NHS complaints procedure and should try to resolve the complaint. If the complainant is still dissatisfied once the NHS complaints procedure has been exhausted, he/she can then complain to the ombudsman.

The ombudsman will not normally become involved unless the complainant has taken up the complaint officially and is still unhappy, for example, because:

- it took too long to deal with the complaint locally
- a panel review was unreasonably refused
- a satisfactory answer to the complaint was not given

The complainant has to send the complaint to the ombudsman no later than a year from the date when he/she became aware of the events that are the subject of complaint. The ombudsman can sometimes extend the time limit, but only if there are special reasons.

Whereas previously, the Health Service Commissioner was predominantly involved in looking at cases of maladministration, often in respect to the handling of a complaint, since March 31, 1996 the ombudsman was also able to investigate complaints about clinical issues in both hospital and general practice.

General Medical Council

Of all the healthcare workers' national regulatory bodies, the best known is almost certainly that of the medical profession, the GMC. There has been a marked growth in GMC complaints and, whereas previously the GMC would write back to the complainant recommending that the NHS complaints procedure had not yet been exhausted, the GMC is now often used as the first stop by a complainant. The GMC will usually take the matter forward if it is felt that there are concerns either about the doctor's conduct, that is, that his/her failing constitutes serious professional misconduct, or that there is significant cause for concern by way of that doctor's performance.

The New Council

The Council is the GMC's governing body, and until 2003 it had 104 members and delegated much of its work, including the consideration of complaints about doctors, to numerous committees.

The new system established a smaller Council on July 1, 2003 consisting of 35 members, 40% of whom were lay people. It is now made up of 19 elected medical members, two appointed medical members, and 14 lay members appointed by the government. This reflects the principle of professionally led regulation in partnership with the public.

The reason for this fundamental change was to produce a council capable of acting more quickly and effectively that included more lay members than before.

By 2002, a record 72 doctors had been erased or suspended from practice and a further 62 had conditions imposed or were reprimanded (previously given an admonishment) by the GMC. The GMC also investigated a record number of 5539 doctors that year, an increase of 4% from the previous year. However, for the first time in seven years the number of complaints made fell, which suggested that there might be a return of public confidence in the profession.

If a doctor is found guilty of a criminal offense within the UK, there is an automatic referral to the GMC. The findings of the court are taken as proved and the case will not be re-heard by the Professional Conduct Committee, although they will allow representation to be made on behalf of the medical practitioner and reach a decision as to whether any additional sanction should be taken against the individual concerned.

Since the inception of the NHS complaints procedure, there has been an increasing tendency for such cases simply to be referred to the GMC as a first stop.

The GMC has legal powers through the Medical Act 1983 (as amended) to act against problem doctors. Until 2004 a decision was taken at an early stage to stream a complaint into one of the three procedures: (1) health; (2) performance; or (3) conduct. Each has, potentially, different possible outcomes and not all can lead to being erased (struck off) from the GMC's register. At that time the cases were heard by members of the GMC Council.

The new system was introduced from 2004, together with a new single complaints process. All complaints now go through the same process; this means that a doctor's fitness to practice will be considered in the round, rather than being "labeled" early on as a health, performance, or conduct case. The same outcomes and sanctions are now available to apply to every case as appropriate. No council members will sit on the panels that decide the case against a doctor and all panelists will be appropriately assessed for suitability.

The reason for this change is to produce a new system to streamline the previous processes and ensure that complaints are processed as promptly as is consistent with achieving fairness.

Not only are doctors personally accountable by way of their medical practice, but they also have certain obligations set out in the GMC document *Management in Health Care: The Role of Doctors*, published in December 1999 that the first consideration for all managers must be the interests and safety of patients. Doctors must take action if they believe that patients are at risk of serious harm by way of a colleague's conduct, performance, or health and it explicitly states in this document that concerns about a patient may arise from critical incident reporting or complaints from patients, and doctors who receive such information have a duty to act on it.

In addition there will now be a license to practice and revalidate. In the old system the GMC's register of doctors was traditionally dependent on a once-only check on a doctor's qualifications. However, in the new system, commencing in 2005, every doctor who wants to practice medicine must not only be registered, but also hold a license to practice from the GMC.

In addition, licenced doctors must be revalidated by the GMC every 5 years. This means that they will be asked to show the GMC that they have been practicing medicine in line with the principles set out in their guidance booklet, *Good Medical Practice*. If they do this, the regulator will confirm that their license will continue.

The changes aim to ensure that doctors are up to date and fit to practice medicine throughout their careers. It also aims to modernize regulation and increase public confidence in doctors.

Council for Healthcare Regulatory Excellence (CHRE)

There is now a statutory overarching body overseeing all the healthcare regulatory bodies, covering all of the UK and separate from government, established in April 2003. Its function is to promote best practice and consistency in the regulation of healthcare professionals by the following nine regulatory bodies:

1. GMC
2. General Dental Council
3. General Optical Council
4. General Osteopathic Council
5. General Chiropractic Council
6. Health Professions Council
7. Nursing and Midwifery Council
8. Royal Pharmaceutical Society of Great Britain
9. Pharmaceutical Society of Northern Ireland.

This body came into being as a consequence of the report of the Bristol Royal Infirmary Inquiry (*Learning from Bristol*, July 2001), chaired by Sir Ian Kennedy, which recommended the establishment of the CHRE (formerly CRHP).

This was implemented in the NHS Reform and Healthcare Professions Act 2002, which was also informed by the NHS Plan for England and the consultation document *Modernizing Regulation in the Health Professions*.

Its functions are to promote the interests of the public and patients in the field of the regulation of health professionals. Another stated aim is to promote best practice in professionally led regulation. An annual report goes to parliament on the CHRE's work, with discretion to report on the performance of individual regulatory bodies and to compare their performance of similar functions. A further role is to promote cooperation and consistency across the regulation of all the healthcare professions, in the interest of patients. In addition, it should develop principles of good regulation and advise ministers across the UK on professional regulation issues in healthcare.

It may also refer a regulator's final decision on a fitness-to-practice case to the High Court (or its equivalent throughout the UK) for the protection of the public. Even in cases where the regulator finds there are insufficient grounds to constitute serious professional misconduct, the CHRE will examine this verdict and consider whether it needs to take action. As a last resort it can order a regulator to change its rules to protection the public (this requires the permission of both Houses of Parliament).

The CHRE is answerable to the Westminster parliament and is independent of the UK Department of Health.

Conclusion

A variety of routes of accountability have been set out but the one that a healthcare worker practicing within the UK is most likely to face is the NHS complaints procedure. As from April 1996 this has almost certainly achieved the purpose of providing a thorough investigation of the issues raised, albeit not always to the complete satisfaction of the complainant. However, the new proposed changes are intended to address reservations expressed by complainants, especially about the independent review process.

The previous confrontational and legalistic process has by and large been dispensed with and, although there are still inherent delays in the system, particularly in the hospital sector, the complainant is usually able to obtain a better understanding of the medical management of his/her care that is within the ethos of clinical governance, allowing doctors to learn from adverse events in order that their practice might subsequently be improved.

Of course, there continue to be safeguards for society, generally where that healthcare worker's conduct may be so serious that regulatory body intervention is justified or his/her performance is so seriously deficient that it is necessary for this to be examined. The system has now been underpinned by the CHRE in order to retain public confidence.

There is no doubt that self-regulation is one of the hallmarks of a profession but the emphasis now is very much that of professionally led regulation, but with a significant lay input, in order to avoid the all-too-prevalent criticism that culminated in an exponential rise in complaints. It appears that the new changes are starting to work in that complaints are no longer rising but society does require an effective legislative backstop to maintain progress in the face of public concern.

See Also

Medical Malpractice: General Practice; Medical Malpractice – Medico-legal Perspectives: Negligence, Duty of Care; Negligence, Causation; Negligence Quantum

Further Reading

Beauchamp TL, Childress JF (1994) *Principles of Biomedical Ethics*, 4th edn. Oxford, UK: Oxford University Press.

Brazier M (2003) *Medicine, Patients and the Law*, 3rd edn. London: Penguin Books.

British Medical Association (2004) *Medical Ethics Today*, 2nd edn. London: BMJ Publishing Group.

Chiswick D, Cope R (eds.) (1995) *Practical Forensic Psychiatry*. Royal College of Psychiatry.

Downie RS, Calman KC (1994) *Healthy Respect – Ethics in Health Care*, 2nd edn. Oxford, UK: Oxford University Press.

Downie RS, Charlton B (1992) *The Making of a Doctor – Medical Education in Theory and Practice*. Oxford, UK: Oxford University Press.

Gee DJ, Mason JK (1990) *The Courts and the Doctor*. Oxford, UK: Oxford University Press.

Gillon R (1986) *Philosophical Medical Ethics*. Chichester, UK: Wiley.

Kennedy I (1988) *Treat Me Right*. Oxford, UK: Clarendon Press.

Kennedy I (1992) *Doctors, Patients and the Law*. Oxford, UK: Blackwell Scientific.

Kennedy I, Grubb A (2000) *Medical Law, Text with Materials*, 3rd edn. London: Butterworths.

Mason JK, Smith RAM (2002) *Law and Medical Ethics*, 5th edn. London: Butterworths.

McLay WDS (1996) *Clinical Forensic Medicine*, 2nd edn. London: Greenwich Medical Media.

McLean SAM, Mason JK (2003) *Legal and Ethical Aspects of Healthcare*. London: Greenwich Medical Media.

White RM, Willock ID (1999) *The Scottish Legal System*, 2nd edn. Edinburgh, UK: Butterworths.

COMPUTER CRIME AND DIGITAL EVIDENCE

E Casey, Stroz Friedberg LLC, Washington, DC, USA

Introduction

Computers can be involved in a crime in three general ways: (1) as a target; (2) as an instrument; (3) and as a source of evidence. Unauthorized access, theft of services, and other offenses defined in many computer crime laws focus on computers as targets. In the past, the term computer crime was associated with this limited set of offenses, but as computer use becomes more prevalent in society, computers are becoming involved in a wider range of crimes and the term computer crime is assuming a broader meaning.

Computers can be directly involved in many types of criminal activity, including terrorism, organized crime, stalking, and child exploitation. For example, sex offenders and obsessional harassers use computers to threaten and control victims, making the computer an instrument of the crime. In addition, due to the nature of digital data and a computer's storage of it, computers can contain evidence relating to crimes. For instance, serial killer Maury Roy Travis sent a letter to a newspaper with a map that showed where a victims' body could be found. Travis was tracked down via a 'cybertrail' comprised of a unique number printed on the map, associated web server access logs, and internet dial-up records that were generated when he connected to the internet to download the map from an online travel website. Investigators searched Travis' home and found incriminating evidence, including victims' blood and videotapes showing a number of the victims being tortured and killed.

The scope of computer crime becomes even broader with the proliferation of mobile devices and equipment with built-in computers such as personal digital assistants, mobile telephones, and computers embedded in cars. A personal digital assistant can contain significant details about a victim or an offender's life and activities. These data are potentially retrievable by others. A mobile telephone can reveal which telephone numbers an individual called or was called from at particular times. Additionally, it may be possible to ascertain the locations of a victim and likely suspect, leading up to a violent crime based on the locations of their mobile telephones. Sensing and diagnostic modules in cars – analogous to the black box on an airliner, recording data such as vehicle speed, brake status, and throttle position during the last five seconds before an impact – are used to investigate automobile accidents.

For forensic purposes, it is generally not computers themselves that are of primary interest but rather the data they contain. Additionally, related data on networks such as the internet and mobile telephone systems can be useful in an investigation. The term digital evidence is used to refer to any data stored or transmitted using a computer that may have probative value. It may support or refute a hypothesis of how an offense occurred or address critical elements of an offense, such as intent or alibi. Given the current ubiquity of digital evidence, it is a rare crime that does not have some associated data stored on or transmitted using computers. It is becoming routine for law enforcement agencies to devote resources to forensic examination of computers in most types of criminal investigation to seek related evidence on computers and networks.

Digital Crime Scene Investigation

When computers are an instrument of a crime or a source of digital evidence, it is useful to think of them as secondary crime scenes. Like a physical crime scene, digital crime scenes can contain many pieces of evidence and it is necessary to apply the same processes to preserve, document, and search the scene. In addition, Locard's exchange principle applies to the digital realm, helping investigators establish continuity of offense and track down criminals. According to Locard's exchange principle, when two entities (e.g., objects, people, locations) come into contact during the commission of a crime, an exchange of evidence occurs. Despite their best efforts to conceal or destroy incriminating digital evidence, criminals who use computers often leave behind digital traces that are useful in an investigation. In past homicide cases, victims' computers contained evidence that led to the murders and evidence on offenders' computers revealed their intent to kill.

In the UK case involving Dr. Harold Shipman, changes he made to computerized medical records on his practice computer system were instrumental in convicting him of killing hundreds of patients. Following Shipman's arrest, police made an exact copy of the hard drive from his computer, thus preserving a complete and accurate duplicate of the digital evidence. By analyzing the computer application Shipman used to maintain patient records, investigators found that the program kept an audit trail, recording changes made to patient records. This audit trail indicated that Shipman had lied about patients' symptoms and made backdated modifications to records to conceal the murders. During his trial Shipman claimed that he was familiar with this audit trail feature and was sufficiently knowledgeable about computers to falsify the audit trail if he had actually been trying to hide these activities. However, the court was convinced that Shipman had altered the records to conceal his crimes and sentenced him to life in prison.

Attributing computer activities to a particular individual can be challenging. Digital evidence can provide a circumstantial link between a person and activities on a computer, but it can be difficult to prove beyond a reasonable doubt that the defendant committed the crime. For instance, logs showing that a particular internet account was used to commit a crime do not prove that the owner of that account was responsible since someone else could have used the individual's account. Attributing a crime to an individual becomes even more difficult when a crime is committed from a publicly accessible computer, such as at an internet cafe or public-library terminal.

Using evidence from multiple independent sources to corroborate each other and develop an accurate picture of events can help develop a strong association between an individual and computer activities. In one stalking case, investigators did not have sufficient evidence to prove that their prime suspect sent a threatening e-mail from a public-library terminal. Therefore, they had to interview witnesses, compare the e-mail with letters that were mailed to the victims by the suspect years earlier, and use other traditional investigative techniques to build a solid case.

As another example, a man accused of possessing child pornography argued that all evidence found in his home should be suppressed because investigators had not provided sufficient probable cause in their search warrant to conclude that it was in fact he, and not an imposter, who was using his internet account to traffic in child pornography (*US v. Grant*, US Court of Appeals, 1st Cir. 2000, available online at http://laws.lp.findlaw.com/1st/992332.html). During their investigation into an online child exploitation group, investigators determined that one member of the group had connected to the internet using a dial-up account registered to Grant. Upon further investigation, they found that Grant also had a high-speed internet connection from his home that was used as a FTP (File Transfer Protocol) server – the type of file-transfer server required for membership in the child exploitation group. Coincidentally, while tapping a telephone not associated with Grant in relation to another child pornography case, investigators observed that one of the participants in a secret online chat room was connected via Grant's dial-up account. Contemporaneous surveillance of the defendant's home revealed that his and his wife's cars were both parked outside their residence at the time. The court felt that there was enough corroborating evidence to establish a solid circumstantial connection between the defendant and the crime to support probable cause for the search warrant. Hence, using multiple independent sources of evidence, it is possible to establish a solid circumstantial link between online activities and an individual.

A Developing Forensic Discipline

From a forensic standpoint, it is necessary to process digital evidence in such a way that it will hold up under scrutiny in court. To address this need, formal principles and methodologies have been developed for processing evidence from a wide range of technologies.

Early approaches to processing digital evidence were developed primarily by law enforcement, with assistance from computer professionals, during the late 1980s and early 1990s in the USA. A number of new terms were created to describe this practice, including computer forensics, forensic computer analysis, and forensic computing. Also, new terms like network forensics, internet forensics, and incident forensics were created to accommodate other technologies. Although certain fundamental evidence-handling principles were applied to computers at this stage, such as maintaining chain of custody, no formalized methodology was developed. The lack of standards for how computers and networks were handled as a source of evidence resulted in a lack of consistency, making it more difficult for the practice to develop into the generally accepted norms of a forensic science discipline.

Several groups were formed to develop standards and a more scientific approach to processing evidence on computers and networks was established. The International Organization of Computer Evidence (IOCE) was established in the mid-1990s "to ensure the harmonization of methods and practices among nations and guarantee the ability to use digital evidence collected by one state in the courts of another state." In 1998, the Scientific Working Group on Digital Evidence (SWGDE) was established to "promulgate accepted forensic guidelines and definitions for the handling of digital evidence." As a result of these efforts, the American Society of Crime Laboratory Directors/Laboratory Accreditation Board (ASCLD/LAB) updated its accreditation manual in 2003 to include standards and criteria for "digital evidence examiners" in US crime laboratories. There are similar efforts to develop digital evidence examination into an accredited discipline under international standards (ISO 17025).

Although the SWGDE developed guidelines for training and best practices, it did not provide a solid methodology that would enable the field to develop into a science. In 2001, the first Digital Forensics Research Work Shop (DFRWS) was held, bringing together knowledgeable individuals from academia, the military, and the private sector to advance the field as a science. One outcome of this workshop was a framework for processing digital evidence and a suggested title for the field: "digital forensic science." Digital forensic science was defined as "the use of scientifically derived and proven methods toward preservation, collection, validation, identification, analysis, interpretation, documentation, and presentation of digital evidence derived from digital sources for the purpose of facilitating or furthering the reconstruction of events found to be criminal, or helping to anticipate unauthorized actions shown to be disruptive to planned operations." The DFRWS workshop also led to the creation of the *International Journal of Digital Evidence* (IJDE), and later the *Journal of Digital Investigation*.

The approach to processing digital evidence developed at the DFRWS was based on traditional methods of the forensic sciences and has focused attention on forensic issues. For instance, more formalized methods of processing computers and networks are being developed that are modeled on physical crime-scene investigation. Researchers and practitioners are developing new techniques and tools for detecting, tracking, and attributing computer crime. Specifications for digital evidence processing tools are being developed to ensure that they address the needs of the forensic science community. In addition, related areas of expertise are emerging to deal with digital evidence from different technologies (e.g., networks, mobile telephones) and to perform specialized tasks (e.g., recovery of deleted or encrypted data, analysis of computer programs).

Digital Evidence

Because any crime can involve a computer, it is important to have a basic understanding of the kinds of digital evidence that might be available. Additionally, a familiarity with the fragility and limitations of digital evidence will minimize the risk of mishandling computers and damaging or misinterpreting the evidence they contain.

At its basic level, digital evidence exists in a physical medium such as a magnetic disk, a copper wire, or a radio signal in the air. Forensic examiners rarely scrutinize the physical medium and instead use computers to translate the data into a form that humans can interpret, such as text, audio, or video. Therefore, examiners rarely see the actual data but only a representation, and each layer of abstraction can lose information and introduce errors. For instance, analyzing the magnetic properties of a hard drive may reveal additional information useful for some investigations (e.g., overwritten data, the cause of damage to the disk). The risk of examining media at this low level is that the act of observing will cause changes that could destroy or undermine the evidence.

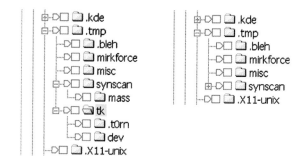

Figure 1 A folder named "tk" contained important evidence related to a computer intrusion investigation. The "tk" folder is visible using a newer version of a digital evidence examination tool (left), but not an older version containing a bug (right).

In fact, it is considered best practice to examine an exact replica of digital evidence to avoid altering the original. However, it can be difficult to obtain an exact and complete copy of a magnetic disk, random access memory (RAM), a copper wire, or a radio signal. For instance, programmatic mistakes (a.k.a. bugs) have been found in tools for collecting digital evidence from hard drives, resulting in only a portion of the data being copied. Bugs have also been found in tools for examining digital evidence on storage media, resulting in an inaccurate representation of the underlying data, as shown in **Figure 1**.

There are many other potential sources of error in digital evidence between the time data are created by a system and the time of preservation and analysis of the evidence. For instance, system malfunction can result in erroneous or missing log entries. In addition, as with other forms of evidence, poor training or lack of experience can lead forensic examiners to mishandle or incorrectly interpret digital evidence.

The multiple layers of separation between a forensic examiner and the original evidence can be problematic from a forensic standpoint. The possibility that important evidence was overlooked, misrepresented, or misinterpreted leaves the door open for criticism and reasonable doubt. To mitigate these risks, experienced digital evidence examiners do not base their conclusions on the results of one tool. For example, making copies of digital evidence with more than one tool reduces the chance that portions will not be collected. In addition, comparing results in multiple tools and validating important findings at a low level reduces the risks of misrepresentation and misinterpretation.

The mutability of digital evidence is another forensic concern. To demonstrate that digital evidence is an exact replica of the original and has not been altered since it was collected, it is common practice to calculate a cryptographic hash (e.g., MD5, SHA1) of the evidence prior to collection. For instance, consider a letter found on a computer containing the sentence "Jane, I want to kill you" that has an MD5 value of 95a2592365b98fcac8c940de3d136943, as shown here:

```
C:\>type letter
Jane, I want to kiss you
C:\>md5sum letter
95a2592365b98fcac8c940de3d136943 *letter
```

By taking such precautions to document the original state of the evidence, any changes in the evidence can be detected quickly using the hash value. For instance, if the aforementioned letter was altered to contain the work "kill" instead of "kiss" this would be reflected in the MD5 value as shown here:

```
C:\>type letter
Jane, I want to kill you
C:\>md5sum letter
ccdcd9ac77345491a6c10609dc3ad338 *letter
```

Although the ephemeral nature of digital evidence has been mentioned, one benefit of digital evidence is that it can persist despite efforts to destroy it. For instance, deletion and formatting often involve removing higher-level "logical" references to the data (e.g., file names, locations of data on disk) but leave data on the physical medium. For instance, when a hard drive containing a Microsoft FAT file system is formatted, the file allocation table (FAT) is obliterated but the data from files remain on the disk and can be recovered. In addition to deleted files, other remnants of data can be found on disks in the form of RAM contents saved to disk by the operating system and temporary files created by some applications.

For instance, Microsoft Word creates temporary files while a document is being edited, creating fragments such as the one shown in uninterpreted form (**Figure 2**).

Among other things, the data on line 4 in this fragment show where the associated document was located and what it was called (C:\Private\Secret1. doc.pgp). The ".pgp" file extension suggests that the original document was encrypted using a program called Pretty Good Privacy (PGP). This example demonstrates the valuable lesson that, even if a document was encrypted, it may be possible to recover portions of its contents in unencrypted form.

The file fragment in **Figure 2** also demonstrates that a Microsoft Word document contains data that are not visible when the file is printed or viewed using Microsoft Word (a.k.a. metadata). In addition to the original file location and name, these metadata can include date–time stamps showing when the file was created and last modified, and can even indicate which computer was used to create the file, and the last ten authors of the document. For instance, the global unique identifier (GUID) value on the last line in **Figure 2** suggests that the document was created on a computer containing a 3COM Ethernet network interface card with address "00-10-4B-DE-FC-E9." Because each network interface card is assigned a unique address, this information is very useful for identifying the source computer. Notably, newer versions of Microsoft Word do not include this address in the GUID value and knowledgeable computer users can alter this address on their computers. If the metadata in a suicide note indicate that it was created after the victim died on a computer other than the victim's, this could indicate that someone else wrote the note.

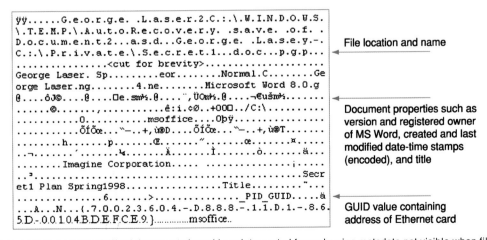

Figure 2 Fragment of a Microsoft Word document viewed in uninterpreted form showing metadata not visible when file is printed or viewed normally.

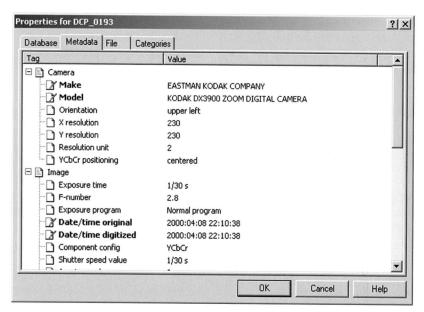

Figure 3 Metadata in photograph from a digital camera extracted using a tool called ACDSee. The metadata includes a time–date stamp created when the photograph was taken. In this instance, the date and time are inaccurate because the camera's clock was not set correctly – this photograph was actually taken in April 2003.

Evaluation of Source and Class Characteristics

Increasingly, offenders are becoming aware of the risks associated with using computers and are taking precautions to conceal their identities and destroy incriminating digital evidence. For instance, some offenders use anonymous internet services to make it more difficult for investigators to find them. Consider a harassment case in which the offender sends the victim threatening e-mail via an intermediate server. Normally the e-mail message would contain information about the computer used to send the message. Specifically, the e-mail header would contain the internet protocol (IP) address of the sender's computer (every computer on the internet is assigned an IP address to enable delivery of data). However, because the harasser sent the message via an intermediate server, the e-mail header will contain the IP address of that server, thus concealing the actual source. For example, headers in the following e-mail sent from a Yahoo! account indicate that the message was sent from an IP address in Japan (210.249.120.210):

> To: Count Rugen
> From: "Inigo Montoya" <inigo_montoya@yahoo.com>
> X-Originating-IP: 210.249.120.210
> Date: Wed, 04 Jun 2003 03:51:45-0000
> Subject: Prepare to die!

However, the sender merely connected to Yahoo! via this computer in Japan. Therefore, additional investigation would be required to determine the actual source of the message. Log files from the intermediate computer, such as those shown below, might contain the IP address of the actual sender's computer (172.16.34.14 in this example):

> **172.16.34.14**, anonymous, 6/4/03, 03:43:24, 210.249.120.210, GET, http://mailsrv.yahoo.com/login.html, 200

> **172.16.34.14**, anonymous, 6/4/03, 03:44:02, 210.249.120.210, GET, http://mailsrv.yahoo.com/inigo_montoya/inbox.html, 200

> **172.16.34.14**, anonymous, 6/4/03, 03:45:27, 210.249.120.210, GET, http://mailsrv.yahoo.com/inigo_montoya/compose. html, 200

> **172.16.34.14**, anonymous, 6/4/03, 03:51:36, 210.249.120.210, GET, http://mailsrv.yahoo.com/inigo_montoya/sent.html, 200

Similarly, it is not safe to assume that a file originated on the computer that it is found on, since it could have been created elsewhere and transferred via a network or cable. Additional investigation is required to determine the actual source of a network connection or piece of digital evidence. In the case of an IP address, the continuity of offense must be established, linking the offender to the crime. In the case of a file, class and individuating characteristics can be used to assess the source. As an example, **Figure 3** shows metadata extracted from a photograph taken with a Kodak DX3900 digital camera.

These metadata could be used to demonstrate that a photograph was likely taken using a suspect's camera, disproving a claim that he downloaded the file from the internet.

If these kinds of metadata are not available in a digital photograph, it may be possible to use other characteristics of a photograph to determine its source. For instance, Europol's Excalibur system uses image recognition technology to search a database of photographs from past investigations for similarities with a given image. If two photographs contain a common component such as a piece of fabric with a distinct design, this may indicate that they were taken in the same place, providing investigators with a lead.

Summary

As computers become more integrated in people's daily lives, investigators are encountering an increasing amount of evidence of witness, victim, and criminal activity in digital form. Even traditional crimes such as homicide and rape can involve digital evidence either directly or incidentally. Something as simple as a murder victim's personal diary on her computer can influence victimology, providing deep insight into her life and the people she interacted with, including the perpetrator and other victims of a serial homicide. In addition, digital evidence on computers and networks has helped identify and apprehend offenders in murder cases. Although some offenders take precautions to conceal, manipulate, or destroy digital evidence, sources may exist of which the offender was not aware or had no control over, particularly when networks are involved. An awareness of the kinds of data that may exist (e.g., deleted files, logs, metadata) and the inherent limitations (e.g., abstraction, mutable, evaluation of source) can help investigators make use of digital evidence.

There is a growing need for reliable methods and trained experts to process digital evidence as it is used in more criminal investigations. Efforts are being made to craft standards of practice and develop this field into a fully-fledged forensic discipline. One such endeavor is to develop a generally accepted training and certification process to help ensure that a crime scene expert who collects digital evidence, a forensic examiner who processes the recovered evidence, and an investigator who analyzes the evidence would all be applying the same principles and standards in their activities, written reports, and in court testimony. Additionally, tools for processing digital evidence are being tested to identify bugs that could introduce errors in the collection or examination stages. Training, standards development, and tool-testing initiatives must keep pace with advances in computer technology, making digital forensics an exciting and rapidly evolving field.

See Also

Children: Sexual Abuse, Overview; Sexual Abuse, Epidemiology; **Internet:** Forensic Medicine; Toxicology

Further Reading

Carrier B (2003) Defining digital forensic examination and analysis tool using abstraction layers. *International Journal of Digital Evidence* 1.

Carrier B, Spafford G (2003) Getting physical with the digital investigation process. *International Journal of Digital Evidence* 2.

Casey E (2002) Error, uncertainty and loss in digital evidence. *International Journal of Digital Evidence* 1.

Casey E (ed.) (2002) *Handbook of Computer Crime Investigation: Forensic Tools and Technologies.* London: Academic Press.

Casey E (2002) Cyberpatterns: criminal behavior on the internet. In: Turvey B (ed.) *Criminal Profiling: An Introduction to Behavioral Evidence Analysis,* 2nd edn. London: Academic Press.

Casey E (2004) *Digital Evidence and Computer Crime: Forensic Science, Computers, and the Internet,* 2nd edn. London: Academic Press.

Hollinger RC, Lanza-Kaduce L (1988) The process of criminalization: the case of computer crime law. *Criminology* 26: 101–126.

CONSENT

Contents

Medical Examination in Custody

C G M Fernie, University of Glasgow, Glasgow, UK

Introduction

Modern-day thinking in medical ethics is that consent should be valid or real. Consent may be explicit or implied, it may be verbal or written, but in the competent adult it should be informed and, certainly, be provided without coercion. Consent is not an endpoint but rather a continuing process based on the mutual respect normally found in the doctor–patient relationship. However, there are circumstances in which a doctor has to work professionally, such as those usually encountered by the forensic physicians (police surgeon), where there is no opportunity to develop this relationship in the traditional manner. Although consent in theory has been provided by the detainee, some may consider this to have been obtained under a degree of duress because of the circumstances in which that consultation takes place. Also, there are a number of situations encountered by the forensic physician, such as those within the provisions of the Road Traffic Act 1988, where, although there may be an apparent freedom of choice, a refusal to participate in the process will constitute an offense (failing sound medical reasons for so doing) if that person does not agree to the proposed examination.

Accountability

The medical profession is becoming increasingly accountable and there are a number of routes through which a forensic physician may have to respond if he/she fails to obtain adequate consent. Principally, these will be alleged medical negligence if the information imparted is not in keeping with the professional standard in place at the time in question, but it is possible that a charge of criminal assault may be faced by that doctor and, should that charge be proven, there will be an automatic referral to the General Medical Council (GMC) for consideration as to whether this constitutes serious professional misconduct. Indeed, a number of complainants are based on that doctor's national regulatory body as a "first stop" when they are dissatisfied as to the way in which a doctor has behaved.

The GMC makes it clear that successful relationships between doctors and patients depend on trust. To establish that trust one must respect patients' autonomy – their right to decide whether or not to undergo any medical intervention even where a refusal to do so would result in harm to that individual or his/her own death. Autonomy is one of the *prima facie* moral principles espoused by Gillon and is surely one of the cornerstones of modern ethical medical practice. Of course, this applies even in the custodial setting.

The GMC specifically recognizes that a doctor must take particular care in order to ensure voluntary decision-making and has identified that persons detained by the police may be particularly vulnerable in this respect. They emphasize that where such patients have a right to decline treatment, the doctor involved has a duty to do his/her best to make them aware of this option and that they are able to exercise this right.

Development of Consent

It is now almost taken for granted in medical practice that before embarking upon a consultation the doctor involved should ask that patient for his/her consent. Some may argue that the interchange between doctor and patient in the custodial setting is not necessarily a consultation in the true sense of the word but because the purposes of that meeting are often not known when it commences, the ethical issues are the ones that cannot be abrogated simply because that doctor is the agent of a third party. Also, different criteria apply in respect to capable and incapable persons and this matter is of particular relevance in the work performed by the forensic physician where over half may be under the influence of illicit substances and a third affected by alcohol.

As long ago as the beginning of the twentieth century, the great American Jurist Cardozo summed up the principle of consent as follows:

> Every human being of adult years and sound mind has a right to determine what shall be done with his own body; and a surgeon who performs an operation without his patient's consent commits an assault, for which he is liable in damages.

Despite this prescient analysis, it was only in the last five years that the GMC recognized the importance of consent being informed, which is a concept initially developed in other jurisdictions within cases such as *Canterbury* v. *Spence* ((1972) (464 F. 2d 772, 780)), where it was held that, although the information imparted by the doctor seeking consent had reached that required to meet the Bolam test it was deemed insufficient by the court.

The GMC does recognize that in an emergency where consent cannot be obtained, one may provide medical treatment to anyone who requires this, provided the treatment is limited to what is immediately necessary to save life or to avoid significant deterioration in that patient's health. This principle applies as much in the clinical forensic setting as in other areas of medical practice. This approach is underwritten by case law and in the Canadian case of *Mulloy* v. *Hopsang* ((1935) 1 WWR 714). It was made clear by this patient that a doctor should not amputate his hand under any circumstances as he wished to consult his own specialist. However, once anesthesia had been administered and an adequate examination undertaken for the hand that had previously been wrapped up, the doctor formed the view that amputation was required and went ahead. When the patient sued in battery, it was held that this management was not justified in the circumstances in that case.

Also, forensic physicians are required to respect the terms of any valid advance refusal which they know about, or that is drawn to their attention. In *Malette* v. *Shulman* ((1988) 63 OR (2d) 243 (Ontario High Court)), the young woman who had been brought into the emergency department whilst unconscious had a card indicating she was a Jehovah's Witness and that she would not consent to a blood transfusion even if that were to the danger of her life. The Court held in favor of the plaintiff, as there really should have been no doubts as to the position.

In the introduction to *Seeking Patients' Consent: The Ethical Considerations,* the GMC stipulates that a doctor is required to respect patients' autonomy, including their right to decide whether or not to undergo any medical intervention even where a refusal may result in harm to themselves or in their own death. Further, this right is protected in law and a registered medical practitioner is expected to be aware of the legal principle set by relevant case law in this area (advice can be obtained from medical defense bodies such as the Medical Defence Union, Medical Protection Society, the Medical and Dental Defence Union of Scotland, or professional associations such as the British Medical Association (BMA), or one's employing organization). Existing case law gives a guide as to what can be considered the minimum requirements of good practice in seeking informed consent from patients.

Although a doctor wishing to visualize the tonsillar area of a patient can presume implied consent should that person open his/her mouth to receive a spatula, it would be rare in the context of clinical forensic medicine that explicit consent would not be obtained through provision of a history, undertaking an examination, and producing a report for the purpose of the court. One of the leading cases in regard to implied consent is that of *O'Brian* v. *Cunard SS Co.* ((1891) 28 N E 266 (Sup. Jud. CT. Massachusetts)), where an immigrant to the USA proffered her arm for smallpox vaccination. However, a comparable type of situation for the forensic physician would be an inebriated individual holding out his/her arm for venous blood sampling under Section 5 of the Road Traffic Act 1988, where that person has been arrested for an alleged drink-driving offense. Whilst the individual's capacity must be in doubt in this situation, it is in the public interest that a sample is obtained and, indeed, with the Police Reform Act 2002 coming into force, it is recognized that where there is an unconscious drunk, in certain specified circumstances it is lawful to obtain a sample from him/her without consent at the time although permission subsequently has to be granted should he/she later recover, albeit a refusal will constitute an offense.

Normally, oral consent is equally valid to written consent (especially where witnessed), but the GMC recommends that written consent should be obtained in cases where providing clinical care is not the primary purpose of the investigation or examination and there may be significant consequences for the patient's employment, social, or personal life. This guidance is of particular relevance in the area in which the forensic physician functions.

This regulatory body reminds doctors that they should use the patient's case notes and/or a consent form in order to detail the key elements of any discussion that takes place with the patient, including the nature of information provided, specific requests by the patient, and details of the scope of the consent given. It may be that the habitual introduction that a forensic medical examiner uses and an explanation as to the use of a report for court purposes would suffice.

Analysis of Informed Consent

In regard to the concept of informed consent, there are three pertinent issues that the forensic physician should consider in deciding upon the adequacy of this:

1. Did that person have capacity in the eyes of the law? In other words, was the patient competent to give consent? The forensic physician may be asked to examine individuals whose age span ranges from newborn to elderly and there will be potential conflict of interest between parent and child or elderly people and their caretakers. Even if adequate information was imparted, did a person under the (significant) influence of alcohol or drugs understand the likely implications that would flow from this decision?
2. Was the individual concerned given appropriate information beforehand – in other words, was the consent truly informed?
3. Was the consent given voluntarily? Voluntariness is probably the most significant ethical worry that the forensic physician is likely to confront, particularly when examining an individual for fitness to be detained or fitness to be interviewed, both categories of which make up the main workload in this subspecialty.

Capacity

The first issue here is, of course, a particular problem given the number of individuals (**Figure 1**) who are affected by either drugs or alcohol in the typical workload of the forensic physician in the UK (**Table 1**).

It is worth noting in respect to alcohol that estimations of the effects of drink are notoriously unreliable under a blood alcohol concentration of 200 mg/100 ml of blood. Whether an individual is significantly impaired from a substance may be even more

Table 1   A year in the life of an urban forensic physician

Persons in custody	468
Sudden death	81
Mental health	39
Child sexual abuse	21
Examination of injuries	18
S4 Road Traffic Act 1988	14
S5 Road Traffic Act 1988	13
Serious assault	13
Rape	13
Nonaccidental injury	10
Murder	11

contentious, and there has been considerable debate as to the appropriateness of the standardized field sobriety testing used in the USA and whether such tests have been truly validated for the purpose for which they are being used in the context of the Road Traffic Act. Given the number of detainees that are under the influence of either alcohol or a substance and that the degree of intoxication may well be underestimated, it seems reasonable to question how legitimate any consent given might be. Considerable work has been undertaken on fitness of the person to be interviewed as a result of concerns such as these and also whether that individual may be suffering from a mental disorder that would affect his/her capacity.

The Codes of Practice to the Police and Criminal Evidence (*pace*) Act 1984 state that: "No person, who was unfit through drink or drugs to the extent that he is unable to appreciate the significance of questions put to him in his answers, may be questioned about an alleged offense in that condition."

The Codes of Practice clarify that "The Police Surgeon can give advice about whether or not a person is fit to be interviewed."

Under Scots Law, this issue is even more problematic in that there is not a statutory equivalent to the Police and Criminal Evidence Act 1984 and much is left to the Force Standing Orders, where, although in practice similar decisions may be taken, it is noticeable that there are considerably fewer cases where there is a requirement to determine fitness to be interviewed as opposed to that found in England and Wales.

Information Imparted

The second point is a matter that varies between individual practitioners and within the joint guidance issued by the Association of Forensic Physicians and the British Medical Association in 1996. This recommends that police surgeons should state explicitly: "Before any information is volunteered, part of their role is to collect any evidence for the prosecution."

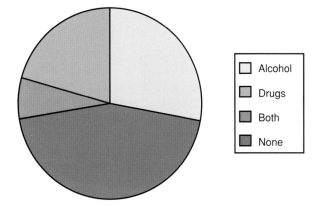

Figure 1   Typical proportions of individuals affected by drugs and/or alcohol.

Alcohol

Drugs

Both

None

The emphasis here is very much on the word "before" as the interim guidelines are prefaced by a note on the legal position in which the view is expressed that the Crown Prosecution Service (CPS) has argued that police surgeons are part of the prosecution team and are therefore obliged to disclose all information to enable the CPS to assess whether it is "material" to their case or not. In contrast, legal advice taken by the Medical Defence Union appears to contradict this belief in that their opinion suggests that police surgeons are only part of the investigating team insofar as they are required to undertake forensic tasks. The ethical dilemma here is that of the dual role where, if the forensic physician is acting as a medical adviser to the victim or suspect, the fact that he/she is supplied by the police does not make him/her their representative. The conclusion is that any information that a doctor obtains in this context is within the ordinary capacity of a medical practitioner and the usual duty of confidentiality will apply. Although this article was classified as being an interim guideline, it is uncertain what its status is until new legislation is passed or it is superseded by case law. However, as a consequence of this document, it seems reasonable to presume that any information volunteered might be used as evidence in the case and that no assurances can be given that confidentiality will be maintained. Thus, in obtaining consent to the examination and provision of a report, forensic physicians should ensure that the person has understood and agreed to this potential lack of confidentiality before any information is collected or an examination undertaken.

Probably the most important aspect to consider in relation to consent and the forensic medical examiner, at least in legal terms, is the issue of whether the consent has been suitably informed. Here, guidance must be sought from case law on the subject generally as the Association of Police Surgeons and the BMA interim guidelines appreciated that specific clarification was not yet available. For the law to accept the validity of the consent obtained, the patient must first have been supplied with adequate information in order to achieve "informed consent." The seminal case in this respect was that of Sidaway in 1985, which gave legal guidance on the doctor's duty to inform the patient on what he or she was proposing (*Sidaway* v. *Board of Governors of the Bethlem Royal and the Maudsley Hospital* ((1984) 2 WLR 778; (1985) AC 871; (1985) AC 871 at 900, [1985] 1 All ER 643 at 663, HL; (1985) AC 871 at 903, [1985] 1 All ER 643 at 665; (1985) 2 WLR at 493)). However, before examining the significance of this case it is worthwhile considering the background that led to it. It seems reasonable to take as a starting point the cases of *Hunter* v. *Hanley* (1955 SC 200, 1955 SLT

213) and *Bolam* v. *Friern Hospital Management Committee* (1957; 2 ALL ER118, [1957] 1 WLR 582), which provide the definition of medical negligence in the UK. It has already been suggested that, although a court may not hold that an action against a forensic medical examiner should be taken in negligence rather than battery, it would seem that its normal reluctance to do so might prevail in this situation.

In the Australian case of *Rogers* v. *Whitaker* ((1992) 109 ALR 625 at 633, [1993] 4 Med LR 79 at 83), concerning a case of sympathetic ophthalmia, the view was expressed that consent is relevant to actions framed in battery or trespass, not in negligence, which is simply a matter of standards. If one does accept that a case against a police surgeon would not be in battery unless the circumstances were exceptional, and an argument has already been put forward that the normal basic rules regarding a traditional medical consultation should apply, then the cases relating to this situation should be those one would usually consider in relation to consent to the examination.

There seems little contention that the position in these cases has, thankfully, moved on from *Hatcher* v. *Black* in 1954 where Lord Denning appeared to endorse a "therapeutic lie."

Thus, British courts continued with the application of the professional standard even though the concept of the "prudent patient" test was adopted in 1972 in *Canterbury* v. *Spence* in an American court. It was said here for the first time that doctors must disclose to their patients any material risk inherent in a proposed line of treatment. By 1980 *Reibl* v. *Hughes* ((1980) 114 DLR (3d) 1) found the Canadian Supreme Court also rejecting the "professional medical standard" in determining how much a doctor must disclose to a patient. Although the court accepted that a particular patient might waive the right to know, voluntarily grasping "the doctor knows best" doctrine, this is unlikely to be applicable to virtually any of the situations encountered by the forensic medical examiner.

However, in the UK there was evolution in *Chatterton* v. *Gerson* ((1981) 3 WLR 1003) where the issue of how much information the doctor should be required to give the patient was once more brought before the courts. It was alleged that, although Dr. Gerson was in no way negligent in his conduct of the surgery, he failed to give his patient sufficient information for her "informed consent." However, Mr. Justice Bristow took the view that, once a patient has been informed "in broad terms of the nature of the procedure which is intended," the consent is real and no action for battery will lie. The contentious issue here is what he meant by his phrase "in broad terms." He clarified this by stating that an action in battery would lie only if a wholly different procedure from the one agreed to was carried out or if the patient's agreement was obtained through fraud. This would very likely be true with the forensic medical examiner, although it is unlikely that a broad consent would suffice if the results of the examination might result in the person incriminating him/herself. The obvious pertinent question is whether there is a difference between therapeutic and nontherapeutic treatments? Mrs. Potts, who won £3000 damages in 1983 after an injection of Depo-Provera, appears to suggest that there is a difference, although this was certainly an emotive controversy at the time.

In Sidaway, the House of Lords did explore at length the doctor's duty to inform patients due to the need for clear legal guidance. There was, however, a three-way division, with only Lord Scarman opting for what was a radical shift at that time, giving consideration to the concept of informed consent. Lord Diplock adopted a decidedly conservative view with the status quo of the Bolam test. Lord Bridge, with whom Lord Keith concurred, and Lord Templeman were more pragmatic in their speeches, taking a middle course. Lord Bridge held that: "A judge might, in certain circumstances, come to the conclusion that the disclosure of a particular risk was so obviously necessary to an informed choice on the part of the patient that no reasonably prudent medical man could fail to make it." Lord Templeman took the view that "the court must decide whether the information afforded to the patient was sufficient to alert the patient to the possibility of serious harm of the kind in fact suffered." Although Lord Scarman also found against Mrs. Sidaway, he did deliver a dissenting judgment when he rejected current medical practice as the test of what the patient needs to be told. His powerful judgment asserted the patient's right to know. The patient's right to an autonomous decision was the factor to which Lord Scarman made the issue of advice given to the patient distinct from other aspects of medical care. The doctor should be liable "where the risk is such that in the court's view a prudent person in the patient's situation would have regarded it as significant." Despite this, Lord Scarman did still feel that the doctor should to some extent be protected by a defense of "therapeutic privilege." This would permit a doctor to withhold information if it can be shown that "a reasonable medical assessment of the patient would have indicated to the doctor that disclosure would have posed a serious threat of psychological detriment to the patient."

Thus, it can be seen from the way that case law developed and affected GMC guidance, the principles considered within Sidaway did subsequently alter the way in which doctors impart information to patients within the UK although, in any event, the Bolam approach was later modified in Bolitho when a court had to deliberate upon competing expert evidence.

Voluntariness

Finally, voluntariness is a contentious issue, and with the Human Rights Act 1998 coming into force there must be particular concern as to whether there is a breach of Article 6, the right to a fair hearing, especially with the increasing likelihood of forensic physicians being regarded as employees with the consequent erosion of independence that was once considered an integral part of this practice. Also, Article 8, the right to respect for one's private and family life, is another principle that may be breached in these circumstances where in reality there is not a true choice of medical practitioner.

Another aspect of consent that has benefited from relevant case law in Gillick and statute (*Gillick v. West Norfolk and Wisbech AHA* (1985) 3 All ER 402), at least in Scotland by way of the Age of Legal Capacity Scotland Act 1991, is that of capacity in regard to the mature minor whom the forensic physician regularly encounters as a suspect in a criminal act. Of course, it is necessary to distinguish between the ability to consent to certain medical treatments that will benefit that individual and an assessment for forensic purposes that may have consequences for their future liberty and here, should there be doubt, the court may determine that any evidence thus obtained is inadmissible.

Conclusion

In conclusion, it is no longer appropriate in the twenty-first century merely to pay lip service to the concept of consent and a failure to comply with this important principle may not only result in civil litigation against a doctor who has fallen below the necessary level by way of a failure to inform the patient adequately, but also, at least theoretically, to face criminal charges of an assault upon that individual's person. Further, with the exponential rise in GMC cases that has become apparent to all medical defense organizations, the reality is that a breach of the GMC's guidance may constitute serious professional misconduct with ramifications including erasure from the Medical Register as a consequence. Where a forensic physician comes into the category of having dual obligations, the possibility of having to account for his/her actions is a practical consideration that should not be underestimated.

See Also

Consent: Treatment Without Consent; Confidentiality and Disclosure

Further Reading

Association of Police Surgeons and British Medical Association (1996) *Interim Guidelines and Confidentiality for Police Surgeons.* London: The British Medical Association.

Gillon R (1986) *Philosophical Medical Ethics*, Ch. 10, p. 60. Chichester, UK: John Wiley.

The Guardian (1983) 23 July, p. 24.

Hatcher *v.* Black (1954) *The Times, 2 July.*

McLay WDS (1990) *Clinical Forensic Medicine,* vol. 6, p. 107. London: Pinter.

Schloendorf *v.* Society of New York Hospital (1914) 105 NE 92.

Treatment Without Consent

C G M Fernie, University of Glasgow, Glasgow, UK

Introduction

Although it is quite clear that consent should be informed and there is both case law and guidance from the General Medical Council (GMC) to support this interpretation, there may yet be circumstances when a doctor, particularly a forensic physician, is placed in a position where he/she has to contemplate treating a patient without consent.

Consideration has already been given to circumstances in which a patient may lack capacity by way of age. Both statute in Scotland and case law in England and Wales by way of the Gillick case (*Gillick* v. *West Norfolk and Wisbech AHA* [1986] AC 112) have assisted considerably in dealing with situations that previously may have caused difficulty because the individual concerned was a minor and so was not legally able to consent.

Capacity

What is more problematic is when a patient is not in a position, whether through short- or long-term incapacity, to indicate agreement to a doctor providing a proposed treatment.

Traditionally, the courts have been charitable to the medical profession in as much as they appear to take the view that medical practitioners recognize comprehending patients. This was the position until 1993 when developing case law formalized the way in which such matters should be considered.

Lord Donaldson's judgment in Re T ((An Adult) (Consent to Medical Treatment) [1993] Fam 95, [1992] 2 FLR 458) concludes with a helpful summary of how to deal with the issue of capacity. The propositions contained in the first four numbered paragraphs govern this case. Those propositions are:

1. Prima facie, every adult has the right and capacity to decide whether or not he/she will accept medical treatment, even if a refusal may risk permanent injury to his/her health or even lead to premature death. Furthermore, it matters not whether the reasons for the refusal were rational or irrational, unknown or even nonexistent. This is so, notwithstanding the very strong public interest in preserving the life and health of all citizens. However, the presumption of capacity to decide, which stems from the fact that the patient is an adult, is rebuttable.
2. An adult patient may be deprived of his/her capacity to decide by long-term mental incapacity.
3. If an adult patient did not have the capacity to decide at the time of the purported refusal and still does not have that capacity, it is the duty of the doctors to treat him/her in whatever way they consider, in the exercise of their clinical judgment, to be in his/her best interests.
4. Doctors faced with a refusal of consent have to give very careful and detailed consideration to what was the patient's capacity to decide at the time when the decision was made. It may not be a case of capacity or no capacity; it may be a case of reduced capacity. What matters is whether at that time the patient's capacity was reduced below the level needed in the case of a refusal of that importance, for refusals can vary in importance. Some may involve a risk to life or of irreparable damage to health and others may not. Those propositions are common ground. It is also common ground that a refusal can take the form of a declaration of intention never to consent in the future or never to consent in some future circumstances, to borrow the words of Lord Donaldson in Re T. That proposition has been confirmed by the judgments and speeches in Bland's case (*Airedale NHS Trust* v. *Bland* [1993] 1 FLR 1026).

Later in 1993, the court evolved a more rigorous three-stage test in assessing a patient's capacity and this was enunciated by Thorpe J in Re C ([1994] 1 All ER 819), when he took the view that the patient must be able to:

- comprehend and retain the relevant information
- believe it
- weigh it in the balance so as to arrive at a choice.

Whilst some patients may permanently lack capacity due to a mental disorder or retardation, others who are normally quite capable of making decisions about their healthcare may be temporarily deprived of it by conditions such as intoxication with drugs or alcohol, unconsciousness, confusion, pains, or, indeed, a phobia of medical treatment.

Comment has already been made that, in order to be valid, the consent provided must be voluntarily given subsequent to the doctor having imparted the relevant information to either that person or whoever has parental responsibility when the individual concerned is a minor.

Autonomy

The importance of autonomy as a concept should not be minimized. One side of the coin is an ability to consent to a proposal in someone who has the requisite capacity, while the other side is refusal of treatment.

Negligence

Although most cases involving treatment without consent will be dealt with through the tort of negligence, an alternative in this situation, albeit it is now out of fashion, would be the tort of battery, which is a type of trespass of the person.

Specific reference to this issue was made in *Chatterton* v. *Gerson* ([1981] QB 432) where it was not thought to be an appropriate way to deal with alleged negligent disclosure of information by doctors provided they had acted in good faith and in the best interests of those concerned.

As Mr Justice Bristow put it in *Chatterton* v. *Gerson*, once a patient has been informed "in broad terms of the nature of the procedure which is intended," the consent is real and no action for battery will lie.

Of course, this begs the question of what constitutes being informed "in broad terms" and this query was addressed when he held that an action in battery would lie only if a wholly different procedure from the one agreed to was carried out or, alternatively, if the patient's agreement was obtained through fraud.

The General Medical Council

In the GMC's publication *Seeking Patients' Consent: The Ethical Considerations*, it specifies that a doctor must not exceed the scope of the authority given by a patient, except in an emergency. Thus, the medical practitioner providing treatment or undertaking an investigation should give the patient a clear explanation of the scope of consent being sought.

This principle applies particularly where:

- Treatment will be provided in stages with the possibility of later adjustments.
- Different doctors (or other healthcare workers) provide particular elements of an investigation or treatment (for example, anesthesia in surgery).
- A number of different investigations or treatments are involved.
- Uncertainty about the diagnosis, or about the appropriate range of options for treatment, may only be resolved in the light of findings once an investigation or treatment is underway, or during the course of treatment, and when the patient may be unable to participate in decision-making.

In cases of this type, it is necessary for the doctor to explain how decisions would be made about whether or when to move from one stage or one form of treatment to another. It is important that there is clear agreement as to whether the patient consents to all or, alternatively, only parts of the proposed plan of investigation or treatment, and whether further consent will have to be sought at a later stage.

Further, the GMC stipulates that, if the patient is unconscious, and if the doctor decides to treat a condition that falls outside the scope of the original consent, that doctor has to consider that he/she may be challenged in the courts, or subject to a complaint to the regulatory body. Consequently, the GMC recommends that the doctor concerned should seek the views of an experienced colleague, if possible, before providing that treatment, and be prepared to justify the decision to go ahead.

An important point is that the patient should be informed what the doctor has done and why, as soon as the patient is sufficiently recovered to be able to comprehend this.

In its guidance contained within *Good Medical Practice*, the GMC makes it clear that in an emergency, a doctor "must offer anyone at risk the treatment you could reasonably be expected to provide."

Doctrine of Necessity

This approach is again backed up by case law in Re F ([1990] 2 AC 1), where Lord Brandon observed:

> In many cases, however, it will not only be lawful for doctors, on the ground of necessity, to operate on or give other medical treatment to adult patients disabled from giving their consent; it will also be their common law

duty to do so. In the case of adult patients made unconscious by an accident or otherwise, they will normally be received into the casualty department of a hospital, which thereby undertakes the care of them. It will then be the duty of the doctors at that hospital to use their best endeavours to do, by way of either an operation or other treatment, that which is in the best interests of such patients.

Having made this point, in their advice on consent, the GMC also advises that, in an emergency, where consent cannot be obtained, you may provide medical treatment to anyone who needs it, provided the treatment is limited to what is immediately necessary to save life or avoid significant deterioration in the patient's health.

It seems that here the emphasis is very much on limiting the treatment to what is required for preservation of life or to avoid a significant deterioration.

The proviso is that, if there is known to be a valid advance directive that the doctor knows about, or that is drawn to the attention of the doctor, the doctor is required to respect this.

This general proposition is supported in case law and if a patient has indicated in advance that he/she has anticipated the examination or treatment and refused that treatment, then the doctor cannot justify proceeding in that situation. This accords with the principle that the wishes of the competent adult patient should be respected.

In the Canadian case of *Malette* v. *Shulman* (1988) 63 OR (2d) 243 (Ontario High Court), a young woman was brought unconscious into the Accident and Emergency department. Despite having a card which clearly stated that she was a Jehovah's Witness and would not agree to a blood transfusion under any circumstances, even if her life were in danger, the doctor proceeded to administer blood. The court held that the doctor had committed a battery. There was no room for doubt and the patient concerned had gone to some trouble to ensure that no doctor should be in doubt of her refusal of blood in any contingency. The argument that this refusal could not be "informed" due to the significant change in her circumstances was rejected by the court. In cases of this type, it is important that necessary treatments are distinguished from those that are merely convenient for the medical staff. In general, it is fairly safe to say that treatment provided while a patient is temporarily incompetent should involve the minimum necessary for health, whereas any treatment that can reasonably be postponed until competence is regained should be deferred.

Despite this, the more recent comparable British case of Re T ((adult)(refusal of medical treatment) [1992] 4 All ER 649, (1992) 9 BMLR 46, CA)

appears to have come to a different conclusion in a not dissimilar scenario. This case involved an adult pregnant Jehovah's Witness in a road traffic accident who signed a form of refusal for a blood transfusion. Subsequently, her condition deteriorated following a cesarean section and the birth of a stillborn baby, and a court order was obtained legalizing a blood transfusion on the grounds that it was manifestly in her best interests. The Court of Appeals, surprisingly, upheld this declaration. This was a fundamental decision by an adult patient with no known mental incapacity who chose to exercise her right to consent or refuse to a proposed treatment. Why was it that the court appeared to authorize involuntary treatment? Effectively, they changed involuntary into nonvoluntary and argued that T's mental state had changed to such an extent that she could not make a valid choice between transfusion and death. The theory was that, if there was doubt as to how the patient was exercising her right of self-determination, that doubt should be resolved in favor of the preservation of life. This was, however, qualified by Lord Justice Staughton who said: "I cannot find authority that the decision of a doctor as to the existence or refusal of consent is sufficient protection, if the law subsequently decides otherwise. So the medical profession ... must bear the responsibility unless it is possible to obtain a decision from the courts."

Other jurisdictions have considered the question of going beyond the stated wishes of the patient with adverse consequences for the doctor in cases such as: (1) *Marshall* v. *Curry* ([1933] 3 DLR 260) (consent was given to an operation to cure a hernia; the doctor removed the patient's testicle; action in battery); (2) *Murray* v. *McMurchy* ([1949] 2 DLR 442) (consent was given to a cesarean operation; the doctor went on and sterilized the patient; the doctor was liable for trespass to the person); and (3) *Mulloy* v. *Hop Sang* (Supreme Court of Manitoba, Appellate Division, 1934. [1935] I WWR 714) (the doctor was told to repair the hand and not to amputate; the doctor performed an amputation, and was held liable in trespass).

Once more, the point is made that the patient should be informed as soon as possible once he/she has sufficiently recovered to understand what has taken place.

Incapacity

With the exceptions of someone fulfilling the criteria within the Adults with Incapacity (Scotland) Act 2000, no one is permitted to consent on behalf of incompetent adults, but it is clearly necessary that those persons are not denied beneficial treatment.

The incompetence may be short-term, for example from anesthesia, sedative drugs, intoxication, or transient loss of consciousness, and in this situation one should consider case law and not just the GMC guidelines previously set out.

Clearly, it is necessary to distinguish between treatments that are essential and those that are simply convenient where the usual approach is that the minimum necessary treatment to preserve well-being is given and any more definitive procedure is deferred until that patient once again achieves competence.

Until the enlightened piece of Scottish legislation alluded to came into force there was major difficulty for those within the caring profession in respect to treatment of patients who are incapaxes, that is, those who are incompetent and are not in a position to give consent to medical treatment even if that is in their own best interests.

It has already been pointed out that the doctrine of necessity provides protection to that care that is required to preserve life but no further, and the dilemma exists in such cases as those with mental disorders who are unable to consent to relatively minor conditions such as dental extractions that would obviously be beneficial but which do not fall into the category of being an emergency.

Unfortunately, the Act alluded to applies only to the Scottish jurisdiction and, thus far, has not been extended to the remainder of the UK. The purpose of this legislation is to provide ways to manage the financial and welfare affairs of people who are unable to manage them for themselves.

The Act provides various methods of intervening (i.e., taking decisions or action) on behalf of an adult. Interventions can cover property and financial affairs, or personal welfare matters, including healthcare. When deciding whether to intervene the statute stipulates that the following principles should be applied:

• The intervention must be necessary and must benefit the adult.
• The intervention must be the minimum necessary to achieve the purpose.
• Account must be taken of the adult's present and past wishes and feelings (and every possible means of communicating with the adult should be taken to find out what these are).
• The views of the adult's nearest relative and primary carer, and of any other person with powers to intervene in the adult's affairs or personal welfare, or with an interest in the adult must be taken into account, so far as it is reasonable and practicable to do so.
• Any skills he/she has must be encouraged.

Consideration should be given whether it would be possible to intervene without using the Act.

Detailed codes of practice have been incorporated into the legislation both in respect to financial management and, innovatively, a welfare power of attorney who must be registered with the Public Guardian.

However, in England and Wales the dilemma still exists in that where a mentally incapacitated individual cannot authorize his/her own treatment, no one else legally has the authority to so do.

Of course, treatment for a mental disorder falls under the Mental Health Act 1983 (there is a Scottish equivalent currently being revised) but this only allows psychiatric treatment as opposed to treatment for unrelated physical illnesses to which that individual is unwilling to agree, even if patently it is in his/her best interests.

In Re F ([1990] 2 AC 1) the House of Lords affirmed there is no inherent jurisdiction to consent to medical treatment where an adult is incompetent but it was possible for the court to issue a declaration making the carrying out of a procedure lawful.

This case, that concerned whether or not a 36-year-old woman with the mental age of a child could be sterilized, considered the salient issues with Lord Brandon's analysis (at 55C-E) as follows:

> At common law a doctor cannot lawfully operate on adult patients of sound mind, or give them any other treatment involving the application of physical force however small ("other treatment"), without their consent. If a doctor were to operate on such patients, or give them other treatment, without their consent, he would commit the actionable tort of trespass to the person. There are, however, cases where adult patients cannot give or refuse their consent to an operation or other treatment. One case is where, as a result of an accident or otherwise, an adult patient is unconscious and an operation or other treatment cannot be safely delayed until he/she recovers consciousness. Another case is where a patient, though adult, cannot by reason of mental disability understand the nature or purpose of an operation or other treatment. The common law would be seriously defective if it failed to provide a solution to the problem created by such inability to consent. In my opinion, however, the common law does not so fail. In my opinion, the solution to the problem which the common law provides is that a doctor can lawfully operate on, or give other treatment to, adult patients who are incapable, for one reason or another, of consenting to his doing so, provided that the operation or other treatment concerned is in the best interests of such patients. The operation or other treatment will be in their best interests if, but only if, it is carried out in order either to save their lives, or to ensure improvement or prevent deterioration in their physical or mental health.

Interestingly, this leading case used the Bolam test (*Bolam* v. *Friern Hospital Management Committee* [1957] 2 All ER 118, [1957] 1 WLR 582), despite criticism by all three judges at the Court of Appeals that it was insufficiently stringent to ascertain if the proposed procedure was in that patient's best interests.

Lord Justice Butler-Sloss concluded that:

In my judgment, that test [Bolam] is too wide. I, for my part, would respectfully adopt the test of a necessary operation set out in the judgment of Neill L.J., as that which the general body of medical opinion in the particular speciality would consider to be in the best interests of the patient in order to maintain the health and to secure the wellbeing of the patient. The criteria for making that medical decision are matters for the medical profession, but the final approval in the category of case including sterilization ought to be by the court.

However, the Lords did adopt the Bolam test despite the reservations expressed by the lower court, although Lord Jauncey concluded:

I should like only to reiterate the importance of not erecting such legal barriers against the provision of medical treatment for incompetents that they are deprived of treatment which competent persons could reasonably expect to receive in similar circumstances. The law must not convert incompetents into second class citizens for the purposes of health care.

He also expressed the important proviso that "convenience to those charged with his care should never be a justification for the decision to treat."

Thus, in Re F, their Lordships made it clear that it was possible lawfully to treat incapacitated adults in England and Wales but the Court of Appeals held that if an irreversible process was contemplated, as a matter of good practice it was highly desirable that a declaration that the procedure was in that patient's best interests should be sought by those caring for the woman or intending to carry out the operation.

Having said this, Lord Brandon at 56D took the view that doctors were not required to do this as "if every operation to be performed, or other treatment to be given, required the approval or sanction of the court, the whole process of medical care for such patients would grind to a halt."

Hunger Strike

Of course, there may be occasions when patients are capable of making decisions on their own but the courts are asked to consider if they might be treated against their will. These instances are typically cases where that individual has either anorexia nervosa or is on hunger strike.

In *Secretary of State for the Home Department* v. *Robb* ([Family Division] [1995] Fan 127) it was held that:

an adult of sound mind and capacity had a specific right of self-determination which entitled him to refuse nutrition and hydration; that that right was not diminished when he was a detained prisoner; that, although that right was not absolute but was to be balanced against potentially countervailing state interests in preserving life, preventing suicide and protecting innocent third parties, there was on the facts no countervailing interest to set in the balance and that, accordingly, since the prisoner was of sound mind and understood the consequences of his decision to refuse hydration and nutrition there was no duty on either the Home Secretary or the prison staff to provide him with nutrition or hydration against his will.

There was an apparently contrasting decision in *R.* v. *Collins Ex p. Brady* (LRM 355) where the view was taken that the decision of Brady to go on hunger strike was a feature or manifestation of his personality disorder and accordingly his force feeding had constituted necessary medical treatment for his mental disorder under s. 63 of the Mental Health Act 1983.

Conclusion

To summarize, it is not that patients who are unable to consent cannot be treated. Certainly, when there is an emergency the doctor who owes the patient a duty of care is ethically required to treat him/her or that practitioner may be guilty of serious professional misconduct with all the potential ramifications that accrue. Provided that the doctor goes no further than necessary to preserve life, he/she is protected by the doctrine of necessity, although case law indicates the limits to this treatment. Where the patient has long-term incapacity and his/her life is not at risk, the management has been made much more straightforward in Scotland. Unfortunately, in England and Wales the previous status quo is maintained and, whilst recent case law is of assistance in that treatment may lawfully be given, where the consequences of that intervention are irreversible the prudent doctor requires to seek advice as to whether an application needs to be made to the High Court, although that is not mandatory. What is essential is that the doctor can justify the treatment being in the patient's best interests even if concern has been expressed that the Bolam test may not be the way to do this.

See Also

Consent: Medical Examination in Custody; Confidentiality and Disclosure

Further Reading

General Medical Council (1998) *Seeking Patients' Consent: The Ethical Considerations*. London: General Medical Council.
General Medical Council (2001) *Good Medical Practice*. London: General Medical Council.

Confidentiality and Disclosure

I Wall, Ruislip, UK

Consent to Medical Treatment

Consent legitimizes otherwise illegal acts of physical contact which would form the basis of the criminal offense of assault and the civil wrong of battery. In addition, consent affirms ethical principles that seek to reflect choice, promote individual autonomy, and ensure the preservation of individual integrity.

Medical paternalism, which endorsed interventions pursuant to the profession's value judgment, has in the past been responsible for denoting consent to an issue of mere procedure rather than one of substance. The emergence of a more sophisticated society means that a respect for self-determination should now form the basis of good medical practice.

Valid Consent

The validity of any individual's act of consent for a proposed treatment depends on him/her having sufficient "capacity," possessing sufficient understanding or "knowledge," and agreeing "voluntarily," that is, not under coercion or subject to undue influence.

Capacity

There is a legal presumption that any person over the age of 18 who is not suffering from a mental incapacity is capable of giving consent for, or refusing, medical treatment unless there is evidence to the contrary.

An individual will only be regarded as having capacity to consent if sufficiently able to comprehend the nature, purpose, and effects of the proposed treatment as well as the consequences of nontreatment. Furthermore the individual must be in a position to retain the information provided, to believe the information, and to be able to balance it in order to arrive at a decision.

The concept of capacity emphasizes the decision-making process within the context of the particular decision the individual purports to make and not the decision itself. Thus, capacity must be commensurate with the gravity of the decision; the more complex the decision, the greater the capacity required to make it.

An individual's capacity to engage in therapeutic decision-making is, ultimately, a question of law and a matter to be decided by the courts.

Adults Lacking Capacity

An adult's decision-making ability may be impaired by a variety of mental and/or physical factors: enduring factors such as severe intellectual impairment, temporary factors such as acute mental illness, or the transient effects of unconsciousness, fear, or intoxication.

There are currently no provisions in England and Wales under which another party, be it next of kin or the courts, may give or withhold consent on behalf of an adult who lacks capacity.

Administering medical treatment in the absence of consent would ordinarily constitute an unlawful act, exposing the treating practitioner to formal legal censure and potentially depriving incapable individuals of the medical care they require. In these circumstances treatment may be justified under the common-law defense of necessity, and may be lawfully provided where it is in the patient's "best interests."

In the case of *F* v. *West Berkshire Health Authority* [1989] 2 All ER 545 the court, faced with an application to sterilize a seriously mentally disabled adult female, stated that, in general, treatment would be in a person's "best interests":

> if, but only if it is carried out in order either to save life or to ensure improvement or prevent deterioration in their physical or mental health.

The concept of best interests is, in this respect, capable of being broadly defined, and could be utilized to justify most types of therapeutic intervention. The court borrowed the peer-group test laid down in *Bolam* v. *Friern Hospital Management Committee* [1957] 2 All ER 118 as the appropriate standard for assessing "best interests" and what was "necessary." These principles conspire to afford the medical profession considerable influence in defining the limits of the "legal" defense of necessity.

The courts are the final arbiters on the issue of best interests and now approach the concept from a wider perspective, requiring an investigation into social, cultural, and religious dimensions, so that it no longer equates simply to best "medical" interests. The Bolam test still remains relevant in providing a basis on which the court can assess the "acceptability" of treatment advocated in individual cases.

The dictates of good medical practice now reflect this judicial holism, and an exploration of an individual patient's premorbid beliefs, values, and feelings forms an essential ingredient in the assessment of consent.

Where the proposed treatment is contentious, such as nontherapeutic sterilization, withdrawal of artificial treatment, or where there is a dispute over the issues of best interests, any decision will require the sanction of the court.

In Scotland, statutory provisions (Adults with Incapacity (Scotland) Act 2000) allow for the appointment of proxies to look after the welfare of incapacitated individuals over the age of 16, and to consent to (but not refuse) medical treatment on their behalf where appropriate.

Emergency Treatment in Adults

In Re F the court recognized the qualitative differences between elective cases involving permanent loss of capacity and emergency situations where there is a temporary loss of capacity. In the latter situation, the doctrine of necessity is strictly limited to treatment that is "reasonably required" in the best interests of the patient. Any further or additional interventions should where possible (or reasonable) be postponed pending recovery of competence, however inconvenient that may be.

Mental Illness and the Mental Health Act 1983

Individuals suffering from a psychiatric illness should not automatically be regarded as incapable of consenting to (or refusing) medical treatment.

Individuals suffering from a defined mental disorder who are the subject of formal detention may be treated without their consent within the confines of s. 63 of the Mental Health Act 1983. While the form of "treatment" permissible has been widely interpreted and extends beyond routine psychiatric treatment, any such treatment must be strictly in respect of the patient's psychiatric condition and not a related physical condition. Additional statutory provisions under the 1983 Act serve to protect the patient's interests in respect of nonconsensual treatment relating to electroconvulsive treatment and "psychosurgery."

Adults Refusing Treatment

As logic would dictate, the law also recognizes the absolute and inviolable right of an individual not to be treated against his/her will. A competent adult has the right to refuse medical treatment even where a refusal appears unreasonable, irrational, and ultimately life-threatening, and refusals that may appear unreasonable to the healthcare professional should not automatically be equated with a lack of capacity or a psychiatric illness.

Where, however, the refusal appears profoundly irrational, or where temporary clinical factors are believed to have reduced the patient's capacity, or where the patient has an insufficiency of information on the consequences of his/her refusal, the practitioner should err on the side of preserving life or preferably seek further guidance from the court concerning the validity of the refusal.

In a series of cases (Re C (Adult: Refusal of Medical Treatment) [1994] 1 All ER 819; Re B (2002) 65 BMLR 149; and *St George's Healthcare Trust v. S* [1998] 3 All ER 673) where pregnant women had refused to consent to cesarean section, the courts expressed their commitment to support the mother's decision, even where the consequences would involve both mother and fetus perishing. The court's simplistic affirmation of general ethical principles of inviolability and self-determination was somewhat undermined by a degree of judicial *legerdemain*. The refusals were overridden by employing the fluid concept of capacity, while influential policy issues remained unaddressed.

Consent to Medical Treatment in Minors

16–17 years of Age

Under section 8 of the Family Law Reform Act (FLRA) 1969, individuals aged 16 years and 17 years (subject to satisfying the general principles in relation to valid consent outlined above) are entitled to consent to medical (and dental) treatment, without reference to those exercising parental responsibility.

In circumstances involving hazardous or complex treatments, good practice dictates the involvement of parents or carers, unless the young person refuses. This consent cannot be overridden by those exercising parental control but can be overridden by the court.

The Under-16s

The capacity of children below the age of 16 to consent to medical treatment depends on whether the child has achieved a sufficient understanding and intelligence to appreciate the purpose, nature, consequences, and risks of a particular treatment (as well as failure to treat), and that he/she has the ability to appraise the medical advice. This developmental concept, which became known as "Gillick" or "Fraser" competence (*Gillick* v. *West Norfolk and Wisbech AHA* [1986] 3 AC 112) is dependent on the child's chronological age, mental age, and emotional maturity, and is a recognition of a child's increasing autonomy with advancing age.

The treating practitioner is entrusted with deciding whether a child is competent and whether the treatment proposed is in the child's best interests, and if of the opinion that the child is competent, the practitioner may proceed without the need to obtain additional parental consent.

In the interests of good practice the practitioner should, however, seek to persuade the child to inform his/her parents in respect of the proposed treatment, especially where such treatment is hazardous or likely to prove permanent.

In Scotland, the Age of Legal Capacity (Scotland) Act 1991 places the "Gillick" ruling on a statutory footing.

Refusal of Treatment (Minors)

Competent minors under the age of 18 may refuse treatment, though their wishes may be overruled by a "person" exercising "parental responsibility" (Children Act 1989), or the courts. In Re R (A minor: wardship consent to medical treatment) ([1991] 4 All ER 177), the court found that a 15-year-old ward of court suffering from mental health problems was not competent to refuse medical treatment. They expressed the view that even if the minor had been "Gillick" competent, the court (or "parent") would have had the power to overrule the decision to refuse treatment, as the power to consent and the power to refuse were qualitatively different. The former required the agreement of either party whereas an exercise of the latter power required both parties to refuse.

In Re W ([1992] 4 All ER 627) a 16-year-old who refused compulsory feeding for anorexia nervosa was deemed competent, though the court held that the FLRA 1969, which appeared to govern this case, did not address the issue of refusals (nor did the Gillick ruling, which was concerned with parental powers) and therefore did not prevent the court from exercising its considerable wardship powers to authorize treatment on the child's behalf. Where treatment is initiated against the child's wishes the court will wish to hear the minor's views (Re M (child refusal of medical treatment) (2000, 52 BMLR, 124)) and where treatment is authorized it is usually restricted to cases where the treatment is in the child's best interests and the child is at grave risk without treatment (Re L (A minor) ((1998) 51 BMLR)). The highly individual nature of theses cases usually requires an application to the court for a ruling on the "legality" of embarking on a particular course of treatment.

Children and Young Persons Lacking Capacity

Treating minors, who by virtue of their age are unable to make decisions about their medical treatment, requires the issue of consent to divest in those exercising parental responsibility. Such treatment, in any event, needs to be in the child's best interests.

Where those exercising parental responsibility refuse to consent on behalf of the child, and that refusal runs contrary to reasonable medical practice as well as the best interests (in the wider sense) of the child, it may be overruled by the courts.

Similarly, a doctor is not required to carry out treatment under parental, or the court's, wishes unless the treatment proposed is both clinically appropriate and in the child's best interests.

Knowledge and the Sufficiency of Information

The act of nonconsensual touching is sufficient to complete the common-law offenses of assault and battery. A failure to provide adequate information or to disclose any attendant risks of a proposed treatment may also vitiate consent and expose the practitioner to an allegation of battery. The courts have, however, indicated that battery is an inappropriate remedy in the context of a failure to disclose risks preferring "negligence" to be the correct action.

The duty to inform, advise, and warn of the risks of a medical procedure is one aspect of the general duty of care practitioners owe to their patients, though for the consent to be legally valid the patient needs to understand the purpose of the procedure in broad terms only (*Chatterton* v. *Gerson* [1981] (1 All ER 257)). In *Sidaway* v. *Bethlem Royal Hospital Governors and others* All ER 1985, 1, the plaintiff had suffered injury as a consequence of a risk inherent in her treatment, of which she had not been informed. She argued that the consent she had given was flawed as she had not received a full and detailed account of the procedure and had not been warned of all possible risks inherent in her treatment. The majority of the House of Lords confirmed that the test of liability in respect of a doctor's duty to warn of inherent risks in treatment was that laid down in Bolam, the quality and quantity of the information provided to a patient including risk warnings was a matter of clinical judgment. Provided a practitioner can demonstrate that he/she has acted in accordance with a practice accepted at the time as proper by a responsible body of medical opinion in relation to what information and what material risks are and are not conveyed, there is no civil liability.

As a matter of law, the court retained the right to overrule medical opinion on disclosure of particular risks where they were obviously necessary for any informed choice, and where a reasonably prudent practitioner would not fail to warn the patient.

The majority of the court concluded that English law did not recognize the doctrine of informed consent.

Informed consent has, however, found favor in other common-law jurisdictions where it is the courts that set the standards of disclosure and not the profession. Individual patients must be provided with information on all "material" or significant risks involved in their treatment.

In this respect the US courts have adopted the "reasonable patient" or "prudent patient" test rather then the "reasonable doctor" test, which is employed in the UK:

> A risk is material when a reasonable person, in what the physician knows or should know to be the patient's position, would be likely to attach significance to the risk or the cluster of risks in deciding whether or not to forgo the proposed therapy (*Rogers* v. *Whitaker* ([1992] 67 AWR 47)).

By this test, duty depends on "materiality" and that is assessed by reference to whether a reasonable person in the patient's position would be likely to attach significance to the risk. The character of the risk is therefore of great importance, thus special risks are more likely to be material as opposed to general risks, but in any event, materiality becomes a matter of law for the court to decide.

Confidentiality

Consent and confidentiality are both fundamental ethical principles of medical practice, founded on respect for individual autonomy. The notion of consent, furthermore, is a necessary starting point when considering disclosure of confidential information.

Patients have a right to expect medical information concerning them to be held in confidence. The duty to keep secret information acquired in the course of professional clinical interactions has venerable origins in the Hippocratic oath. The periodic enshrinement in international conventions (Declarations of Geneva (1947), Lisbon (1995), and Sydney (1968 and 1983)) that the duty has subsequently enjoyed is an explicit recognition of a professional undertaking prohibiting disclosure.

The duty of confidentiality, as an integral part of the diagnostic process, finds justification in "consequentialist" reasoning. Sufficient trust, it is argued, must inhabit the doctor–patient relationship in order to allow the unencumbered passage of sensitive information not only to ensure the integrity of the diagnostic process, but also to assuage patient concerns that details of embarrassing activities or criminal behavior will not be broadcast.

Legal Duty

A general duty of confidence arises by operation of the common law when a person discloses information to another in circumstances where there is a legitimate expectation that all identifiable information should not be disclosed (*Hunter* v. *Mann* ([1974] 1 QB 767)).

While the civil law provides a modicum of protection in the form of injunctive relief in respect of threatened breaches, the civil remedies available for the completed act are largely inadequate. Article 8 of the European Convention on Human Rights establishes a general requirement to protect the privacy of individuals and preserve the confidentiality of their health records, and while its provisions are enforceable through the courts, the jurisprudence awaits full exploration in the UK.

The law does not always reflect the appropriate ethical standards contained in professional codes of conduct. It is as an ethical concept that the duty of confidence purportedly finds its greatest protection under the auspices of the bodies that oversee professional conduct and standards. In the UK all practitioners must submit to the authority of the General Medical Council (GMC) and a failure to adhere to the strict rule of confidentiality may result in censure for serious professional misconduct.

Disclosure

The duty of absolute confidentiality, if it ever existed, is now much eroded. There are a number of exceptions to the ethical duty that may make the disclosure of confidential information appropriate, though should disclosure take place, it must be both lawful and ethical.

Disclosure with Consent

Where disclosure of confidential medical information does occur, general principles indicate that the "explicit" consent of the patient should be sought and only the minimum information sufficient for the purpose divulged.

An explicit request for nondisclosure should ordinarily be respected unless exceptional circumstances operate, such as where the patient's medical condition poses a threat to others or where the patient lacks competence and disclosure of relevant medical information is essential to the patient's medical interests.

Where patients have consented to healthcare, they are normally content for information to be disclosed to other members of the healthcare team who are under similar professional obligations. Where, however, the purpose is not directly concerned with the healthcare of a patient, it would be inappropriate to assume this "implicit" consent.

Disclosure in Connection with Judicial Proceedings

Disclosure must be forthcoming in both civil and criminal proceedings when ordered by a judge or certain tribunals; the doctor–patient relationship does not attract the privilege enjoyed by lawyers, allowing them to refuse to divulge certain confidences.

Where there is concern that disclosure of sensitive and irrelevant information may be ordered, or where information about third parties may be imparted, the doctor is entitled to make the appropriate representations. Ultimately, however, the court is the final arbiter on this matter, and a doctor's refusal to comply with judicial directions carries with it the prospect of being found in contempt.

The doctor has a legal obligation to cooperate with a coroner's judicial investigation of sudden or suspicious death.

Disclosures in the Public Interest

The notion of "public interest" provides a legal and ethical justification for the disclosure of confidential information under a variety of circumstances where the perceived benefits to society are seen to outweigh the doctor's individual duty of confidence.

Under common law, clinicians are permitted, but not obliged, to disclose personal information to assist the police in the investigation of serious crime in circumstances where a failure to disclose information would put the patient, or someone else, at risk of death or serious harm. The decision to disclose rests on balancing the competing public interests in the provision of a confidential service with the public interest in maintaining law and order.

A variety of public interest statutory exceptions to the nondisclosure rule exist in respect of criminal activities such as prevention of terrorism, and medical undertaking such as abortion and communicable disease reporting. In respect of the former, however, individual clinical information should not normally be forthcoming.

The positive duty imposed on doctors to provide information to the Drivers and Vehicle Licensing Authority (DULA) in the UK, where it is suspected that a patient is driving a vehicle contrary to medical advice, is based on the interests of protecting the public at large from the potential danger posed by this activity.

Where disclosures in the public interest are judged to be appropriate, they should be proportionate and limited to relevant details. Wherever possible the issue of disclosure should be discussed with the individual concerned and consent sought. Where this is not forthcoming, the individual should be told of any decision to disclose against his/her wishes.

Public interest considerations apply in respect of disclosures to statutory bodies involved in the collection of data necessary for planning and delivery of healthcare strategies and in respect of the valuable public health information passed to disease registries, though again, in general, patient consent for disclosure should be sought. In England and Wales the Health and Social Care Act 2001 now governs situations where it would be impossible or impracticable to obtain informed consent, where excluding those who refuse may detract from the essential value of the research, or where anonymized information is not sufficient.

Section 60 provides a legislative power to ensure that patient-identifiable information can be used without patient consent, subject to approval by the Patient Information Advisory Group – an independent statutory body. This statutory protection for disclosure provided without the consent is, however, only in respect of activities with a medical purpose, where the interests of public welfare outweigh issues of privacy.

Disclosure after a Patient's Death

The legal obligation to keep personal information confidential is extinguished on a patient's demise, though the ethical obligation survives.

In the event of a patient's death there is an obligation to disclose information in respect of National Confidential Enquiries, to assist the coroner in inquest proceedings, in death certification, public health surveillance, to relatives who request further information on the circumstances of death, or under The Access to Health Records Act 1990.

Audit, Teaching, and Research

Where identifiable information is to be disclosed for purposes whose aims are to benefit patient welfare such as research, epidemiology, financial audit, or administration, the express consent of the patient must be sought prior to disclosure. Patients should be provided with the appropriate information in relation to the utilization of their personal data, and given the opportunity to object to disclosure. In general, administrative and financial data should be maintained separately from clinical data and should be made anonymous.

The publication of case studies or medical photography in media within the public domain requires the explicit consent of the patient. Where such material is to be employed as a teaching resource then provided features likely to identify the patient are removed, their use is not prohibited.

While the use of confidential patient information in medical research and public health surveillance is not directly associated with the healthcare that patients receive, their purposes are undoubtedly extremely important and the benefits they endow on society are incontrovertible.

Clinicians cannot, however, assume that patients who seek healthcare are content for their information to be used in these ways; indeed a disclosure to research workers may involve a breach of confidentiality (as well as transgressing the provisions of the Data Protection Act) even where the researchers may be medical practitioners themselves.

Statutes Expressly Protecting Confidentiality

There are strict regulations preventing the disclosure of identifying information obtained within the UK National Health Service, in respect of the examination or treatment for any sexually transmitted disease (including human immunodeficiency virus (HIV) and acquired immunodeficiency syndrome (AIDS)). While these conditions are of a particularly sensitive nature, the pragmatic basis for the restrictions rests on the understanding that the absence of confidentiality may discourage patients from seeking help, thereby facilitating the spread of infection.

Strict confidentiality provisions were deliberately drafted into the Human Fertilization and Embryology Act 1990 to ensure that the confidentiality of any person receiving licensed fertility services in the UK would be fully protected.

Inspecting Medical Records

The extent to which patients can access confidential clinical information about themselves is now largely governed by statute.

The Access to Medical Reports Act 1998 allows patients to see insurance and employment reports written about them by the doctor responsible for their usual medical care. This will afford the patient the opportunity to ensure that the report does not perpetuate potentially misleading statements.

The Access to Health Records Act 1990 gives patients, as well as a number of duly authorized third parties; access to manual health records made after the Act came into force. The Data Protection Act 1998 permits access to all manual health records whenever made, subject to specified exceptions.

The principal purpose of the Data Protection Act is to safeguard fundamental privacy rights by providing a framework that governs the processing of identifying information such as patients' records, whether electronic or paper.

The legislation is complex, but in summary it contains eight Data Protection Principles which state, *inter alia*, that all data must be processed fairly and lawfully, obtained and used only for specified and lawful purposes, and must be accurate, and where necessary, kept up to date. Patients have a right to be informed about the nature of the data held on them as well as its destination, and to consent to such use where appropriate.

Subject to certain criteria, the Act provides certain exemptions to its provisions for research purposes (s. 33 Data Protection Act). This is not a blanket exemption and, in this respect, there appears to be a degree of controversy over the interpretation of the precise scope of the Act and its potential to hamper legitimate research.

Inspection may be resisted in respect of all these Acts if disclosure is judged harmful to the patient's physical or mental health, or where the information relates to a third party.

See Also

Autopsy: Medico-legal Considerations; **Consent:** Medical Examination in Custody; Treatment Without Consent

Further Reading

Gillon R (2000) *Philosophical Medical Ethics.* London: Wiley.

GMC (1998) *GMC Guidelines on Patient Consent, Seeking Patients' Consent; the Ethical Considerations.* Available online at: www.gmc-uk.org.

GMC *Confidentiality; Protecting and Providing Information* (2004). Available online at: www.gmc.org.uk.

Mason JK, McCall Smith RA, Laurie GT (2002) *Law and Medical Ethics,* 6th edn. London: Butterworths.

Mental Health Act (1983) Department of Health and Welsh Office, Codes of Practice (1999) London: Stationery Office.

Michael D (1998) *Textbook on Medical Law,* 2nd edn., chapter 6. London: Blackstone Press.

Reference Guide to Consent for Examination or Treatment. Department of Health; Chapter 1. Available online at: www.doh.gov.uk/consent. BMA and The Law Society, Assessment of mental capacity: guidance for doctors and lawyers, 1995. Available online at: www.bma.org.uk.

Royal Liverpool Children's Inquiry ('Alder Hey') (2001) Available online at: www.rlcinquiry.org.uk.

Consent, Clinical Trials   *See* **Clinical Trials:** Legal Aspects and Consent

Consent, Body Cavity Searches   *See* **Body Cavity Searches, Practical Issues and Consent**

COURT SYSTEMS

Contents

Jewish (Halacha) Law

J Levinson, John Jay College of Criminal Justice, New York, NY, USA

Introduction

Source

A summary of the rulings on victim identification in Halacha (Jewish law) can be found in the *Shulchan 'Aruch* (codex of Jewish law) *Even HaEzer*, chapter 17. The basic sources of this summary are from the Talmud. They are supplemented by extensive rabbinic responsa literature that applies Talmudic principles to specific situations.

Purpose

These laws were developed to guide rabbinic courts in resolving matters of personal status. For example, according to Jewish law a woman cannot remarry unless her husband gives her a bill of divorce or dies. Laws regarding victim identification are meant to prove the death of a husband when no remains or unidentified remains are found. Another less common application is to prove the death of a wife; the widower can divorce her and marry another woman, but it is only once his ex-wife has died that he can marry her sister. Thus, conclusive proof of death is needed in such a circumstance. Proof of death is also important in inheritance cases.

Testimony

The norm in Jewish law is that two proper witnesses present testimony before a rabbinic court of at least three judges; only then can a ruling be made. In most cases of victim identification the testimony of one person (with no conflicting interest) is sufficient. Hearsay testimony is also allowed for victim identification. This easing of restrictions is done to facilitate the remarriage of women.

No Remains Found

Jewish law does not recognize mere disappearance for a specified period of time as a basis to assume or declare death. When no remains of a person are found, death can still be proven by showing that the missing person was in a situation from which there was no escape. A modern application would be proving that a person was definitely on board a flight that crashed under circumstances that did not allow any survivors.

Remains Found – Personal Recognition

Identification can be made by personal recognition. That is to say, a person looks at a body and testifies that he or she recognizes the face. There are, however, certain requirements before such an identification can be valid.

Time

The victim must be dead for no longer than 3 days; after that time changes in the face can prevent accurate identification. There is an unresolved question of whether 3 days means an exact 72 h, or whether part of a day is considered the entire first day. There is also Talmudic discussion about whether 3 days is dependent upon climate, with more time allowed in colder temperatures. A modern application is whether refrigeration of a body extends the time limit. The general tendency is to be strict in answering these questions so that there is no doubt about the identification.

If the victim is pulled out from water, personal recognition must be made within the first hour since changes are more rapid.

Condition

The face must have three parts present: forehead, nose, and cheeks. This is similar to the modern practice of covering eyes to prevent identification, for example on television. These three parts of the face cannot be reconstructed, since the result is not necessarily accurate and is heavily dependent upon the work of the mortician. Nor can there be extensive damage (including charring and burning) of any of these parts of the face.

Pictures

It is generally accepted that there cannot be personal recognition based upon pictures – neither stills nor video. One reason is that they are only two-dimensional and lack depth. Pictures, however, are an accepted means of recording marks or characteristics on the body; this includes X-rays.

Witness

The person making the identification must be unbiased and of sound mind. The latter is particularly difficult to judge, since it can be difficult to recognize the traumatic reactions that a person undergoes when he or she views the body of a close friend or relative.

Although there is validity to personal identification, there have been errors. In the modern era rabbinic courts have shown a tendency to prefer identification by technical means whenever possible.

Remains Found – Characteristics or Marks

Introduction

Characteristics or marks can be classified into three groups: simple, medium, and absolute. A simple mark is one that is so common that it has no value for identification. For example, the presence of a beard would be a simple mark. An absolute mark is something so uncommon that it is found in fewer than 1 in 1000 persons; it can be the sole basis of an identification. (There is an unresolved debate whether one is talking about any population sample of 1000 persons, or whether this is 1000 apparently similar persons; for this reason there is a tendency to require much larger numbers.) A medium mark is exactly what the name infers – something in the middle. There is extensive literature concerning the question of whether two medium marks can constitute the equivalent of an absolute mark.

This discussion of marks relates to an incident with an open population; that is to say, the victim to be identified could theoretically be anyone in the world. There are different considerations when dealing with a closed population. In the 1990s, a helicopter crashed with five passengers aboard. This was an incident with a closed population. Thus, although the sex of a victim would normally be a simple mark, it was sufficient to identify the only female aboard.

Fingerprints

These have been recognized as an absolute mark. There is no discussion in Jewish law concerning the number of identification points required. The decisions of competent local police are accepted.

DNA

This is a relatively new and controversial subject. Assuming that experts in properly equipped laboratories do the comparisons, responsa in Jewish law accept DNA as a reliable negative (nonidentification). That is to say, "A" is not related to "B" is accepted without reservation.

Acceptance of positive identifications is much more qualified, since DNA for identification was first discovered in 1985 and widely introduced only in the 1990s. The most widely accepted opinion on positive identification is that DNA is a very important medium mark that still requires at least some more supporting evidence. This is further qualified by requiring that the sample that is to be compared with the postmortem DNA should be an antemortem sample from the victim or a DNA sample from a biological relative of the first order (parent, sibling from both parents, or child).

Scars

The scars left from a common operation are considered a medium mark at best. Scars from an accident are random and can often be considered an absolute mark.

Odontology

Dental comparisons are considered an absolute sign when, in the opinion of a qualified forensic odontologist, there is sufficient uniqueness of formations or dental work to constitute an identification. Jewish law is very specific that teeth missing in the mouth upon postmortem examination do not constitute a characteristic or mark, since they may have fallen out at any time, including upon death.

Tattoos

Unique tattoos, for example the numbers tattooed by Nazis on the arms of concentration-camp inmates, are absolute marks. The tattoos often given to hundreds, if not thousands, of sailors on a ship are of lesser importance.

Fractures

The mere presence of a fracture is of questionable importance, except to exclude an identification. Since fractures are random, and bones break differently, an X-ray of a fracture is of strong importance.

Malformations

Anomalies or significant birth defects are generally considered absolute marks.

Identification by Property

In theory it is possible to identify a body based on property; however there are significant restrictions.

First, one must be absolutely certain that the property belonged to the deceased. This is relatively simple with clothing that is worn. Property found next to a body is not automatically associated with the deceased.

There is no reason to worry that property on a body is stolen, unless there are significant reasons to suspect such.

Only property not loaned to other persons is considered as a basis of identification. There is significant responsa literature concerning clothing as a basis for identification. In the past centuries, clothing was often made for a person, and that person never gave it away. However, that is far from present reality. Today clothing is routinely given to charity or to friends when it no longer fits or is out of style. The responsa regarding clothing are, therefore, not considered relevant to modern western society.

Another modern question of property involves the identification of bodies found in vehicles after traffic accidents. The mere presence of a body in a vehicle is insufficient to determine that the deceased person was the owner. It is common to lend cars to others.

An example of property not lent to others is dentures. Other examples are dependent upon the customs of society.

Autopsy

Any acts not routinely done to a living person (e.g., autopsies) and performed upon a cadaver are a violation of the honor of the deceased and are prohibited. Notwithstanding, there are instances when autopsies are permitted: to obtain information that can save the life of another person; to enable the arrest and prosecution of a murderer; and to identify a body. Hence general autopsies are prohibited.

If, for example, an autopsy is permitted to remove a bullet, that removal must be done as directly as possible, leaving the rest of the body intact.

Autopsies to identify a body are a last resort and not a general procedure to be implemented on a routine basis.

Burial and Mourning

Burial

According to Jewish law, deceased Jews are buried on a timely basis in a Jewish cemetery. It is certainly permissible to delay burial so that the body can be accurately identified.

Burial includes all remains recovered, including blood spilt as part of death (for example, a victim's blood after a shooting or bombing). For this reason blood-stained clothing is not laundered and is buried with the deceased.

Each body is buried in its own grave. Mass graves are not allowed in Jewish law except in cases with no practical choice, such as under war conditions. This applies to the head and the majority of limbs and torso; some opinions are that it applies to all significant parts of the body. After a mass casualty incident, there are often unidentified remains such as blood, skin, and tissue fragments; these miscellaneous remains can be buried in a mass grave.

Jewish law does not recognize symbolic graves containing dirt from the scene of a disaster or pieces of an airplane. When there are no remains to be found, there is no grave.

Jews are buried in simple shrouds made of plain and undecorated white cloth. An exception is soldiers who fall in battle and are buried in their uniforms. The Israeli Rabbinate has ruled that civilians who are killed in terrorist attacks are to be buried in their clothes and not in shrouds.

There is no requirement for a coffin. When a coffin is used, it is of simple wood with no metal. An advantage of a coffin is that it gives no visual indication of how much of the body was recovered for internment. This is particularly important when only partial remains are recovered after incidents such as fire or bomb explosion.

If a body is buried in a temporary grave, the custom is not to remove it for reburial for at least 11 months.

Mourning

The customs of mourning fall upon the parents, siblings, children, and spouse of the deceased. After the death of a relative, the mourners occupy themselves with preparations for the funeral. In mass casualty situations, this includes providing information for victim identification. The week of mourning begins either at the time of the funeral or at the moment of despair that the body will be recovered.

Note

This entry is a summary of the most common decisions in Jewish law. It should absolutely not be used as a basis to make decisions in Jewish law. Some of the decisions are written in couched language, since they are dependent upon specific application.

Further Reading

Karo J ben Ephraim (1488–1575) *Shulchan Aruch (codex of Jewish law): Even Ha-'Ezer.* (Many editions are available. There is no translation into western languages.)
Levinsohn A, Levinson J (1999) *Aspects of Disaster Victim Identification in Jewish Law: Part I.* Jerusalem: Israel Police Rabbinate.
Levinson J (2001) *An Halachic Reconsideration of Victim Identification*, pp. 55–57. Jersualem, Israel: ASSIA (Shaarei Tzedek Medical Centre).

Sharii'ah Law

H A N El-Fawal, Mercy College, Dobbs Ferry, NY, USA

Introduction

The purpose of this article is to provide a Muslim perspective on the Sharii'ah (pronounced sha-ree-aah), often referred to as Islamic law. In part, it is intended to clarify some of the misconceptions popularized since the eleventh century in the West, propagated with insufficient research by the popular media, and dramatized on the big screen. The article will review the sources of Sharii'ah and the authority provided by these sources. It will also review the

organization of the Sharii'ah legal system, the crimes that are the scope of this system, and the provisions of the penal code. How Sharii'ah law impacts on the forensic sciences, or relies on it, will also be addressed. In addition, the impact of Sharii'ah on the role of government and the guarantee of human rights will be touched upon to shed light on contemporary Islamic societies. This is not a religious treatise, although it may seem so at times, since Islam does not separate church and state. It does illustrate why, for the Muslim, Sharii'ah cannot be divorced from its scriptural and spiritual sources. The reader is cautioned from concluding that Islam operates as a theocracy, since for 90% of Muslims, Ahl As-Sunnah w-al-Jama'ah, known in the west as Sunni Muslims, this is not the case. Rather, it is incumbent on all Muslims to seek knowledge and understanding in general and of their religion in particular.

Definitions

Sharii'ah literally means "the way" and according to some "the way to water … the source of all life." In point of fact, this latter definition is quite illuminating since Sharii'ah is about the preservation of life. The Muslim philosopher Ibn Khaldoon points out that the purpose of a legislative system is to preserve the well-being of the individual and of the society of which the individual is part. We, therefore, find that Sharii'ah encompasses 'Aqeedah (beliefs), 'Ebadah (ritual worship), Adaab (morals and manners), Mu'amalat (transactions and contracts), and 'Uqubat (punishments). In this regard, the purpose of Sharii'ah is to protect the individual's and society's life, family, property, religion, and intellect. For the Muslim, these are indisputable rights and practices guaranteed by revelation, the *Quran*, and by the practice carried out by the Messenger Mohammed.

Sources of Sharii'ah

There are four sources of Sharii'ah law. The first two take precedence over all others, and none is ever to be considered above or in conflict with the first. These are the *Quran*, the Islamic revelation; the *Sunnah*, referring to the sayings and practices of the Messenger Mohammed; *Ijmaa'*, the consensus of the Islamic scholars/religious authority; and *Qiyas*, referring to the drawing of analogy from sanctioned precedence as formulated through *Ijtihad*, the exertion of one's reasoning in light of the *Quran* and *Sunnah*.

The *Quran*

For the Muslim, the *Quran* is the verbatim revelation received by the Messenger Mohammed over a

23-year period beginning in 609 through 632 CE. The *Quran* was written down as it was revealed during the messenger Mohammed's lifetime. It has not been revised or edited since its revelations, as witnessed by the historical record and extant manuscripts in Arabia, Egypt, Turkey, and Uzbekistan. It is also preserved by oral recitation, since it is the essential means of performing the five daily ritualistic prayers of its 1.4 billion adherents worldwide. The *Quran* is recited *in toto* during the Muslim fasting month of Ramadan, is recited daily in mosques, and is broadcast on radio and television. It has a place in every Muslim gathering, wedding, or even business transaction. In this regard, it has been continually recited, without interruption, for over 1400 years. The language of revelation is Arabic, the language of recitation is Arabic, and the language of prayer is Arabic. Whether in China, the UK, or South America, the *Quran* remains Arabic. Commentary and interpretations exist in an individual's own language, but because, for the Muslim, this is the verbatim word of God, no translation will do it justice. The *Quran* is organized into 114 chapters (surah) of decreasing length. Each chapter has a title and numerical designation. For brevity we will be using the numerical designation of chapter and verse (ayah).

It is estimated that about 11% of the *Quran* deals with strictly legal matters such as penal law for transgressions, debts, international relationships, rights of individuals, and inheritance. Nevertheless, most Muslims would recognize the *Quran*, as a whole, as Sharii'ah since even in its historical narratives of earlier civilizations and prophets, it aims at providing a spiritual and moral guide as to consequences or rewards for a particular action and not history for history's sake. Because Sharii'ah is rooted in revelation, the Muslim perceives an unnatural dichotomy in the much-touted separation of church and state.

In order to establish, maintain, and protect society, the *Quran* emphasizes five major aspects:

1. knowledge of God, as the creator, provider, and ultimate arbitrator
2. knowledge of one's origin, purpose, and role in society
3. knowledge of the blessings bestowed upon one (in Islam this does not simply refer to material possessions, but extends to talents, responsibility, and family). All of these are considered trusts for which one is accountable
4. knowledge of one's ultimate fate. This refers to the rewards or consequences of our actions, in this life and the hereafter, for which we, as creatures of free will, are responsible

5. correcting and improving the human lot. This refers to the five purposes of Sharii'ah: preserving freedom of faith, family, property, life, and intellect.

The nature of *Quranic* legislation has been characterized as being inclusive, shammel, e.g.,

"We have neglected nothing in the Book (6:38)" and "We have sent down to you the Book as an exposition of everything, a guidance, a mercy, and glad tidings (16: 89)."

It includes an exposition of international relationships, war, contracts, debts, inheritance, divorce, and judicial punishment. A second characteristic is the establishment of generalities, 'Ummum, that allow for adaptability to time and place, e.g., "and they conduct their affairs by mutual consultation (shurah) (42: 38)." This is usually interpreted as pertaining to the governance of the Islamic society, whether as community, city, or nation. It does not lay down the system of government, but rather establishes the major principle that must be found in government. To the vast majority of Muslims, and in contradiction of popular opinion, this is a principle that lays down a foundation for an Islamic democracy, but not necessarily a western-style democracy. Another characteristic aiming to establish a just and equitable society is the *Quranic* appeal to one's humanity and emotions. For example:

O you who believe! Avoid suspicion of one another, indeed some suspicions are sins. And spy not, nor backbite one another. Would one of you like to eat the flesh of his dead brother? You would hate to do so, so do not backbite. So fear and obey God. Indeed God is the one who forgives and accepts repentance. He is the most merciful (49:12).

This is an admonishment against suspicion of others, and bearing false witness. The verse makes it repugnant to do so by the analogy of cannibalism, for false witness may lead to the injust loss of livelihood, property, or life of another.

The fourth major characteristic of the *Quranic* narration is the appeal to one's intellect and sense of justice

O you who believe! Stand firmly for God as just witnesses, and let not the enmity and hatred of others make you avoid justice. Be just! That is nearer to piety, and fear God. Indeed God is acquainted with all that you do (5:8). ... And come not near the orphan's property, except to improve it, until he/she comes of age, and give full measure and full weight with justice. We do not burden any person with more than he/she can bear. And when you give your word (in witness), say the truth even if a near relative is concerned, and fulfill the Covenant with God. This He commands you, that you may remember. This is my straight path so follow it and do not follow other paths, for they will lead you away from

His path. Thus He directs you that you may become righteous (6: 152–153).

The *Sunnah*

The term *Sunnah* refers to the sayings, *Hadith*, of the Messenger Mohammed, as well as his actions, or actions which he approved. *Seerah*, which is considered part of *Sunnah*, describes his biography. The authority of the *Sunnah* as a basis of Sharii'ah is based on several *Quranic* injunctions, e.g.:

> O you who believe! Obey God and obey the Messenger and those of you in authority. If you differ in anything among yourselves, refer it to God and His Messenger if you indeed believe in God and in the Last Day. That is better and more suitable for a final determination (4: 59) … Indeed in the Messenger of God you have a good example, for whoever desires to meet God and the Last Day, and remember God much (33: 21) … what the Messenger has commanded take it, and what he forbids, abstain from it (59: 7) … But no, by your Lord, they cannot truly believe unless they make you judge in all disputes between them, and find no resistance against your decisions and accept them in full submission (4: 65).

This role for the Messenger Mohammed is eloquently voiced by his wife, 'Aishah, one of the major narrators of *Hadith*, when she said, "He was the *Quran* walking" – in other words, the embodiment of its precepts.

Many western writers have analogized the collection of *Ahadith* (plural of *Hadith*) with that of the New Testament gospels in that they are based on the narration of the messenger's companions. However, the canon of traditions in Islam began to be collected at the end of the seventh century, when many of these companions were still alive. Furthermore, they were transmitted and written in their original language, and they did not require an assembly similar to the Council of Nicea in 325 CE to be accepted into the canon of Islamic practice.

A *Hadith* is composed of two sections, the *Assnad* (transmitters) and *Matn* (text). Five criteria must be met for a *Hadith* to be accepted in Sharii'ah and become a source of legal statute. These are given as follows:

1. continuity in the chain of transmitters (*Ittisal Assnad*) refers to a verifiable chain of narrators who heard the *Hadith* in question from the transmitter before him
2. integrity (*'Adalah*) of the transmitters refers to their being practicing Muslims and not of ill repute or dubious morality
3. soundness of the transmitter's memory, and accuracy of his writings

4. conformity of the *Hadith* in content and transmitters with other *Ahadith* dealing with the same topic
5. the absence of defects (*'Illah*) that may come to light on further examination.

The care in establishing the veracity of *Ahadith* gave rise to what is known as the science of *Hadith* biography ('illum Ar-Rijal), a virtual investigation of narrators, their conduct, and their reputation. In many respects it was more intense than the "background check" run before the appointment of government officials to office in the USA.

Even after having met these criteria, not all *Ahadith* are considered equal. There are two distinct categories of *Ahadith*:

1. The recurrent *Hadith* (*Al-Hadith Al-Mutawatir*) is definitive in its certainty with no doubt that it originated with the messenger. To establish this, four criteria must be met:
   a. The *Hadith* is narrated by at least four independent narrators.
   b. It is impossible for them to have concurred in a lie.
   c. The chain of transmitters is identical.
   d. Narration is dependent on more than memory alone.
2. The nonrecurrent *Hadith* (*Al-Hadith Al-Ahad*) applies to those that do not meet the four criteria of the recurrent *Ahadith*. The categories include:
   a. The well-known *Hadith* (*Mash-hur*) is one narrated by at least three narrators.
   b. The strong *Hadith* (*Aziz*) is one narrated by at least two narrators.
   c. The rare *Hadith* (*Gharib*) is one narrated by one narrator.

The nonrecurrent *Ahadith* may also be classified as to whether it is traceable to the messenger (Marfu'), to a companion of the messenger (Mawquf), or to a companion of a companion of the messenger (Maqtu').

For the purpose of Sharii'ah only those *Ahadith* called sahih (authentic), having met all five criteria, or hasan (good), having met the five criteria, except that only the condition of the soundness of the transmitter's memory or accuracy of his writings is satisfied. The most authentic of the *Hadith* collection is sahih (authentic) *Al-Bukhari*, completed before 870 CE when Al-Bukhari died.

Ijmaa' (Consensus), Qiyas (Analogy), and *Ijtihad* (Informed Reasoning)

Ijmaa' is the consensus of those scholars versed in Islamic studies. The concepts and ideas dealt with may not be found explicitly in the *Quran* or *Sunnah*;

however, this consensus cannot have precedence or deviate from the general directive of Sharii'ah to preserve life, family, property, religion, and intellect. Jurists can examine *Ijmaa'* to formulate and create new innovative means of dealing with crimes and social problems associated with social development. It may also deal with the place and practices of immigrant Muslims in a non-Muslim society.

Qiyas refers to analogy with similar, but not identical, situations confronting the Islamic society. Qiyas, *per se*, is nor explicitly found in the *Quran, Sunnah,* or *Ijmaa'*. It relies on *Ijtihad*, the informed reasoning of the judge, and allows for the development of new case law. For example, in the USA, much debate goes on about copyright and the internet and whether material on the internet belongs in the public domain. *Ijtihad* may reason that downloading material for personal use may not be theft, but blatant plagiarism, profiting, or freely distributing such material at the cost of the author would be. Alternatively, using the internet to access the bank account of someone would not necessitate *Ijtihad*, because this sophisticated form of theft is not explicitly mentioned in the *Quran*, or *Sunnah* does not change the nature of the crime as theft.

The informed opinion of a respected jurist may be used as a basis for new case law. This is not unlike the deliberations of the Supreme Court in the USA in attempting to reach a consensus and use legal precedence from earlier rulings. There are, however, differences. The Supreme Court does not usually reach a consensus, partially due to partisanship, but publishes a majority and a dissenting opinion. Furthermore, while it may rely on precedent, it is not bound by revealed text as Sharii'ah is.

Despite the fact, that Ijmaa' and Qiyas may rely on consensus and informed reasoning of a group of jurists or an individual jurist, respectively, there is precedence in the *Quran* and *Sunnah* for the practice of seeking the opinion of experts in a given field. In the *Quran* we find: "So ask those who know, if you know not (16: 43)." The Messenger Mohammed, appointing a governor to Yemen, asked him: "What will you do if a matter is referred to you for judgement?" The governor-to-be answered: "I will refer it to the Book of God," and then was asked: "And if it is not there?" The governor-to-be answered: "I will refer it to the Sunnah," and then was asked: "And if it is not there?" The governor-to-be answered: "Then I will make Ijtihad to arrive at a judgement." The Messenger smiled and patted him on the chest, stating: "Praise to God who has guided the messenger of His Messenger to that which pleases Him."

Since *Ijtihad* does rely on informed reasoning, it is in this that forensic sciences contribute. Forensic accounting and computing provide a new dimension to uncovering theft, fraud, and other crimes. One is reminded of the admissibility of e-mail in stock fraud on Wall Street and in divorce procedures. Forensic toxicology, anthropology, dentistry, and pathology are of evidentiary value to jurists. DNA technology has come into acceptance, although it may not necessarily supplant eyewitness accounts. Some jurists are hesitant in encouraging routine autopsy, if there are more acceptable lines of evidence. However, Matwali Sha'rawy, a renowned Muslim scholar, is of the opinion (following *Ijtihad*) that such dissections are sanctioned to prove a crime.

What has been discussed above is collectively known as Usul Al-Fiqh (Sources of Knowledge). Fiqh is the aggregate of legal proofs, and evidence that will lead to certain knowledge of Sharrii'ah ruling or at least to a reasonable assumption concerning same, as well as the manner by which such proofs are adduced and the status of the adducer. It deals with the manifest aspects of human conduct, as opposed to the inner spiritual aspects. Between 719 and 850 CE there arose several Schools of Jurisprudence (Madhaahib). Four of these, named after their scholars, predominate in the Muslim world. They are Al-Haneefiyah, Al-Maalikiah, Al-Shaafi'eyah, and Al-Hanbaliyah. Many of the other schools were absorbed by these. It is important to point out that these are not sects, but schools of legal thought. In point of fact, the overlap of opinion is greater than 75%, while divergence in opinion is not in regard to criminal law, but in the details of civil and ritualistic practice.

The Sphere of Sharii'ah Law and Islamic Society

The principle of conduct for the Muslim is permissibility of all things, unless they are explicitly prohibited or discouraged in clear-cut sources. What is forbidden is referred to as Haram, what is discouraged is Makruh (literally, detested), and what is permitted is said to be Halal. It is interesting to note that what is Haram is often referred to as Munkar, literally meaning that which is denied by civilized society, and what is Halal is referred to as Ma'rouf, literally meaning that which is acknowledged by civilized society. A *Hadith* states: "God has prescribed certain obligations for you, so do not neglect them. He has set limits, so do not transgress them. He has prohibited certain things, so do not do them; and He has kept silent concerning other thing out of mercy for you, not out of forgetfulness, so do not question them." In another *Hadith*, the Muslim is instructed: "Whoever of you sees a Munkar, let him change it with his hand (if in a position of authority), and if he cannot, with his tongue (advising, critiquing, protesting), and if he cannot, then with his heart (prayer), and that is the weakest of faith."

We should also bear in mind that unanimously, with good reasoning, Islamic jurists agree that whatever is conducive to an act that is Haram is itself Haram. For example, Islam prohibits sex outside the sanctity of marriage; it therefore prohibits men and women from wearing suggestive or revealing clothing, nudity, and pornography, which may encourage such practices. Justifying obscenity as constitutionally protected freedom of speech is contrary to Islamic practice. Similarly, Islam prohibits racial discrimination, therefore the freedom of hate speech à la Ku Klux Klan is not acceptable.

Categories of Crimes in Sharii'ah

It has been argued that a requirement of a viable legal system is to be inclusive of both fixed and variable elements in its penal postulates. Indeed, this is the case of Sharii'ah. Crimes are classified into three categories based on the punishment associated with them. These categories are:

1. Hadd (plural Haddud, which literally means limits) are the most serious. These include capital offenses where there is no plea-bargaining and no commuting of sentence by the judge. The crime and associated punishment are decreed by God alone in the *Quran*. However, there is a provision of qesas (equitable justice of retribution, reparation, or restitution).
2. Al-Ta'zeer: crimes that deal with the rights of the community (e.g., pollution, cheating).
3. Al-Mukhalafat (fines): crimes that deal with the right of the state and its ability to run the state (e.g., traffic violations, industrial compliance).

Ta'zeer Crimes

These are less serious Hadd crimes, and are often analogized with misdemeanors of common law. Because these are not explicitly mentioned in the *Quran* or *Sunnah,* there is significant judicial flexibility in sentencing. Countries like Egypt have codified many of the associated punishments, while Arabia leaves it to judicial discretion. It is recognized that societies change in time and place. Islamic judges have much more flexibility than their common-law counterparts. Since Sharii'ah places an emphasis on societal interest, punishment may be judged to be appropriate in preventing a future "greater evil" to society. The specific punishment is determined by the judge on an individual basis, with the emphasis that he/she does not exceed God's commands. Punishments may include counseling, fines, public or private censure, confiscation of property, detention, or corporal punishment. Who has not seen a judge (and occasionally police officers) reduce a charge, or a fine, or revoke a license at his/her own discretion and insight into the specific defendant, despite the legal statutes?

The definition of some Ta'zeer crimes is found in the *Quran* and/or *Sunnah*, and in addition, many countries define others through their legislative process. Some of these crimes include bribery, selling defective goods (including cheating and fraud), usury, and selling drugs or intoxicants. Sharii'ah judges are free to punish based upon local norms, customs, and informal rules. The judge determines the appropriate punishment that will likely deter others from similar crimes and rehabilitate the offender. From contemporary headlines we are not strangers to so-called "white-collar" crimes. Do they do harm to society? Do they deny people their savings and earnings beyond the normal risks of business? The fate of such perpetrators, in Sharii'ah, is not likely to be a slap on the wrist. Since this is a Ta'zeer crime, the guilty party may be freed under judicial supervision in order to make restitution to the victim(s) of the fraud and/or community services that address the wrong done to society.

Although punishment for Ta'zeer crimes is typically less stringent than for Hadd crimes, if the offender in Ta'zeer crimes is determined to be a repeat offender who poses a threat to the well-being of society and is perceived to be beyond rehabilitation, a stronger punishment, including capital punishment, may be applied. For example, a drug dealer who kills through his "product" and profits not only corrupts society, but may use violence as a means to an end, thereby accelerating the harm done to society. Such an individual, or organization, would be perceived in Sharii'ah as being in open rebellion against God and society. The *Quranic* injunction is then:

> We ordained for the Children of Israel that if anyone killed a person, not in retaliation for murder, or to spread mischief in the land, it would be as if he killed all of mankind. And if anyone saved a life, it would be as if he saved all of mankind. Indeed there came to them Our Messengers with the clear evidence, but many continued to exceed the limits. The recompense of those who wage war against God and His Messenger and do mischief in the land is that they should be killed, or crucified, or have their hands and feet cut from opposite sides, or exiled from the land. That is their disgrace

in this world, a great torment is theirs in the Hereafter. Except for those who repent before you establish power over them. Indeed God is Oft-Forgiving, Merciful (5: 32–34).

In the USA, the baseball analogy of "three strikes and you're out" is used indiscriminately for repeat offenders, many of which are minorities. Similarly, the Rockefeller mandatory drug sentencing law is used. One has to wonder at the lack of flexibility given to the American judiciary: such flexibility is an inherent characteristic of Sharii'ah, except in capital crimes.

Judges in Sharii'ah

A *Hadith* says: "Whoever God tests by letting him become a judge, should not let one party of a dispute sit near him without bringing the other party to sit near him. He should fear God in how he sits, his looking at both of them, and his judging between them. He should take care not to look down at one as if the other is in a higher station. He should be careful not to address one and not the other, and he should be careful of both of them." In another Hadith: "Judges are three, two in Hell and one in Heaven. One who knows the truth and judges by it is in Heaven. One who knows the truth and does not judge by it is in Hell. The one who does not know the truth and judges between the people in ignorance is also in Hell."

This introduction illustrates the weight of responsibility placed on being a judge in Sharii'ah, the least of which are knowledge of the law and impartiality. This is significant, since there is no jury system in Sharii'ah. It is crucial to recognize that, although judges are appointed by the government, specifically the Head of State, the judiciary is independent of the government. Qualifications of the person to be appointed a judge are that they be knowledgeable of legal injunctions in the *Quran* and *Hadith*, the opinions of the early companions of the Messenger Mohammed and later scholars of jurisprudence, what they agreed upon and differed in, be knowledgeable of the nuances in language and of qiyas. As to restricting the position of judge to a particular gender, according to the majority school of Islamic jurisprudence, Al-Haneefiyah, women are not restricted from becoming judges of civil or commercial matters. Indeed, Omar Ibn-El-Khattab, the second successor (Khalifah) to the Messenger Mohammed, appointed a woman to oversee trade in the markets of Medina. In addition, the ninth-century scholar, Al-Tabarii, was of the opinion that there are no restrictions in women becoming judges of any category. There are

three types of judge (singular Qadi; plural Qudaa) in Sharii'ah:

1. Qadi 'Aam (General Judge) who settles disputes between people, dealing with both civil and criminal cases. Only one judge can hear a given case and his decision is binding. Other judges can be referred to in consultation, but they do not deliberate or interfere. All disputing parties, or their proxies, and witnesses must be present and in attendance with the judge in court. The types of cases heard and decided by the Qadi 'Aam include:
   a. Munaza'at: disputes between people (e.g., property disputes)
   b. Huquq: rights
   c. Wilayah: guardianship of orphans and their possessions
   d. Tanfeedh Al-Wasiyah: probate and execution of wills
   e. Waliiy Amr: guardianship of those who do not have family or other qualified guardian
   f. Iqamat Al-Hadud: capital crimes
   g. Misalih An-Nass: public interest, like building projects that impact on the community and its prosperity (e.g., determining right-of-way for a railroad)
   h. Tassaffahi Shuhud: investigation and verification of witnesses eligible for deposition
   i. Taswaia fi Al-Hukm bain Al-Qawi wa Al-Da'eef: adjudication between the strong and weak.

   A Qadi 'Aam may specialize in one or more of these areas. A judge's ruling is final and can only be reversed by that judge. The exception is a ruling that is contrary to Sharii'ah according to the *Hadith*: "Anything not derived from our teaching is a reject." Reversal here is instituted by Qadi Madhaalim (see point 3 below).

2. Qadi Muhtasib (Judge of Standard Compliance) is a judge who regulates the performance of trade and commerce in the interest of the consumers. For example, he/she ensures the compliance with manufacturing, weights, and measures, so the public is not subject to fraud. This applies to the common rights and expectations of society. The Qadi Muhtasib has the right to adjudicate an offense on the spot to see that it is corrected, and does not require a court. There is no specific plaintiff, since here the judge represents the public, and is in effect the plaintiff and judge. It may take place in the marketplace, in a trading house, wherever he/she finds an infraction against the public interest. The Qadi Muhtasib may also appoint deputies to help perform the judge's task providing they have proper knowledge and

training, similar to the Qadi Muhtasib. The analogy to the Qadi Muhtasib is the inspectors of Board of Standards.

3. Qadi Madhaalim (Judge of Grievance and Injustice) is responsible for removing any injustice or grievance perpetrated by the state, including the Head of State, against any individual citizen or noncitizen. The precedence for this is exemplified by a *Hadith* where the Messenger Mohammed, speaking as Head of State, says: "If I took money from someone, here is my money, and if I whipped someone (unjustly), here is my back." It should be made clear that, contrary to popular belief and contemporary practice, the Head of State according to Sharii'ah is an employee of the society. Therefore, among the mandatory duties of the Qadi Madhaalim is removal of the Head of State or any civil servant of that state that has perpetrated an injustice against an individual or society. Qadi Madhaalim may remove cabinet members, governors, and county executives, even if the Head of State may object. This court would also look into unlawful taxes, government price-fixing, and bribery. In point of fact, Qadi Madhaalim does not need a plaintiff or for a complaint to be filed. This is a court whose sole mandate is to look into abuse of power. Is it any wonder that in contemporary society many governments shy away from Sharii'ah?

There is one last type of judge in Sharii'ah – Qadi Al-Qudaa (Judge of Judges), who is responsible for the compliance of other judges in terms of qualification and their application of Sharrii'ah. Qadi Al-Qudaa may appoint or remove judges based on their conduct and compliance with the law.

Sharii'ah and Human Rights

In the West, what we are not told is that before the Magna Carta (1215 CE), the American Constitution (1787 CE), and in the late twentieth century the Universal Declaration of Human Rights, there were the *Quran* and *Sunnah* (609–632 CE) guaranteeing human rights. Below are some examples, and by no means an exhaustive catalog.

Sharii'ah and the Sanctity of Life and Property

According to *Quranic* injunction:

O you who believe. Eat not your property among yourselves unjustly, but trade by mutual consent between you. Do not kill yourselves or each other. Surely God is Most-Merciful to you (4: 29) ... and do not kill anyone which God has forbidden, except in truth (justice). This

He has commanded, perhaps you may understand (6: 151; also see 5: 32 above).

And in Hadith: "Your lives are and properties are forbidden to one another till you meet your Lord on the Day of Resurrection."

Specifically referring to nonMuslims or those under treaty with the Muslim state: "Anyone who kills a person from among the people with whom there is covenant will not smell the fragrance of Paradise. Regarding property: It is Haram for a Muslim to take so much a stick without permission of its owner."

Sharii'ah and the Sanctity of Honor, Privacy, and Human Dignity

According to *Quranic* injunction:

O you who believe! Let not one group scoff at another group, it may be that the latter is better than the former, nor let one group of women scoff at another group of women, it may be that the latter are better than the former. Do not defame one another, nor insult one another by labels [nicknames]. How repugnant is this after belief. Whoever does not repent [desist] is an oppressor. O You who believe! Avoid suspicion of one another, indeed some suspicions are sins. And spy not, nor backbite one another. Would one of you like to eat the flesh of his dead brother. You would hate to do so, so do not backbite. So fear and obey God. Indeed God is the One Who forgives and accepts repentance. He is the Most Merciful. O Mankind! We have created you from male and female, and made you into nations and tribes that you may know one another. Indeed the most honored among you in the sight of God is the most pious. Indeed God is All-Knowing, All-Aware (49: 11–13) ... O you who believe! Do not enter houses other than your own without seeking permission and greeting those within them. That is better for you, perhaps you will remember. And if no one is there, still do not enter without permission. And if you are asked to withdraw, then do so. That is purer for you. God knows all that you do (24: 27–28).

As for *Hadith*, we have some examples. Regarding slander the Messenger Mohammed said: "Backbiting is saying something about your brother, in his absence, which he dislikes. When asked what if what is said is true? If it is true, it is backbiting. If it is untrue, you have slandered him." When reprimanding someone who uttered something critical of another in that person's absence, he said: "You have spoken something such that if it were mixed with the water of the ocean would have polluted it." Regarding spying and suspicion, he said: "He who pulls the curtain and looks into a house without permission granted to him has committed an offense," and "The ruler who sows suspicion among the people corrupts them." Regarding gossip and false witness, he said: "The most evil among God's servants are those who go about spreading gossip, dividing those who love one another, and desiring to defame those who are innocent."

Sharii'ah and the Opposition to Tyranny

According to *Quranic* injunction:

> God does not like to hear the public utterance of evil, except by someone who is oppressed. Indeed God is All-Hearing, All knowing (4: 148).

Abu-Bakr, the successor and Head of State after the Messenger Mohammed, said: "Cooperate with me when I am right, but correct me when I commit an error. Obey me when I obey God and His Messenger, but turn away from me when I deviate."

It is a given, according to Sharii'ah, that the individual will receive equal and fair justice, and that the individual will also receive the services of the state, without resorting to bribery or gifts. In the *Quran*, for example, we read: "And do not consume one another's property unjustly (stealing, robbing, deceiving), nor give bribery to those who govern (rulers and judges), that you may knowingly consume a portion of people's property sinfully (2: 188)."

The Messenger said: "God's curse is on the one who offers a bribe, and the official who accepts it." He also said: "God has cursed the one who offers the bribe, the one who receives it, and the one who arranges it." It is not likely that the "contributions" of Political Action Committees (PAC) and lobbyists would be endorsed in an Islamic state. We read reports on how bribery is business as usual in "Islamic countries." Sharii'ah denounces that as being anti Islamic.

Sharii'ah and the Freedom of Religion

One of the most frequently recited verses in the *Quran* states unequivocally:

> There is no compulsion (coercion) in religion. Indeed the right path becomes distinct from the wrong path (2: 256).

This flies in the face of the illusion of the Arab galloping with the *Quran* in one hand and sword in the other. As Bernard Lewis points out in the *Jews of Islam*, this could only be true if all Arab swordsmen were left-handed, because a Muslim would never handle the *Quran* with his left hand. In point of fact, respect for other religions, particularly People of the Book (the *Quranic* term for Jews and Christians), was long practiced in Islam. Karen Armstrong, in *Holy War*, indicates that the concepts of antisemitism (many Arabs would argue that they could not be antisemitic since they are Semites themselves) did not exist until the introduction of Anglo-French literature

in the late nineteenth and early twentieth centuries. NonMuslim populations were not obligated to serve in the Islamic army or to pay zakat, the obligatory alms required by every Muslim. They were, however, required to pay a jizyah (tax) to support the efforts of the state for protection. Furthermore, they were not obligated to Sharii'ah in their own civil laws. These populations are known as Ahl Al-Dhimmah (People of Covenant or Trust). The Messenger said: "On the Day of Resurrection I shall dispute with anyone who oppresses a person from among the People of a Covenant, or infringes on his right, or burdens him with a responsibility beyond his strength, or takes something from him against his will."

Conclusions

Sharii'ah law provides a framework that, if implemented as intended, should ensure justice in contemporary Muslim societies. It is a grave mistake to think that what is often espoused in the name of Sharii'ah is a reflection of its sources. And if the reader asks whether Sharii'ah exists today as it was designed and established over 1400 years ago? The answer is a resounding "No!" Are there parts of Sharii'ah in practice? Typically in civil law, such as marriage and inheritance. This does not preclude the fact that some countries pay lip service to practicing Sharii'ah. Much of the criticism leveled at contemporary Muslim societies as violation of human rights, repression, and oppression, as well as the characterization of Sharii'ah as being "archaic fanaticism" is a critique of governments or groups that would not exist if Sharii'ah existed. Repressing the voices of criticism against inequality, bribery, nepotism, and despotism is to have effectively abrogated Sharii'ah, even if those in authority clothe their actions as Islamic.

Sharii'ah, as outlined in its sources, is a viable legal system offering solutions for those who view justice as a divinely ordained right and that humanity is not a dichotomy of spiritual and secular, body and soul. The condition that is established, and deviated from in the past centuries, is succinctly stated:

> Indeed God commands that you should render trusts to those to whom they are due, and that when you judge between people, that you judge with justice. How excellent the teaching He has given you. Indeed God is All-Hearing, All-Seeing. O you who believe! Obey God and obey the Messenger, and those who are in authority (when they satisfy the conditions of justice). If you differ in anything among yourselves, then refer it to God (*Quran*) and the Messenger (*Sunnah*). This is if you believe in God and the Last Day. That is better and more suitable for a final determination (4: 58–59).

See Also

Court Systems: Law, China; **Judicial Punishment**

Further Reading

Al-Qaradawi Y (1989) *The Lawful and Prohibited in Islam.* Indianapolis, IN: American Trust Publications.
Armstrong K (2001) *Holy War.* New York: Anchor Books.
Asad M (1987) *This Law of Ours.* Gibraltar: Dar al-Andalus.
Azami M (1977) Isnad and its significance. In: *The Place of Hadith in Islam*, pp. 41–53. Indianapolis, IN: Muslim Student Association.
Bassiouni MC (1982) *The Islamic Criminal Justice System.* Dobbs Ferry, NY: Oceana Publications.
Bucaille M (1979) *The Bible, the Quran and Science.* Indianapolis, IN: American Trust Publications.
Doi A (1997) *Shari'ah: The Islamic Law.* London: Ta-ha.
El-Awa M (1980) *On the Political System of the Islamic State.* Indianapolis, IN: American Trust Publications.
Hassanain MM (1990) *The Criminal Law Policy in Islamic Legislation.* Riyadh: Institute of Islamic and Arabic Sciences in America.
Hofmann M (1992a) Islamic jurisprudence. In: Benerji C, Hofman M (trans.) *Islam, the Alternative*, pp. 102–109. Beltsville: Amana Publications.
Hofmann M (1992b) Human rights. In: Benerji C, Hofman M (trans.) *Islam, the Alternative*, pp. 110–115. Beltsville: Amana Publications.
Holy Quran (1999) Abd Allah, Yusuf Ali (trans.). Indianapolis, IN: American Trust Publications.
Kamali MH (1999) Law and society, the interpretation of revelation and reason in the Shariah. In: Esposito JL (ed.) *The Oxford History of Islam*, pp. 107–153. Oxford, UK: Oxford University Press.
Qutb S (1980) Islamic approach to social justice. In: Ahmad K, Azzam S (eds.) *Islam – Its Meaning and Message*, pp. 117–130. Leicester, UK: The Islamic Foundation.
Sahih Bukhari (1994) Muhsin Khan M (trans.) Saudia Arabia: Darrussalam.
Von Denffer A (1983) *'Ulum Al-Quran: An Introduction to the Sciences of the Quran'* Leicester, UK: The Islamic Foundation.

Law, China

Z Gaoling and H Youyi, Peking University, Beijing, China

An Overview of Court Systems in China

The court system of the People's Republic of China derives from the trial mechanism in the revolutionary bases and has been remodeled several times. In 1949, the following courts were set up: (1) the Supreme People's Court in the capital; (2) subcourts of the Supreme People's Court in administrative districts; (3) courts in provinces and counties; and (4) subcourts of province's courts in districts. In 1954, the administrative districts were eliminated, and the people's courts were reorganized into four levels: (1) in the capital, the Supreme People's Court; (2) in districts, intermediate people's courts; (3) in counties, grassroots-level courts; and (4) special people's courts. The current court system has been established in line with the Constitution of the People's Republic of China (1982) and the Organic Law of the People's Courts (1983).

Organization and Functions of the Courts

The current Chinese court system consists of local courts, special courts, and the Supreme Court: the Supreme Court supervises the local and special courts. Local courts are established in the administrative divisions, while special courts are set up where necessary. The Supreme Court is responsible for and reports to the national People's Congress and its Standing Committee. Local courts are responsible for the local People's Congress and its Standing Committee. Lower people's courts are supervised by the higher people's court (**Figure 1**).

Local Courts

Local courts are divided into three levels: primary, intermediate, and higher.

The primary courts sit in counties, autonomous counties, cities without administrative districts, or administrative districts of cities. They are responsible for trying minor criminal, civil, and administrative cases as courts of first instance.

Intermediate courts are set up in prefectures, cities directly under provinces, autonomous regions, and municipalities directly under the central government (henceforth referred to as municipalities). The intermediate courts try the first-instance cases under their jurisdiction, first-instance cases transferred by primary courts, cases appealing the verdict and decisions of primary courts, and first-instance cases transferred from courts at higher level according to law.

The higher courts are set up in provinces, autonomous regions, and municipalities. They try first-instance cases under their jurisdiction, first-instance cases submitted for trial by lower courts, cases of appeal against judgments made by lower courts, and protested cases submitted by prosecutors in accordance with the procedures of trial supervision.

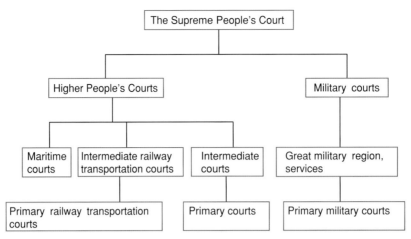

Figure 1 Organization of people's courts.

Special Courts

Special courts are set up in special departments for particular cases wherever necessary. Currently, China has special courts handling military, maritime, and railway cases. The military courts deal with violation of military duties and criminal cases involving servicemen in the Chinese army. The maritime courts handle cases related to maritime affairs. Railway transportation courts deal with criminal cases that occur along rail lines and aboard trains, and cases of economic dispute related to railway transportation.

The Supreme People's Court

The Supreme People's Court is the highest judicial body in China. Its main responsibilities include: (1) dealing with cases that have a significant impact on the judicial system of the whole nation; (2) cases of appeal against the judgments of higher courts and special courts; (3) cases of protests filed by the Supreme People's Procuratorate in accordance with legal procedures; (4) supervising the administration of justice by local people's courts and special courts at all levels; and (5) giving a judicial interpretation of questions concerning special applications of law in judicial proceedings.

The Major Principles and Systems of the Courts

The Major Court Principles

According to the Constitution and related laws, the organization and functions of the courts in China are governed by the following major principles:

- The courts exclusively exercise the judicial power of the state.

- The courts exercise judicial power independently in accordance with the law, taking facts as the basis and the law as the criterion.
- All citizens are considered equal before the law.

The Major Court Systems

The main systems relating to organization and functions of the courts in China are as follows.

System of open trials The courts try all cases publicly, except those involving state secrets, individual privacy, or minors.

Defense system The accused is entitled to the right to defend him/herself. A defendant may also be represented by a lawyer or by a close relative or guardian.

System of second instance as final In trying cases, the courts apply the system whereby the second instance is final, except those first-instance cases handled by the Supreme Court and cases heard by primary courts in accordance with civil procedures.

Withdrawal system Criminal procedure law states that, in any of the following situations, a member of the judicial, prosecutorial, or investigative personnel shall voluntarily withdraw, and the parties to the case and their legal representatives shall have the right to demand his/her withdrawal:

- if he/she is a party or a near relative of a party to the case
- if he/she or a near relative has an interest in the case
- if he/she has served as a witness, expert witness, defender, or agent *ad litem* in the current case
- if he/she has any other relations with a party to the case that could affect the impartial handling of the case.

The other two procedure laws on civil and administrative cases have similar provisions.

System of trial supervision This is a special system for the court to reexamine judgments and rulings that have already taken effect and have been found to contain errors in establishing the facts or application of laws. It is a remedy to the system of second instance as final.

Criminal Trial

The Procedure of Trials of First Instance

Trials of first-instance criminal cases are a public prosecution initiated by the people's procuratorates or a private prosecution initiated by the complainant. A criminal case is under the jurisdiction of the people's court in the place where the crime is committed. If it is more appropriate for the case to be tried by the People's Court in the place where the defendant resides, then that court may have jurisdiction over the case.

Procedures of first instance can be classified into ordinary and summary procedures.

Ordinary procedure of first instance Criminal cases of first instance are generally tried in a people's court by a collegiate panel. Trials of cases of first instance in the Primary and Intermediate People's Courts are conducted by a collegiate panel composed of three judges or of three judges and people's assessors. Trials of first-instance cases in the Higher People's Courts or the Supreme People's Court are conducted by a collegiate panel composed of three to seven judges or judges and people's assessors.

There are five stages in the ordinary procedure of first instance: (1) open court session; (2) courtroom investigation; (3) court debate; (4) the defendant's final statement; (5) deliberation, and pronouncement.

When evaluating articles, bodies, and corpses in reference to crimes, professional experts should be appointed by the courts. Independent judicial evaluation bodies should be established in the Supreme Court, Higher People's Courts, and possibly some Intermediate People's Courts. Courts may appoint these judicial evaluation bodies. In a particular situation and following the principle of respecting litigants' choice, combined with the appointment of people's courts, the litigants from both parties may request other individuals to evaluate. If parties cannot reach an agreement after negotiation, an expert person will be selected from the list of judicial evaluation bodies and who meet evaluation requirements. For people's courts without judicial evaluation bodies, full-time judicial evaluation personnel may be provided by judicial executive management bodies. For contested medical evaluations of personal injuries that need reevaluation, or medical evaluation on mental disease, hospitals appointed by the people's government in the provinces should carry out the evaluation. Judicial evaluation of mental diseases committees is set up in provinces, autonomous regions, municipalities, districts in the four municipalities, and cities with administrative districts. The committee comprises related officials in charge and experts in people's courts, people's procuratorates, public security, judicial, and health organizations. They are responsible for checking evaluators, organizing evaluation groups, and supporting the evaluation. In criminal cases, the task of judicial evaluation of mental diseases is to verify:

- whether the defendant suffers from a mental disease
- which kind of mental diseases the defendant is suffering from
- the relationship between mental disease and harmful behavior
- whether the defendant is criminally responsible
- the defendant's mental state during the lawsuit
- whether the defendant is fit to stand trial
- the defendant's mental state while serving a sentence
- suggestions on legal measures that should be taken.

After evaluating, the evaluator should write a conclusion, sign his/her name, and affix a special evaluation seal.

Summary procedures of first instance Summary procedure is only applied in primary courts. Summary procedures are not limited by rules in ordinary procedure. The people's court (**Figure 2**) may apply summary procedure to cases that are only to be handled upon complaint, and minor criminal cases, that are tried by a single judge.

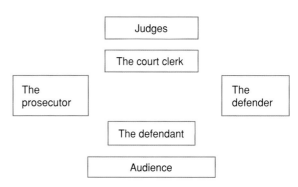

Figure 2 A plan of a courtroom.

Procedure of Second Instance

Criminal procedure of second instance is followed after an appeal by the defendant, the private prosecutor, or legal representatives, or a protest of the people's procuratorate at all levels. In the trial of a case appealed by a defendants legal representative, or defendants near relative, the people's court of second instance may not increase the defendant's sentence. A people's court of second instance will conduct a complete review of the facts determined and the application of law in the judgment of first instance and will not be limited by the scope of appeal. A people's court of second instance forms a collegiate panel and opens a court session to hear an appeal case. However, if, after consulting the case file, interrogating the defendant, and heeding the opinions of the other parties, defendants, and agents *ad litem*, the collegiate panel thinks the criminal facts are clear, it may rule that no court session is to be opened. A people's court of second instance opens a court session to hear a case appealed by a people's procuratorate.

Procedure for Review of Death Sentences

Death sentences are subject to approval by the Supreme People's Court. When necessary, the Supreme Court may delegate to the Higher Courts the power of approving death sentences in crimes that seriously undermine public security and social order. A case where an Intermediate People's Court has imposed a death sentence with a two-year suspension of execution is subject to approval by a Higher People's Court. Reviews by the Supreme People's Court of cases involving death sentences, and reviews by a Higher People's Court of cases involving death sentences with a suspension of execution are conducted by collegiate panels, each composed of three judges.

Procedure for Trial Supervision

A party or the defendant's legal representative or near relative may present a petition to a people's court or a people's procuratorate in regard to a legally effective judgment; however, execution of the judgment is not suspended. If the president of a people's court at any level finds a definite error in a legal judgment with regard to the facts or application of law, he/she refers the matter to the judicial committee to handle and determine a retrial. If the Supreme People's Court or a higher-level people's court finds a definite error in a legal judgment of a lower-level people's court, it has the power to bring the case up for trial itself or may direct a lower-level people's court to conduct a retrial. If the Supreme People's Procuratorate finds a definite error in a legal judgment of a people's court at any level, or if a higher-level people's procuratorate finds a definite error in a legal judgment of a lower-level people's court, it has the power to present a protest to the people's court at the same level against the judgment in accordance with the procedure for trial supervision.

Civil Trial

In general, trials of civil cases of first instance are under the jurisdiction of the people's court in the place where the defendant has his/her domicile or in the place of his/her habitual residence.

Ordinary Procedure of First Instance

Civil cases of first instance are tried in a people's court by a collegiate panel consisting of both judges and assessors or of judges alone. The collegiate panel must have an odd number of members.

Trial procedures in courts are as follows: open court session; courtroom investigation; court debate; judgment; or conciliation.

The organization and entrusting of judicial evaluation are the same as in criminal cases. In civil cases, the task of judicial evaluation of mental disease is to verify:

- whether the person suffers from a mental disease
- which kind of mental disease the person is suffering from
- the influence of mental disease on the person's ability to express him/herself
- whether the defendant has civil capacity
- the defendant's mental state during mediation and trial
- whether the defendant is fit to stand trial.

As with the evaluation of cases involving medical malpractice, medical societies of cities with administrative districts, prefectures or cities directly under provinces, autonomous regions, and municipalities are responsible for organizing the first judicial evaluation of cases involving medical malpractice. If necessary, China's Medical Society may organize an evaluation of difficult, complicated, and nationally influential and controversial medical malpractice cases. Medical societies responsible for organizing the evaluation of medical malpractice should set up a database of experts. Experts from related professions who participate in the evaluation of medical malpractice are chosen at random from the database by hospitals and patients under the direction of medical societies. An expert evaluation group operates under the collegiate system. The number in the evaluation group should be odd. Where cause of death and degree of disability are concerned, legal medical experts should be chosen at random from the database to participate in the evaluation.

Summary procedure, second instance, and procedure for trial supervision are generally the same as in criminal cases.

Special Procedure

When a people's court handles cases concerning the credentials of voters, the proclamation of a person as missing or dead, the determination of a citizen as incompetent or with limited capacity for civil conduct, and the determination of a property as ownerless, the provisions of special procedure apply. With respect to a case tried in accordance with the procedure, the judgment of first instance is final. A collegiate panel of judges is formed for the trial of any case involving the credentials of voters or any important, difficult, or complicated case; other cases are tried by a single judge.

Procedure for Hastening Debt Recovery

When a creditor requests payment of money or negotiable securities from a debtor, if certain requirements are met, he/she may apply to the basic people's court that has jurisdiction for a payment warrant.

Procedure for Public Invitation to Assert Claims

Any holder of a bill which may be endorsed to someone else according to regulations may, if the bill is stolen, lost, or missing, apply for public invitation to assert claims to the basic people's court in the place where the bill is to be paid.

Company Bankruptcy Repayment Procedure

If an enterprise as a legal entity has serious losses and is unable to repay its debts, the creditors may apply to a people's court to declare bankruptcy, and the debtor may also file at a people's court to declare bankruptcy.

Procedure of Execution

Legally effective judgments in civil cases, as well as judgments relating to property in criminal cases, are carried out by the people's court that tried the case in the first instance. Other legal documents, that are to be executed by a people's court as prescribed by law, are carried out by the people's court in the place where the person subject to execution has his/her domicile or where the property subject to execution is located (**Figure 3**).

Administrative Trial

If citizens, lawyers, or an organization consider that their lawful rights and interests have been infringed upon by a specific act of an administrative organ or its staff, they have the right to bring a suit before a people's court. Administrative divisions of

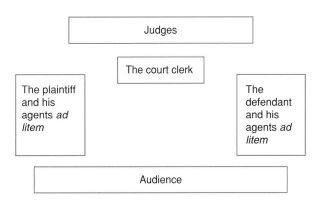

Figure 3   A plan of a civil courtroom.

the people's courts handle administrative cases. Special people's courts do not have administrative divisions to handle such cases.

When people's courts handle administrative cases, they may apply the Administrative Procedure Law (1989) and the interpretations of the Supreme People's Court; if there are no specific regulations, they may apply the regulations of the Civil Procedure Law (1991).

Range of Cases Accepted

People's courts only check whether the actual administrative act is legal and do not check the legality and reasonableness of the abstract administrative act. The people's courts do not accept suits in any of the following matters:

- acts of the state in areas such as national defense and foreign affairs
- administrative rules and regulations or decisions and orders with general binding force formulated and announced by administrative bodies
- decisions of an administrative organ on awards or punishments for its personnel or on the appointment or relief of duties of its personnel
- specific administrative acts that, as provided by law, are finally decided by an administrative body.

Evidence Providing Responsibility

In administrative procedure, the defendant has the burden of proof for the specific administrative act he/she has undertaken and provides the evidence and regulatory documents in accordance with which the act has been undertaken. In the course of legal proceedings, the defendant does not by him/herself collect evidence from the plaintiff and witnesses.

Mediation

In handling administrative cases, a people's court does not apply conciliation, as the people's court only affirms whether an actual administrative act is legal. But if citizens, lawyers, or organizations suffer damage because of an infringement upon their lawful rights and interests by a specific administrative act of an administrative body or the personnel of an administrative body, they have the right to claim compensation.

Making Judgments

After hearing a case, a people's court makes a judgment according to the varying conditions.

Qualifications of Judges, Public Procurators, and Lawyers

Judges

Judges must have the following qualifications:

- be a citizen of the People's Republic of China
- be at least 23 years of age
- support the Constitution of the People's Republic of China
- be of good political, professional, and moral standing
- be in good health
- be a graduate of law from an institution of higher learning
- alternatively, be a nonlaw graduate from an institution of higher learning with indepth knowledge of law, and two years of work experience
- have a Master's or PhD degree in law and one year's work experience
- have a Master's or PhD degree in another major, but with indepth knowledge of law, and one year's work experience.

With a degree, candidates who aim to be judges in higher people's courts and the Supreme People's Court need three years' work experience; those with a postgraduate qualification must have two years' work experience.

Judges must sit national judicial examinations held in a unified way across the nation to gain their judicial credentials. Those who have a criminal record or who have been dismissed from public office are not eligible to become a judge.

Procurators

The qualifications of procurators are generally the same as those of judges.

Lawyers

An individual must pass the national judicial examination if he/she wants to be a lawyer. A graduate of law from an institution of higher learning or a graduate of other subjects from an institution of higher learning with indepth knowledge of law must also pass the judicial qualification examination.

Lawyers wishing to set up in practice must also have a lawyer's business license. According to the Law on Lawyers and Legal Representation, a lawyer's business license can be gained with the following qualifications: having a lawyer's credentials; having worked as a trainee in a law office for a full year; and demonstrating good behavior.

A lawyer's business license will not be granted in the following circumstances:

- if the candidate is incapable of civil action or restricted from performing civil conduct
- if the candidate has a criminal record – however, those who have committed a negligence crime are an exception
- if the candidate has been discharged from public employment or has had a lawyer's business license revoked.

Court Reform

The developing court system in China has had many problems and has been unable to keep abreast of legal changes in other countries. In view of these problems, the Supreme Court is exploring judicial reform. Court reform will be carried out in the following four ways: (1) extending judicial democracy; (2) strengthening the judge's independence; (3) improving judicial prestige; and (4) improving the quality of judges.

Extending Judicial Democracy

The Supreme Court hopes that a perfect people's assessors system may make China's judicial system more democratic. In order to perfect the people's assessors system, the Supreme Court has drafted *Decisions Concerning Perfecting the People's Assessors System (Draft)* and submitted it to the Standing Committee of the National People's Congress for review. It has made specific demands as to the conditions for being an assessor, the choosing procedure, the range of trials attended, and an assessor's rights and obligations. The Supreme Court hopes that the people's assessors system will be well implemented to prevent judges from acting arbitrarily.

Strengthening the Judge's Independence

China's management system for judges is a typical administrative system. Court presidents and divisional chief judges decide on judges' promotions. The judicial committee has a right to override a judge's opinion on a certain case. The Supreme Court expects to strengthen the trial function of a collegiate panel and a judge's independence, by reforming the trial procedure and emphasizing an adversarial system. It also hopes that introducing court presidents and chief judges of divisions to be presiding judges may make the collegiate panel more independent. At the same time, the Supreme Court hopes to standardize the judicial committee's function. As it is the highest judging organization in a court, the judicial committee is expected to discuss serious, difficult, and complex cases submitted by the collegiate panel to the court president and not to interfere with the collegiate panel when it handles specific cases.

Improving Judicial Prestige

The prestige of China's courts has been threatened in two ways: first, that cases cannot be handled for a long time, and second, that judgments are difficult to implement. For the first problem, the Supreme Court separates simple cases from complicated cases and applies the summary procedure to simple cases. The Supreme People's Court, the Supreme People's Procuratorate, and the Ministry of Justice have issued *Suggestions Concerning Applying the Summary Procedure to Public Prosecuting Cases* (2003) and *Regulations Concerning Applying the Summary Procedure to Civil Cases* (2003) in order to improve the efficiency of judging civil cases and lighten the burden for litigants. As for the second problem, China requires that governments at all levels support and assist courts at different levels. The Supreme Court has submitted Article 313 in Criminal Law (1997) on the crime of refusing to execute judgments to the National People's Congress for practicable interpretation. It hopes that the penalty for a criminal offense will guarantee that the execution is carried out. The Supreme Court coordinates with different ministries and commissions in order to guarantee that departments at different levels cooperate fully when executing judgments. At the same time, the Supreme Court has provided courts at different levels with many personnel and equipment in order to guarantee the efficiency of execution.

Improving the Quality of Judges

It was only in 2001 that the Judges' Law (2001) stipulated that if a person wants to be a judge, he/she must have a qualifying certificate. At present, some judges are still not formally educated in law. Overall, the standard of judges is not very high. In addition, for a long time, the function of a clerk and a judge has been confusing and not clear-cut. National judges' colleges have now strengthened judges' training. The Supreme Court has taken many measures towards improving the quality of judges by making a public appraisal and choosing "model judges" and dismissing some judges who have broken the law. For the confusing function of a clerk and a judge, the Supreme Court, the Ministry of Organization, and the Ministry of Personnel have issued *Managing Ways of Clerks in People's Courts* (2003) and established separate management for clerks.

See Also

Court Systems: Sharii'ah Law; Law, United Kingdom; Law, United States of America

Further Reading

Liu J, Zhang L, Messner SF (2001) *Crime and Social Control in a Changing China*. West Port, CT: Greenwood Press.

National People's Congress (1982) *Constitution of the People's Republic of China*. Beijing, China: China Legal Publishing House.

National People's Congress (1989) *Administrative Procedure Law of the People's Republic of China*. Beijing, China: Law Press.

National People's Congress (1991) *Civil Procedure Law of the People's Republic of China*. Beijing, China: China Legal Publishing House.

National People's Congress (1996) *Criminal Procedure Law of the People's Republic of China*. Beijing, China: China Legal Publishing House.

Standing Committee of the National People's Congress (1983) *Organic Law of the People's Courts of the People's Republic of China*. Beijing, China: Law Press.

Standing Committee of the National People's Congress (1983) *Organic Law of the People's Procuratorates of the People's Republic of China*. Beijing, China: Law Press.

Standing Committee of the National People's Congress (1996) *Lawyer Law of the People's Republic of China*. Beijing, China: Law Press.

Standing Committee of the National People's Congress (2001) *Judges' Law of the People's Republic of China*. Beijing, China: China Legal Publishing House.

Standing Committee of the National People's Congress (2001) *Public Procurators' Law of the People's Republic of China*. Beijing, China: China Legal Publishing House.

Zhou J (1998) The people's courts of the People's Republic of China. *Crime and Justice International*: 19–25.

Law, Japan

T Sawaguchi, Tokyo Women's Medical University, Tokyo, Japan

The Legal Systems and Courts of Law in Japan

Japan is a unitary state that has a unitary legal system.

In Japan, a system of law in the early modern age evolved from continental origins, particularly from the German law: Anglo-American concepts were introduced in 1948 after World War II. At the end of this article, detailed information on the historical background of the law and judicial system in Japan is summarized.

The judiciary system is divided into criminal and civil sections in Japan. The interrelationship among the criminal, civil and family courts in Japan is shown in **Figures 1–3**.

The Japanese court adopts an inquisitorial system with no jury. The opinions of experts are neutral.

Types of Court in Japan

The Summary Court

There are 437 summary courts spread throughout Japan. Civil cases and civil claims for amounts not exceeding 900 000 yen come under the jurisdiction of these courts. Minor offenses, such as those involving theft or embezzlement, also fall under the jurisdiction of the summary courts.

The penalties handed out by these courts are usually fines or light punishment. Imprisonment not exceeding 3 years is rarely handed out by the summary courts. Cases that are considered to be outside the jurisdiction of the summary courts must be transferred to the district courts.

Several proceedings for summary disposition of civil and criminal cases are possible in the summary courts. The summary courts also offer conciliation proceedings for citizens concerned with the civil law. For these proceedings the judge and more than two conciliation commissioners help to reach an agreement and hear the arguments of both sides. The results of conciliation are recognized to have the same effect as a final binding judgment.

All cases in a summary court are handled by a single summary court judge.

The Family Court

The family courts and their branch offices are located at the same sites as the district courts and their branches. Local offices of the family courts share facilities with the summary courts. The family court system is composed of about 200 judges, 150 assistant judges, and 1500 family court probation officers.

Family disputes as well as all related domestic affairs (e.g., divorce and cases of juvenile delinquency involving youths under 20 years of age) are handled at the family court. All criminal cases of juveniles must first be sent to a family court. Juvenile cases are handled by a single judge who utilizes reports prepared by the family court probation officers and medical officers whose specialty is psychiatry.

The District Court

There are 50 district courts and about 200 branches in Japan. About 900 judges and 500 assistant judges serve at the district courts, which generally have original jurisdiction. However, in civil cases, they also have appellate jurisdiction against judgments of the summary courts.

In a district court, cases are handled either by a single judge or by a collegiate body of three judges. The collegiate court is required in appellate cases.

The High Court

The high courts are located in eight major cities in Japan and their six branch offices are distributed throughout Japan. Almost 300 high court judges, including eight presidents, serve on the high courts. The presidents of high courts are appointed by the cabinet.

A high court has jurisdiction over appeals against judgments by the district and family courts. In criminal cases originating in the summary courts, appeals come directly to the high court. A civil case that originates in a summary court must be appealed first to a district court, then to a high court.

Cases in a high court are usually heard by three judges.

The Supreme Court

The Supreme Court is the highest court in Japan. It is vested with rule-making power and is the highest authority of judicial administration. The chief justice and 14 justices serve on the Supreme Court. The chief justice is appointed by the Emperor as designated by the cabinet. To assist the justices of the Supreme Court, judicial research officials are selected from the judges who serve on the inferior courts.

The Supreme Court exercises appellate jurisdiction from a high court and may overrule a decision by a district or family court. Criminal cases handled by a summary court are also judged in the Supreme Court.

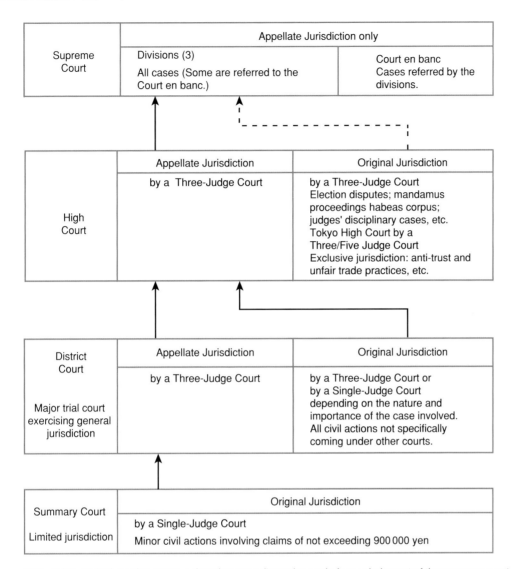

Supreme Court	Appellate Jurisdiction only	
	Divisions (3) All cases (Some are referred to the Court en banc.)	Court en banc Cases referred by the divisions.

High Court	Appellate Jurisdiction	Original Jurisdiction
	by a Three-Judge Court	by a Three-Judge Court Election disputes; mandamus proceedings habeas corpus; judges' disciplinary cases, etc. Tokyo High Court by a Three/Five Judge Court Exclusive jurisdiction: anti-trust and unfair trade practices, etc.

District Court Major trial court exercising general jurisdiction	Appellate Jurisdiction	Original Jurisdiction
	by a Three-Judge Court	by a Three-Judge Court or by a Single-Judge Court depending on the nature and importance of the case involved. All civil actions not specifically coming under other courts.

Summary Court Limited jurisdiction	Original Jurisdiction
	by a Single-Judge Court Minor civil actions involving claims of not exceeding 900 000 yen

Note: 1) Where both parties agree, a 'jumping appeal' may be made from a judgment of the summary court to the high court or from a judgment of the district court to the Supreme Court.

2) Where a summary court case involves constitutional questions, a special appeal may be made from a judgment of the high court to the Supreme Court.

Quoted from "Justice in Japan" The General Secretariat, the Supreme Court of Japan ed. Reproduced with permission.

Figure 1 Jurisdiction and procedure of Japanese courts: civil cases.

Historical Background of Japanese Legal System

From the Ancient to the Heian Era

According to *Nihonshoki*, which was the first historical document compiled in 720 AD, justice was first administered in the fourth century by Emperor Ingyo, the ancestor of the present emperor of Japan. *Jushichijo Kempo* (Seventeen Maxims), the oldest written code in Japan, was promulgated by Prince Shotoku.

As the fundamental law of the nation, it was applied to officials and people.

The centralization of power and bureaucratic governing structure under the Emperor was established by the Great Reform of Taika in 645. Ritsuryo, the form of which came from China, was enacted to centralize power. The term Ritsuryo comprises ritsu, signifying a criminal code, and ryo, all other regulations, including the law of national organization, administrative law, and civil codes.

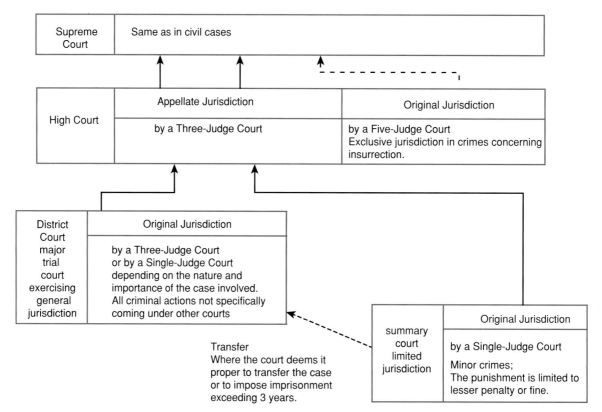

Figure 2 Jurisdiction and procedure of Japanese courts: criminal cases.

Note: A direct appeal may be made to the Supreme Court from a judgment of the district court or the summary court in which the court decided unconstitutionality of law, ordinance, etc.

Quoted from "Justice in Japan" The General Secretariat, the Supreme Court of Japan ed. Reproduced with permission.

There were two kinds of judicial proceeding under Ritsuryo. One was by oral presentation, in which a lawsuit was instituted when a plaintiff complained to the local authority having regional jurisdiction in the defendant's domiciliary area. In the other, a judgment was recorded and an action was instituted when an accusation was made by an injured person or the general public to the authority having jurisdiction in the place where an alleged crime had been committed. The judgment was based on a confession.

From the Kamakura Era to the Edo Era

In the history of Japan, the Samurai-family Feudal Era, the so-called Sengoku, Kamakura, Muromachi, and Edo, are important. The Emperor delegated an authority to the Shogunate at Kamakura under the government by Bakufu. Shogun is a general of Samurai-family Feudal Era in Japan. Shogunabe is a duty of Shogun. The Samurai-family Feudal Era lasted from this time until the Tokugawa Era.

In the Kamakura Era, Goseibai Shikimoku (Shogunate ordinance) was enacted and promulgated by the Shogunate in 1232 AD. Civil cases were tried at a documented hearing and appeals were possible when the defendants disagreed with the judgment. In criminal trials, the procedure was almost identical to that used during the Ritsuryo period except that torture in felony cases was banned and few appeals were allowed.

After the Kamakura Shogunate, the Muromachi Shogunate was established. However, the authority of the Shogunate declined gradually and the Shugo-daimyo, the local authority in each province, exercised power by administering his domain as he saw fit, so the former legal order was eroded. This era is called Sengokujidai (the civil-war era of 1467–1573). During this period, many codified local laws were developed by each Shugodaimyo.

Sengokujidai came to an end with national unification under Hideyoshi Toyotomi in 1590. The Edo Shogunate was founded by Ieyasu Tokugawa, who succeeded Hideyoshi Toyotomi. The decentralization of power was accomplished by establishing a unique relationship between the Shogunate and Han, which is the subordinate local unit.

Under the Edo Shogunate, Bukeshohatto was enacted as customary laws. In the initial stage of this

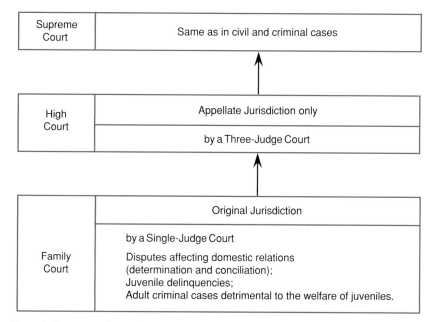

Supreme Court	Same as in civil and criminal cases
High Court	Appellate Jurisdiction only
	by a Three-Judge Court
Family Court	Original Jurisdiction
	by a Single-Judge Court Disputes affecting domestic relations (determination and conciliation); Juvenile delinquencies; Adult criminal cases detrimental to the welfare of juveniles.

Note: A direct appeal may be made to the Supreme Court from a judgment of the Family Court in which the court decided unconstitutionality of law, ordinance, etc.

Quoted from "Justice in Japan" The General Secretariat, the Supreme Court of Japan ed. Reproduced with permission.

Figure 3 Jurisdiction and procedure of Japanese courts: family cases.

era, justice was carried out according to Bukesho-hatto. As the unitary code of criminal law, Kujikata Osadamegaki, promulgated in 1742, formed a basis of justice under the Edo Shogunate. The official judicial court, the so-called Hyojyosho, and its performance were defined by this code, which included the organization of a police system. A magistrate's office was called Bugyosyo. A trial was conducted on the basis of a documentary hearing or oral presentation. In a criminal case, a decision was rendered only on the confession of the accused. Confessions obtained through torture could also constitute evidence.

Before the Promulgation of the Meiji Constitution

The feudal age of military ascendancy continued for about 700 years. In 1867 the last Shogun, Yoshinobu Tokugawa, restored the supreme power of the Emperor as the ruler of the nation.

In 1868, Seitaisho was promulgated. Seitaisho is the basic statute in Meiji Era after Tokugawa Era which was the last Samurai-family Feudal Era. The basic principles of the form of government were shown in Seitaisho. The cabinet, the so-called Dajokan, was divided into three branches: legislative, the judiciary, and administration. However, the separation of these three branches was not complete at this time.

In 1871, all civil and criminal affairs were under the jurisdiction of the Ministry of Justice. At that time, the nationwide judicial system included five types of courts: (1) the temporary courts of the Ministry of Justice; (2) Courts of the Ministry of Justice; (3) branch courts; (4) prefectural courts; and (5) local courts. The Supreme Court was created in 1875 as the highest appellate court and the independence of the judiciary was established.

The Code of Criminal Law, patterned after the Napoleonic Criminal Code, was promulgated in 1880 and in use until 1907.

Under the Meiji Constitution

The constitution of Japan was promulgated in 1889. Since then, Japan has adopted a constitutional parliamentary monarchy. Under this constitution, three independent bodies exist: (1) the National Diet, which has the power of legislation; (2) the cabinet, which has administrative power; and (3) the courts, which have judicial power. The independence of each separated power was not complete and was subordinate to the emperor. The jurisdiction of the courts was limited to ordinary, civil, and criminal suits. For special cases, the administrative court was used and courts martial were held.

The Code of Civil Procedure and the Code of Criminal Procedure, modeled after the German system, were enacted in 1890. The courts were organized in the following manner: Supreme

Court, Court of Appeals, District Court, and Local Court.

Civil procedure was handled by an adversary system. Appeal to an immediate appellate court was a continued trial and only legal problems could be finally appealed under the Code of Civil Procedure.

Under the Code of Criminal Procedure, official prosecutions were organized. Appeals to an immediate appellate court were handled as a new trial. Legal and factual problems and a penalty that was considered unjust could be brought to a higher court.

The Minister of Justice, a member of the cabinet, had the administrative authority in judiciary and judges were under his influence. However, the independence of the judicial branch was defined under the constitution.

Japanese Medicolegal System

Historical Background

In Japan, the practice of forensic activities, such as a postmortem examination, was active even during the Edo period. Instead of physicians, low-level officials of the then feudal government (Bakufu), such as the secret police (Okappiki) and constables (Doshin), engaged in these activities. During this period, medicolegal textbooks from China were used mainly as guidebooks. Meanwhile, western medicine was beginning to be introduced by Dutch physicians. In 1862, a Dutch army surgeon, Pompe Van Meerderfort, gave lectures on forensic medicine in Nagasaki.

The practical aspect of forensic medicine is closely related to the legal system of the country. The legal system used on the European continent was transplanted to Japan after the Meiji Restoration, while criminal laws were strongly influenced by German law. Following the end of the Second World War, the Anglo-Saxon and American legal systems were introduced into Japan. Their effects were particularly eminent in the Criminal Procedure Act. The introduction of the philosophy of a trial based on evidence resulted in an extensive change in court procedures. Corresponding to these changes in the legal system, regulations and the system of forensic medicine in Japan underwent changes. During the Meiji period, German legal medicine prevailed, while, after World War II, the system of medical examiners was introduced from the USA. Thus, the Japanese forensic medical system has assumed a legislative form that is unique in the world, with features of two contrasting systems blended into one.

The following are the notable events in the history of forensic medicine in Japan during the Meiji period: in 1875, Wilhelm Doenitz gave a lecture on legal medicine at Tokyo Medical School (the present Tokyo University Medical School); in 1888, Kuniyoshi Katayama, who had completed his medical studies in Germany, established the Department of Forensic Medicine at Tokyo University Medical School and started giving lectures on legal medicine. Since then, departments of forensic medicine have been created in many other universities. In 1914, the Japanese Society of Legal Medicine was founded. Currently, legal medicine is taught at almost all university medical schools and the courses specially designated for forensic medicine number 80 in all. During the Meiji and Taisho periods, activities related to criminal identification were performed by special technologists and parttime physicians affiliated to Metropolitan Police Headquarters and the Ministry of Home Affairs. After the end of the Second World War, with the modification of the Criminal Procedure Act in 1949, the Institute for Scientific Investigation (the current Scientific Police Institute) was founded at Metropolitan Police Headquarters for criminal identification. Currently, the identification section at each prefectural police headquarters has a laboratory for scientific investigation for actual identification and research. During the Meiji and Taisho periods also, criminal autopsies were conducted in the department of forensic medicine at a university medical school; and inquests on deaths were conducted by a parttime police surgeon. In 1948, under a directive from the US occupational forces, a medical examiner system was established in several cities that were designated by ordinance and all administrative autopsies and inspections were conducted by medical examiners. However, as indicated in the next section, the medical examiner system in Japan is somewhat different from that of the USA. In spite of the presence of a medical examiner system, criminal autopsies are still conducted in departments of forensic medicine at various university medical schools.

Medical Examiner System in Japan

The medical examiner system in Japan differs from its counterpart in the USA.

First, medical examiners in the USA have a legal authority (mainly the power to conduct investigations) equal to or greater than the police, whereas in Japan, similar authority (especially that involving corpses) is only given to the Public Prosecutor's Office. Medical examiners and students of forensic medicine at university medical schools have no such authority.

Second, there are multiple coroners' offices in each US state and a coroner is assigned to each district under his or her jurisdiction. In Japan, there are no facilities equivalent to a coroner's office. The Japanese medical examiners are employees of municipal governments and are not legally empowered in the same way as their counterparts in the USA.

Third, an autopsy is conducted at the medical examiner's office in Japan (especially in the city of Tokyo) on the body of a person who died in unnatural and suspicious circumstances and that involved in a criminal act. In the 23 wards at the center of the city of Tokyo, these autopsies are performed by forensic pathologists in the departments of forensic medicine of university medical schools. In Osaka, Kobe, and Yokohama, where medical examiner's offices are located at university medical schools, physicians specializing in forensic medicine at each medical school act as medical examiners and perform both criminal autopsies of corpses found under unnatural and suspicious circumstances and those who died from an unnatural cause.

Fourth, the medical examiner's system is not prevalent throughout Japan. Currently, medical examiners reside in the medical examiner's office or medical examiners' headquarters which are only located in the central part of Tokyo, Yokohama, Osaka, and Kobe. Handling of bodies found in unusual and suspicious circumstances is independently determined in the following three administrative areas: (1) the area with the existing medical examiner's system; (2) one where there is no medical examiner's system and a criminal autopsy (that should otherwise be performed by a medical examiner) is conducted as the so-called "autopsy under the agreement of family"; (3) and the other, the area where there is no medical examiner's system or the practice of autopsy under the agreement of family. The administrative differences among these three areas are faithfully reflected in the percentage of autopsies performed. In those prefectures where there is no medical examiner's system, parttime physicians employed by a local police station (local practitioners in many instances) preside at a postmortem inspection of bodies that were found in abnormal circumstances.

A corpse found in abnormal or suspicious circumstances and the handling of such bodies are defined in article 21 of the Japanese medical practitioner's law, under Report of Unusual Cases: "A medical practitioner shall, in a case where he has found anything unusual on examining a dead body or a stillborn baby of four months or more in gestational age, report it to the police authorities within 24 hours."

However, the law does not clearly stipulate the details of "unusual." One may presume that it is up to an individual physician to determine whether the circumstances are unusual or not; and there is a problem of individual differences among physicians in determining what is unusual. In 1994, to avoid ambiguity, the Japanese Society of Legal Medicine published a guideline for identifying death under unusual circumstances. According to this guideline, death under unusual circumstances is outlined as follows:

1. Death due to external causes (regardless of whether the patient had been treated; and if treated, how long he or she had been under a physician's care)
   a. Unexpected accidents
      i. Traffic accidents: death due to accidents involving various means of transportation (automobiles, as well as all others, such as bicycles, trains, and ships). The victim may be the operator of the vehicle, a passenger, or a pedestrian. Accidents include all types (e.g., driver error and a collision involving a single vehicle)
      ii. Falls of all types: death due to a fall on to a flat surface, from steps, stairs, or from a building
      iii. Drowning: drowning of all types, including in the ocean, river, lake, marsh, pond, swimming pool, bathtub, and a puddle
      iv. Fatal injuries caused by fire and flame: death due to a fire (all types of death due to fire, including fatal burns, carbon monoxide poisoning, airway burns, and their combinations); and death due to burns through contact with a flame or highly heated substance
      v. Asphyxiation: fatal asphyxiation due to causes such as compression of the neck or the thoracic region, airway obstruction, the presence of a foreign body in the airway, or anoxia
      vi. Poisoning: death due to ingestion, injection, or coming into contact with a drug or poison
      vii. Exposure to an abnormal environment: exposure to abnormal thermal environments (e.g., heatstroke and freezing), sunstroke, and caisson disease (dysbarism and barotrauma)
      viii. Electrocution or being struck by lightning: death due to electrocution at a work site, a short circuit, or being struck by lightning
      ix. Other accidents: death due to external causes involving all other types of accidents not listed above
   b. Suicides: death due to the wish and action of the deceased, regardless of the means of committing suicide. Examples include strangulation,

jumping from a height, throwing oneself into a path of an oncoming train, self-infliction of wounds by using a sharp or blunt instrument, self-drowning, and ingestion of a poison

c. Homicide: all deaths due to injuries inflicted by another, regardless of a homicidal intention on the part of the assailant. The homicidal means are not limited: examples include strangulation, obstruction of the nose and mouth, injuries inflicted by a sharp or blunt instrument, burning by fire-setting, and poisoning

d. Death due to external causes under unknown circumstances (death may be caused by an accident, suicide, or homicide). No restrictions are placed on the means responsible for the death

2. Death due to complications or sequelae from injuries of external causes. Examples include bronchopneumonia developing from head injuries or poisoning caused by sedatives; interstitial pneumonia and pulmonary fibrosis subsequent to Paraquat poisoning; septicemia, acute renal failure, multiple organ failure, and tetanus subsequent to external injuries, poisoning, and burns; fat embolism associated with fractures

3. Incidents that are suspected to be involved in (1) or (2) above, including instances in which there is a slight suspicion of a cause-and-effect relationship between the external cause and death or such a cause-and-effect relationship is not evident

4. Unexpected death related to a medical action or a suspicion that the death may have been due to a medical action. This includes an unexpected death that occurred during or relatively soon after a medical action, such as an injection, anesthesia, surgery, diagnostic procedure, or delivery; a death possibly related to a medical action; and a sudden death of unknown etiology that occurred during or relatively soon after a medical action. The presence of errors in medical actions or questions of negligence are unrelated to this category

5. Deaths without any evident cause:
   a. Discovery of a body after death has occurred
   b. Unexpected sudden death of a person who has been seemingly healthy up to then
   c. Death of a patient who sought medical care for the first time but expired shortly after the examination before a diagnosis was established
   d. Death of a patient who had been treated at a medical facility but it is not clear that he/she expired from the disease for which he/she had been treated (when the patient expired within 24 h of the final treatment and it is difficult to conclude that he/she died from the disease from which it had been known he/she suffered)
   e. Others in which the cause of death is unknown: instances where it is uncertain whether a death was caused by an illness or an external cause.

When a death under an unusual circumstance is reported, the police conduct an investigation and postmortem examination to determine whether it was a natural death (death due to an illness), noncriminal death (e.g., suicide or accidental death), or an unnatural death (i.e., one in which there is a suspicion of criminal involvement). Article 1 of the Guidelines for Handling Corpses Found in Unusual Circumstances (the 1975 Regulation) classifies corpses handled by the police into the following three types:

1. Bodies of those who were killed in a criminal act: those that exhibit clear evidence that the subject died as a consequence of a criminal act.
2. Bodies found in unnatural circumstances: The Criminal Procedure Act, article 229, item 1, defines those who succumbed and were found in unnatural circumstances as follows: "If there is a person who expired in an unnatural circumstance, or a dead body that is suspected to be in an unnatural circumstance, a public procurator of the district or local public procurator's office having jurisdiction over the place where it is found shall make the postmortem inspection."
3. Bodies of those who expired without involvement of criminal acts: bodies in which it is objectively evident that the deaths were due to noncriminal causes. It is understood that bodies found in unnatural circumstances are only those in which the involvement of a criminal act cannot be established. The postmortem examination defined by article 229 of the Criminal Procedure Act is conducted to obtain clues to investigate a possible criminal act and it is designed to gather all evidence so that a criminal act causing a death may not escape detection by the police.

Therefore, there is no need to conduct such an examination on those bodies with or without obvious criminal involvement: only the bodies found in unnatural circumstances are subjected to criminal investigation. The bodies of persons who evidently suffered from a criminal act are immediately inspected and examined at the site by police officers, according to the specifications of the Criminal Procedure Act and Criminal Investigation Code. At the same time, investigative activities, such as the issuance of a permit to identify the victim and assign a professional to conduct an autopsy (criminal autopsy), are initiated. When no criminal involvement is indicated, administrative processing based on the Family Registration Act and regulations on the handling of corpses are considered to be sufficient. In Japan, article 192 of the Criminal Law and article 229 of the Criminal Procedure Act stipulate that bodies found in unusual circumstances cannot be buried without a postmortem examination.

Secret burial of a person who died an unnatural death: a person, who without a postmortem examination buries another who has died an unnatural death, shall be punished with a fine of not more than 50 yen or a minor fine (Criminal Law, article 192).

Postmortem inspection: if a person dies in an unnatural circumstance, or a dead body is found with a suspicion of an unnatural death, a public procurator of the district or local public procurator's office having jurisdiction over the place where the body was found shall make a postmortem inspection (Criminal Procedure Act, article 229).

4. A public procurator may cause a secretary in the public procurator's office or a police official to take such measures as noted in the preceding paragraph. These regulations require a public prosecutor's inspection and examination of the body (a comprehensive procedure, normally called a criminal autopsy, including a death scene investigation, to determine if the person in question was killed in the performance of a criminal act) accompanied by a postmortem inspection by a medical doctor (external examination of the body to establish the cause of death, the time that had elapsed after death, and whether the death was due to a natural or unnatural cause). The definition of "a person who died under an unnatural circumstance," as cited in article 192 of the Criminal Law, is more comprehensive than that described in article 229 of the Criminal Procedure Act: the former includes all those found in unnatural circumstances (even when it is obvious that the persons were not involved in criminal acts but the cause of death was not established) and may also include some that are the subject of an administrative autopsy (examination required by administrative regulation, conducted on bodies found in unnatural circumstances and those also found in unnatural circumstances but where no criminal act is suspected. The examination is conducted for purposes such as a contribution to public welfare and general hygiene). The person who dies in an unnatural circumstance cited in article 229 of the Criminal Procedure Act refers to an individual who is found dead in unnatural circumstances, where there is a suspicion of

criminal involvement. Therefore, the requirement of this article does not apply to a death in unnatural circumstances where the involvement of a criminal act is evident, a death due to natural disasters, such as floods and lightning, drowning while swimming, unquestionable cases of suicide, and accidental deaths due to carelessness. In other words, this law requires a postmortem inspection of those bodies that were found in unnatural circumstances and where there is a suspicion of criminal involvement. Major criminal acts, especially vicious homicidal acts, arson, and rape culminating in a homicide, violence, and fatal injuries caused by a violent crime constitute criminal deaths.

At a postmortem inspection, a physician conducts the inspection and renders a medical judgment. The physician who inspected a body that had been found in an unnatural circumstance confirms or determines the cause of death, and submits a record of the inspection to the attending police officer and a report on the inspection to the survivor of the victim. In this instance, the inspection is conducted by a medical examiner in those areas where the medical examiners' system exists (23 wards in the center of Tokyo, Yokohama, Osaka, and Kobe) and by a physician assigned by the police in other areas (a police surgeon who is primarily employed to care for the health of the detainees or a general practitioner).

When a natural death or death not involved with a criminal act is proven and a cause of death is established through inspection, the surviving family members submit the inspection report and a notice of death to the municipal office and make arrangements for burial or cremation.

When the cause of death cannot be determined through inspection, an autopsy is conducted. In those areas where the medical examiner's system exists, a medical examiner conducts the autopsy (this is called an administrative autopsy). In areas where there are no medical examiners' systems but there is a system for conducting autopsies with the agreement of the family, the department of forensic medicine of a university medical school does the autopsy. However, the budget allocated to autopsies by the local municipal government is not always sufficient so it may not be performed in all cases of a death under unnatural circumstances or with unknown etiology. An autopsy under the aforementioned conditions is rarely performed in areas where neither a medical examiner's system nor the system of autopsy under the agreement with a family exists. If an autopsy is absolutely necessary, steps are taken to resort to a judicial autopsy. An administrative autopsy is performed by a medical examiner in accordance with article 8 of the Autopsy and Body Preservation Act:

> Inspection and autopsy by a medical examiner: the metropolitan or prefectural governor having jurisdiction over a place stipulated by cabinet order shall, with regard to a corpse suspected to be affected by a contagious disease, intoxication, or disaster or a corpse from an unknown cause of death in that place, appoint a medical examiner to clarify the cause of death that has not been clarified even after the examination, by performing its dissection, provided that, with regard to a corpse found in an unnatural circumstance or suspected to be from an unnatural death, the examination or dissection shall not be performed until a postmortem inspection under article 229 of the Code of Criminal Procedure Law is carried out. The examination or dissection under the preceding paragraph shall not affect an autopsy for inspection or gaining expert evidence under the Code of Criminal Procedure.

If the death has occurred in an unnatural circumstance or has been caused by a criminal act, the judicial authority shall investigate to discover how the death occurred or on whom the responsibility rests. As part of this investigative activity, an autopsy is necessary. In accordance with articles 165 and 168 of the Criminal Procedure Act, an autopsy is conducted:

> An investigation is made to find the cause of death and other pertinent facts; and an expert opinion based on these findings is submitted. (Expert testimony: The court may order persons of learning and experience to give expert testimony. Expert testimony, a necessary measure: A permit; an expert may, when it is necessary with respect to expert testimony, enter a dwelling, or residence, building, or vessel under guard, examine the body, dissect a corpse, exhume a grave, or destroy things by obtaining permission from the court. The court shall, in granting permission … issue a permit setting forth therein the name of the accused, the offense, the place to be entered, the body to be examined, the corpse to be dissected, the grave to be exhumed, or the things to be destroyed, the name of the expert, or such other matters as are specified by the rules of the court. The expert shall show the permit to the person subjected to the measures …)

The procedure is called a judicial autopsy. There are no regional differences in this procedure.

See Also

Court Systems: Sharii'ah Law; Law, China; Law, United Kingdom; Law, United States of America; **Crime-scene Management, Systems:** Continental Europe; United Kingdom; United States of America; **Death Investigation Systems:** Japan

Further Reading

Abe N (2001) *The Complete Illustrated Guide to Japanese Systems: Politics, Economics, Law and Order*, pp. 166–202. Tokyo, Japan: Kodansya.

Misawa S, Honda K (1996) History of the medicolegal system in Japan. *Forensic Science International* 80: 3–10.

Nagano T, Miyake B (1996) The present situation of forensic sciences of police in Japan and the National Research Institute of Police Science. *Forensic Science International* 80: 11–22.

Shoji M (1996) History and present status of the Tokyo Metropolitan Medical Examiner System. *Forensic Science International* 80: 23–31.

Tsunerari S (1986) Forensic medicine in Japan. *American Journal of Forensic Medicine and Pathology* 7: 219–223.

Law, United Kingdom

I Wall, Ruislip, UK

Introduction

Laws are rules that seek to guide and regulate orderly behavior in a collective society. The agencies responsible for the creation and enforcement of these rules form the collective enterprise known colloquially as "the law."

The legal systems of England and Wales are fully fused. In Scotland, by way of contrast, historical forces have shaped a distinct legal tradition, which draws upon English common law and Roman law influences.

Sources of Law

In England and Wales the two principal sources of law are Parliament, and the decisions of judges in the courts of law. Increasingly, however, rule-making powers are now the subject of delegation to other bodies.

Judicial Law

Often referred to as "common law" or "case law," this form of evolved, case-precedent law is based on the corpus of decisions made by judges in courts. Until the seventeenth century, it was the preeminent source of law in the UK, and while "statute law" has since superseded it in terms of volume, case law still enjoys an important role. Judicial law seeks to apply rules of law to particular factual situations and occasionally, in novel situations, to extend and develop the law. Judges therefore perform both an adjudicative and a "legislative" role.

Consistency and fairness are maintained to a certain extent by the "doctrine of precedent," which ensures that the principles enunciated in one court will normally be binding on judges of inferior courts in subsequent cases. Under the principle of *stare decesis*, the decision of the House of Lords is binding on the lesser courts but not themselves. Decisions of the Court of Appeal are binding on inferior courts and to a limited extent on themselves in civil cases and to a lesser extent in criminal cases. A decision of the Divisional Court binds inferior courts. Clearly for such a system to operate there must be an appropriate and adequate system of reporting cases. Though bound to follow the provisions of statutory law, the courts have always exercised a role in interpreting statutory language, sometimes with the effect of thwarting Parliament's intention.

Branches of Law

The common law in the UK is divided into a number of specialist areas, each with its own language, procedures, and substantive rules of law and evidence. The two principal categories are civil law and criminal law. Civil law is concerned with the resolution of disputes between private individuals. It is the aggrieved party who undertakes the legal action or suit, and remedies are usually financial. Criminal law, on the other hand, is concerned with the relationship between individuals and the state. The focus of the state's coercive powers is the elimination of behavior of which it disapproves by the proscription of punitive sentences.

There is an overlap between these two main jurisdictions such that a criminal offense will often have an equivalent in the civil jurisdiction (for example, the offense of assault and the civil wrong of trespass, respectively).

An Adversarial System

The conduct of criminal and civil litigation is adversarial in nature. The court's final adjudication is based upon the strength of the opposing arguments presented before it, and "truth," therefore, is not a matter of principal concern.

Some jurisdictions utilize an inquisitorial approach whereby the tribunal itself embarks upon, and sets the agenda and parameters of, its own fact-finding exercise.

The Prosecution of Offenses

The Crown Prosecution Service (CPS) is responsible for the conduct of all criminal prosecutions commenced by the police in England and Wales.

The head of the service is the Director of Public Prosecutions, who is superintended by the Attorney General, a member of the government. The Attorney General and the Solicitor General are both political appointees and have final responsibility for enforcing criminal law, in addition to their advisory role to the government. Responsibility for the independent public prosecution service in Scotland lies with the Procurator Fiscal and the Crown Office. The Crown Office is led by the Lord Advocate, in whose name all prosecutions are brought, and the Solicitor General for Scotland.

The Court System

The court system is similarly split into civil and criminal jurisdictions, and the courts are arranged in hierarchical tiers reflecting precedent and expertise. Most business is transacted in the lower or "inferior" courts, operating as trial courts of first instance, with the superior courts functioning in an appellate capacity.

The Criminal Courts of England and Wales

The Magistrates' Courts

Magistrates' courts are local courts, and are the lowest of the courts in the criminal hierarchy. They hear 95% of all criminal offenses, including all minor "summary" offenses, as well as the less serious examples of offenses "triable either way" (offenses such as assault, criminal damage, and theft). In respect of "either-way" offenses, the magistrates will decide whether to remit the case to the crown court for trial on indictment or to hear the case summarily themselves. The accused must consent to the summary trial of an either-way offense but cannot insist on one, and where the accused elects trial by judge and jury at crown court, the magistrates will undertake committal proceedings to ensure that the crown has a *prima facie* case.

The 30 000 or so lay magistrates or justices of the peace are not legally qualified; they are unpaid and are drawn from the local community. Magistrates sit as a "bench" of three, assisted on matters of law by a legally qualified Clerk to the Justices, who does not participate in the outcome of a case. In metropolitan areas, 100 legally qualified, salaried District Judges (Magistrates' Courts) sit alone.

The Crown Court

The Crown Court is a single court that sits in a number of different "tiered" centers throughout England and Wales, and has exclusive jurisdiction over trials on indictment.

Indictable offenses are classified according to their gravity to ensure their allocation to an appropriately experienced judge. High Court judges will hear the most serious cases such as murder, while circuit judges, who are the typical Crown Court judges, will hear most less serious cases. Recorders are parttime judges who hear the least serious cases and combine their role with private legal practice.

Unlike the Magistrates' Courts, where the justices act as tribunal of "fact and law," the roles are split in the Crown Court between the judge as arbiter of law, and jury as tribunal of fact.

The Crown Court has a criminal appellate function in respect of appeals from magistrates' courts against conviction on a legal issue, or sentence.

The Queen's Bench Division of the High Court exercises an appellate role, "by way of case stated" in respect of criminal appeals from magistrates' courts and Crown Courts where there is dissatisfaction over points of law or issues of jurisdiction.

Court of Appeal

The Criminal Division of the Court of Appeal hears appeals against conviction and sentence from the Crown Court.

The court comprises the Lord Justices of Appeal and is presided over by the Lord Chief Justice and the Vice-President of the criminal division.

An appeal to the court requires permission or "leave," a matter that will usually be ruled on by a single Lord Justice after considering a transcript of the crown court proceedings.

Appeals will only be allowed where the initial conviction was unsafe (Criminal Appeals Act 1995) as a consequence of a procedural or a legal error.

The court has the power to allow the appeal and to acquit the appellant or to order a retrial. The Attorney General can refer a case to the Court of Appeal where there is concern over the interpretation of a point of law that has resulted in an acquittal, or where a sentence has been passed that is considered too lenient.

The House of Lords

The House of Lords, sitting in its judicial capacity, is the supreme criminal court in England and Wales, and hears appeals from the Court of Appeal involving a point of law of general public importance, though this is not a requirement for a civil appeal. (Interestingly, the Scotland Act 1998 treats rights granted under the European Convention on Human Rights as "devolution issues" and so criminal cases raising human rights issues are, with leave, appeallable to the Privy Council.)

An appeal to the House requires leave and the cases heard are not by way of retrials, as evidence is considered by the three or five of the Lord Justices of Appeal (Law Lords) in written form only.

The Civil Courts in England and Wales

The magistrates' court exercises a significant, though more limited, role in the civil sphere, where its jurisdiction relates to matrimonial issues and licensing for the gaming and liquor industry.

County Courts

Above the magistrates' court are the 230 or so County Courts situated throughout England and Wales. Here, in the presence of a Circuit Judge or District Judge, 90% of all civil disputes are heard annually.

The manner in which each case is dealt with depends on the monetary value of the case, so that time spent (and therefore costs) are proportionate.

The High Court

The High Court has unlimited civil jurisdiction, and hears cases that involve more complex legal issues or where high monetary values are involved. It sits principally in the Royal Courts of Justice in London, but increasingly, much business is conducted in provincial High Court District Registries.

The High Court itself comprises three divisions, and each division exercises both first-instance and appellate jurisdictions. The Chancery Division specializes in matters of bankruptcy, trusts, and tax, and has an appellate jurisdiction in respect of bankruptcy petitions from the county courts. The Family Division specializes in matrimonial issues, matters relating to minors, and probate; while the Queen's Bench Division, whose judges sit under the auspices of the Lord Chief Justice, deals with general civil matters.

The High Court's "puisne" judges usually sit in the absence of a jury when hearing a case at first instance, but as a bench of two or three as an appellate "Divisional Court." The Divisional Court of the Queen's Bench is a distinct entity that exercises a supervisory appellate jurisdiction by way of judicial review over inferior courts and tribunals, and in respect of certain jurisdictional appeals from Magistrates' Courts and County Courts.

Civil Division of the Court of Appeal

The Civil Division of the Court of Appeal also sits at the Royal Courts of Justice and hears appeals on matters of law (and therefore are not retrials) from the three divisions of the High Court, the Divisional Court, the County Courts, and certain tribunals.

It is presided over by the Master of the Rolls, and courts of two, three, or five judges are normally constituted from the Lords Justices of Appeal, depending on the importance of the case.

The time constraints on appeals to the House of Lords mean that, in practical terms, the Court of appeal is the final Appellate court for urgent cases.

To ensure that only cases of a complexity appropriate to the standing of the court reach there, all classes of cases require permission to appeal.

Where a case has already been heard on appeal at a lower court there is no longer a right to appeal to the Court of Appeal unless the case raises important legal issues (Access to Justice Act 1999).

House of Lords

This is the supreme appellate civil court for Great Britain and Northern Ireland. The vast majority of appeals originate in the Court of Appeal, though certain cases may "leapfrog" directly from the high court. Appeals are heard by either five or seven The Lords of Appeal in the Ordinary.

Special Courts

Youth Courts

Youth Courts are special magistrates' courts, established to deal with persons under the age of 18. There is an assumption that all criminal offenses involving juveniles will be tried here (with notable exceptions, such as homicide).

The bench comprises justices who have particular experience in dealing with juveniles. The Youth Courts are held in the same building as the adult magistrates' court, but differ from the magistrates' court in that the language and setting of the courtroom are less formal and their proceedings are private affairs with restrictions on public access and media reporting.

Coroners' Courts

These ancient courts are unique to English law as their proceedings are inquisitorial in nature. The coroner's jurisdiction is over certain categories of unexplained or unnatural deaths, and inquests are held to determine the "how, when, and where" of death and not to apportion blame or to give an opinion on criminal or civil liability.

Coroners are either lawyers or medical doctors with legal qualifications. It is usual for inquests to be held in the absence of a jury, though the coroner may empanel one in high-profile cases.

Scotland does not have a coroners' court; instead the Procurator Fiscal deals with unexpected deaths, and where circumstances require, a public fatal accident inquiry may be held.

The Judicial Committee of the Privy Council

This court, sitting in London, is composed principally of Law Lords. It exercises an important appellate role in respect of civil and criminal cases arising in the 24 Commonwealth territories and six independent republics within the Commonwealth who have retained the option to appeal to "Her Majesty in Council."

Acting in this capacity, the decisions of the Judicial Committee are not binding in domestic law, though they are highly persuasive.

The court also exercises a jurisdictional role in matters relating to the legality of the operation of powers devolved to the legislative and executive authorities established in Scotland, Wales, and Northern Ireland, and in this capacity its decisions are binding on the House of Lords.

Finally the court also has a domestic appellate jurisdiction in respect of decisions of disciplinary committees of certain professional bodies governing medical, dental, and veterinary professions.

The European Court of Justice

The European Union's judicial power resides in the European Court of Justice, which sits in Luxembourg. It has responsibility for ruling on the interpretation or application of the treaties and legislation of the European Union in disputes between member nations, or member nations and European institutions.

Referrals to this court can arise from any domestic UK court or tribunal, except the House of Lords (Article 177 of the European Economic Community Treaty).

The European Court of Human Rights

Sitting in Strasbourg, France, this court is one of the institutions of the Council of Europe, an agency distinct from the European Union. The Council of Europe was established in 1949 with the aim of defending human rights; under its auspices the European Convention on Human Rights was drawn up, and the European Court of Human Rights was established. The European Court of Human Rights is entrusted with the responsibility of enforcing the obligations of member states under the convention, and its jurisdiction lies where there is an allegation that guaranteed rights and freedoms have been infringed.

A Supreme Court

The incumbent government has advanced proposals to establish a supreme court for the UK. This, it is anticipated, would address issues of judicial independence pursuant to Article 6(1) of the European

Convention on Human Rights, as well as assuageing the discomfort exhibited by European courts in relation to the interpretation of legislation by judges who have had a role in its enactment.

One further aspect of this desire to achieve a tangible separation of powers is the proposed abolition of the ancient office of the Lord Chancellor and the establishment of a new Department of Constitutional Affairs and an "independent" Judicial Appointments Committee that would assume responsibility for the appointment of judges.

The putative court would assume ultimate appellate jurisdiction for the UK (except criminal cases arising in Scotland), and it would act as a constitutional court, assuming responsibility for devolutional issues currently undertaken by the Judicial Committee of the Privy Council.

The Scottish Courts

Scottish Criminal Courts

Scotland has a three-tier criminal court system. The High Court of Justiciary is Scotland's supreme criminal court. Under the auspices of the Lord Justice General, the Lord Justice Clerk and the 25 judges known as Lords Commissioners of Justiciary, the court exercises first-instance jurisdiction in respect of grave crimes by way of solemn procedure, in which a judge and jury sit. The High Court also acts in an appellate capacity, hearing appeals from courts of "inferior" jurisdiction.

Below this is the sheriff court, which exercises a wide criminal jurisdiction in all but the graver criminal offenses. There are six sheriffdoms in Scotland, each headed by a Sheriff Principal. The Sheriff Court has an extensive workload dealing with over 60% of criminal cases.

At the bottom of the court hierarchy are the 30 District Courts. They are broadly similar to the magistrates' courts of England and Wales, and sit locally under the auspices of lay magistrates assisted by a legally qualified assessor or convenor. The District Court deals with lesser criminal offenses by way of summary procedure in which only a judge (or bench) sits.

Scottish Civil Courts

The Court of Session is Scotland's supreme civil court. Sitting in Edinburgh, it consists of 32 judges, known as Lords of Council and Session, and is divided into an Inner House and an Outer House.

The Inner House is itself divided into the First and Second Divisions, of equal authority, and exercises an appellate role in respect of cases originating in the Outer House, Sheriff Courts, and certain tribunals.

The Outer House functions as the court of first instance in respect of a wide range of civil matters, usually in the absence of a jury.

The Sheriff Courts deal with the majority of civil cases and they have a jurisdiction broadly similar to the Outer House.

The Courts

The institutionalization of the process of arbitration and dispute resolution is a common feature of developed legal traditions.

The hierarchical court system in England and Wales has evolved from Anglo-Norman times and has been shaped by both constitutional forces and peculiar legal rules such as the doctrine of precedent.

The English common-law tradition has spread beyond its shores so that its court structures are now reflected in other jurisdictions.

See Also

Court Systems: Jewish (Halacha) Law; Sharii'ah Law; Law, China; Law, Japan; Law, United States of America

Further Reading

Gary S, David K (2001) *The English Legal System*, 5th edn. London: Cavendish.
Human Rights (2000) *The 1998 Act and the European Convention*. London: Sweet and Maxwell.
John S (2000) *Emmins on Criminal Procedure*, 8th edn. London: Blackstone Press.

Law, United States of America

R T Kennedy and T L Sanchez, New Mexico Court of Appeals, Albuquerque, NM, USA

Introduction

The USA comprises a national government, including 50 state governments, sovereign Native American tribes, and US territories. Thus, it is a paradox to apply the term "court system" to the USA when discussing the structure of the courts, as that term implies a single, unified system. This article will provide a general overview of the US's court system, its interrelation, general development, and the commonality of procedure and evidence law between the disparate jurisdictions.

Although the general structure of US courts is similar among various jurisdictions, there are also practical differences within any given forum. This article will generally discuss: (1) the background and formation of the US and its courts; (2) the branches of government; (3) sources and types of laws; (4) the federal and state judiciary and their jurisdiction; and (5) the interplay between federal and state court jurisprudence.

Background

The USA emerged from 13 autonomous colonies that had enjoyed broad powers of self-determination for over a century prior to securing their independence from the UK. Though diverse, they possessed similar institutional structures, legal doctrines, and political constructs predicated upon English law. Upon declaring independence, they became individual independent states possessing republican governments with their own written constitutions that were adopted by the consent of their citizens.

Upon independence, the 13 original states derived their existence from the consent of their citizens to be governed. When the colonies united under the Constitution, they did so as representatives of their citizens. The underlying sovereign authority in the USA therefore belongs to and emanates from the people. When a national government formed, the people, represented by the states, ceded the power and authority to do so by allowing the formation of a national government by adopting and ratifying a national constitution. Through the US Constitution, states yielded some sovereignty to the national government, and established the framework within which the national government was created.

Branches of Government

The Constitution defined and enabled the new US government. It created and delegated powers to three branches: legislative, executive, and judicial. Each branch possesses power over the functions of the other; this system is referred to as "checks and balances" between the branches of government. This structure is duplicated in the individual states' governmental structure.

Article I of the Constitution established a legislature (Congress), composed of two houses, the House of Representatives and the Senate. Article II established the Office of the President, as the executive branch that carries out the laws enacted by Congress. These articles enumerate the powers given to each branch and provide a framework for their exercise of these powers.

Article III established the judiciary. The US Supreme Court is the only court created by the Constitution.

Congress is given the power to create lower-level courts. One of Congress' initial pieces of legislation was the Judiciary Act of 1789. It established lower federal courts – the district courts and circuit courts. All states have their own constitutions. Their governmental structure is uniquely similar to that set forth in the US Constitution. The US Constitution organizes and distributes national governmental power. It confers the power to form a government. The Constitution also establishes the structure to which government must adhere. The Constitution confers upon the Congress the power to make law. Article VI, Section 2 of the Constitution provides that the US Constitution and laws created pursuant to it are the supreme law of the land, "and the Judges in every state shall be bound thereby." This provision establishes the supremacy and uniting force of federal law among the states, and perhaps more importantly, makes the Federal Constitution enforceable in all courts. Federalism is also a system of dual sovereignty, with the national government being limited by the existence of the states. Today, each state is also governed by its own constitution which serves as the ultimate law of the state. A state constitution may grant greater protection than the federal constitution but no less protection.

The US government combines the features of both a unitary state and a federation. The Constitution limits the federal government's power to those stated in the document, and reserves for the states those powers not ceded by them in the US Constitution. The judiciary is no exception to these limitations. Judicial powers and obligations are inherently vested in both national and local governments.

Legal Framework

There are four main types of law in the US: (1) constitutional law; (2) common law; (3) statutory law; and (4) regulatory law. Each originates from a different source and serves a different purpose.

Constitutional Law

Constitutional law is the body of principles which apply in the interpretation and construction of constitutions. The law of constitutions is considered fundamental law, which is applied to statutes and other legislative acts. In the USA, constitutional law is derived from English jurisprudence. Its rules and principles have grown out of the development of the USA and the individual states. Constitutional law is the supreme law, expressed in written form, by which all private rights must be determined and public authority administered.

Common Law

The original colonies' legal system was founded in English common law. Common law is derived from the courts resolving disputes and creating legal decisions, of which the holdings are then binding on all lower courts. Trial courts' decisions are reviewed by appellate courts for error. Appellate decisions exist to resolve issues and establish legal precedent from which to govern the conduct of the courts in future cases. The principle that precedent decisions are to be followed by the courts is called *stare decisis*.

Supreme courts, both state and federal, review decisions of lower courts and are the final arbiters of their constitutions and the laws created by their respective governments. The US Supreme Court is the court of last resort for cases arising under the US Constitution and federal laws. Its decisions are binding in all federal jurisdictions. States must conform their rulings to those of the US Supreme Court. The US Supreme Court's decisions are "authoritative" and must be followed. State Supreme Court decisions are only binding within that state's jurisdiction, but are frequently cited as persuasive authority by other states in the absence of their own law on a particular issue.

Statutory Law

Statutes are the product of their representative legislative branches of government. For the USA, this power rests with Congress. Each state also has its own legislative body to pass laws for governing affairs within its borders. Statutory law defines criminal offenses and establishes a body of law through which public, governmental, and private affairs are governed. Disputes concerning statutory law are decided by the courts, which have the power to decide relationships between individuals, individuals and the government, or parts of the government itself. Statutory law is limited by combined or separate state and federal constitutional power. Legislatures cannot exceed their constitutional authority to act, nor can they pass laws inimical to rights or duties that are constitutionally secured. Laws passed by the US Congress generally regulate national or interstate matters, and are binding upon the states on matters within their purview. The states may not legislate matters to control the federal government.

Administrative/Regulatory Law

When legislation is passed, the executive branch of government implements it into law. The US Constitution establishes the Office of the President as the executive office of the USA. States generally have governors. The executive branch institutes suboffices, agencies, or departments to carry out its functions.

For example, agencies and departments may have police and prosecutorial powers to enforce criminal laws or regulatory and enforcement power over commerce and the environment. Legislatures delegate some power to the executive agencies to make rules governing these functions within legislated boundaries. This "quasilegislative" function is limited by enabling legislation, as state legislatures themselves are limited by the Constitution. Additionally, many agencies create "quasijudicial" agencies to resolve disputes arising in the administration of the laws, which are subject to judicial review.

Foundations of the US Court System

Judicial Review

In the 1803 case of *Marbury* v. *Madison*, 5 US (1 Cranch) 137 (1803), the US Supreme Court held that laws passed by the Congress could be interpreted against the Constitution by the courts, and if the Constitution and the laws were in disagreement, the laws are pronounced as invalid. The Supreme Court held part of the Judiciary Act itself could not be enforced, because it gave the Supreme Court powers beyond those conferred by the Constitution. Chief Justice Marshall stated, "It is emphatically the province and duty of the judicial department to say what the law is." Even though Congress may have believed it was acting properly in passing the law, that was not the issue.

The Adversarial System

Courts in the USA employ an adversarial system. This requires individuals to present their dispute to a neutral fact-finder. The litigants, without assistance, guidance, or direction from the court, accomplish the work of collecting evidence and preparing it for presentation to the court. Failure to present one's case properly, or preserve issues of dispute for appeal, generally results in losing the case. The adversarial system is believed best suited for dispute resolution. This method permits the court to examine opposing facts, determine the truth, and resolve disputes. The USA inherited this tradition from English common law.

Federal and State Courts

United States Courts: Structure

The constitutional provision for a Supreme Court and granting of power to Congress to establish the inferior courts creates the judicial branch. The Constitution provides that "The Judicial Power of the US, shall be vested in one Supreme Court, and in such inferior courts as the Congress may from time to time ordain and establish" (Article III, Section 1). There are three levels of federal courts. Specialty courts also exist. Jurisdiction is determined by federal statute, except with regard to the Supreme Court, whose jurisdiction derives from the Constitution.

The US Supreme Court is composed of a Chief Justice and eight associate justices. It is the court of last resort for the USA. It is the highest supervisory court in the USA, and has final authority over all US courts, both state and federal, concerning matters of federal law and the US Constitution. Its jurisdiction extends to those subjects enumerated in Article III of the Constitution. While the Supreme Court has the power to review and dictate states' application of federal law, it may not review state decisions based on "adequate and independent" state grounds.

Federal judges, including US Supreme Court Justices, are nominated by the President and "hold their [o]ffices during good [b]ehavior," after confirmation by the US Senate, unless they resign or are impeached and convicted by the US Congress. The Supreme Court sits *en banc* with all nine justices participating. Each justice of the Supreme Court oversees one or more circuit courts, with jurisdiction to act in emergency matters within those circuits. The Supreme Court, with Congressional approval, also makes procedural rules for the lower federal courts.

As the nation's highest court, the Supreme Court chooses the cases it hears, usually by granting a writ of certiorari. Once the Supreme Court decides a constitutional case, its decision is virtually final. Only through a subsequent Supreme Court opinion invalidating its previous ruling or a rarely enacted amendment to the Constitution itself, which requires ratification by three-fourths of the states' legislatures, can a constitutional decision of the Supreme Court be abrogated. When the Supreme Court interprets a statute, and Congress does not agree with the interpretation, the opinion governs, but Congress can enact another statute addressing the court's decision.

Below the US Supreme Court are 13 circuit courts of appeal. These intermediate appeals courts review decisions of the district courts, specialty courts, and administrative agencies in their circuits (**Figure 1**). These courts are created by Congress' power to establish inferior federal courts. Circuit courts have panels of three judges, though they can sit *en banc*, which means that all of the judges in the circuit participate in the decision.

The circuit court is the forum provided by law to review for error district court judgments and administrative agency decisions. A party who disputes the lower court or agency's ruling has a right to appeal. The Court of Appeals for the federal circuit sits in Washington, DC. It has national jurisdiction to hear appeals in specialized cases, including intellectual

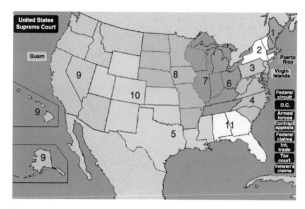

Figure 1 Map of federal judicial circuits.

property and decisions from the Court of International Trade and Court of Claims.

As an intermediate appellate court, circuit courts interpret the law. Their decisions are binding in matters of federal law within the geographical areas of the circuit. If a circuit's interpretation or application of federal law conflicts with the decision of another circuit, the US Supreme Court may resolve these disputes. US district courts exercise original trial jurisdiction of the federal courts. There are 94 US district courts. Each district is contiguous with one state's boundaries, with more populous states having subdistricts. There are also district courts in US territories that are not states. District courts also include additional courts such as adjunct magistrate and bankruptcy courts within their jurisdictions, to handle limited matters.

State Courts: Structure

As in the federal system, each state has a judicial branch of government. The head of the judicial branch is typically the court of last resort or the chief judge or justice of that court. Because there are a number and variety of state courts, it is necessary to discuss general court organization. State court structure parallels the federal court system. State courts are organized into trial courts, which are typically courts of general jurisdiction that decide disputes by examining the facts in each case. Appellate courts review the trial court's application of the law to those facts as established in the trial court. Trial courts may also have limited jurisdiction over a statutorily or constitutionally defined area of the law. They often exercise some form of appellate review over outcomes in limited-jurisdiction courts or decisions by administrative agencies.

Limited-jurisdiction trial courts exist in most states and typically have criminal jurisdiction over misdemeanor offenses and ordinance violations. Limited-jurisdiction courts typically have jurisdiction over civil cases where the claims are under a fixed maximum amount. Appellate courts are also divided into either intermediate appellate courts, which hear initial appeals, or courts of last resort (typically called supreme courts) which have final jurisdiction over appeals.

State court judges are typically elected by voters in their states to serve for a fixed term. Depending on the state, judges may be selected in partisan and nonpartisan elections or by appointment by the state's governor. Once selected, a judge may face partisan or nonpartisan reelection or retention elections if he/she decides to remain in office past the fixed term. Qualifications for service as a judge are set by state statutes and constitutions. To qualify for office, judges must typically meet age and residency requirements and possess specific legal credentials. Most states have an official evaluation process which is responsible for evaluating judicial performance, conduct, and judicial recommendations.

The judicial branch is governed by rules of court procedure, which may be formulated by the state's highest-level court and its state legislature, including a combination of statutory and constitutional authority. States have central offices to handle administrative responsibilities for their courts. Some states have also established state–federal judicial councils to address issues of jurisdictional overlap and other matters of common concern between these two parallel judicial branches.

Appellate courts review issues that were raised and preserved during the lower court proceedings concerning issues of law, procedure, evidence, results, and error. Appellate courts may also create broad public policies through their interpretation of the law and public policy. All losing parties have the right to a review of their case in an appellate court. Each case is entitled to be reviewed only once by the appellate court. After the losing party appeals to an intermediate appellate court, their right to appeal is considered protected. A further appeal may be made to the state's highest court. The court of last resort, in its discretion, chooses the cases it wants to consider and decide. However, under certain limited circumstances (e.g., death-penalty cases), cases are appealed directly to the state's highest court. Cases that are accepted by this high court are typically complex and implicate public policy considerations.

Jurisdiction

The state and federal court systems are similar in design and function. One of the important distinguishing characteristics between them is jurisdictional requirements to file a cause of action. Jurisdiction is "[a] government's general power to exercise authority over all persons and things within its territory." With a few exceptions, state courts have general jurisdiction over all cases arising within the state. Federal court jurisdiction is limited only to cases enumerated in the Constitution and those provided for by Congress. These include cases in which the USA itself is a party, cases involving federal statutory or constitutional law, and cases between citizens of different states that meet diversity of citizenship requirements with a specified amount in damages. Courts must have either personal jurisdiction over the defendant or have in *rem* jurisdiction over the *res* or thing situated in the state in order for the case to be properly before it.

Conclusion

Despite the existence of many legal jurisdictions and sources of law in the USA, common legal traditions, structure, and continuing interdispersment of ideas have created a diverse, unified, and consistent court system in the USA. This diversity illustrates how the interrelationships between federal and state law and courts can be complicated, even for experienced practitioners.

See Also

Court Systems: Sharii'ah Law; Law, China; Law, United Kingdom

Further Reading

Baker TE (1995) A catalogue of judicial federalism in the United States. *South Carolina Law Review* 46: 835–875.

Ballentine JA (1969) *Ballentine's Dictionary*, 3rd edn., p. 253. Rochester, NY: Lawyers Co-Operative.

Calabresi G (2003) Madison lecture: federal and state courts: restoring a workable balance. *New York University Law Review* 78: 1293–1308.

Farrell NS (1997) Congressional action to amend federal rule of evidence 702: a mischievous attempt to codify Daubert *v.* Merrell Dow Pharmaceuticals, Inc. *Journal of Contemporary Health Law and Policy* 13: 523.

Federal Judicial Center (1997) *Reference Manual on Scientific Evidence* (www.fjc.gov/newweb/jnetweb.nsf).

Federal Judicial Center (2000) *Reference Manual on Scientific Evidence*, 2nd edn. (www.fjc.gov/neweb/jnetweb.nsf).

Federal Judicial Center website: http://www.fjc.gov/newweb /jnetweb.nsf.

Geyh CG (2003) Judicial independence, judicial accountability, and the role of constitutional norms in congressional regulation of the courts. *Indiana Law Journal* 78: 153–221.

Imwinkelried EJ (1999) Whether the federal rules of evidence should be conceived as a perpetual index code: blindness is worse than myopia. *William & Mary Law Review* 40: 1595–1596.

Jay J, Hamilton A, Madison J (1961) Wright BF (ed.) *The Federalist*, (1787–8). Boston, MA: Harvard University Press.

Jonakait RN (1996) Text, or ad hoc determinations: interpretation of the federal rules of evidence. *Indiana Law Journal* 71: 551–591.

Kelly AH, Harbison WA, Belz H (1983) *The American Constitution, Its Origins and Development*, 6th edn. W. W. Norton & Company Ltd.

National Center for State Courts website: http://www.ncsonline.org.

Virginia Law Review (1992) *National Conference on State–Federal Judicial Relationships* Rev. vol. 78 No. 8, 1655–1902 Charlottesville, Va: The Virginia Law Revision Association.

Rottman DB, Flango CR, Cantrell MT, Hansen R, LaFountain N (2000) *Bureau of Justice Statistics*. St. Paul, MN: State Court Organizations.

Wright CA, Graham KW Jr (1978) *Federal Practice and Procedure*, 2nd edn., vols. 21–26A. St. Paul, MN: West.

COURTS, REPORT WRITING

M Solon, Bond Solon, London, UK

Definitions

More healthcare practitioners today are preparing evidence and supplying it in court, if by court is meant any legal forum where evidence is heard (e.g., a coroner's court, civil and criminal courts, public inquiries, and disciplinary hearings).

This article gives practical advice on how to prepare written evidence. Although the document format may vary between courts, the basic principles are the same. The report should be written for an intelligent reader who does not have specialist knowledge, and the document should have everything the reader may need to understand the issues discussed. In fact, well-written evidence can save the writer from the unpleasant experience of cross-examination. The intention should be to help the reader with precision and clarity rather than including complex descriptions.

Healthcare practitioners will either be witnesses of fact or expert witnesses. Witnesses of fact give evidence of what they saw, heard, and did in the course of an incident. Such a witness would have been part of the actual events and probably would have made contemporaneous notes. The witness will not be asked to express an opinion on what happened but may have to justify why a procedure was utilized. The witness of fact should try to recreate for the court the events as they happened.

An expert witness is independent of the case and assists a judge or tribunal to understand technical issues and expresses a professional opinion on these issues. The technical expert is case- and issue-specific and is entitled to express an opinion by way of his/her qualifications and experience relevant to that issue. The expert's duty is to the court and not to the party who pays the fee. Like the witness of fact, the expert witness should aim to give accurate, complete, and honest evidence.

Criminal cases involve the state trying to prove that a crime has been committed. Because this can involve an individual's liberty, the level of proof required is high. The case must be proved beyond reasonable doubt. The defense will try to raise doubts and obtain an acquittal. The defendant will be found either not guilty or guilty and if guilty, will usually be punished.

Civil cases generally involve disputes over money. An individual or organization wants money from another for something that happened or did not happen. Because the case is between private parties, the level of proof required is less than in criminal cases, that is, on a balance of probabilities, was something more likely than not? There is no element of punishment but the court will try to put the parties back into the same position had the dispute not arisen.

Both civil and criminal proceedings are adversarial. This means that the parties test each other's evidence to find the truth, with the judge (or jury in a criminal trial in a crown court) as decision-maker. All the evidence of witnesses, including expert witnesses, will be tested in cross-examination, if the written evidence is not agreed before.

Written Evidence for Criminal Proceedings

This section considers the procedure for preparing written witness statements of fact for criminal proceedings; describes the rights of the police in reference to a patient undergoing medical treatment and the implications for a healthcare professional treating the patient; explains the reasons for the appointment of healthcare professionals as expert witnesses for the criminal courts; and reviews the preparation of expert reports for criminal proceedings.

Who is Responsible for Prosecutions in England and Wales?

The prosecution of criminal offenses is controlled by the Crown Prosecution Service (CPS), a body set up by act of parliament in 1985 that became fully operational in October 1986. The CPS receives the evidence concerning a crime and makes the decision as to whether or not to proceed with charging an individual.

Who Provides the Evidence to the CPS?

The police gather the evidence and present to the CPS to decide on charges. In the case of injuries sustained by a victim, the police normally approach the healthcare professionals who examined and treated the victim to obtain statements in relation to a possible offense. In these circumstances, the healthcare professional is providing clinical evidence regarding the injuries received or information on specific aspects of the care the victim was given. While the victim may generally describe the injuries suffered, he/she is not in a position fully to know the extent of injuries or, more specifically, the treatment required. The reason why healthcare professionals are required to describe the injuries and their treatments is because they have both the skills and the knowledge that a layperson neither has nor has access to.

A description of the injuries received and the necessary treatment given to the patient indicates the seriousness of the injuries. When this information is presented to the CPS, it may influence the charge that a person faces and therefore influence the sentence pronounced, if found guilty.

In these circumstances, the healthcare professional is a "witness to fact." He/she recalls what was observed or heard during or following an incident. A witness of fact will be required to discuss facts only as remembered or recorded in his/her notes.

The Nature of the Request to Provide a Statement

For doctors, most requests for statements regarding patients who have been treated in a hospital are coordinated through an administrative channel. The police will request a statement from the doctor(s) involved in the case. In serious cases, particularly where evidence such as clothes, personal effects, or samples are taken by the police, other healthcare professionals may be asked to give a statement outlining their involvement in the case. In these circumstances, the most important part of collecting the evidence linking a suspect to the crime may be the circumstances of the crime. It is important for the prosecuting authorities to show an uninterrupted and complete record of the movement of a piece of evidence, including all the individuals who touched it. This is needed to show whether the evidence was tampered with or remained unchanged until a forensic scientist was able to examine it.

Most statements are compiled from the clinical notes made about a patient. These notes should be made at the time of contact or shortly after contact. It is important that all clinical records are dated and signed by the person writing them. When compiling notes, in the midst of trying to treat a patient, it may be difficult to remember that the most important thing asked in the future may be clinically insignificant during that first examination.

With some serious offenses, particularly murder, a statement may be requested shortly after the event, when the memory of the event is still clear. However, it is not unusual for a statement request to be delayed by weeks or sometimes months.

In such cases, memory is likely to have faded and the only records of involvement and findings are the written notes made at the time. This again emphasizes the importance of good note-taking. If the contemporaneous notes are unclear or brief, or if one is unable to remember a particular patient, the temptation to add anything that cannot be clearly remembered should be avoided.

In most criminal cases, medical evidence takes the form of written evidence, and the legal profession tries not to involve healthcare professionals in the court hearing. However, if the statements give cause for concern, either by the prosecution or the defense, the writer may be required to appear in court. Thus, there is always the possibility that by the time of the court appearance the memory may have faded further.

Requirements before Writing a Statement

Before preparing a statement it should be ensured that all the relevant clinical records are available. A witness to fact, who has been personally involved, should be able to clarify the position. While some clinical records may be available, there may be specific problems in obtaining all the notes. It is important that the statement is made from notes taken and, if the practitioner is unable to provide a complete history of the treatment (e.g., if the patient was transferred to another team), details should not be added to the statement that cannot be confirmed in court.

Patient consent for disclosing clinical data from medical records must be checked. In most cases, the police obtain consent for the release of medical records when taking a witness statement from the victim, and the consent may be appended to the request. It is necessary to have written consent, and this should be retained with a copy of the statement. If no consent is available, the police officer concerned should be requested to obtain consent.

If the patient has subsequently died and consent cannot be obtained, there are some circumstances where clinical details may be divulged as a matter of public interest. However, it would be better for the healthcare professional to discuss with either his/her professional organization (e.g., in the UK, the Medical Defence Union or Royal College of Nursing) or the statutory body regulating practice (e.g., General Dental Council) before releasing this information to the prosecuting authorities.

Procedure for Preparing a Statement

While hand-written statements are acceptable, type-written statements are preferable, as this saves transcription errors later. Sometimes the police ask for statements and will write the statement on behalf of the healthcare professional. Alternatively, the statement may be written by a healthcare professional and in such cases the police may be requested to return the statement.

To comply with court proceedings, most statements are written on standard paper. This includes a standard declaration known as a "Section 9 declaration" (**Figure 1**). This is part of the Criminal Justice Act 1967, and statements in this form are acceptable to the court. Such statements can be read out in court and have the same weight as personal appearance for giving evidence, provided both sides agree to the contents of the report.

What Should the Statement of a Doctor Ideally Contain?

The first part of the statement should show the doctor's name and qualifications (without abbreviations). It should include the position held and the relevance to the reason for the report. Although not essential, some indication of experience, time since qualification, further examinations, and any specialist knowledge can aid the legal team to assess the contents of the statement. The statement should then identify the victim by name and date of birth (not by address). The doctor should note the date, place, and time he/she examined the victim, and the availability of records. Many notes, particularly relating to emergency treatment, do not include all these details, and sometimes the exact timing of events may be important in the case. Therefore, if not included in the medical statements, this may lead to the practitioner being called to court.

The victim's medical complaint and the reason for treatment can be recorded. This is not known *a priori* because in general the doctor was not present at the incident. The narration by the victim amounts to hearsay; therefore, as such it cannot be taken as factually correct and, in most instances, the doctor would be unable to recite the victim's narrative in a criminal court.

Witness   Statement

(C.J. Act 1967, s9; M.C. Rules 1981, r.70)

(Magistrates Courts Act 1980 s102)

Statement of .... Age ....

This statement (consisting of pages each signed by me) is true to the best of my knowledge and belief and I make it knowing that, if it is tendered in evidence, I shall be liable to prosecution if I have wilfully stated in it anything which I know to be false or do not believe to be true.

Dated ....

Signed ....

Figure 1 Format of standard declaration.

Civil Cases

A healthcare professional may also be involved in a civil case. The process of preparing reports and a template for the production of such reports are discussed with a view to assist the healthcare professional in analyzing the evidence prepared for the other party in the litigation.

Many people who sustain injuries seek compensation. The injuries may be the result of an accident or clinical negligence. To show both the injuries received and the subsequent effect on his/her life, the patient or client will normally approach a solicitor to act on his/her behalf, and this solicitor will probably instruct an independent healthcare professional to assist in the preparation of the case and to provide clinical evidence for the court.

In this instance, the healthcare professional is being asked to act as an independent expert witness. The most important part of assessing the letter of instruction is the healthcare professional's decision that he/she is an appropriate person to prepare this report. This means that he/she must have the expertise to prepare the report and to give an authoritative opinion on the questions asked by the lawyer. Unless the solicitor has a practice exclusively in personal injury, he/she may be unaware of the difference in the medical specialties, such as between a neurologist and neurosurgeon, or between the role of a physiotherapist and that of an occupational therapist, when assessing continuing care needs.

For a claimant to prove that a healthcare professional was negligent in giving or refusing the claimant treatment, he/she must show:

1. that there was a duty of care
2. that there was a breach of that duty
3. that the breach of duty resulted in damage
4. that the damage was a direct result of the breach of duty (causation).

To establish each of these, there is a need for expert evidence, and the defendant health authority or individual practitioner (normally through his/her professional indemnity insurer) will also have obtained expert opinion.

Often the experts used to establish each of these parts of negligence are from differing specialist areas, and it is important that healthcare professionals involved in this work realize this.

The injury the claimant has suffered may be similar to injuries sustained in accidents where the negligence is from another source (e.g., road traffic accident (RTA)), and the type of report produced in this instance is similar to that produced for personal injury claims (known as a condition and prognosis report).

However, the report that considers the alleged breach of duty – the liability report – is completely different. A healthcare professional must have some knowledge of the legal background involved. The same report may cover causation. In such cases the expert chosen to give an opinion on liability must work in the same discipline and area of expertise as the healthcare professional against whom the allegation is made.

It is also important that the expert has knowledge of the work environment of the alleged allegation. For instance, if, as a result of an accident, a patient has suffered brain damage and it is alleged that the hospital where the patient was first admitted did not treat the patient properly, the expert chosen to prepare a report should be from the same discipline as that of the admitting hospital's head of the injury team and should work in a similar type of establishment.

Similarly, if the allegation is against a physiotherapist in private practice, the report should be submitted by a practitioner in a similar field. The following points must be considered before agreeing to prepare a report.

What Happens if This Initial Contact is Outside the Expertise of the Healthcare Professional?

If it is felt that the area requiring an expert opinion is outside the field of expertise of the healthcare professional, the case should not be accepted. If it is accepted, and the practitioner is subsequently asked to attend court, the required expertise will be found to be lacking and a great deal of time and money will be wasted. It is far better to inform the solicitor, after reading the letter, that the request falls outside the practitioner's expertise, and explain to the solicitor exactly where the area of expertise lies. The healthcare professional could suggest to the solicitor the name of someone personally known who is in the appropriate field. However, if such a recommendation is made, the expert may create problems for him/herself if the suggested expert does not meet the requirement or produces an inadequate report.

It is appropriate to estimate the best time to prepare a condition and prognosis report. If the injuries were sustained recently, the claimant may not have recovered fully and a definitive opinion on long-term prognosis may not be possible. The instructing solicitor has to be informed by the expert if it is felt that this is the wrong time to prepare the report. There may be a legal, rather than clinical, reason for the report at this time.

Once the expert has decided that he/she is appropriately qualified to prepare the report, and is willing to do so, an acknowledgment should be sent to the instructing solicitors indicating the terms of business. This should include an estimate of the fee and the terms on which payment is to be made following invoice submission. Also, the letter should inform the solicitor of the timeframe necessary to prepare the report. All documents required for the report or, where necessary, the authority to obtain these from the person who holds them, should be requested. A flexible approach with regard to the timing will allow the solicitor and the expert a chance to discuss this if there are any questions. Finally, the number of copies of the report needed should be confirmed.

Sometimes in civil cases one expert (known as a single joint expert) is instructed to prepare a report by both parties to save time and costs and to assist in an early settlement or decision. This is more common in smaller claims and is rare in clinical negligence disputes, particularly for liability and causation reports. Here the judge will need to know the spectrum of medical opinions within which lie the actions of the allegedly negligent practitioner.

Obtaining Clinical Records

Most hospitals and general practitioners charge for photocopying notes and copying X-rays. In a complex case, these may be required by a number of experts. The costs of multiple copies for each expert can become high. Therefore, many solicitors now obtain the relevant records themselves, copy, paginate, and file, and send copies to the expert for the preparation of the report. If, however, the solicitor asks the expert to obtain the records, it is important that these records are sought as early as possible. For these records to be disclosed to the expert, the request must be accompanied by the patient consent (or consent of the parent or legal guardian, if the patient is a minor). The UK Law Society and British Medical Association produced a revised model consent form in 2003 which is available on their websites at http://www.lawsoc.org.uk and http://www.bma.org.uk/.

The Type of Records to be Obtained

Records from hospitals include medical, nursing, and other clinical records, and there may be relevant general practitioner records covering the medical history before the incident. If there are complex considerations, other records from rehabilitation services may need to be obtained and reviewed. Accident reconstruction and police reports may be helpful in preparing a report in an RTA case, depending on the questions being asked. The claimant's statement may also be helpful but the expert should be aware that the statement may not be in a final form, ready for disclosure to the other parties, and

therefore it may not be appropriate to quote from the statement in the report.

Examination of the Patient or Investigation of Needs

While the format of the examination is similar to assessments made by healthcare professionals, during their normal clinical role (and similar standards of care must be exercised in the examination), the result of the investigation must be precise, with documentary evidence, to produce an independent assessment of the patient's clinical state and his/her needs. The expert's examination of the claimant should be recorded in contemporaneous notes. This is crucial, as these notes may be taken into court and used to refresh the memory. Notes made at a time distant from the event cannot be used and the healthcare professionals must rely on memory alone.

If standard further investigations are necessary, most solicitors will not worry about a small additional charge. If, however, complex assessments are deemed necessary following an initial examination, it is prudent to obtain consent from the solicitor before proceeding.

There is a difference between an expert acting on behalf of the claimant and one acting on behalf of the defendant insurers. Many claimant solicitors now request that even simple X-rays of their client are not taken by an expert acting for the defendant, without the express consent of the solicitor. In this context, the courts have interpreted Article 8 of the European Convention of Human Rights, the right to a private and family life, as requiring good reasons for repeated medical examinations of a claimant and for the disclosure of clinical records. The exceptions are those obviously relevant to the treatment of the particular injury or to a closely related previous medical condition.

Preparing the Report

Many legal and expert witness organizations have produced a standard format for medical reports. In this age of technology there is no excuse for unprofessional reports.

In summary:

1. The report should contain information about the expert and his/her qualifications to produce the report.
2. The purpose of the report should be stated, instructions should be summarized accurately, and the issues to be addressed should be outlined at the beginning. These may be used in the opinion section of the report as paragraph headings.

3. The historical aspects of the case should be laid out using references to documentary evidence and the patient's memory.
4. The expert's examination and/or any investigations should be described, together with any further tests, and their results.
5. Finally, the expert should provide his/her opinion and conclusions and the CPR (Civil Procedure Rules) statement of truth should be attached to the report.

As appendices, the expert's letter of instruction, a list of the documents received and considered, and any supporting material to back up the opinion, such as articles from medical journals, should be included.

A brief résumé should be attached to the report.

Formalities to be Completed before Sending the Report

Prior to submission to the solicitor, the report should be read at least twice – the first time to look for obvious errors, and again to check for clarity, plain English (with minimal medical jargon or addition of a glossary), veracity of conclusions, and consistency in style.

The number of copies needed should be prepared, each copy signed with the date, and sent with a fee note to the instructing solicitor(s).

Who Will See the Report?

The report will initially be seen by the instructing solicitor, who will show it to the client and discuss it with him/her. When the contents of the report are accepted, a barrister may be asked for an opinion on the case, particularly in complex clinical negligence disputes. The barrister will review all the evidence, including the medical reports, and advise on the next steps. After proceedings have been issued, the evidence used to support the case will be given to the other party in the case (i.e., disclosed). This disclosure will include the expert reports. At this stage, the reports will be seen by the solicitor for the other party, possibly the party him/herself, and the barrister and expert advising the other party. If the case cannot be resolved without a trial, the judge will see the reports as part of the evidence presented to the court, by the parties to the action. In legal terms, this evidence forms "the trial bundle."

What Can Happen to the Report After it Has Been Initially Submitted?

The next stage depends on the contents of the report and for whom it is written. If the report is prepared on behalf of a claimant, the solicitor is likely to show the claimant the report. The claimant may wish to comment on the contents and the solicitor would then send a copy of these remarks to the expert, particularly if the patient feels that there are omissions or errors in the factual part of the report.

Procedure to Modify the Report (if Asked)

Some comments on the submitted report may be of a factual nature, and, unless there is evidence from other sources, for example, written clinical records, that do not support the comments, amendments can be made. If the facts alter the basis upon which an opinion is made, then the opinion can be legitimately changed.

If, however, the comments dispute the conclusions, unless there is a factual error leading to that conclusion, the expert must not forget that he/she is an independent witness. If the alterations requested cannot be supported, based on the factual evidence, including the expert's clinical findings, the report should not be modified, but the expert should explain why he/she believes the conclusions are correct. Finally, it is the author and signatory of the report who may have to defend its contents in a court witness box.

Much has been said about solicitors attempting to rewrite expert reports and influence the conclusions of reports. It is becoming clear that, although the judiciary are trying to stop the partisan expert, they do not wish to stop genuinely held opposing views between practitioners.

In the new world of "openness," many previously privileged documents are being disclosed, including the letter of instruction to the expert from the solicitor.

What Happens When the Solicitor Seeks Comments on the Report from the Other Side?

Sometimes the other side will have expert evidence from another practitioner. When this is disclosed, the instructing solicitor will send a copy to the expert asking for comments. The time taken to read the report from the other side, to reread one's own notes and report, and to prepare a detailed response is chargeable and the expert should raise an invoice with the comments, detailing the time involved.

It is important to evaluate the information logically and methodically as both experts look for common ground and areas of disagreement; it is then easier for solicitors to crystallize any area of conflict within the evidence.

Preparation of Reply with Comments

It is important to reread the earlier report, particularly if some time has elapsed between the preparation of the report and the request for comments. Any investigation or examination that has occurred and the date of that examination in relation to the expert's own examination of the claimant should be noted.

There are two distinct routes for comments. First, are the conclusions justified, based on the examination that the other expert carried out (i.e., if the expert was given the same facts, would he/she reach the same conclusions?). Are the facts at variance, even allowing for the passage of time, with the evidence collected by the expert? If the answer to this last question is yes, then this simple fact cannot be disputed, and it may be appropriate to ask the instructing solicitor for a reexamination of the claimant to ascertain whether his/her clinical status has changed since the initial examination. If, following reexamination, a change has been observed, and the conclusions drawn are now similar to those of the expert from the other side, then the medical evidence is likely to be agreed and the expert should indicate this agreement with the contents of the report.

Second, are the conclusions drawn different from what the expert would have aimed at given a similar factual basis? If the second condition applies, then there will be a disagreement between the medical experts. In this instance, it is important to provide support for any conclusions drawn in the report.

The expert should not feel intimidated by the expert from the other side, for example, his/her status in the profession. If the expert believes in his/her opinion and can support it with documentary evidence, he/she should feel secure in this position.

What Form Should the Comments on the Report from the Other Side Take?

For the sake of clarity, any comments made by the expert should be written in a report form, using the paragraph numbers given in the expert's own report as well as those used in the report from the other side. The expert should provide a point-by-point explanation of the background and opinion whether in support or rebuttal of the other expert's conclusions. If the report appears to be lacking in factual information, this should be questioned in the response, backed up by information justifying the expert's own conclusions, rather than those of the opposing expert. Initially, this will be sent to the expert's instructing solicitor and barrister, and may possibly be disclosed if the arguments made are persuasive.

If the matter still cannot be resolved, then the parties may proceed to put formal written questions to each other's experts to clarify aspects of their reports. Such points must be answered within a short time (usually a few weeks), and the experts may be required to discuss the differences between their reports with a view to removing these differences if possible.

The questions raised on the other expert's report, the formal exchange of written questions and answers, and a note of the experts' discussion may all be useful to the barrister when preparing the case for the court.

Medical Negligence Liability, Written Evidence

The written evidence in medical negligence liability cases has the following goals:

1. to give an outline of the procedures in clinical negligence
2. to show how an appropriate report is commissioned on liability
3. to give an outline of the preparation of such a report
4. to give advice regarding the final report for disclosure
5. to help respond to written evidence from the other party.

The Initial Letter

Most requests to undertake a liability report commence with a letter (**Figure 2**) from a solicitor asking if the expert is prepared to act and including brief details about the case.

Example Letter of Approach

Procedure to be followed if a request for preparation of clinical negligence report is received First, the letter should be read thoroughly and the expert should ask him/herself the following questions:

- Do I know anyone who may be involved in this litigation?
- About what am I being asked to give an opinion?
- Do I know enough about the area in question and the procedures at the time of the alleged incident?
- Does the solicitor asking for an opinion appear to know what he/she is doing?

Having looked at this list of questions, an initial response to the request can be made. The possible responses include the following:

Dear Sir

    I have been instructed by Miss Smith to pursue a claim against the War Memorial NHS trust for alleged medical negligence and you have been recommended to give an expert opinion.

    In brief, my client instructs me that she attended the War Memorial hospital on several occasions over a period of weeks having, on occasions, attended herself and, on other occasions, being referred by her GP to various specialists. On each occasion, she was discharged home until on the last when she was admitted complaining of abdominal pain and severe vomiting.

    She complained that she was not admitted or appropriate investigations carried out and as a result she had to be admitted as an emergency case for surgery to be carried out.

    I confirm that I have in my possession the complete hospital and GP records of my client and these have been ordered and paginated.

    Before we can instruct you formally, we need to know your fee so that we can seek specific authority from the Legal Aid Board.

    In addition to an estimate of your fees and your timescale for preparing the report, we would be grateful that there is no conflict of interest in dealing with this matter and that you have not previously been instructed to prepare expert evidence in this case on behalf of any other party.

    Once we have received specific authority from the Legal Aid Board, we can formally instruct you and forward the medical records to you.

Yours faithfully

Figure 2 Example letter of approach.

- This request falls within the area of expertise. If so, and there is no conflict of interest, then a letter can be sent stating that the expert is prepared to give an opinion and the terms and conditions.
- If this falls within the expertise but there is a conflict (e.g., if the expert personally knows the person against whom the allegation is being made), the solicitor should be informed about the conflict of interest. The solicitor will appreciate an honest refusal due to conflict.
- After reading the letter, if it is felt that the allegations concern areas outside the expert's professional area, or if the expert belongs to a different professional discipline within the same clinical area (e.g., nursing rather than medical), then this should be explained to the solicitor, explaining what the areas of expertise are.
- Finally, if the practitioner thinks that the questions asked may be within his/her area of expertise but has doubts, further details may be requested from the solicitor.

Having received a letter of instruction, some immediate actions should be undertaken to smoothe the subsequent management of the case. All the notes should be briefly checked to ensure that the solicitor has provided all the relevant papers for preparation of the report. After reading the extent of the clinical and other material, the time estimated for preparation of the report should be checked. It should be kept in mind that a detailed evaluation of the contents of these records will only be possible when the actual report is prepared. This will take place according to the timetable agreed with the solicitor. If any records or other material appear to be missing, the solicitor must be informed immediately. If the quantity of material is much greater than expected according to the initial letter and if it is felt that the estimate given to the solicitor was an underestimate, a letter should be sent to the solicitor explaining why the estimate was incorrect and a revised estimate, including the reasons for the change, should be communicated. Before commencing any work on the report, the expert must wait for the solicitor to agree to this revision. At this stage, it is important that all the records are present and that the estimate is approximately correct: a diary note should be prepared indicating the schedule to prepare the report, and this should be kept to.

Preparing the Report

There are three parts to a liability report:

1. What happened (the historical narrative)?
2. What should have happened (the expected standard of care)?
3. What went wrong (the breach of those standards)?

While every expert has his/her own system of setting out reports, the above outline shows one method of dividing opinion from facts. It displays to the solicitor and others the clarity of thinking in the report.

Reading the Factual Documents

The factual documents may include not only copious clinical records, but also statements from witnesses of fact from the party who has instructed the expert. There may also be some correspondence from the defendant trust if the claimant has followed the complaints procedure before initiating legal proceedings. Finally, if there has been a death and an inquest has been convened, witness statements used in that forum may be available.

Clinical Records

The clinical records should not be read with the benefit of hindsight. Once the diagnosis or treatment is clear, many things may appear to be below acceptable care if viewed with that knowledge. However, the healthcare professional works within an area where there is often no exact right or wrong, and incomplete information may be available at the commencement of contact between the patient and the healthcare worker. It is important for the expert witness reading the records to put him/herself in the place of the healthcare professional receiving the information as documented in the records. The expert witness should view the subsequent actions of the healthcare professional in the light of the information that was obtained at the time.

It should be appreciated that the information in the notes may be in conflict with the evidence of the witness statements in the case, particularly the proof of evidence from a claimant. When reading the clinical records, it is advisable to maintain a healthy skepticism about the total truth of these records. Records and statements from witnesses should be read, noting any similarities or differences between them and the written records.

Writing the Narrative

The narrative section of the report can be written once all documents have been read. If there are two different accounts of the circumstances, both should be recorded in the report as alternative explanations, without, at this stage, commenting on the differences.

If there are reports from other experts that inform the narrative, particularly about an area outside the expert's field, a brief summary of this part of the circumstances should be given, as no opinion regarding that part of the case will be sought from the expert.

Defining the Standard of Care

Having read and recorded the narrative section of the report, the next logical step is to define the acceptable standard of care for any patient presenting to a healthcare professional of equal grade at that particular time with the same problem.

Within this, there may be a variety of similar standards that could be adopted, according to the interpretation of various factors found in the history and initial assessment of the patient. At this time, any relevant texts, current at the time of the incident, should also be consulted for an authoritative view of acceptable standards of care. Sometimes, the relevant guidelines produced by statutory bodies may also be helpful.

Writing the Opinion

The opinion is often the most difficult part of a report to write. First, the facts may be in dispute – the patient and the healthcare professional may have different perceptions of the consultation between them. It should be remembered that it is not for the expert witness to define the facts of the case but only to define whether the standard of care was acceptable.

If there are two differing accounts, then an opinion must be given for each set of facts. The expert witness must remain objective in his/her report. If there was an acceptable standard of care in some parts of the treatment but not others, it is necessary for the expert to acknowledge this. It should be stated that the expert witness feels that some of the allegations have not been substantiated by medical records. However, the expert witness may find that the overall standard of care was below an acceptable level.

Each part of the case should be dealt with logically and in sequence, as often the series of events that occur is additive, and it is the total package of care the patient received that was unacceptable.

Writing the Conclusions

Having the report, the expert should compile a summary of the main facts plus his/her opinion. This should be brief and positioned at the beginning of the report.

Appendices

Any literature used to help form the opinion should be copied and appended to the report. In addition to the relevant section, the title page and publication details should also be supplied as information for the legal team and, after exchange, to allow the expert on the other side to see the literature review.

A single-page résumé of the expert should be appended to the report.

See Also

Expert Witness: Qualifications, Testimony and Malpractice; Medical; Daubert and Beyond

ISBN 0-12-547970-0

9 780125 479707